Cinemeducation

VOLUME 2

Using Film and Other Visual Media in Graduate and Medical Education

Edited by

MATTHEW ALEXANDER
Professor of Family Medicine
University of North Carolina School of Medicine

PATRICIA LENAHAN
Adjunct Faculty
USC School of Social Work
The University of Southern California

ANNA PAVLOV
Assistant Clinical Professor of Family Medicine
David Geffen School of Medicine at UCLA
Director of Behavioral Science
Pomona Valley Hospital Medical Center, Pomona, California

Forewords by

SUSAN BAILEY
OBE, FRCPsych
President, The Royal College of Psychiatrists

JOSEPH E. SCHERGER
MD, MPH
Vice President, Primary Care and Academic Affairs
Eisenhower Medical Center
Rancho Mirage, CA

Radcliffe Publishing
London • New York

Radcliffe Publishing Ltd
33–41 Dallington Street
London
EC1V 0BB
United Kingdom

www.radcliffepublishing.com

Every effort has been made to ensure that the information in this book is accurate. This does not diminish the requirement to exercise clinical judgment, and neither the publisher nor the authors can accept any responsibility for its use in practice.

British Library Cataloguing in Publication Data

A catalogue record for this book is available from the British Library.

ISBN-13: 978 184619 507 5

Typeset by Darkriver Design, Auckland, New Zealand
Printed and bound by Cadmus Communications, USA

Index

Index

Contents

Contents

Contents

Foreword by Susan Bailey

Films have been used for educational purposes for a long time. However, it is only in the last quarter of a century that a more structured approach has emerged to studying film in the context of health-care delivery and to using film to educate the physicians of the future. It is now evident that training in a myriad of aspects of medical care can be provided by identifying selected clips and highlighting various aspects of doctor-patient interaction, working with families, response of patients to acute and chronic illnesses, and response of helping professionals and loved ones to the sick. While efforts have been made to include medical humanities in undergraduate and postgraduate medical education, many educators are looking for methods to increase and integrate their use into the existing medical curriculum. This book is a welcome contribution that brings together an impressive number of enthusiasts who write about using films with illustrative clips to teach a wide variety of subjects ranging from what movies mean to the viewer and the teacher to family functioning and the impact of specific diseases. In so doing, the book encourages teachers and students alike not only to learn but also to have fun at the same time. There is no doubt that films are made to be enjoyed and to make money (and may be "too entertaining") but they are a reflection of cultural values and nuances and, as such, they provide rich teaching material. The editors are to be congratulated on the comprehensive selection of topics and the high quality of material compiled. I hope this book will be widely read and used.

Professor Susan Bailey, OBE, FRCPsych
President, The Royal College of Psychiatrists
March 2012

Foreword by Joseph E. Scherger

Everyone learns from movies. No other art form recreates life as vividly as film, with its people and settings vast in opportunities for presenting human experience. Good movies enrich us and are long remembered. Bad movies make us angry at the distortion and missed opportunity.

Using film and other visual media as an educational tool is easier now than ever before in the digital age. Segments of film are readily sliced and readily available in almost any classroom. This second edition of *Cinemeducation* greatly expands the scope of situations and experience by presenting an amazing array of films and other visual media for medical education. Many new authors have been added to provide additional expertise for guidance and recommendations.

The editors of this text are behavioral scientists who have spent their careers in medical education. They have assembled an international group of contributors from five continents. They represent various medical and health disciplines. They know physicians and other health-care professionals and the many human situations presented in the medical setting. They are well grounded in ethics and they understand the struggles experienced by patients and caregivers. Bringing these situations to life through film is analogous to being in a candy store of delicious opportunities for teaching.

A major strength of this book is the outstanding organization of its major parts. After an overview by lead author Matthew Alexander, the text dives deep into human experience. Family functioning and health are covered throughout the life cycle. Many specific disease states are covered, including substance abuse, gambling, dealing with tragedy, diabetes, heart disease, other chronic illness, and even having babies. Mental health problems are covered in detail. Some films portray health-care professionals both positively and negatively and these are presented with rich detail. A wide variety of specialties and different health careers are covered. All of these converge on the common ground of compassion in the medical experience.

While most of this book covers movies, other visual media are also discussed. Reality television is a newly recognized art form and it provides a rich amount of experience in medicine. Documentaries of health professionals and situations have expanded. YouTube puts almost anything on the Internet for illustration and this book helps sort that out for medical education. Finally, even music has become visual through video presentation.

The second edition of *Cinemeducation* will go a long way to bringing film and other visual media into mainstream medical and graduate health education. Using these illustrations has never been technically easier, yet the number and quality of options from which to choose has never been greater. This book is a library unto itself and will serve as a valuable and fun resource for medical educators.

Joseph E. Scherger, MD, MPH
Vice President, Primary Care and Academic Affairs
Eisenhower Medical Center
Rancho Mirage, CA
March 2012

Preface

It has been 7 years since the publication of *Cinemeducation: A Comprehensive Guide to Using Film in Medical Education* (2005). During this time, there have been countless movies released – some of them outstanding, some mediocre, and many somewhere in the middle. Simultaneously, there has been expanded interest in (and application of) cinemeducation to medical and graduate education. These developments are discussed in detail in Chapter 1 of this new volume.

Other changes have occurred, as well, since 2005. Entire series of television shows are now available on DVD and through the Internet; YouTube has become a phenomenon, growing to such gargantuan proportions that some estimate it would take a million years to view all the content found there; Netflix and streaming video provide new modes of offering visual content to audiences; and video games are widely popular, recently surpassing cinema in terms of both total sales and frequency of use. All these developments make it evident that the public's appetite for visual media of all varieties is as strong as or stronger than ever.

Cinemeducation, Volume 2: Using Film and Other Visual Media in Graduate and Medical Education is entirely new in content, although we have tried to keep the same format as the first volume. The impetus of writing this new volume arose, in part, from the desire to encourage the use of all types of visual media in medical and graduate education. Consequently, in Chapter 1 we have broadened our definition of cinemeducation to reflect a broader vision, and we dedicate entire chapters in this new volume to reality television, mainstream television, documentaries, and YouTube. Given that so many of our students have come of age "plugged into" these new formats, we are very excited to promote the use of these formats in cinemeducation.

Volume 2 is applicable to multiple disciplines/specialties in medical and graduate education. In fact, many of the chapters in *Volume 2* are written by physicians for use within their medical specialties (i.e. surgery, obstetrics, pediatrics, cardiology, oncology, and sports medicine). Chapters geared toward allied health professionals such as pharmacy, nurse, dietary, palliative, veterinary, and pastoral care providers and educators are also included in *Volume 2* and are written by providers in these areas.

Other chapters in this new volume cover topics dear to the hearts of mental health educators: the Myers-Briggs Test, empathy, psychotherapy, the Enneagram, couple therapy, and depth psychology. A few chapters – one on disaster health and another one on military issues – are particularly timely, given the current state of affairs worldwide. Contemporary films are used to address special "repeat" topics such as sexuality, grief, aging, addiction, and trauma. We also include chapters that allow educators to use visual media to teach a host of other cutting-edge and useful topics such as medical malpractice, ethics, and international medical missions. Like the first book, the chapters, with one or two exceptions, provide detailed information for the educator regarding scene location, movie and scene description, and suggested discussion questions, all of which allow for the seamless introduction of cinemeducation into any curriculum.

As much as possible, we have incorporated diversity in every chapter, recognizing that culture, race, gender identity, aging, and ethnicity are important aspects of all health issues. We also have attempted to promote diversity among the collaborators, to encourage multidisciplinary collaboration and to support multinational participation in authorship. We have encouraged all contributors to use new films (those that have been released since 2005) rather than older films, although some classics have made their way into this volume.

From our perspective, *Volume 2* is a perfect companion to the first book, as both books cover mostly different topics, showcase different movies/video clips, and include alternative media-based approaches. In both volumes, the emphasis has been on US films that by and large emanate from Hollywood. There are, however, some independent films used and a few foreign films.

We are extremely excited about the utility of both books and hope that you, the reader, find them to be a user-friendly guide to enhance your teaching/educational efforts. The discussion questions that follow each listed scene are intended to assist the educator in initiating discussion. These questions are by no means exhaustive. It may be that questions listed for other scenes within a chapter may be appropriately used as additional questions for a selected scene(s). Answers to the discussion questions are provided in only a few chapters of this volume and so we recommend that educators consult the full references provided at the end of the chapters for more information about the topic at hand.

Please know that we may have missed your favorite film or a film more ideally suited to teach the particular topic than what has been provided. Like sand blown in the desert, there are always new films being released, not to mention many undiscovered gems. We apologize for any unintended omissions. In addition please note that we have multiple authors from across the world. While most of the films cited are consistent with the US audience format, some counter times may differ by region. Also, movies cited by authors using Netflix may include counter times but not chapter numbers.

Copyright protection is a concern that continues to be raised in professional meetings pertaining to cinemeducation, despite new developments such as streaming videos and YouTube clips, which would seem to make the issue less urgent. As we stated in the first volume, the use of movies for teaching purposes is protected in the United States under the Fair Use Doctrine (more information available at: www4.law.cornell.edu/uscode/17/107). Other countries, however, do not have laws pertaining to fair use of copyrighted material. In the United Kingdom, for example, institutions often obtain an Educational Recording Agency license (www.era.org.uk), which allows them to record and use TV/radio broadcasts for teaching. Institutions also obtain separate licenses to permit them to use commercial film for teaching. More information about copyright guidance pages for a number of UK higher education institutions can be obtained from the Loughborough University website (available at: www.lboro.ac.uk/library/skills/crightpages.html). Much depends, it would seem, on the licenses to which institutions subscribe, and it will certainly vary from country to country.

Technologies now exist to readily allow scenes from rented or purchased DVDs to be embedded in PowerPoint presentations or burned onto one disk for easier educational applications. It is best to work with technical support services if you are unfamiliar with these rapidly evolving technologies. For an excellent overview of new US copyright laws (e.g. 2010) as they pertain to decrypting and repurposing copyrighted content in the context of higher education, we encourage those interested to read "Movie clips and copyright," a 2010 article by Steve Kolowich (available at: www.insidehighered.com/news/2010/07/28/copyright). As always, we encourage cinemeducators to check with local legal resources to answer questions about the appropriate use of copyrighted material in their own educational settings.

Caveats being duly noted, we are delighted to welcome you now to sit back, eat some popcorn, and enjoy the (educational) show as you peruse *Volume 2* with an eye toward using many of the clips offered in your respective educational settings!

Matthew Alexander
Patricia Lenahan
Anna Pavlov
March 2012

About the Editors

Matthew Alexander, PhD, MA, is Professor of Family Medicine at the University of North Carolina School of Medicine, the first psychologist to have achieved this distinction. He is Director of Behavioral Medicine in the Department of Family Medicine at Carolinas Medical Center, Charlotte, North Carolina, and has an active clinical psychology practice, specializing in individual and couple therapy. Dr. Alexander has had a long interest in medical humanities, and he coined the term "cinemeducation," which is now a Google search-engine word. He is a distinguished public speaker who has spoken in Europe and throughout the United States on the use of cinema as a teaching tool. His articles on cinemeducation have been published in such professional journals as the *International Review of Psychiatry*; *Family Medicine*; *Families, Systems and Health*; and the *Annals of Behavioral Science and Medical Education*. Dr. Alexander resides in Charlotte, North Carolina, with his wife, Elaine, and their two children, Ethan and Natalie. Dr. Alexander is also an accomplished musician who performs regularly in the southeastern United States and has recorded five CDs of original music on Caravan Records. More information about him can be found by visiting his websites (www.alexandertherapy.com and www.alexandertunes.com).

Matthew Alexander
Professor of Family Medicine
Department of Family Medicine
Carolinas Medical Center
Charlotte, NC
Email matthew@alexandertherapy.com

Patricia Lenahan, LCSW, LMFT, BCETS, received her AM degree from the University of Chicago School of Social Service Administration. She is licensed both as a clinical social worker and as a marriage and family therapist in California and she is also a state-certified domestic violence advocate. She served as Health Sciences Associate Professor at the University of California Irvine School of Medicine and Director of Behavioral Medicine for the Department of Family Medicine for many years. While at the University of California Irvine, Ms. Lenahan was the content theme coordinator for the medical school in the areas of diversity, sexuality, and family violence.

Ms. Lenahan also taught gerontology courses at the California State University

Fullerton's gerontology certificate program and served as faculty for the American Society on Aging's substance abuse and gambling in aging program.

Presently, Ms. Lenahan is adjunct faculty at the University of Southern California's School of Social Work where she teaches courses in the practice and health concentrations as well as electives in domestic violence and sexuality.

In addition to coediting the first volume on cinemeducation, Ms. Lenahan has published in the areas of family violence, sexuality, and diversity. She has lectured on these topics at national and international conferences in Europe, Asia, and Africa. Ms. Lenahan enjoys adventure travel, photography, and working with her therapy dog, Maeve.

Patricia Lenahan
Adjunct Faculty
University of Southern California
School of Social Work
Irvine, CA
Email plenahan@usc.edu

Anna Pavlov, PhD, is a licensed clinical psychologist with a specialty in health psychology. She has worked in graduate medical education since 1992 when she was a postdoctoral fellow in primary care health psychology at the Michigan State University College of Human Medicine, Flint Campus. Dr. Pavlov has been the Director of Behavioral Science at UCLA-affiliated Pomona Valley Hospital's Family Medicine Residency Program since 1998. Her clinical and teaching interests are in lifespan health, physician well-being, and psycho-oncology. Dr. Pavlov is coinvestigator on a study of depression during pregnancy and the postnatal period. She lives in Southern California and enjoys time with her family, travel, reading, film and theater.

Anna Pavlov
Assistant Clinical Professor of Family Medicine
David Geffen School of Medicine at UCLA
Director of Behavioral Science
Pomona Valley Hospital Medical Center, Pomona, CA
Email anna.f.pavlov@pvhmc.org

Contributors

Jonathan Alexander, MD, FACC, FAHA
Clinical Professor of Medicine
University of Vermont Medical School
Clinical Assistant Professor of
  Medicine
Yale University School of Medicine
Director of Nuclear Cardiology and
  Cardiac Rehabilitation
Danbury Hospital
Danbury, CT
Email Jonathan.alexander@
  wcthealthnetwork.org

Matthew Alexander, PhD, MA
Professor of Family Medicine
Department of Family Medicine
Carolinas Medical Center
Charlotte, NC
Email matthew.alexander@
  carolinashealthcare.org
Website www.alexandertherapy.com

Corisande Baldwin, MD
Department of Medicine
University of British Columbia
Vancouver, BC, Canada

Snezana Begovic, MD
Faculty, Pomona Valley Hospital
  Medical Center
Family Medicine Residency Program
Pomona, CA
Email Snezana.begovic@pvhmc.org

Dinesh Bhugra, MA, MSc, MBBS,
  FRCP, FRCPsych, MPhil, PhD
Professor of Mental Health and
  Cultural Diversity
Institute of Psychiatry (King's College
  London)
London, England
Email Dinesh.bhugra@kcl.ac.uk

Allison K. Bickett, MS
Department of Family Medicine
Carolinas HealthCare System
Charlotte, NC
Email aaknotts@uncc.edu

Pablo González Blasco, MD, PhD
Scientific Director, SOBRAMFA
Brazilian Society of Family Medicine
São Paulo, Brazil
Website www.sobramfa.com.br

Kelly Breen Boyce, PsyD
Assistant Professor of Counseling
Gordon-Conwell Theological Seminary
Charlotte, NC
Email Kboyce@gcts.edu

Gregory P. Brown, MD
Associate Professor, University of
  Nevada School of Medicine
Residency Training Director, Psychiatry
  Las Vegas Department of Psychiatry
University of Nevada School of
  Medicine
Las Vegas, NV
Email gpbmd93@embarqmail.com

Contributors

Dennis J. Butler, PhD
Professor, Department of Family and
  Community Medicine
Medical College of Wisconsin
Milwaukee, WI
Email dbutler@mcw.edu

David Carl, MDiv, BCC
Executive Director
Pastoral Care and Education
Carolinas HealthCare System
Charlotte, NC
Email david.carl@carolinashealthcare.
  org

Amy E. Cassidy, MSN, ACNP-BC
Mayo Clinic Hospital
Phoenix, AZ
Email Amycassidy02@gmail.com

Suzanne Classen, MSW
Clinical Social Worker
University of California, Irvine
Irvine, CA
Email sclassen@uci.edu

Henri Colt, MD, FCCP
Professor of Medicine
University of California, Irvine
Irvine, CA
Email hcolt@uci.edu

Lauren M. Consonni, DMD, MPH
Family Dentistry
Avon, CT
Email lconsonnidmd@gmail.com

LaTasha K. Crawford, VMD, PhD
Pathology Post Doctoral Fellow
Department of Molecular and
  Comparative Pathobiology
Johns Hopkins University School of
  Medicine
Baltimore, MD
Email lcrawf12@jhmi.edu

Peter Cronholm, MD, MSCE
Assistant Professor, Department of
  Family Medicine and Community
  Health
Associate Program Director and the
  Director of Community Programs
Department of Family Medicine and
  Community Health
Penn Medicine
Philadelphia, PA
Email peter.cronholm@uphs.upenn.edu

Greg Dahlquist, MD, FAAFP
Program Director, Pomona Valley
  Hospital Medical Center
Family Medicine Residency Program
Pomona, CA
Email greg.dahlquist@pvhmc.org

Gary Fontan, MD
Department of Family Medicine
Kaiser Permanente
Claremont, CA
Email Fontan2@aol.com

Anne Geary, BS
Certified Enneagram Consultant
Geary Associates, Consulting
Charlotte, NC
Email anne@geary.net

Kim Goodman, MSW, LCSW
Associate Professor Clinical Field
  Faculty
University of Southern California
School of Social Work
Los Angeles, CA
Email kwgoodma@usc.edu

Renee Hickson, MD
Assistant Professor, Family and
  Community Medicine
Tulane University
New Orleans, LA
Email rmathis@tulane.edu

Hans House, MD, FACEP
Associate Chair for Education
Department of Emergency Medicine
University of Iowa
Iowa City, IA
Email Hans-house@uiowa.edu

Dawn Joosten, PhD, LCSW
Clinical Assistant Professor
University of Southern California
School of Social Work
Los Angeles, CA
Email joosten@usc.edu

Tracy R. Juliao, PhD, LP, NCC
Owner & Licensed Health Psychologist
Total Health & Wellness
  Associates, PLLC
Farmington Hills, MI
Email docjuliao@gmail.com

Michael Kahn, LPC, JD
Email michael@reeltoreal.biz
Website www.michaelkahnworkshops.
  com

Meghann Kaiser, MD
Fellow in Trauma and Surgical Critical
  Care
R. Adams Cowley Shock Trauma
  Center, University of Maryland
Baltimore, MD
Email mkaiser@uci.edu

Gurvinder Kalra, MD
Assistant Professor of Psychiatry
Lokmanya Tilak Medical College &
  Sion General Hospital
Sion, Mumbai, India
Email kalragurvinder@gmail.com

Darin Kennedy, MD, FAAFP
Assistant Professor of Family Medicine
Department of Family Medicine
Carolinas Medical Center
Charlotte, NC
Email darin.kennedy@
  carolinashealthcare.org

Amanda Kotis, DMD, MA
Private Practice
Charlotte, NC
Email amandakotis@gmail.com

Kevin Krause, BA
Studio Page, Paramount Pictures
Hollywood, CA
Email Kevinmkrause@gmail.com

Patricia Lenahan, LCSW, LMFT,
  BCETS
USC School of Social Work
Adjunct Faculty
Orange County Academic Center
Irvine, CA
Email plenahan@usc.edu

Karen Likar Manookin, DDS
Private Practice
Email kmanookin@gmail.com

Susan Fleming McAllister, MD, PhD
Physician, Family Medicine
Mississippi Physician Services
MEA Clinics
Jackson, MS
Email susanmcallister@yahoo.com

Douglas McGeachy, MPA, Doctoral
  Student
Commander, Santa Ana Police
  Department
Former Marine
Santa Ana, CA
Email dmcgeachy@santa-ana.org

Contributors

Michael Metal, BS
USC School of Social Work
Graduate Student in the Military
  Sub-Concentration
Orange County Academic Center
Irvine, CA
Email mmetal@usc.edu

Graziela Moreto, MD
Professor of Family Medicine Program
University Nove de Julho
International Programs Director
  SOBRAMFA
São Paulo, Brazil
Email graziela@sobramfa.com.br
Website www.sobramfa.com.br

Rohit Pai, MD, BSc
Internal Medicine Resident,
  Department of Medicine
University of British Columbia
Vancouver, BC, Canada
Email r.pai@utoronto.ca

Anna Pavlov, PhD
Assistant Clinical Professor of Family
  Medicine
David Geffen School of Medicine at
  UCLA
Director of Behavioral Science
Pomona Valley Hospital Medical
  Center
Family Medicine Residency Program
Pomona, CA
Email Anna.f.pavlov@pvhmc.org

Shay Phillips, PharmD, BCPS
Carolinas HealthCare System
Elizabeth Family Medicine
Assistant Professor
Department of Family Medicine
Charlotte, NC

Leslie L. Pitt, MA, LMFTA
Behavioral Health Intern
Elizabeth Family Medicine
Charlotte, NC
Email pitt.leslie@gmail.com

Layne Prest, PhD, LMFT
Assistant Clinical Professor
University of Washington
Behavioral Scientist, PeaceHealth
  Southwest Family Medicine
Vancouver, WA
Email lprest@swmedicalcenter.org

David E. Price, MD
Clinical Assistant Professor of Family
  Medicine
Associate Director, Primary Care Sports
  Medicine Fellowship
Department of Family Medicine
Carolinas Medical Center
Charlotte, NC
Email david.price@carolinashealthcare.
  org

James Pruett, PhD, DMin
Director of Training
Integrative Pastoral Psychotherapy
  Training Program
Department of Pastoral Care and
  Education
Carolinas HealthCare System
Charlotte, NC
Email James.pruett@
  carolinashealthcare.org

Silvia Quadrelli, MD, PhD
Thoracic Oncology Center, Buenos
  Aires British Hospital
University of Buenos Aires
Buenos Aires, Argentina
Email silvia.quadrelli@gmail.com

Lawrence Raymond, MD, ScM
Professor of Family Medicine
University of North Carolina at Chapel
  Hill
Director of Occupational and
  Environmental Medicine
Carolinas HealthCare System
Charlotte, NC
Email Larry.raymond@
  carolinashealthcare.org

Jo Marie Reilly, MD
Associate Clinical Professor, Family
  Medicine
Keck School of Medicine of USC
Los Angeles, CA
Email jmreilly@usc.edu

Jeffrey M. Ring, PhD
Director of Behavioral Sciences and
  Cultural Medicine
Family Medicine Residency Program
White Memorial Medical Center
Los Angeles, CA
Email ring@usc.edu

Kimberly Romig, LCSW, ACHP-SW
Behavioral Health Coordinator
PIH Family Practice Residency
  Program
Whittier, CA
Email kromig@pih.net

Anthony L. Rostain, MD, MA
Director of Education, Department of
  Psychiatry
University of Pennsylvania Health
  System
Professor of Psychiatry and Pediatrics
Perelman School of Medicine at the
  University of Pennsylvania
Email Rostain@mail.med.upenn.edu

Katrina Saunders, MA, LLPC, NCC
Primary Care Health Psychology
  Therapist
Doctors' Hospital of Michigan
Pontiac, MI
Email kvsaunde@oakland.edu

Laura J. Schrader, MD
Family Medicine Physician
Lakeside Family Physicians
Denver, NC
Email lauraschrader@live.com

H. Russell Searight, PhD, MPH
Associate Professor of Psychology
Lake Superior State University
Sault Sainte Marie, MI
Online Bio www.lssu.edu/faculty/
  hsearight/

David Stanley, NursD, MSc
Associate Professor of Nursing
University of Western Australia
School of Population Health
Crawley, Western Australia
Email David.Stanley@uwa.edu.au

John D. Stokes, MD
Assistant Clinical Professor of
  Medicine
Department of Internal Medicine
  Division of Endocrinology
University of Illinois College of
  Medicine
Champaign, IL
Email stokesjhnd@aol.com

Edward Thibodeau, DMD, PhD
Associate Dean, Assistant Professor
Department of Oral Health and
  Diagnostic Sciences
University of Connecticut School of
  Dental Medicine
Farmington, CT
Email Thibodeau@nso.uchc.edu

Contributors

Nigel E. Turner, PhD
Scientist, Centre for Addiction and
  Mental Health
Social Epidemiological Research
Assistant Professor, University of
  Toronto
Department of Public Health Science
Toronto, ON, Canada
Email NigelTurner@camh.net

James Tysinger, PhD
Distinguished Teaching Professor
  and Vice Chair for Professional
  Development
Department of Family and Community
  Medicine
The University of Texas Health Science
  Center at San Antonio
San Antonio, TX
Email tysinger@uthscsa.edu

F. Scott Valeri, MD, FACC
Sanger Heart and Vascular Institute
Charlotte, NC
Email scott.valeri@carolinashealthcare.
  com

Danielle Vanier, BS
Department of Psychology
Lake Superior State University
Sault Sainte Marie, MI
Email dvanier@lssu.edu

Dael Waxman, MD
Associate Professor of Family Medicine
Department of Family Medicine
Carolinas Medical Center
Charlotte, NC
Email Dael.Waxman@
  carolinashealthcare.org

Crystal Wilson, MD
Baylor Family Medicine at Lake Ridge
Grand Prairie, TX
Email crystalwilsonmd@gmail.com

Leslie Wind, PhD, LCSW
Clinical Associate Professor
Director, Orange County Academic
  Center
University of Southern California
Irvine, CA
Email wind@usc.edu

Roger Y. Wong, MD, FRCPC, FACP
President, Canadian Geriatrics Society
Clinical Professor and Assistant Dean
  Postgraduate Medical Education
Faculty of Medicine, University of
  British Columbia
Head, Geriatric Consultation Program
  Vancouver General Hospital
Vancouver, BC, Canada
Email rymwong@interchange.ubc.ca

Anthony Zamudio, PhD
Associate Professor of Clinical Family
  Medicine
USC Family Medicine Residency
  Program
California Hospital
Los Angeles, CA
Email azamudio@usc.edu

PART I

Overview

Let's Look at the Data: A Review of the Literature

Matthew Alexander

ALL INDICATIONS SUGGEST THAT CINEMEDUCATION IS HERE TO STAY. The use of film as a bona fide teaching tool appears to be occurring everywhere, from film-based, state-sanctioned continuing education classes for psychologists and social workers[1,2] to common utilization as an adjunct to psychotherapy.[3–5] Some residency programs have a regular "movie night" in which films are watched in their entirety and then discussed for learning purposes.[6] Entire courses are being offered based on movies that shed light on various aspects of the medical profession.[7] A recent issue of the *International Review of Psychiatry* was devoted to cinema, showcasing the worldwide appeal of film as a teaching tool and featuring authors from India, Denmark, New Zealand, Australia, and Canada (as well as prominent medical educators from the United States and the United Kingdom).[8] A few chapters in this landmark issue highlighted non-English-speaking films, such as those from Malaysia or from specific Indian cultures (Kannada, Tamil Nadu, Hindi), that are useful in graduate and medical education programs. Also, it's no longer just film that is being used for teaching; many educators are now using clips from televised medical dramas in their medical and graduate programs.[9,10]

No less a mainstream publication than the *Wall Street Journal* recently devoted the front page of their Personal Journal section to a story about the use of popular movies and television shows to teach medical students, residents, and mental health learners about the diagnosis and treatment of common medical and psychiatric problems.[11] The wide assortment of genres used to teach such topics is surprising. The article included the following:

- vampire flicks, particularly from the *Twilight* series, to teach about neurosis, emotional immaturity, and self-esteem as well as such diseases as Wilson's disease and the eating disorder Pica
- television shows such as *The Sopranos* to teach about psychological dysfunction and professional ethics[12]

- animated movies such as *Winnie the Pooh* (2007) to teach about obsession, mood disorder, and cognitive impairment
- classic movies such as *Gone With the Wind* (1939) to teach about narcissistic personality disorder
- children's movies such as *Charlie and the Chocolate Factory* (2005) to teach about schizotypal personality disorder.

The term "cinemeducation," now a Google search engine word, was first used in 1994 to describe the use of clips of popular movies on videotape to educate family practice residents in the psychosocial aspects of medical care.[13] The definition was updated in 2005 to include the use of movie clips or whole movies to help educate learners about biopsychosocial-spiritual aspects of health care.[14] Given the evolution of formats utilizing "moving" images in education, a new definition is proposed for cinemeducation; namely:

> The use of movies, television, YouTube, music videos or documentaries, either in their entirety or in short segments, to educate graduate and medical learners in the biopsychosocial-spiritual-ethical aspects of health care.

This definition is meant to be inclusive of other terms for similar approaches, including "tele-education,"[15] and "medicinema."[16]

Cinemeducation is an integral part of the broader field of medical humanities. Medical humanities is an interdisciplinary field for scholarship and teaching which embraces the use of the creative arts to educate medical learners about the human condition. The assortment of creative modalities used in the medical humanities is exhaustive, including painting, cinema, poetry and prose, music, dance, cartoons, and theater. Lest one think that such approaches are outside the mainstream, it is important to note that approximately half to three-quarters of all medical schools have programs in medical humanities.[17,18]

As has been previously reported in the literature, there are unique advantages to drawing on movies and television to educate graduate and medical learners.[19-21] Such advantages include, but are not limited to, the following:
- easy access to riveting case studies not protected by HIPAA (Health Insurance Portability and Accountability Act of 1996) guidelines
- easy access to the broadest possible spectrum of diagnostic conditions
- winning the attention of new generations of students raised in a video culture
- inspiring awe and introspection
- making learning fun
- strengthening the bond between student and teacher
- time efficiency (a clip may only last 3 minutes and yet it may stimulate an hour's worth of discussion)
- engaging both hemispheres of the brain, verbal and nonverbal

- increasing memory and recall
- promoting empathy.[22]

In addition to all these benefits, there are practical advantages as well; namely, that movies and television shows are easy to access and show. They are also inexpensive to buy. Thanks to technology available on any PC or Mac, video clips are increasingly, if not ubiquitously, embedded in PowerPoint presentations. Entire seasons of such popular television shows as *House*, *ER*, or *Grey's Anatomy* are available for purchase. Movies are easily downloaded or ordered overnight via Netflix (www.netflix.com). Having replaced videocassettes, DVDs allow educators to easily go to the movie chapter containing the scene to be shown. Technologies such as Blu-ray enhance the visual experience even more.

Cinemeducation has been used to teach a broad and compelling list of subjects in graduate and medical education. MEDLINE currently identifies nearly 6000 articles on the use of film in medicine, some dating back to the late 1940s. A literature search of articles published since 2000 on this topic surfaced a dizzying array of teaching applications using film or television including, but not limited to, the following areas: (1) schizophrenia,[23] (2) child psychiatry,[24] (3) psychosocial formulation,[25] (4) medical professionalism,[26] (5) grief,[27] (6) empathy and altruism,[28] (7) couple dynamics,[29,30] (8) family systems theory,[31,32] (9) Asperger's disease,[33] (10) psychosis,[34] (11) addiction medicine,[35] (12) end-of-life issues,[36] (13) pharmacology,[37] (14) logotherapy,[38] (15) ethics and moral reasoning,[39] (16) gender stereotypes,[40] (17) organizational behavior,[41] (18) countertransference,[42] (19) multicultural awareness,[43] (20) qualitative research,[44] and (21) psychiatric diagnosis.[45] Many of these peer-reviewed articles appear in such prestigious medical and psychological journals as *Academic Medicine*, *Academic Psychiatry*, and the *Family Journal*.

Just as there is a broad assortment of topics appropriate for cinemeducation, there are also many different ways to "cinemeducate." Clips from movies or television shows can be used to trigger group discussion, "anchor" teaching points during a lecture, form the basis of a role-play, motivate and inspire learners, re-energize a class whose energy has "dropped," or provide the basis for an ongoing project. Medical educators have even asked students to make short documentary movies, for example, to deepen their understanding of chronic illness.[46]

Of course, there are caveats to consider when using popular film and television for educational purposes.[47] As Neil Postman[48] points out in his book *Amusing Ourselves to Death*, television and movies don't require the viewer to have any previous knowledge in order to effectively entertain. Both mediums dispense with the notions of sequence and continuity, notions that are essential to education. Consequently, cinemeducation works best with advanced learners who have already acquired sufficient book knowledge and experience to bring to the discussion. Movies and television also contain stereotypes to which educators need to be sensitive, even though such stereotypes themselves can become fodder for productive discussion.

Finally, cinemeducators must acknowledge that the essential mission of popular media is to entertain, not to teach; however, this too is a benefit, since film and television, designed as they are to entertain, are very compelling and succeed to the extent that they pull the viewer in. Still, the entertainment must "ring true" to effectively hold the audience's attention. As noted psychiatrist and author Glen Gabbard has stated,[12] movies work precisely because they realistically portray our subconscious anxieties and conflicts. Movies that don't get their portrayals of the human condition right usually don't "make it." However, even when a movie doesn't get it right, this too can be used as a teaching point. For example, in the movie *A Beautiful Mind* (2001), John Nash, the schizophrenic protagonist, is portrayed as having visual rather than auditory hallucinations even though auditory hallucinations are more often the norm in schizophrenia. A skilled cinemeducator can easily use an inaccuracy like this to his or her teaching advantage.

It is, of course, always important to be aware that certain students, because of prior life experience, may find watching certain scenes traumatic. In such rare cases, students should be encouraged to inform their instructors after the viewing and, if necessary, seek counseling. It is also important to choose scenes carefully. Cinemeducation works best when the scenes chosen are relatively short (usually less than 10 minutes), self-contained (having a clear beginning and end) and inoffensive (unless purposely chosen for that purpose).

In a recent address, John Frey, Professor of Family Medicine and a thought leader in medical eduction, stated that "strong visual components will dominate verbal components in the education of future health care professionals."[49] Such a prediction is a powerful endorsement of cinemeducation, a technique which relies heavily on visual components. However, what is the actual science supporting cinemeducation? Studies of learning provide consistent support for what is called the dual coding theory;[50] that is, students are more likely to recall and comprehend material presented visually and auditorily rather than by either approach alone. Such findings are consistent with what is called the pictorial superiority effect,[51] a finding that memory is enhanced if concepts are presented as pictures rather than words.

While most published articles in this area report strong subjective and qualitative support for cinemeducation, the fields most commonly associated with this approach (nursing, psychiatry, psychology, family medicine, internal medicine, and undergraduate medicine) have supplied few quantitative studies supporting it. One such study did find that internal medicine residents exposed to a teaching curriculum based on the television shows *Grey's Anatomy* and *House* significantly improved their understanding of effective communication and increased their level of comfort in addressing clinical scenarios.[10] However, the study was not randomized, lacked a control group, and ultimately relied heavily on subjective assessment. The same is true of another study that asked graduates of a family medicine program to evaluate their experiences with cinemeducation.[52] While the study revealed positive impressions of cinemeducation, both quantitatively and qualitatively, there were clear limitations in the study design.

The problem of demonstrating the efficacy of cinemeducation is one shared with the broader field of medical humanities. Here too, most studies rely on small sample sizes and learner self-reports that fail to answer important questions such as whether or not changes brought about by arts-based curricula are observable by objective evaluators, and whether or not these changes make an actual change in clinical performance as assessed by patients.[17] In the final analysis, quantitative studies will be desirable, in addition to more detailed qualitative findings, to demonstrate that cinemeducation is an effective, if not superior, approach when compared with other, more traditional forms of medical education such as role-playing, standardized patients, and the old-fashioned lecture.

As we wait for the hard science to catch up with widespread practice, cinemeducators will nevertheless continue to cinemeducate. This book is designed to broaden the appeal of cinemeducation to as many medical and graduate specialties as possible. Thank you for reading and, more importantly, we hope you enjoy your classroom time at the movies!

References

1 Delson N. *SPA Film: Once Were Warriors* [online course]. Sacramento, CA: National Association of Social Workers California Chapter. Available at: www.socialworkweb.com/nasw/choose/details.cfm?course_number=1297 (last accessed 12/01/11)

2 Kahn M. Reel Therapy Too: ethical and professional challenges in small communities [workshop]. Charlotte, NC: Charlotte Area Health Education Center; May 15, 2010. Available at: www.michaelkahnworkshops.com (last accessed 4/14/12)

3 Alexander M. A Day in the Life of a Cinemeducator. In: Tischler, V, editor. *Mental Health, Psychiatry and the Arts: a teaching handbook.* Oxford: Radcliffe Publishing; 2010. pp. 25–32.

4 Woltz B. *Cinema Therapy: using the power of movies in the therapeutic process* [online course]. Sebastopol, CA: Zur Institute. Available at: www.zurinstitute.com/homeonline.html (last accessed 4/14/12)

5 Wolz B. *E-Motion Picture Magic: a movie lover's guide to healing and transformation.* Centennial, CO: Glenbridge Publishing; 2005.

6 Kalra G. Psychiatry movie club: a novel way to teach psychiatry. *Indian J Psychiatry.* 2011; **53**(3): 258–60.

7 Glasser B, Clark M. *7AAEM651 Medicine on Screen: doctors and medical care in fiction films, 1920s–present* [course]. London: King's College London. Available at: www.kcl.ac.uk/artshums/depts/english/modules/2011-12/level7/7aaem651.aspx (last accessed 4/14/12)

8 Bhugra D, Gupta S. Special issue on cinema. *Int Rev Psychiatry.* 2009; **21**(3): 181–2.

9 Pavlov A, Dahlquist GE. Teaching communication and professionalism using a popular medical drama. *Fam Med.* 2010; **42**(1): 25–7.

10 Wong RY, Saber SS, Ma I, *et al.* Using television shows to teach communication skills in internal medicine residency. *BMC Med Educ.* 2009; **9**: 9.

11 Beck M. Fictional stars, real problems. *Wall Street Journal.* June 8, 2010: D1, D8.

12 Gabbard G. *The Psychology of 'The Sopranos': love, death, desire, and betrayal in America's favorite gangster family.* New York, NY: Basic Books; 2002.

13 Alexander M, Hall M, Pettice Y. Cinemeducation: an innovative approach to teaching psychosocial medical care. *Fam Med*. 1994; **26**(7): 430–3.

14 Alexander M, Lenahan P, Pavlov A. Preface. In: *Cinemeducation: a comprehensive guide to using film in medical education*. Oxford: Radcliffe Publishing; 2005. p. xiv.

15 Lim EC, Seet RC. In-house medical education: redefining tele-education. *Teach Learn Med*. 2008; **20**(2): 193–5.

16 Miksanek J. Book and Media Reviews: *Medicinema – Doctors in Films. JAMA*. 2010; **303**(16): 1652.

17 Shapiro J. A sampling of the medical humanities. *Journal for Learning through the Arts: A Research Journal on Arts Integration in Schools and Communities*. 2006; **2**(1). http://repositories.cdlib.org/clta/lta/.http://repositories.cdlib.org/clta/lta/ (last accessed 4/14/12)

18 Rodenhauser P, Strickland MA, Gambala CT. Arts-related activities across U.S. medical schools: a follow-up study. *Teach Learn Med*. 2004; **16**(3): 233–9.

19 Charon R. Narrative medicine: form, function, and ethics. *Ann Intern Med*. 2001; **134**(1): 83–7.

20 Berk R. Multimedia teaching with video clips: TV, movies, YouTube and mtvU in the college classroom. *Int J Technol Teach Learn*. 2009; **5**(1): 1–21.

21 Alexander M, Waxman D, White P. *What's Eating Gilbert Grape?* A case study of chronic illness. *J Learn Arts*. 2007; **2**(1): Article 13.

22 Blasco PB, Moreto G, Roncoletta A, *et al*. Using movie clips to foster learners' reflection: improving education in the affective domain. *Fam Med*. 2006; **38**(2): 94–6.

23 Rosenstock GJ. Beyond *A Beautiful Mind*: film choices for teaching schizophrenia. *Acad Psychiatry*. 2003; **27**(4): 117–22.

24 Zerby SA. Using the science fiction film *Invaders from Mars* in a child psychiatry seminar. *Acad Psychiatry*. 2005; **29**(3): 283–8.

25 Mersch D. Psychosocial formulation training using commercial films. *Acad Psychiatry*. 2000; **24**: 99–104.

26 Lumlertgul N, Kijpaisalratana N, Pityaratstian N, *et al*. Cinemeducation: a pilot student project using movies to help students learn medical professionalism. *Med Teach*. 2009; **31**(7): 3327–32.

27 Furst BA. Bowlby goes to the movies: film as a teaching tool for issues of bereavement, mourning and grief in medical education. *Acad Psychiatry*. 2007; **31**: 407–10.

28 Shapiro J, Rucker L. Why going to the movies can help develop empathy and altruism in medical students and residents. *Fam Syst Health*. 2004; **22**(4): 445–52.

29 Alexander M. The couple's odyssey: Hollywood's take on love relationships. *Int Rev Psychiatry*. 2009; **21**(3): 1–6.

30 Shepard DS, Brew L. Teaching theories of couples counseling: the use of popular movies. The Family Journal. 2005; **13**(4): 406–15.

31 Alexander M, Waxman D. Cinemeducation: using film to teach family systems. *Fam Syst Health*. 2001; **18**(4): 455–62.

32 Stinchfield TA. Using popular films to teach systems thinking. *The Family Journal*. 2006; **14**(2): 123–8.

33 Sharp BW. Napoleon Dynamite has Asperger's? Gosh, it's called cultural competence, you freakin' idiots. *Acad Psychiatry*. 2007; **31**(3): 248.

34 Raballo A, Larøi F, Bell V. Humanizing the clinical gaze: movies and the empathic understanding of psychosis. *Fam Med*. 2009; **41**(6): 387–8.

35 Cape G. Movies as a vehicle to teach addiction medicine. *Int Rev Psychiatry*. 2009; **21**(3): 213–17.

36 DiBartolo MC, Seldomridge LA. Cinemeducation: teaching end-of-life issues using feature films. *J Gerontol Nurs*. 2009; **35**(8): 30–6.

37 Ventura S, Onsman A. The use of popular movies during lectures to aid the teaching and learning of undergraduate pharmacology. *Med Teach*. 2009; **31**(7): 662–4.

38 Melton A. Using movies to teach principles of logotherapy. *Int Forum Logother*. 2005; **28**(2).89–92.

39 Champoux JE. At the cinema: aspiring to a higher ethical standard. *Acad Manag Learn Edu*. 2006; **5**(3): 386–90.

40 Bonds-Raacke J. The psychology of Disney and fairytale movies. *J Instruct Psychol*. 2008; **35**(3): 232–4.

41 Holbrook Robert L. OB in a video box: using *Remember the Titans* as a microcosm for the organizational behavior course. *J Manage Educ*. 2009; **33**(4).

42 Edwards J. Teaching and learning about psychoanalysis: film as a teaching tool with reference to a particular film, *Morvern Callar*. *Br J Psychotherapy*. 2010; **26**(1): 80–99.

43 Rorrer A, Furr S. Using film as a multicultural awareness tool in teacher education. *Multicultural Perspectives*. 2009; **11**(3): 162–8.

44 Saldana J. Popular film as an instructional strategy in qualitative research methods courses. *Qual Inq*. 2009; **15**(1): 247–61.

45 Pearson Q. Using the film *The Hours* to teach diagnosis. *J Humanist Couns*. 2006; **45**(1): 70–9.

46 Shapiro D, Tomasa L. Patients as teachers, medical students as filmmakers: the video slam, a pilot study. *Acad Med*. 2009; **84**(9): 1235–43.

47 Greenberg HR. Caveat actor, caveat emptor: some notes on the hazards of Tinseltown teaching. *Int Rev Psychiatry*. 2009; **21**(3): 241–4.

48 Postman N. *Amusing Ourselves to Death: public discourse in the age of show business*. New York, NY: Penguin Books; 1985.

49 Frey J. Keynote address to University of North Carolina Statewide Department of Family Medicine. Wildacres Retreat, Little Switzerland, NC; November 15, 2011.

50 Clark JM, Paivio A. Dual coding theory and education. *Educ Psychol Rev*. 1991; **53**(2): 445–59.

51 Nelson DL, Reed VS, Walling JR. Pictorial superiority effect. *J Exp Psychol Hum Learn*. 1976; **2**(5): 523–8.

52 Alexander M. A graduate survey of cinemeducation. In: Alexander M, Lenahan P, Pavlov A, editors. *Cinemeducation: a comprehensive guide to the use of film in medical education*. Oxford: Radcliffe Publishing; 2005. pp. 183–7.

2

Teaching Us What It Means to be Human: Why Movies Move Us

Matthew Alexander

This chapter is adapted from the keynote presentation for the Association for Medical Humanities, Leicester, England, on July 11, 2011

I am delighted to have been asked to speak here today. The invitation to deliver this keynote address to the Association for Medical Humanities is a wonderful opportunity for me to share with you a topic of great personal and professional interest while also making a journey "across the pond." For the past 20 years, I have been using clips from popular movies to teach psychology and behavioral medicine to family medicine residents, graduate students in counseling and health psychology, medical students, and a broad array of practicing health-care professionals. The use of movies and movie clips to teach health professionals is known by the term "cinemeducation."[1]

Much has been written about why cinemeducation is an effective way to teach health-care professionals about the biopsychosocial-spiritual aspects of their chosen careers.[2-4] Movies, for one, provide ready-made case studies. Unlike real patients, the privacy of the screen character needs no protection. Also, through movies and movie clips, students can be exposed to a wider range of disorders than they are likely to encounter in real life. Because learners have no relationship with the screen characters, they are freer to explore their honest reactions to them. Movie clips are short and can provide effective triggers to stimulate many minutes, if not hours, of didactic interchange.

Finally, movies are fun. Even though I have now seen my teaching clips dozens of times, I never tire of them. They continue to entertain and provide a wonderful platform from which to teach. At its core, cinemeducation works because movies work. Learners and teachers enjoy cinemeducation because they enjoy movies.

But movies are more than just entertainment. At their best, popular movies offer a universally compelling experience that speaks to our collective need for connection, reflection, and wisdom. As Glen Gabbard, a professor of psychiatry and psychoanalysis at Baylor College of Medicine in Houston, Texas, has said, "Students … can sometimes learn as much about what it means to be human from studying popular films and novels as they can from sitting with a patient."[5] Of course, good literature, theater, music, and art also teach us what it means to be human. Are movies any different? I believe they are.

I consider cinema to be the great art form of our era and that as a humanities-based teaching tool it is without peer. I wish to use this keynote opportunity to explore why this is so. In order to accomplish my objectives, I will use Dr. Gabbard's splendid observation as a stepping-off point. What can movies teach us about the human condition? Do they ultimately provide an accurate or distorted portrayal of our existence? If movies teach us what it means to be human, exactly how do they manage to do this? Why do moving pictures move us so deeply?

I believe these are important questions. After all, as health-care professionals and educators we are intimately involved in the human condition, the frailty, the longing, the humor, and the tragedy. If movies can help foster a better understanding of our lives, while simultaneously being entertaining, then it seems that we are all better off.

Of course, not all movies are created equal; there are great, bad, and mediocre movies. Or perhaps I should say, there are good, bad, and ugly movies. Bad movies are boring and clichéd. Ugly movies promote stereotypes, play on our worst impulses, and inculcate unrealistic expectations. Perhaps the most egregious aspect of Hollywood filmmaking has to do with its romanticized view of relationships; this idealization of love confuses fantasy with reality and in so doing unwittingly promotes a "grass is greener" mentality. Good movies, on the other hand, provide meaningful, real-world insights. Such films offer new visions, provide fresh ways of seeing our lives and inspire nobility and courage. Then, of course, there are also the great movies that transcend time and space and remain with us long after the final credits.

If it is not clear already, let me state for the record that I have a bias. While I am not financially tied either to Hollywood or to Bollywood, I do *love* movies. This is not to say that I don't love other art forms. I do. But I simply place movies in a category all their own. As much as I love music (and as a musician myself and an attendee of the original Woodstock Festival in 1969 I believe I am in a unique position to comment on the power of live music) I still love movies more. I am not, unfortunately for my wife, a big fan of the theater, but take a theatrical production and turn it into a movie (e.g. *Glengarry Glen Ross*, 1992) and I am all in. I admire a great painting and I enjoy the occasional visit to the art museum, but it can't hold a candle to watching Scarlett Johansson walking through a London art gallery in one of my all-time favorite movies, *Match Point* (2005)!

So, yes, I love movies. But while I am in a confessional mode, let me admit to another bias. I love movie stars. Not just the beautiful ones, for obvious reasons, but also the rugged ones who show me how to be strong, and the vulnerable ones who, in their screen roles, teach me how to gracefully endure suffering. As Joseph Campbell said in his famous series of interviews with Bill Moyers, movie stars are like gods in that they can inhabit two places simultaneously. Campbell said, "There is something magical about films. The person you are looking at is also somewhere else at the same time. That is a condition of the god. If a movie actor comes into the theater, everyone turns and looks at the movie actor. He is the real hero of the occasion. He is on another plane. He is a multiple presence."[6 (p. 15)]

So, for example, if Albert Finney were to walk into the theater where *Before the Devil Knows You're Dead* (2007) is playing, everyone would turn their heads and burst with excitement to be in Finney's actual presence. While television creates celebrities about whom we love to gossip, movies create large mythic figures. We are in awe of these celebrities and we often strive to emulate them.

Why the difference? Perhaps it is due to the fact that while we watch television in our home, movies are often watched in what Campbell refers to as "a special temple" – that is, the movie theater. Despite the proliferation of movies on DVD and in other formats, there is still a huge market for seeing movies in the movie theater, where such larger-than-life impressions are formed.

Clearly, I am not alone in my love of movies and movie stars. Movies are a very popular form of entertainment. Why are movies so popular? Certainly, there is the escapism factor. The lights go down, the projector starts whirring and our own lives recede into the background until the lights come back on. Have you ever walked out of a movie theater and felt totally disoriented as you attempt to readjust to reality? I know I have.

Movies gross huge numbers. *Star Wars: Episode IV – A New Hope* (1977), a classic escapist-type movie, has made $775 103 103 in total box office sales since its release.[7] This figure is through June, 2009, not adjusted for inflation and *excludes* DVD rentals and sales. A recent Reuters poll looked at why we go see movies, and it found that at least one in four moviegoers seek out movies primarily for escapism. This effect is universal, with 67% of moviegoers in Turkey and 61% of East Indians seeking out movies for escapism.[8]

Perhaps another reason why we love movies so much is that they help us compare our life choices with those portrayed on the screen. Sooner or later in life, we are all faced with certain profound choices: Do I stay with my spouse or do I leave? Can I be a better parent than my parent? Why can't I be happier? Movies address such questions, and in so doing they prompt us to consider (and reconsider) our own choices by providing us with examples of successful and unsuccessful resolutions to our core dilemmas. Literature certainly does this also. It's just that movies provide a more visual, time-efficient, and, some may argue, entertaining exposure to the resolution of human dilemmas than books.

In fact, a night out at the movies can often have a life-changing impact. I recently suggested to a couple with whom I was working that they reconnect by having a fun evening out. They were struggling with the aftermath of an affair, were trying to decide whether or not to stay together, and seemed to be making progress toward reconciliation. Unfortunately, the movie they chose to see that night was *Eat Pray Love* (2010). This movie is considered by some to be the ulti-mate divorce movie. My couple was deeply influenced by the story of Elizabeth Gilbert, as played by America's sweetheart Julia Roberts, who decides to abruptly leave her unhappy marriage to tour the world. They left the theater in silence but were soon engaged in a heated argument in which they shared how disgruntled they were with each other. Whether or not the movie was the turning point, the couple soon decided to separate. Perhaps this was ultimately the right choice for them. However, I wonder if they had instead seen a different movie that night, perhaps *Life is Beautiful* (1997) or *Slumdog Millionaire* (2008), whether or not they would still be together.

Perhaps we simply love movies because they provide us an opportunity to be voyeurs and peek into another's life and personal thoughts for a couple of hours. Movies offer us, the viewer, a rare opportunity to inhabit two places at the same time. They provide us with an optical illusion; what we are seeing looks very real and three-dimensional but it is merely the rapid progression of two-dimensional film frames being run quickly together. We sit in our seat, inhabiting our own body and mind, while simultaneously having a bird's-eye view of someone else's life. In a movie, we can see behind the closed curtain, peer into the bedroom, and share the most intimate thoughts and emotions of the lead characters. We break through the masks that humans wear and ever so briefly inhabit another's life. Come to think of it, watching movies is the next best thing to being a therapist!

Maybe we love movies because they help us bond. Going to a movie with someone you love provides a powerful shared experience. Couples often enjoy going to the movies simply for the opportunity to discuss the movie afterward. It may have helped my wife, Elaine, decide to marry me knowing that after we saw our first movie together (*With Honors*, 1994), we both agreed the movie was terrible. (I know for a fact that her decision wasn't based on the car I was driving at the time.)

While couples can bond over a shared piece of literature, this process is less immediate. I have a long personal history of bonding through movies. As a child in New York City, I would go to the movies every Saturday morning with my friends in the gilded movie palaces of the 1950s. My mother loved movies and we would often attend them together during the long hot summers. I took my seventh-grade sweetheart on my first real date to see *How the West Was Won* (1962) and somehow found the courage to take her hand in the darkness of the theater. And how can I forget the connection I felt with my children upon watching *Pinocchio* (1940) and *Dumbo* (1941) with them for the first time?

While all these are valid ways of explaining our affinity for the movie-watching experience, I don't think they go deep enough. Is there more at play here? Why do movies move us so deeply? What is happening on the subconscious, subliminal level? How do movies achieve their power? To address these questions, I will focus on two key elements: process (how a movie is made) and content (what a movie is about).

A first step in understanding the process aspect of movie "magic" is to recognize that humans are, and always have been, storytellers. The earliest stories are encrypted onto stone walls in the manner of cave drawings. However, most early storytelling occurred in the oral tradition: humans telling stories to one another, often around a fire late at night. On a subliminal level, the movie-watching experience mirrors that of the ancient storytellers. When the lights go down and the movie starts to flicker on the silver screen, we are unknowingly experiencing the deeply rooted pleasure of sitting around an ancient fire, somewhere deep in the night, waiting for the storyteller to begin her story.

There is an art to the successful storyteller; she must start by bringing her audience in, perhaps by lowering her voice or painting a fantastic, over-the-top scene for her audience. She must make the most of nonverbal communication, perhaps waving her arms or clenching her fist while telling her story. She must keep the story moving along, provide original and compelling details and end on a high note that often pulls together disparate elements and teaches a moral lesson.

So it is with movies. They have to start with a bang. No one, by the way, opens a movie better than James Bond; if you are in doubt about this, please watch the opening scene of *Casino Royale* (2006) starring Daniel Craig. Movies must then move quickly along, keep us interested in the story and characters and, finally, inspire us with a meaningful conclusion at the end. Like the storyteller, actors and actresses are masters at fine-tuning their nonverbal expressions for maximum impact.

The director and movie editor work together to pace the movie and the screenwriter hones the dialogue to keep the audience invested and, it is to be hoped, enlightened. All these professionals work together synergistically; truly the sum of all their talents is greater than their individual contributions. In their synergy, modern moviemakers have a distinct advantage over the solo storyteller.

Of course, the story itself must not just be compelling; it must also be accurate. Glen Gabbard has stated that movies "have to tap into subconscious anxieties and conflict in the audience or we wouldn't see them."[5] However, such portrayals must be correct or audiences will be disappointed and the movie will in all likelihood fail. Screenwriters and actors often consult with psychiatrists to make sure their portrayals of mental illness are true. For example, a worldwide expert on obsessive-compulsive disorder, Dr. Jeffrey Schwartz, was a paid consultant for the movie *The Aviator* (2004).[9] Dr. Schwartz's job was to ensure that both the screenwriter and the actor playing Howard Hughes (Leonardo DiCaprio) provided accurate portrayals of Hughes's legendary obsessive-compulsive disorder.

One of the best ways to understand "how" a movie works is to see it twice. In fact, this was a requirement in a semester-long class I took at Harvard University on French cinema. During the first viewing, we were drawn in by the story, oblivious to how the movie achieved its impact. However, during the second viewing we could step back and observe the subtle ways in which the multiple talents of the director, actors, editors, screenwriters, and cinematographers worked together to create the desired effect. Freed from having to follow the plot line, we could pay attention to things like camera angles, nuances in facial expressions, scene editing, and the use of light and shadow.

The synergy of word with image, geography with spoken word, and photography with music is an important part of what makes movies move us on a deep, subliminal level. What would the tragic love story depicted in the movie *Doctor Zhivago* (1965) be without the beautiful "Lara's Theme"? What would the movie classic *Lawrence of Arabia* (1962) be without the images of long sandy desert that stay rooted in one's mind? What would *Casablanca* (1942) be without the subdued lighting of Rick's Café? And what would a suspenseful Alfred Hitchcock or Claude Chabrol masterpiece be without taut editing? All these elements are necessary in creating a powerful movie experience, one that can have strong emotional resonance.

Interestingly enough, as a cinemeducator, I watch movie clips over and over again. Each time I see the clip, I notice another way in which the multiple elements that make up a movie work together. I am doing in my professional life what I learned to do as a student of cinema all those many years ago.

However, movies don't just tug at our heartstrings. Movies can actually teach us to slow down and be more mindful about the world around us. Mindfulness, a very "hot" topic in psychological circles these days, occurs when we pause long enough to use our five senses to orient ourselves fully to the present moment. Movies teach us to be mindful through visual attention to detail.

A recent example of this comes from the Academy Award–winning movie, *Up in the Air* (2009). This movie tells the story of Ryan Bingham, as played by George Clooney, who is a "downsizing expert" hired to fire people from their jobs. In order to do his job, Bingham spends his professional life flying cross-country, from distressed company to distressed company, carrying out his dirty work. He is a commitment-averse male when it comes to relationships and actually considers air travel to be the best part of his job. In the movie, there are repetitive close-ups of Bingham packing and unpacking his suitcase. Watching scenes like these subliminally teach us in small ways to become more mindful. Perhaps we never before saw the beauty in the mundane task of packing for a trip. Perhaps, like Bingham, we will pack a little more intentionally next time we travel, taking greater care to neatly fold our clothes and paring them down to what is essential, as we see Clooney do.

There is a powerful movie clip that beautifully illustrates the point that movies, through their close attention to visual detail, can help us see the divine in the mundane. The movie *American Beauty* (1999) has a scene that anyone living in a city has likely witnessed dozens of times … a plastic bag caught in the wind. But while we have seen it, we most likely have never "seen" it … until now.

Movie images, like these, stay in our mind for a long time. As the Chinese say, a picture is worth a thousand words. Who among us can forget some of these movie images: Burt Lancaster and Deborah Kerr embracing in the ocean waves in *From Here to Eternity* (1953), Tom Courtney catching his breath while he stalls at the finish line during *The Loneliness of the Long Distance Runner* (1962), or

Humphrey Bogart saying a wistful goodbye to Ingrid Bergman in *Casablanca* as the last flight from Vichy-controlled Casablanca leaves for the continent? When it comes to memory, images rule. They remain with us long after the spoken word is forgotten.

In terms of their content, movies explore universal experiences and emotions. Such common, universally relevant, themes include (1) the role of chance in our lives (e.g. *Match Point*; *Sliding Doors*, 1998), (2) the importance of human traits such as defiance (e.g. *Defiance*, 2008; *Braveheart*, 1995), (3) courage (e.g. *Breaker Morant*, 1980) and persistence (e.g. *Hoosiers*, 1986; *The Blind Side*, 2009), (4) the mystery of death (e.g. *Ghost*, 1990; *Defending Your Life*, 1991; *Always*, 1989; *The Lovely Bones*, 2009), and (5) the corrosive impact of regret (e.g. *La Strada*, 1954; *Sophie's Choice*, 1982).

Many of these universal themes are built upon powerful archetypes rooted deep within the human psyche. An archetype is an elementary idea that is universal. In Jungian psychology, an archetype is defined as a primitive mental image inherited from the earliest human ancestors and present in the collective unconscious.[10] In ancient times, storytellers taught "wisdom" through fables that involved characters built upon these fundamental archetypes. When movies work well, they work with such elementary ideas, or archetypes, to which our collective psyche resonates.

Movies are the ideal medium for exploring archetypal themes. As Jung suggested in his book *Man and His Symbols*,[11] archetypes are recognized in image and emotion, both of which are readily evoked in the cinema. Because archetypes reside in the unconscious, they have a "particular potential for significance and may be feared or revered as mysterious signifiers of things beyond our complete understanding."[12] No wonder that movies dealing with these archetypal themes can move us so deeply.

The most common archetypal story seen in movies is the transformation story. In this story, the lead character makes a journey from selfishness to selflessness and, in so doing, has a "change of heart." This compelling narrative shows up again and again in literature, of course, but for the reasons already discussed, it is shown even more powerfully in movies – think *A Christmas Carol* (1938, 2009) and *Scrooge* (1951), *It's a Wonderful Life* (1946), *The Doctor* (1991), or even the recently released comedy *Gulliver's Travels* (2010).

A recent movie built around the transformation story is *Gran Torino* (2008), a hugely successful American drama, produced and directed by Clint Eastwood, who also stars in the film. Eastwood plays Walt Kowalski, a widower and bitter Korean War veteran who lives in a Detroit neighborhood that has seen a dramatic influx of immigrants from Southeast Asia. Kowalski feels alienated from these immigrants. In the movie, we see Eastwood's character transform from an angry and racist man to one capable of great love, generosity, and self-sacrifice.

The animated movies *Up* (2009) and *Despicable Me* (2010) are also splendid examples of the transformation story. In both movies, an older man who is alone and bitter becomes a changed person because of his involvement with children.

Even though I am very consciously aware of this transformation theme as it appears in literature and movies, I was still in tears by the end of *Despicable Me*, a movie that I saw under duress upon multiple requests from my 7-year-old daughter, Natalie. In this movie, the wicked Gru wishes to steal the moon and take over the world. To further his evil ambitions, he adopts three girls whom he plans to discard after his plot succeeds. In the course of the movie, however, he learns to be a loving father and to forego his evil ambitions. In other words, he is transformed. Perhaps I cried because in some ways this is my story; I too am a formerly reluctant and late-in-life dad who has been forever changed for the better by being a parent. However, I think the success of the movie speaks to the power of this transformation narrative, not just for me but for all of us, whether we are aged 7 or 97.

Perhaps the all-time best movie about transformation is the brilliant *Groundhog Day* (1993) starring Bill Murray. In this American comedy (with deep spiritual undertones), Murray plays Phil Connors, a selfish Pittsburgh TV weatherman, assigned to cover the annual Groundhog Day event in Punxsutawney, Pennsylvania, an annual assignment he has come to hate. When Connors and his team are trapped in the town overnight because of a snowstorm, Connors finds himself having to live the same day over and over until he finally realizes that the essence of living is to love and give to others. It is only after he is able to live according to these principles that he can start living new days again.

The hero's journey is another common archetypal theme in literature and movies. A hero, as Joseph Campbell states, is one who has given his or her life to something bigger than oneself.[6] The hero often embarks on a hero's journey in which he goes away, gains some larger insight about life, and returns to his community to share this insight. In a broader sense, we are all on a hero's or heroine's journey through life.

A powerful cinematic example of the hero's journey is embodied in the movie *The Shawshank Redemption* (1994), recently rated as one of the 100 top American movies of all time by the American Film Institute. This movie was adapted from a Stephen King novella entitled *Rita Hayworth and Shawshank Redemption* and tells the story of Andy Dufresne, a banker who spends nearly 20 years in a state prison, wrongly accused of murdering his wife. In this movie, Dufresne is able to overcome considerable big house cruelty to manage a brilliant escape in which the "bad guys" are punished and the good guy is freed. When we see Andy reunited at the end of the movie with his fellow former inmate, Red, on the beach at Zihuatanejo, we all identify with his heroism, resilience, and courage.

Another good example of the hero's journey occurs in the movie *Any Given Sunday* (1999). In this Oliver Stone movie, Al Pacino plays the world-weary Tony D'Amato, the head coach of a professional football team, who gives a pep talk to his team prior to a pivotal game. In this talk, D'Amoto shares a lifetime of hard-won experience gleaned from his own hero's journey.

Men and women play out many archetypal roles other than the hero. Some common archetypes for both men and women are King/Queen, Warrior, Magician,

Lover, Wise Old Man/Crone, and Youth/Maiden. Because these archetypes are unconscious, we may not be aware of their presence in our own lives. Movie and literary characters, however, can bring them to life. The archetypes represent human qualities and potentials beyond their narrow designation. For example, because the Magician archetype involves the communication of hidden knowledge, it can be seen in a multitude of professionals – namely, writers, psychotherapists, filmmakers, physicians, performers, teachers, or innovators.

Each archetype has an adult or realized form in which the best elements of that archetype are actualized. Think of King Arthur, perhaps, as a fully realized version of the King archetype. Each archetype has, as well, a shadow form. The archetype of the Shadow, a mainstay of Jungian psychology, consists of the darker qualities that the ego rejects but which exist nonetheless. If unrecognized, shadow elements can take hold of the ego and lead it on a destructive path. Think of Darth Vader as a great example of a shadow representation of the Warrior archetype.

Interestingly enough, two movies about the Magician archetype were recently released within months of each other. In *The Illusionist* (2006), Edward Norton plays Eisenheim, a man who uses his extraordinary magical skills to reconnect with and free his childhood love who has been imprisoned in her royal house in Vienna. Eisenheim represents the mature form of the Magician archetype. In the same year, the *The Prestige* (2006), was released. In this movie, Hugh Jackman plays Robert Angier, a magician bitter over the death of his wife at the supposed hands of another magician, Alfred Borden, as played by Christian Bale. The film tells the story of these two men's rivalry centered on the mastery of a magic trick involving the creation of a human double. The tragic truth of the trick, called the Transported Man, involves the double disappearing and being drowned offstage every night the trick is successfully performed. Angier represents the immature, destructive form of the Magician archetype.

By portraying the realized and shadow aspects of archetypes, movies, and of course literature, help us reflect upon and learn from the successes and mistakes of the characters. If we are wise, we can choose to aspire to the realized form of each archetype rather than its shadow counterpart.

In their brilliant book *King, Magician, Warrior, Lover*,[13] authors Robert Moore and Douglas Gillette suggest a tripartite model. In their model, shadow archetypes consist of not one but two elements, an active and an inactive form; in the active form, the dark energies are directed outwardly and in the passive form they are directed inwardly.

Let us take the Warrior archetype for example. The mature Warrior knows that the real war is within. This warrior acts as an energy source for us to be assertive about our lives and shows considerable self-discipline so as to harness his powers to live in service to others. As defined in this way, the Warrior archetype can be seen in a variety of roles: politician, father, environmental activist, defense lawyer, soldier, and so on. No greater portrayal of the mature Warrior archetype exists in my mind than that of Robert De Niro in the *The Deer Hunter* (1978). In this film, Robert De Niro plays Michael, who portrays the fully realized Warrior – loyal, brave, and fiercely protective. In an opening clip, we are introduced to Michael and his penchant for killing a deer with one shot, certainly the most humane way to kill prey.

However, by the end of *The Deer Hunter*, one of Michael's fellow soldiers, Nick, as played by Christopher Walken, is involved in an addictive form of masochism, Russian roulette, played out for hire in the dark alleys of Saigon right before its fall. This behavior is a result of posttraumatic stress disorder and represents the passive form of the Warrior shadow, where the warrior energy is turned masochistically inward.

A more recent example of the Warrior shadow turned masochistically inward occurs in *The Wrestler* (2008). *The Wrestler* stars a resurrected Mickey Rourke as Randy "The Ram" Robinson, a professional fighter 20 years past his prime. After a disastrous falling-out with his daughter and girlfriend, Randy commits what amounts to suicide by returning to the ring, despite his cardiologist's strong entreaties for him to retire. At the end of the movie, "The Ram," in tears, salutes the crowd and engages in his trademark maneuver, "The Ram Jam," against his opponent despite the presence of serious chest pain. The fact that the screen goes to black after the execution of this diving stunt implies that it is fatal.

In another movie, *The Great Santini* (1979), we see Robert Duvall play Bull Meechum, a marine officer who is sadistic in his dealings with his family. In one scene, we observe Meechum's shadow Warrior emerge in its destructive fullness during a basketball game with his son. This is the full realization of the active shadow of the Warrior archetype.

There certainly are many female cinematic examples of this tripartite model of archetypes. One common female archetype is the Crone (Wise Woman).[14] We see the mature form of the Crone played out in the classic movie *Harold and Maude* (1971), in which Maude, as played by Ruth Gordon, befriends the suicidal teenager Harold (Bud Cort) and mentors him about life, love, and happiness. The sadistic version, or active shadow, form of the Crone can be seen in the movie *Notes on a Scandal* (2006), in which Dame Judi Dench plays Barbara Covett who covets a relationship with the younger Sheba Hart, as played by Cate Blanchett. Hart is manipulated and secretly undermined by Covett so that Covett can possess the younger woman sexually. The masochistic, or passive shadow, form of the Crone archetype can be seen in *The Last Picture Show* (1971), through the character of Ruth Popper, the coach's wife, who is shown early in the movie to be melancholic, lonely, and lost. Cloris Leachman played Popper in the film and won an Academy Award for her performance.

All these images and portrayals have deep meaning to us because they represent universal archetypes embedded in our unconscious minds. By seeing both the realized and shadow forms of each archetype, viewers are able to discern how others either find or lose their way in life and, in so doing, be more aware of their own choices. Because these archetypal stories and characters are brought to our awareness through the talents of the finest actors, directors, cinematographers, and screenwriters and because they occur in a darkened theater that simulates a dream state, they are powerful and profound. Process and content work together seamlessly.

In 1964, Marshall McLuhan, a Canadian educator, philosopher, and scholar, made the declaration that "the medium is the message."[15] McLuhan observed that the way in which information is shared, e.g. via TV, film (or iPod), has a greater impact on our collective consciousness than the content itself that is being shared. When it comes to movies, however, I would argue that the synergistic interplay between content (what the movie is about) and process (how the movie is made) is the message. Movies move us because they tell universal stories through a powerful medium that simulates real life and builds upon our ancient memories of the earliest storytellers. Movies show us what it means to be human in a manner uniquely fashioned to have a deep and lasting impact on our soul. At their best, movies are waking dreams full of great import and potent longing, capable of evoking our deepest yearnings for joy, human connection, and transcendence. In this light, I would like to conclude my keynote presentation with one of the most exhilarating scenes in recent movie history, the closing railroad station scene of *Slumdog Millionaire*. Long live the cinema!

References

1 Alexander M, Hall MN, Pettice Y. Cinemeducation: an innovative approach to teaching psychosocial medical care. *Fam Med*. 1994; **26**: 430–3.

2 Alexander M. A review of the literature. In: Alexander M, Lenahan P, Pavlov A, editors. *Cinemeducation: a comprehensive guide to using film in medical education*. Oxford: Radcliffe Publishing; 2005. pp. 3–7.

3 Bhugra D, Gupta S, editors. Special issue on the cinema. *Int Rev Psychiatry*. 2009; **21**(3): 181–2.

4 Blasco PB, Moerto G, Roncoletta A, *et al*. Using movie clips to foster learners' reflection: improving education in the affective domain. *Fam Med*. 2006; **38**(2): 94–6.

5 Beck M. Fictional stars, real problems. *Wall Street Journal*. June 8, 2010: D1, D8.

6 Campbell J. *The Power of Myth*. New York, NY: Doubleday Books; 1988.

7 Vaux R. *How Much Money Did Each Star Wars Movie Make?* Mania.com. Available at: www.mania.com/much-money-did-each-star-wars-movie-make_article_116389.html (last accessed 4/14/12)

8 Reuters Life. *Escape to the Movies? 1 in 4 people do: poll*. March 5, 2010. Available at: www.reuters.com/article/.../us-movies-poll-idUSTRE6243N0201003... (last accessed 4/14/12).

9 Royal College of Psychiatrists. *The Aviator*. Available at: www.rcpsych.ac.uk/mental healthinfo/mindsonfilmblog/theaviator.aspx (last accessed 12/01/11)

10 Munafo RP. *Archetypes in Literature*. Available at: http://mrob.com/pub/std/archetypes. html (last accessed 4/14/12).

11 Jung C. *Man and His Symbols*. New York, NY: Doubleday; 1964.

12 Changing Minds. *Jung's Archetypes*. Available at: www.changingminds.org/explanations/ identity/jung_archetypes (last accessed 12/01/11).

13 Moore R, Gillette D. *King Warrior Magician Lover: rediscovering the archetypes of the mature masculine*. New York, NY: Harper Collins; 1990.

14 Conway DJ. *Maiden, Mother, Crone: the myth and reality of the triple goddess*. Llewellyn Publications; 1994.

15 McLuhan M, Fiore Q. *The Medium is the Message*. New York, NY: Simon & Schuster; 1989.

3

Diving Deep:
Jung's Layers of the Psyche

Gregory P. Brown

CARL JUNG AND SIGMUND FREUD BOTH CONCLUDED THAT HUMAN beings have an unconscious level of being not immediately available to awareness. While some layers of the unconscious could reveal themselves with gentle self-reflection, deeper layers could require years of depth therapy to unearth. Jung and Freud agreed that clients could live fuller lives if therapists assisted them in bringing unconscious forces to consciousness. However, while Freud believed that successful treatment would relieve patients of the misery of neurosis (allowing them to love and to work), Jung believed that making the unconscious "conscious" would allow clients to embark upon a journey toward wholeness.

A key component of Jung's approach to the unconscious was his delineation of archetypes, or elementary principles, which are revealed through personal and universal symbols. Some common archetypes identified by Jung are the Persona, the Shadow, the Syzygy (Anima/Animus), and the Self. Once clients can successfully integrate these archetypes into their consciousness, they are freer to make choices in their lives.

All the World's a Stage: The Persona

The Persona refers to our public face or mask. The recognition of the Persona emerges when we experience a gap between who we really are internally and the presentation we give to our friends, coworkers, family, and intimate partners. When this discrepancy enters awareness, we often perceive a need for change or growth in life.

The Matrix (1999; Keanu Reeves, Laurence Fishburne): This movie tells the story of Thomas Anderson (Reeves), a computer programmer living a traditional life before opening himself to a deeper level of Self, known as Neo.

1 (Ch 3, 0:07:05–0:09:42) Anderson awakens to find a computer console beckoning him to "follow the white rabbit." He takes this as a clue and allows his curiosity to lead him out of his apartment to a party where he meets Trinity (Carrie-Anne Moss).

    a. In what ways do you play an expected role in your own life? Do you experience a dissonance between this expected role and who you feel you truly are?

    b. Have you ever experienced a life adventure set off by a set of interesting coincidences? Please elaborate.

2 (Ch 6, 0:17:07–0:20:47) During this interview with the "agents," Neo is terrified to find reality "bending" in an unexpected manner.

    a. Have you ever had experiences that altered your view of what was real? Did such experiences cause you to think differently about yourself?

    b. How do you conceptualize experiences in which reality is altered (i.e. as a statistical abnormality, a psychopathology, an opening to change, or a calling from a deeper level of being)?

3 (Chs 8–9, 0:25:13–0:29:45) Morpheus (Fishburne) offers Mr. Anderson/Neo (Reeves) the choice to look deeper into his life. Neo accepts this invitation and in so doing he affirms awareness of his Persona and accepts a call to deeper personal growth. As an aside, the word "Morpheus" relates to sleep. The metaphor of sleepers awakening from dreams to reality is commonly used to describe the process of individuals deepening their awareness of the Persona to embrace a deeper sense of self.

    a. How do psychotherapy patients exhibit their Personas in session? How might you encourage your patients to manifest their real selves in the world?

Hearts of Darkness: The Shadow

The Shadow represents the inner aspect of a person that is rejected or despised. Individuals tend to deny that Shadow impulses are part of who they are. The personal Shadow tends to focus around such traits as greed, hatred, jealousy, and revenge. The collective Shadow of a society, if unintegrated, can lead to fascism, war, and abandonment of long-held values.

The Lord of the Rings: The Two Towers (2002; Special Extended Version; Ian McKellen): Tolkein's epic tale reveals a host of archetypal images and themes. The character of Gandalf (McKellen) provides an example of the enormous benefits of integrating one's Shadow.

1 (Disk 1, ch 1, 0:00:50–0:03:44) The Balrog, a mythical beast of fire and destruction, personifies all that Gandolf is not. To deal successfully with the Balrog, Gandolf must confront his own Shadow.

    a. What do you imagine your Shadow looks like? (Hint: personal Shadows usually take the form of behaviors or attitudes that we dislike in others.)

     b. Societies and cultures have collective Shadows. What is our culture's current collective Shadow?

     c. What makes acknowledgment of the Shadow so difficult? Contrast the process of acknowledging and integrating one's personal Shadow with that of identifying and confronting one's Persona?

2 (Disk 1, ch 15, 0:53:13–0:55:28) Following his death, Gandalf the Grey is reborn as Gandalf the White. This scene displays Gandalf's transition from gray to white as a death-rebirth experience brought about by the integration of his Shadow.

     a. Why did Gandalf's transformation require the temporary death of his ego?

     b. How might you acknowledge Shadow elements in your own life? How might you most effectively work with therapy patients to help them access Shadow material?

     c. What is the difference between acknowledging and integrating Shadow elements in one's self and succumbing to evil?

Some Like it Hot: The Syzygy

The Anima is the female aspect of the psyche contained within the male. Likewise, the Animus is the male aspect of the psyche contained within the female. The Anima and Animus are collectively referred to as the Syzygy, a Latin term meaning conjunction. Until these archetypal aspects are integrated into our awareness, we tend to project our Anima or Animus upon members of the opposite sex, thereby limiting our ability to make free choices.

The Anima as Healer

Lady in the Water (2006; Paul Giamatti): Cleveland Heep (Giamatti) is the caretaker of The Cove, an apartment complex separated from the world. The Cove serves as a safe holding environment for a group of tenants, all of whom are involved in some form of life transition. Story (Bryce Dallas Howard) arrives from within the waters of a brain-shaped pool on the premises. Her connection to the unconscious is demonstrated both by her living in the water and by her saving Cleveland after he falls into the water.

1 (Ch 9, 0:33:45–0:37:46) In this scene, Story discovers Cleveland's past life trauma in which his family was brutally murdered in their home. Cleveland, a former physician, has blocked these memories and lives a sheltered existence in The Cove. Story also meets Vick Ran (M. Night Shyamalan) whom she motivates to complete an unfinished book.

     a. Prior to Story's discovery, Cleveland is portrayed solely as manager and caretaker of the Cove. What changes occur in your perception of Cleveland now that he is identified as a physician?

     b. What is it about Cleveland's traumatic past that prevented him from continuing his work as a physician?

     c. What are the helpful and the destructive aspects of isolation following a major life trauma? What parts of Cleveland did he have to isolate to protect himself from the pain of his family's loss?

2   (Ch 12, 0:46:10–0:49:00) Cleveland leaps into the pool to find the healing force hidden in Story's cave located under the pool. This action symbolizes his attempt to face his unconscious, a dangerous journey illustrated by the fact that he is nearly trapped in the process. Historical aspects of the unconscious are illustrated in Story's cave, which is cluttered with items that she has gathered from the community over time.

     a. Cleveland now wants Story's help rather than wanting her to disappear. What inner change does this represent within Cleveland?

     b. Have you treated patients who became lost, or drowned, in unconscious material? How do they get a "breath of air"? What treatment approaches are most effective in such situations?

     c. How might your own Anima/Animus appear to you?

3   (Ch 23, 1:32:00–1:37:12) A group has assembled to heal Story so that she can return to her world. Cleveland discovers, to his surprise, that he himself must play the role of healer. His heartfelt sacrifice ultimately heals both Story and him. This symbolic integration of the feminine unconscious element is characteristic of a positive interaction with the Anima.

     a. How did Cleveland finally release the pain of the death of his family?

     b. What healed Story?

     c. What healed Cleveland? Might he now return to medicine? If so, would his experiences with Story make him a better doctor?

     d. In what ways is healing different from "treating"? How does the concept of wholeness and integration differ from the concept of symptom control? How does change manifest in each?

     e. Have you worked with clients who have successfully integrated Anima/Animus elements? Please describe your approach.

Animus as Teacher

The integration of the Syzygy may be a harrowing sequence with the danger of losing the ego to the archetypal energy.

The Phantom of the Opera (2004; Emmy Rossum, Gerard Butler): Christine (Rossum) finds herself transformed in the caverns below the opera house. Her teacher, the Phantom (Butler), had helped to hone her vocal skills, but then he attempts to steal her away so as to keep her for himself.

1   (Chs 8–10, 0:29:22–0:41:00) Christine's descent into the unconscious with the Phantom is both frightening and alluring at the same time. Christine's experience, and subsequent integration of archetypal elements, provides her with the capacity to become the new star of the opera. The image of water represents the unconscious depths of this process.

     a. How does the death of Christine's father and her relationship with the

Animus figure of the Phantom parallel Cleveland's loss and relationship with his Anima as previously discussed?

    b. In what way was Christine not whole prior to her contact with the Phantom?

    c. How would you (females) imagine your Animus might appear to you?

2 (Chs 32–33, 2:01:17–2:07:19) Christine has been captured by the Phantom and returned to the underworld, where he plans to trap her. She redeems herself and him by an act of love rather than engaging in rejection or aggression. This choice to include and integrate the Phantom frees her and her lover from perpetual imprisonment.

    a. What makes integration of the Animus the greatest challenge for Christine?

    b. How is integration of the Syzygy different from integration of the Shadow or of the Persona?

    c. In terms of either yourself or a patient, what would be the result fighting the Syzygy component of the psyche compared with integrating it?

Steps Toward Wholeness: The Self

Jung described dream sequences that demonstrate symbols of wholeness. He believed these dream symbols would only manifest themselves after the Persona, Shadow, and Syzygy were fully integrated into the psyche. These symbols would often take the form of mandalas or other symmetrical figures. Jung considered these symbols as representative of the completion of the individuation process, his description for becoming whole.

The Ninth Gate (1999): Dean Corso, played by Johnny Depp, begins the movie as a crass, materialistic book trader. Through deciphering mysteries within a series of books, he transforms into a spiritual seeker. Corso is cleansed by water and purified by fire in the early phases of the movie, a sequence common to Western esoteric traditions. The final scenes demonstrate the entire Jungian sequence of integrations.

1 (Ch 25, 1:51:17–1:51:56) Corso is offered and then refuses a large sum of money to return to New York. His refusal allows him the opportunity to embark upon a journey of inner transformation. Corso's choice embodies the successful integration of the Persona.

2 (Ch 27, 1:57:08–2:02:50) Corso spars with Boris Balkan, played by Frank Langella, in an attempt to gain the knowledge Balkan has sought. He tricks Balkan into self-destruction through engaging Balkan's pride. This interchange allows Corso to integrate the Shadow elements of his personality.

3 (Ch 28, 2:03:35–2:06:25 [NB: mature content]) Corso sexually unites with "The Girl," played by Emmanuelle Seigner. "The Girl" was perceived as enigmatic and unapproachable by Corso earlier in the film because Corso had not yet integrated either his Persona or Shadow. "The Girl" then provides him

with the final clue on his journey that facilitates the integration of the Anima (Syzygy).

4 (Ch 29, 2:07:52–2:08:49) Corso has completed each of the steps of integration, and enters the castle filled with a glowing, divine light. This represents the integration of the Self, or inner Divine quality of wholeness.

   a. What transformed Corso from an opportunistic book trader into a spiritual seeker?

   b. What do you imagine Corso's new life may be like after entering "the light"?

   c. What would an experience of inner wholeness mean to you? What might it be like? What might it be like for clients you see in psychotherapy?

The Whole Sequence

As a review, a single scene from *The Lord of the Rings: The Fellowship of the Ring* (2001) demonstrates the integration of each of the aforementioned archetypes.

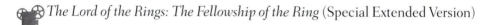 *The Lord of the Rings: The Fellowship of the Ring* (Special Extended Version)

1 (Disk 2, ch 12, 0:54:35–1:00:13, immediately followed by disk 2, ch 14, 1:06:15–1:06:43) Frodo, played by Elijah Wood, awakens from sleep to have an interaction with Galadriel, played by Cate Blanchett.

   a. Identify the element of the scene that represents the Persona.

   b. Identify the element of the scene that represents the Unconscious.

   c. Identify the element of the scene that represents the Shadow.

   d. Identify the integration within Frodo that occurs if Galadriel is assumed to be his Anima.

   e. Identify the integration within Galadriel that occurs if Frodo is assumed to be her Animus.

   f. What is the symbol of the Self in this scene? Why? (Hint: it is in the second clip.)

   g. How are Galadriel's words regarding being a "ring-bearer" symbolic of the journey of psychotherapy? Have clients discussed a feeling about their journey of transformation similar to that shared by Frodo?

Summary

The transpersonal journey of the characters in these movies changed them in ways they could not have imagined prior to embarking upon these paths. The acts of transformation within these films follow a Jungian interpretation of personal growth from ego to Self, moving through a series of integrating steps. The acceptance, acknowledgment, and wholeness engendered by integration of the

Persona, the Shadow, the Syzygy (Anima/Animus), and the Self are representative of Jung's path of Individuation.

1   How did Neo, Gandalf, Cleveland, Christine, Frodo, Galadriel, and Corso change? Why? Would a behavioral description or cognitive elaboration do any of these inner transformations justice? Why or why not?

2   Jung considered these steps of integration as part of psychotherapeutic change. Have you noted similar experiences or patterns within yourself? Have you noted similar types of transformation in patients?

3   Does this model imply a different perspective towards the development of symptoms than the model you now use to treat patients? In what way?

4   Jung described ego inflation as a risk of this work (essentially confusing ego for Self). Which characters in these clips run the greatest risk of ego inflation? Why? How is such a potential pitfall best managed?

5   What aspects of this archetypal model might be appropriate in your practice? In your interactions with patients? In exploring yourself?

6   Please discuss the role of dream study in helping patients work with archetypal themes. The role of active imagination?

Further Reading

- Campbell J. *The Hero with a Thousand Faces*. Princeton, NJ: Princeton University Press; 1949.
- Edinger E. *Ego and Archtype*. Boston, MA: Shambhala; 1992.
- Jung CG. *Man and His Symbols*. New York, NY: Doubleday Press; 1964.
- Stein M. *Jung's Map of the Soul*. Chicago, IL: Open Court Publishing; 1998.
- Wilmer HA. *Practical Jung: nuts and bolts of Jungian psychotherapy*. Brooklyn, NY: Chiron Publications; 1987.

PART II

Family Functioning and Health

4

Two to Tango:
Couples in the Cinema

Matthew Alexander & Anthony Zamudio

THE HIGH EXPECTATIONS THAT AMERICANS HAVE FOR THEIR ROMANTIC relationships motivate many to seek couple counseling. In fact, millions of Americans attend couple therapy, and approximately 40% of engaged couples attend some form of premarital therapy.[1] It is estimated that approximately 80% of therapists offer couple therapy to their clients.[2]

All of these factors underscore the importance of high-quality education for couple therapists, whether in practice or in training. Cinemeducation offers a rich tool for such education. After all, when it comes to couples in the cinema there are myriad movies suitable for teaching and illustrating all aspects of the "couple odyssey."[3,4] This chapter cites some favorites.

While the movies used here deal primarily with heterosexual unions, the insights gleaned from them are applicable to same-sex pairings.

The Couple's Journey

Stage One: Infatuation – "I'm so glad I found you"

Ira and Abby (2006; Chris Messina, Jennifer Westfeldt): A couple meet, fall in love, and marry in a very short period of time, setting them up for multiple relationship challenges.

1   (Ch 2, 0:10:54–0:19:05) Ira and Abby meet at a Manhattan health club. Within moments they "fall in love" and soon thereafter decide to marry.
   a. While clearly an exaggeration, what elements of infatuation does this clip illustrate?
   b. What are some personal differences that the couple is glossing over?
   c. What are the benefits of long versus short periods of dating prior to making a long-term commitment to another person?
   d. Do logic, passion, or a combination of both provide the best basis for

making a decision to commit to a long-term relationship? Which of these is the best predictor of long-term success?

About Last Night (1986; Rob Lowe, Demi Moore): Danny's (Lowe) and Debbie's (Moore) relationship progresses from a one-night stand to casual dating and, eventually, to their living together. During the dating phase, differences in their respective interests are exposed. Moving in together, in turn, leads them to struggle about communication, the importance of friendships, and past relationships and commitment.

1   (Chs 7–8, 0:24:06–0:28:50) In these scenes, we observe Danny and Debbie in the dating phase of their relationship, where they share respective interests, engage in passionate sex, and disclose life dreams. Their time together infringes on work and availability for close friends such as Joan (Elizabeth Perkins) and Bernie (James Belushi).

   a. Danny likes to spend his free time watching baseball and Debbie prefers visiting art museums. Do differences like these become a source of growth for couples or do they become barriers to satisfaction?

   b. Which is more important for long-term success in coupling: shared interests or shared values?

   c. The couple has gratifying sex. Is good sex always present in the early parts of a relationship? Can sex become a major resource in helping a couple tolerate differences and difficulties in the relationship?

   d. Joan is angry over Debbie's neglect of their friendship since her involvement with Danny. Is Joan being unreasonable, given the "honeymoon phase" of Debbie's relationship? When should partners set limits and prioritize time with friends apart from their love interests?

2   (Chs 11–12, 0:36:00–0:41:15) Danny and Debbie's relationship progresses from dating to living together in Danny's apartment with strong disapproval and negativity from Debbie's friend, Joan. The couple must readjust and reorder Danny's household and separate practical from sentimental belongings.

   a. Does marriage make the process of living together easier or harder than being unmarried partners?

   b. Is it best for couples planning to cohabit to move into neutral territory, such as a new residence, or into one partner's current residence?

   c. What impact, good or bad, does living together have prior to marriage? Is living together prior to marriage a predictor of divorce?

   d. Couples often fight about each other's stuff in the early parts of their relationship. How can you help couples navigate differences about "stuff"?

Stage Two: Disillusionment and Power Struggle – "I can't believe you don't see things my way"

Ira and Abby (see earlier description)

1   (Ch 8, 0:42:48–0:46:31; ch 9, 0:48:34–0:49:18) In these scenes, we see Ira and Abby have their first fight as their personality differences begin to emerge. We then see them seek out a couple therapist (Jason Alexander) for help in resolving these conflicts, only to have the conflicts escalate upon leaving the couple therapist's office.
    a. In what ways are Ira and Abby now entering the power struggle phase of their relationship?
    b. How can one prepare newlyweds for the inevitable disappointment and tension that occurs once they realize that their partner is, indeed, different from them? Is there a role for premarital counseling in this regard?
2   (Ch 9, 0:51:00–0:55:00) In this scene, Ira finds out that Abby has not told him about her previous marriages. He becomes very angry and agitated by this revelation and creates a scene in front of both sets of parents.
    a. How are attachment wounds in relationships – such as lies, neglect, and betrayal – best worked through? What is likely to happen to Ira and Abby if this disagreement is swept under the proverbial rug?
    b. What are the vulnerable emotions that underlie Ira's reaction to these revelations?
    c. What does this scene say about the importance of trust in committed relationships?
    d. How do you help a couple regain trust after betrayal?
    e. Is there a difference between lies of omission and lies of commission?

Fools Rush In (1997; Matthew Perry, Salma Hayek): This is a romantic comedy about an uptight New Yorker, Alex Whitman (Matthew Perry), and an independent, free-spirited Latina, Isabel Fuentes (Salma Hayek). The couple's one-night stand leads to pregnancy and sudden marriage resulting in a wake-up call when personality differences, extended families, and cultures clash.
1   (Ch 13, 0:40:59–0:44:03) In these scenes, Isabel's father confronts Alex over his daughter's marriage outside the Catholic Church. Nonetheless, Isabel and Alex continue to make plans about their future but soon discover important differences are emerging between them.
    a. What does the scene illustrate about challenges brought about by a couple's religious differences?
    b. When are conflicts over beliefs, values, and lifestyle most likely to surface in a committed relationship?
    c. What is the best way for couples to negotiate important decisions such as where to live, how many children to have, what religion to practice etc?
    d. Is this couple at risk for divorce? What are common risk factors for

divorce? Would marrying someone with a similar background help reduce conflicts and stress over differences?
  e. What psychological characteristics and/or circumstances allow couples to tolerate and even thrive with differences?

Blue Valentine (2010; Michelle Williams, Ryan Gosling):The film shows the dissolution, over time, of the relationship between Dean Pereira (Gosling) and Cindy Heller (Williams), who meet, fall in love, marry, and ultimately divorce. Dean, a high school dropout and Cindy, a premed student, fall in love and then marry soon after finding out that Cindy is pregnant from a previous boyfriend. She works at a medical clinic and he is a house painter who likes to drink alcohol.
1 (0:50:16–0:53:49; 0:53:50–0:57:17) In these two scenes (which run back to back), we first see the couple as they are falling in love. In the second scene, we see them many years later, discussing their disintegrating marriage during a failed romantic getaway at a motel.
  a. What elements of infatuation are evident in the first clip?
  b. What do you make of the song sung during the first clip? Is it a harbinger of things to come? Why do people often "hurt the ones they love"?
  c. What are some of the lifestyle and value differences between the couple that are unacknowledged by them at the beginning of their relationship? Is their infatuation an example of opposites attracting? Do these two clips support the premise that opposites attract, then polarize, and then repel?
  d. What are the different values espoused by Dean and Cindy during the second clip? How well do they express their value system to the other? Is their value clash reparable?
  e. Is it true that couples often "grow apart" as they age? How can this development be handled in a way that allows couples to stay together rather than break up?
  f. The couple is consuming alcohol as they talk. Is it a good idea for couples to have serious conversations about their relationship while drinking?
  g. What is the role of alcohol in troubled marriages? Does alcohol treatment have to occur before couples can benefit from couple therapy? If so, what is the best language for the therapist to use to encourage the chemically dependent partner to get treatment without alienating him/her and losing the couple?

Stage Three: Reconciliation, Acceptance, Co-Creation – Together, Warts and All

A Single Man (2009; Colin Firth, Julianne Moore): The story of a gay English professor, George Falconer (Firth) whose longtime partner Jim (Matthew Goode) dies in a motor vehicle accident. The movie shows Falconer's grief process over the course of 1 day in his life.
1 (Ch 16, 0:47:55–0:50:50) In this scene, Falconer flashes back to an evening when he and his partner are at home, reading and listening to music.

a. Comment on the level of intimacy demonstrated in this clip.
b. How does this clip reveal the couple's acceptance of each other?
c. The couple appears very nonreactive. How might a more reactive couple be portrayed in the same scene?
d. Can couples be intimate even when they are not talking? If so, how? Are certain types of emotional intimacy more typical of women? Of men?
e. Are there ways this scene might have played out differently if a heterosexual union were portrayed? If a lesbian relationship were portrayed?

Ira and Abby (see earlier description)

1 (Ch 16, 1:34:56–1:37:30) In this scene, Ira and Abby decide to divorce (for the second time) and, paradoxically, embrace a more honest love for each other.
a. In what way does this scene reflect each partner's deep acceptance of the other, flaws and all?
b. How is acceptance of one's partner different from resignation?

51 Birch Street (2005): In this film Doug Block documents his parents' 54-year marriage with real-life interviews. During the movie, his mother, Mina, and father, Mike, discuss their history and their views of marriage. When Doug's mother dies unexpectedly, his father quickly marries a former secretary. Doug unexpectedly discovers his mother's diaries, which help him understand the complexities and compromises of his parents' marriage.
1 (Ch 11, 1:05:10–1:07:10) Doug asks his father if he misses his deceased wife. His father describes his marriage to Doug's mother as a "functional" rather than "loving" association and he discusses phases of marriage.
a. Is it possible for spouses to discover or rediscover "love" in the latter phase of marriage? What about with a new partner after a spouse's death?
b. How common are "functional associations" in couples married 5, 10, or 50 years?
c. Did Mike and Mina reach a successful goal by staying together for the sake of the kids? In what ways might their children have suffered by their staying together? What if they had divorced?
d. How do you counsel couples who are not sure that they wish to stay married for the sake of the kids?

The Story of Us (1999; Bruce Willis, Michelle Pfeiffer): This is a movie that tells the story of a couple going through a painful separation.
1 (Ch 17, 1:23:00–1:31:00) In this scene, Katie (Pfeiffer) realizes all the shared history connecting her with Ben (Willis) as she tearfully announces her decision to stay with him.
a. What does Katie's monologue say about the value of shared history to couples?

b. How can one encourage couples to stay together during the bad times so that they can reach Stage Three (i.e. reconciliation, acceptance, and co-creation) of the couple's journey?

c. How might Katie's monologue be used with couples contemplating divorce?

Specific Issues

Reentry/Reconnection

About Last Night (see earlier description)

1 (Ch 13, 0:46:33–0:47:47) Danny arrives home after a stressful workday. The scene illustrates common communication problems between couples.

a. How can a partner's initial greeting at the end of the working day create either distance or contact? What are best ways for couples to re-enter each other's lives after being apart?

b. How does this scene speak to issues of boundaries and the importance for couples to balance alone time with together time?

Division of Labor

The Break-Up (2006; Vince Vaughn; Jennifer Aniston): This romantic comedy/drama tells the story of Brooke (Aniston) and Gary (Vaughn), a Chicago couple living together who turn to their friends for advice after a serious fight.

1 (Ch 4, 0:18:47–0:24:50) This scene shows Gary and Brooke fighting over cleaning the dishes after a dinner party. The scene not only illustrates issues around division of labor but also touches on the critical importance of emotional regulation in managing conflict and the presence of gender issues in heterosexual unions.

a. What does this scene illustrate about gender and division of labor? What are the current trends regarding division of labor in heterosexual couplings? How can you help couples resolve issues related to division of labor?

b. What does this scene illustrate about "emotional hijacking" (i.e. the process by which this fight over the dishes unexpectedly turns into a fight about the entire relationship)? How does anger lock couples into positions that they must then justify?

c. What skill set (i.e. pattern interrupt: soft start-up) would have helped this couple avoid the negative escalation of their fight?

d. How does this scene reflect the importance of respect to men and connection to women?

2 (Ch 16, 1:18:38–1:22:13) In this scene (which should be shown after the previous scene above), Brooke has had her hopes for reconciliation dashed when Vince doesn't show up at a concert to which she invited him. She is devastated and Gary attempts to make amends. In the process, they discuss

how they got to be so far apart and revisit the argument about the dishes that led to their separation.

a. How is this discussion different from their initial fight? Why did it not occur during the night of their fight? What skills do couples need to be able to de-escalate fights before they turn toxic?

b. Was the original fight really about division of labor or about the security of the couple's emotional connection? How would a "reframe" such as this help a couple better understand conflicts about division of labor?

c. Comment on Gary's nonreactivity and how this helps facilitate the conversation. How can therapists encourage couples to be a "nonanxious" presence for each other?

d. Comment on the role of appreciation in successful couplings.

e. How would you respond to Brooke's assertion that Gary is just "who he is" and is incapable of change?

f. Is it fair to expect your partner to be a mind reader? Was Gary oblivious or was Brooke too vague about her initial expectations about the dishes?

g. What does this scene say about the "five love languages"?[5] What is Brooke's love language? Gary's?

Masturbation

Couples Retreat (2009): In this movie, four couples attend an island retreat; however, only one of them is prepared to do the requisite couples counseling that is part of this "bargain" package.

1   (Ch 9, 0:45:10–0:47:30) Here we see a husband getting ready to masturbate while his wife is in the shower. It is clear that there is considerable emotional tension between the two of them.

a. Is masturbation "normal" in committed relationships? Are there gender differences in frequency of masturbation in marriage?

b. In what ways can masturbation keep a couple apart? Together?

c. How would you encourage couples to discuss masturbation and determine their own ground rules about it?

d. Are there ways to make masturbation a "couple" activity? Pros and cons of this approach.

Male Fixation on Youth

American Beauty (1999; Kevin Spacey, Annette Bening): This film tells the story of Lester Burnham (Spacey), a depressed, married, suburban dad who develops an infatuation with his teenage daughter's best friend, Angela (Mena Suvari).

1   (Ch 4, 0:13:50–0:17:13) In this scene, Burnham (Spacey) is "dragged" by his wife to his daughter's cheerleading performance at a high school gym. There he becomes fixated on young Angela.

a. Why are men so prone to developing infatuations with younger women/girls?

    b. How would you counsel a man considering leaving his wife for a younger woman? The movie *It's Complicated* (2009) offers some perspective on this question.

    c. Discuss the difference in time perspective that occurs during the scene. Is Burnham's slowed-down perspective typical of how a person with sex addiction might view the performance?

Loss of Spontaneity

The Story of Us (see earlier description)

1   (Ch 5, 0:22:50–0:24:19) In this scene, Ben (Willis) and Katie (Pfeiffer) are about to make passionate love when Katie remembers that the tooth fairy has not put money under their daughter's pillow.

    a. How does this scene speak to the relative difficulty women have disengaging from their family commitments in order to lose themselves in passion? How much of this trait can be traced to brain differences between the genders?[6]

    b. This scene shows the couple early in their marriage. How might continued differences about sexual spontaneity play out later in their relationship? How can couples best handle the loss of sexual spontaneity that frequently occurs when they have children?

Creating a Family

Making Grace (2005; Ann Krsul, Leslie Sullivan [as themselves]): This film is an intimate portrait of a lesbian couple's relationship and their efforts to conceive a child. This documentary chronicles their unique emotional journey from sperm donor anxieties to daughter Grace's first birthday.

1   (0:07:41–0:08:26) Leslie discusses the couple's differences in anxiety level regarding being pregnant, getting pregnant, and being a parent, with Ann being the more anxious of the two.

    a. Discuss some of the ways partners express their own and tolerate their respective partner's anxiety, stress, and/or moods.

    b. Was Ann's level of anxiety likely pre-existent before the pregnancy and becoming a parent? Are there times when pregnancy and parenting help alleviate rather than exacerbate anxiety? Are there times when pregnancy and parenting bring a couple together rather than push them apart? What pre-existing factors might account for these differences?

2   (1:05:23–1:07:02) Leslie and Ann talk about the intense stress having a child places on a relationship. "Any problems you had before are only magnified as are problems that you have in your own personal self. You're working with incredible sleep deprivation. You end up fighting more." The couple share that they've probably had their worst fights since becoming parents.

    a. If Leslie and Ann sought your consultation prior to their pregnancy, what forms of education, and community resources would you provide to help

them better manage stress from sleep deprivation, lifestyle changes, and/
or unresolved personal issues associated with becoming a parent?
  b. How can a couple therapist help partners work though important conflicts
  related to differences in parenting styles?
  c. What are the societal pressures that lesbian and gay couples confront
  when forming a family? How would you counsel such couples to help
  them cope with these pressures?

Emotional Reactivity

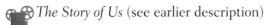*The Story of Us* (see earlier description)

1   (Ch 13, 0:56:40–1:00:36) Here, Ben and Katie are returning from a long trip
to Italy. What starts out as a loving evening soon turns disastrous.
  a. How do Katie and Ben trigger each other?
  b. From an emotional standpoint, what is this fight really about?
  c. Why do reactive couples throw the proverbial "kitchen sink" at each other
  when they are flooded emotionally?
  d. What skills does this couple need to develop in order to have more productive disagreements?

Blue Valentine (see earlier description)

1   (Ch 13, 1:22:34–1:31:13) Cindy and her husband, Dean, have gone overnight
to a motel as part of a last ditch effort to salvage their marriage. Cindy is called
away from the motel early in the morning by her medical clinic. She leaves
without informing Dean, who then comes to her workplace drunk and has a
violent disagreement with her and a doctor with whom she works.
  a. Map the process by which Dean emotionally escalates. What are his triggers? Discuss Dean's cascade of emotions. Is shame an internal factor in
  his becoming so angry (i.e. the shame-rage connection)? In what way does
  Cindy telling Dean to be a "man" escalate his rage?
  b. Given that Dean was drunk, what might have Cindy done differently to
  de-escalate the situation (i.e. not address their issues when he's been
  drinking; acknowledge her culpability in the current situation; reflect at
  a later time on the wisdom of staying in the relationship if he continues
  to drink; and so forth)?
  c. What is the role of alcohol in domestic violence?
  d. Dean hits the doctor, who he believes is having an affair with his wife.
  Is physical violence (or the thought of violence) common when men feel
  betrayed by their partners? How about for women when they discover
  infidelity?
  e. How is the altercation between Dean and Cindy another good example
  of emotional hijacking (i.e. emotions running people rather than people
  running their emotions)? What techniques and/or advice would you give

to help Dean and Cindy more effectively discuss their differences?

    f. The implication at the end of the movie is that this couple will divorce. When is divorce "justified"? When do couples break apart prematurely and end a relationship that might be salvageable? Is it best to stay together for the kids? What would you tell a couple who asks you if they should stay together for the kids?

Affairs

Match Point (2005; Jonathan Rhys Meyers, Scarlett Johansson): Tennis pro Chris Wilton (Rhys Meyers) starts an affair with his brother-in-law's ex-girlfriend, Nola Rice (Johansson), while married to heiress Chloe Hewett (Emily Mortimer).

1 (Ch 12, 0:58:44–1:01:23) In these two scenes, we see Wilton first having breakfast with Chloe who is trying to conceive a child with him. He avoids a sexual encounter with her and then goes to see his mistress, Nola Rice, with whom he has passionate sex.

    a. Contrast the staid nature of the relationship between Wilton and his wife with the passionate nature of the relationship between Wilton and his mistress.

    b. What is the impact that trying hard to conceive a child has on a couple's sexuality?

    c. How does this scene speak to issues relating to infidelity such as secret lives, betrayal, and sexual compulsion?

    d. How do you feel watching these two clips? With whom do you identify?

Toy Story 3 (2010; Tom Hanks, Tim Allen, Joan Cusack): This is the third installment of the popular *Toy Story* series.

1 (Ch 18, 0:48:17–0:52:24) In this scene, we find out the truth about Lotso, the abusive teddy bear in charge of the toys at the daycare center. His previous owner has abandoned him, replacing him with an identical bear. This experience embitters him deeply.

    a. What does this scene say about what it feels like to be replaced by an attachment figure – say, for example, when a partner leaves the relationship for another partner? Is the feeling of being replaceable less or more intense than that brought about by the actual abandonment?

    b. How does this scene relate to issues that arise in couples upon the discovery of infidelity? What is the best way to address issues of neglect, betrayal, and replacement in individual and couple counseling?

Please Give (2010; Catherine Keener, Oliver Platt): This movie focuses on the lives of Alex (Platt) and Kate (Keener), married co-owners of a retro-furniture store in New York City, and their teenage daughter (Sarah Steele), and on the lives of two sisters, Rebecca (Rebecca Hall) and Mary (Amanda Peet), whose grandmother lives next door to Alex and Kate.

1 (Ch 9, 0:59:44–1:01:25) Mary and Alex are having an affair. In this scene, we see them in bed discussing the pros and cons of infidelity.
   a. Are most affairs about unmet needs, boredom or opportunity?
   b. Can affairs sometimes improve marriages? If so, how?
   c. What percentage of married couples stay together after the discovery of an affair? Of those who seek counseling, what percentage report a healthier marriage after therapy? What steps, in general, need to be taken to help a couple work through issues related to infidelity?

Remarriage

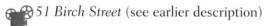*51 Birch Street* (see earlier description)

1 (Ch 4, 0:17:30–0:22:10) Three months after Mina's death, Doug's father travels to Florida, reconnects with his former secretary, Carol (aka Kitty) and marries her. This wedding scene shows Doug making the toast. He notes the newlyweds' lengthy 9-second kiss, something Doug and his sisters don't recall their father or mother ever doing.
   a. What are the statistics about the longevity of second marriages? Are outcomes different based on the circumstances (i.e. widowed versus divorced)?
   b. What are the many challenges entailed in remarriage – for the children, for the parent, and for the step-parent?
   c. Is a second marriage emotionally easier for men or women after becoming widowed?
   d. Is kissing something only newlyweds do? In what way might kissing be more intimate than intercourse?

Two-Career Households

Why Did I Get Married? (2007; Tyler Perry, Jill Scott): Four married couples gather annually for a weeklong reunion. A painful revelation of infidelity in Mike's (Richard T. Jones) and Sheila's (Scott) marriage causes the other couples to reveal indiscretions and painful forms of dishonesty in their respective marriages.

1 (Ch 2, 0:4:03–0:6:20) This scene shows Terry (Perry) and Diane (Sharon Leal) driving to the weeklong retreat. Terry, a pediatrician, tries to keep Diane, an attorney, engaged in conversation while she takes business calls and text messages from her law firm. Terry explodes and criticizes his wife's 12-hour workdays and subsequent reduced time for their daughter. Diane defensively attacks her husband's similarly long work hours and characterizes him as controlling.
   a. Contrast the conflicts which occur in dual income partnerships versus those that occur in single income partnerships.
   b. What are some coping strategies that help couples manage the stress of having dual careers, particularly as their situation impacts the children?

   c. How does defensiveness create a barrier for effective problem solving? What are antidotes to defensiveness?

   d. What is the impact of communication technology (i.e. Facebook, email, text messages, pagers, and so forth) on family life? What are ways to help couples manage the "24/7" office so as to protect family time?

Beyond Heterosexism

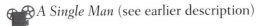*A Single Man* (see earlier description)

1 (Ch 20, 1:03:25–1:06:25) In this scene, Falconer and close female friend Charlotte (Julianne Moore) console each other over Jim's death with dinner and excessive drinking. Charlotte expresses her love for Falconer and wish that they'd had a "real relationship." She suggests his love and 16-year relationship with Jim was a "substitute for something else." George confronts Charlotte's failed 9-year marriage that ended in divorce. She apologizes and admits wishing she'd had "that kind of love" (referring to that between Falconer and Jim) with her ex-husband. She further admits never having "that kind of love" with anyone.

   a. What psychological models promote Charlotte's perspective that same-sex relationships are deficient in the expression and experience of "real love"?

   b. What types of difference might exist in the expression and experience of love in same-sex versus opposite-sex relationships?

   c. How might the process of grief and loss be different for same-sex partners versus opposite-sex partners?

References

1 Davis R.L. *More Perfect Unions: the American search for marital bliss.* Cambridge, MA: Harvard University Press; 2010.

2 Lepore J. Fixed: the rise of marriage therapy and other dreams of human betterment. *The New Yorker.* March 29, 2010.

3 Alexander M. The couple's odyssey: Hollywood's take on love relationships. *Int Rev Psychiatry.* 2009; **21**(3): 183–8.

4 Shepherd DS, Brew L. Teaching theories of couples counseling: the use of popular movies. *Fam J.* 2005; **13**(4): 406–15.

5 Chapman G. *The Five Love Languages: how to express heartfelt commitment to your mate.* Chicago, IL: Northfield Publishing; 1992.

6 Brizendine L. *The Female Brain.* New York, NY: Random House; 2006.

5

The Kids are Not All Right: Adolescents Facing Challenges and Disappointments

Anthony L. Rostain

CLINICIANS WORKING WITH ADOLESCENTS MUST LEARN TO UNDER-stand the interplay among key variables affecting this critical stage of development including genetic influences, temperament and personality traits, intellectual differences, family and peer relationships, and the role of culture in determining normative and non-normative behaviors. In our society, this time period, from 10 to 20 years of age, is viewed with a mixture of positive and negative attitudes. In most cultures, adolescence marks the transition from childhood to adulthood. It is a time of change; of rapid intellectual, emotional, and physical growth; and of new expectations and responsibilities.

Among the many challenges facing adolescents are understanding pubertal changes, searching for a personal set of values, gaining competencies to assume social roles (e.g. problem solving, decision making, examining alternatives), acquiring social interaction skills, and searching for self-definition. Indeed, one of the hallmarks of adolescence in the United States is a preoccupation with the self, and with achieving a sense of self-worth. The term "self-concept" is used to describe the ways in which individuals view themselves and assess their strengths and weaknesses. Self-concept is far from static or linear. It is complex, multidimensional, constantly changing, and differentiated along multiple aspects of the self, including physical appearance, academic achievement, athletics, friendships, sexual and romantic involvements, family relationships, employment, and global self-worth. Adolescents are able to evaluate themselves along these (and other) dimensions and can differentiate who they are from who they would like to be, and who others think they are.

Even in the best of circumstances, with strong family support and positive individual attributes ("resilience"), this is a complicated process. It becomes even more difficult when adolescents must confront less-than-favorable social-environmental conditions (e.g. family dysfunction, parental divorce, economic hardship, physical abuse) or personal-developmental differences. The films selected for this chapter illustrate youths facing challenges and disappointments in their search for self-definition and meaningful connections with others. They provide intimate glimpses into the web of family and peer relationships that profoundly affect every facet of an adolescent's life, and offer rich material for discussions about clinical approaches to teens and families facing life crises.

Family Dysfunction

Little Miss Sunshine (2006; Abigail Breslin, Greg Kinnear, Toni Collette, Alan Arkin, Paul Dano, Steve Carell): This film examines the dynamics of a zany, complicated family, the Hoovers, as they drive from Albuquerque, New Mexico, to Redondo Beach, California, so that 7-year-old Olive (Breslin) can participate in a beauty pageant. Facing a series of obstacles and setbacks (including the untimely death of Olive's paternal grandfather [Arkin]) the Hoovers manage to make it there just in time for the contest. This ensemble piece is quick-paced and simultaneously moving and funny. Alan Arkin won an Academy Award for Best Performance by an Actor in a Supporting Role (2007), and the film also received an Oscar for Best Writing, Original Screenplay.

1 (Ch 6, 0:25:28–0:29:03) The Hoovers stop in a restaurant for breakfast. Olive (Breslin) happily orders waffles "à la mode," but her choice of a dish with ice cream raises concerns from her father (Kinnear) who warns her that she might not want to eat something so fattening. Olive's mother (Collette), brother (Dano), uncle (Carell), and grandfather (Arkin) try to defuse the father's criticism.
   a. How does Olive's father approach his daughter's choice of ice cream?
   b. How do family members respond to the father's warning that if Olive eats ice cream she will get fat?
   c. How might repeated negative comments by Olive's father about her food choices and her body influence her eating behavior and her body image?
   d. What are the most common risk factors for the development of eating disorders in adolescent girls?
   e. What would you recommend to Olive's father regarding his approach to her eating behavior?
2 (Ch 11, 0:44:08–0:45:56) Olive and her grandfather share a room in the motel where they are rehearsing part of her dance routine. As he puts her to sleep, she expresses anxiety about the upcoming beauty pageant.

    a. How does Olive's grandfather respond to her when she asks if he thinks she's pretty? How does he address her fear about losing the contest?

    b. What are Olive's greatest fears? Where do these come from? How would you address her anxieties if she were in your office?

    c. What role do grandparents play in children's lives?

3 (Ch 16, 1:05:32–1:11:52) Olive's 15-year-old half-brother, Dwayne (Dano), is in open rebellion against his family. He refuses to speak to anyone and communicates strictly by writing down his replies to their questions. Suddenly, his dream of going to the Air Force Academy and becoming a jet pilot is dashed when he discovers that he is color-blind.

    a. Comment on Dwayne's emotional outburst. What's going on in him during this scene? Why does he express so much anger at his family?

    b. Comment on how Dwayne's mother responds to his emotional outburst. What does she do that seems to help him the most?

    c. How does Olive approach her brother? What is his response? What leads him to apologize?

    d. How would you counsel parents to handle their adolescent when he or she is experiencing emotional turmoil?

    e. How would you approach Dwayne if his parents brought him to you for counseling?

4 (Ch 20, 1:22:55–1:25:00) Dwayne and his uncle are on a pier overlooking the Pacific. Dwayne expresses a wish to sleep until he's 18 so he can avoid all the "crap" of adolescence. His uncle responds by sharing insights about the meaning of suffering.

    a. How does Dwayne make use of his uncle's comments?

    b. What are the major challenges of adolescence?

    c. What are positive and negative ways in which adolescents face the challenge of forming an identity?

    d. What risk factors and protective factors should be assessed when evaluating an adolescent who presents in a state of emotional crisis?

Divorce and Adolescence

The Squid and the Whale (2005; Jeff Daniels, Laura Linney, Jesse Eisenberg, Owen Kline, William Baldwin, Anna Paquin): This autobiographically based film (nominated for an Oscar in 2006 for Best Writing, Original Screenplay) explores the impact of parental separation/divorce on the lives of two brothers: Walt (Eisenberg), aged 16, and Frank (Kline), aged 12. The boys are distressed by their parents' decision to break up as they struggle to adjust to the new realities of a problem-ridden joint custody arrangement. While their parents, Bernard (Daniels) and Joan (Linney), try to portray the separation as amicable, the reality is that they are engaged in an ongoing emotional battle that deeply and differentially affects their sons.

1 (Ch 2, 0:11:05–0:15:13) Bernard and Joan break the news to their sons that they are separating. The boys protest the decision and pose many questions about the future.

   a. What does this couple do right in terms of having the "divorce" discussion with their children? What do they do wrong? How do you counsel couples who want your advice on how to tell their children that they are divorcing?

   b. What are the immediate reactions that Walt and Frank have to the news of their parents' impending separation? What are the questions that are most pressing to them?

   c. Comment on the way in which the two boys take opposing sides. How common is this in families experiencing divorce?

   d. What would you counsel Bernard and Joan to do during the immediate postseparation period so as to minimize their sons' emotional distress?

   e. A friend of Walt's comments: "Joint custody blows." What are the pros and cons of joint custody arrangements? What factors predict successful and less-than-successful joint custody?

2 (Ch 3, 0:16:37–0:18:39) Walt and Frank arrive for the first time at their father's new place. While Walt is fine with it, Frank is clearly upset and thinks it's inadequate. He confronts his father and his brother.

   a. What do you make of Bernard's response to his son's protests about the new house? What might you counsel him to do regarding Frank's displeasure about it?

   b. Why are Walt and Frank fighting? What do you make of their differing views of their parents?

   c. How can parents make it easier for their children to accept the realities of a postdivorce family?

3 (Ch 4, 0:19:57–0:24:43) Walt learns from his father that his mother cheated during their marriage. He then confronts his mother and leaves her home to stay with his father. On the phone with Frank, he learns of other extramarital relationships that their mother has carried out. Frank acts out by drinking beer and masturbating in the library.

   a. What is the impact on children of hearing about their parents' marital infidelities?

   b. How would you counsel parents about sharing the intimate details of their lives with their children?

   c. How do you explain Frank's behavior? What would be your approach to counseling his parents were they to come to you for assistance?

   d. What are the major predictors of postdivorce adjustment for children and adolescents?

4 (Ch 7, 0:37:10–0:41:55) Frank runs away from his father's home after an argument and returns to his mother's house. He discovers his mother has been entertaining someone: his tennis coach, Ivan (Baldwin). On the way to picking him up, Bernard insists to Walt, "It's my night," to which Walt responds, "Ever think we could ease up on whose night is whose?" Joan then

explains the situation with Ivan to Frank and tries to engage her estranged son in a conversation.

    a. How does Bernard appear to his sons when he insists on keeping to the joint custody schedule?

    b. How do children typically react when learning about new relationships their parents are having?

    c. At what point is it appropriate for children to be introduced to a parent's new significant other?

    d. What is "parental alienation syndrome"? How does it affect postdivorce family relationships?

5   (Ch 10, 0:59:18–1:02:10) Walt is sent to a therapist after being caught plagiarizing a song. Initially defensive, he begins to connect with the therapist.

    a. Comment on how the therapist responds to Walt's initial challenging questions.

    b. What is Walt's insight when asked to recall positive early memories?

    c. How might individual psychotherapy help an adolescent cope with parental divorce?

    d. What is the value of family therapy in postdivorce families? What conditions need to be met in order for therapy to be effective?

Parental Death, Emotional Abuse, and Depression

The Secret Life of Bees (2008; Dakota Fanning, Paul Bettany, Jennifer Hudson, Queen Latifah, Alicia Keys, Sophie Okonedo): Set in the summer of 1964, this film tells the story of Lily Owens (Fanning), a 14-year-old girl who lives with her abusive single father T. Ray (Bettany) in racist South Carolina. Lily is searching for answers to questions she has about her mother, whom she accidentally shot and killed when she was 4 years old as her parents were having a violent argument. The movie explores a critical moment in her life when she runs away from her home, along with Rosaleen her nanny (a fugitive from the town's racists) (Hudson) to find a place she associates with her mother.

1   (Ch 1, 0:03:50–0:05:15) Lily serves breakfast to her father and mentions that her birthday is the next day. She asks her father to tell her about her mother. He replies with a story about how her mother was "a lunatic about saving bugs" and proceeds to squash a roach on the kitchen floor.

    a. What do you imagine is the impact of her father's insensitivity on Lily?

    b. What is the emotional impact of a mother's death on a young child? How might it affect the child's sense of self-worth?

    c. What are the long-term consequences of a parent's death on a child's development? How do the surviving parent's attitudes and behaviors influence this process, and in what ways?

2   (Ch 3, 0:06:58–0:10:17) Lily sneaks out to dig up a hidden box with mementos of her mother including her gloves, her photo, and a small picture of a

black Mary. She looks up at the starry sky and talks to her mother while holding these precious items against her navel. Suddenly her father appears, grabs her, and hauls her back to the house, where he punishes her by making her kneel down on raw grits.

   a. Comment on Lily's ritual of digging up these reminders of her mother. What is the significance of her holding them against her belly?

   b. How might the onset of puberty affect a girl whose mother died when she was young? What would this adolescent be most in need of during this critical phase of development?

   c. What is the impact of Lily's father's abusive behavior on their relationship? Why might he be acting so harshly toward her?

   d. How does harsh parental discipline (including abuse) affect a child's sense of him- or herself? How would you intervene in this family if Lily's father brought her to your office for counseling?

3 (Ch 4, 0:12:30–0:17:16) Racists confront Lily and Rosaleen in town. Rosaleen gets badly beaten and arrested, while Lily's father takes Lily home. Lily confronts him when he tries to discipline her. He grabs her and tells her that her mother never really cared about her. Lily decides to run away, stopping at the hospital to rescue Rosaleen.

   a. How does the racist nature of the culture surrounding them affect Lily and Rosaleen's relationship?

   b. What does her father's complicity with the town's racists mean to Lily?

   c. What is the source of Lily's father's cruelty? Could her involvement in her mother's death be a continuing factor in their relationship?

   d. Comment on how Lily responds to her father's claims about her mother not loving her. What is the impact of his statements on Lily?

   e. What happens to a child if a surviving parent expresses bitterness toward a parent who has died?

4 (Ch 7, 0:25:54–0:29:04) The Boatwright sisters (Latifah, Keys, Okonedo) take Lily and Rosaleen in. August (Latifah) welcomes them, but June (Keys) is more suspicious of Lily's story, which is largely fabricated. The girls discuss their impressions of the sisters (whom they are surprised to see are so cultured) and express relief at being safe at last.

   a. What is Lily's explanation for fabricating a story? Comment on her need for secrecy.

   b. What is the significance of having "safe havens" for people to escape from abusive relationships and situations?

   c. Lily comments: "I feel like I'm where I'm supposed to be. I really do. I just need some time to figure out why." To what is she referring? What is Lily looking for?

   d. What is the role that racial inequality plays in creating stereotypes about African-Americans being less cultured and less educated than Caucasian Americans?

5 (Ch 19, 1:19:08–1:26:47) Lily shows August a picture of her mother and

learns that August knows about Lily's mother and actually was her nanny when she was young. This is a pivotal scene in which Lily confesses that she was responsible for her mother's death. August tells Lily about her mother's life, including her courtship and marriage to Lily's father, her depression, and her departure from the family.

a. What questions does Lily have about her mother and her parents' relationship? How are these addressed by August?

b. Comment on Lily's fantasy that she was with her mother when her mother came to stay with the Boatwright sisters. What is the function of this fantasy? What happens when she learns the truth?

c. As she smashes several honey jars, Lily cries out: "Why didn't you love me?" Comment on this statement and what it says about Lily's sense of herself.

d. How does Lily's guilt about her role in her mother's death play into her sense of being unlovable? How would you address this if you were her therapist?

e. What do you imagine were the causes for Lily's mother's depression? How might it have affected Lily? What is the significance of maternal depression in family life? How might you screen for it in your practice?

6 (Ch 20, 1:26:49–1:29:56) August brings Lily a box with some of her mother's possessions. One of them is a photo of Lily and her mother together.

a. How do these objects help Lily come to terms with her life story?

b. From what you can observe, comment on the relationship between Lily and August. How does it transform Lily's life?

c. Comment on how "forgiving oneself" is a fundamental aspect of developing a healthy identity.

d. How can mentors and "surrogate parents" help young people confront parental loss? How might therapists play a role?

e. What experiences, if any, have you had with recovering from the loss of an important relationship? Who helped you most through the process?

Asperger's Syndrome and the Building of Social Skills

Napoleon Dynamite (2004; Jon Heder, Efren Ramirez, Tina Majorino, Emily Dunn, Haylie Duff): This extremely popular teen comedy set in Idaho traces the adventures of a nerdy high school student as he tries to find friends, gain acceptance, and go out on a date. Through caricature and exaggeration, it paints a portrait of high school existence through the eyes of a social misfit whose "geeky" appearance and behavior set him up for ridicule and harassment by fellow students. An additional discussion question has to do with psychiatric diagnosis: i.e. does Napoleon fit the diagnosis of Asperger's syndrome or not? (See Levin and Schlozman's[1] article for a thoughtful discussion of this topic.)

1 (Ch 2, 0:03:42–0:07:16) Napoleon (Heder) rides the bus to school, recites

current events and gets laughed at, tries to impress his classmates, and endures teasing and bullying.

   a. How does Napoleon try to impress other students? What are their reactions?

   b. What aspects of Napoleon's appearance and behavior demonstrate his social atypicality?

   c. How aware is he of his "difference"? What might he say about the basis for his troublemaking friends?

   d. Comment on the teasing and bullying that socially awkward students often endure in school?

2 (Ch 7, 0:17:35–0:21:02) Napoleon makes friends with Pedro (Ramirez), a new student at the school. They talk about asking someone to the upcoming dance. Napoleon lies to Pedro about having a girlfriend. During lunch, he goes over to befriend a girl who is sitting alone.

   a. Why does Napoleon lie to Pedro about having a girlfriend? Comment on the role of lying and making up stories as a means for gaining social acceptance.

   b. What qualities do Napoleon and Deb (Majorino), the girl he approaches, have in common? How does Napoleon try to make her comfortable?

   c. What social skills are required for teenagers to succeed at making friends?

3 (Ch 11, 0:34:14–0:36:30) Pedro asks Deb to the dance and she accepts. Napoleon complains to him that he doesn't have the skills to get a girl to go out with him. He tries to impress a girl by drawing a picture of her.

   a. How does Napoleon react when he learns his friend asked Deb to the dance?

   b. How much are one's skills involved in getting a date versus one's appearance and personality traits?

   c. How is Napoleon's experience and way of responding to social ostracism similar or different from that of most teenagers?

   d. If Napoleon were one of your patients, how would you counsel him regarding dating and finding a girlfriend?

4 (Ch 13, 0:48:15–0:53:10) Napoleon invites Trisha (Dunn) to go to the dance with him, but once there, she dumps him to be with her friends. At Pedro's invitation, Napoleon dances with Deb and strikes up a conversation with her.

   a. What are some of the feelings that Napoleon might be experiencing at the dance? What does he do to manage his nervousness and his feelings of rejection?

   b. What are the "rules" by which teenage boys and girls are supposed to negotiate their attractions to one another?

   c. Comment on the dress, looks and behaviors of Pedro's cousins who give Napoleon and his date a ride to the dance. What were some of the cliques in your high school?

   d. What are the major determinants of teen culture? How do these influence adolescent behavior and identify formation?

5 (Ch 14, 1:00:45–1:02:48) Pedro decides to run for class president. Napoleon

observes a classmate being harassed by a bully. He offers the student "protection" from Pedro. Outside school, when the same bully approaches him, Pedro's cousins show up and intervene on his behalf.

   a. Why does bullying occur? What is the role of "machismo" in male adolescent development?

   b. What are the effects of bullying? How should school staff address bullying?

6 (Ch 17, 1:16:30–1:23:29) Summer Wheatly (Duff) and Pedro present presidential speeches. During the skits section, Napoleon surprises everyone in the school by dancing artfully to a disco number.

   a. Contrast the speeches and skits of the two candidates.

   b. What is the significance of Napoleon's dance performance? Have you ever experienced something similar in your life?

   c. In what ways can socially "different" teens gain acceptance from their peers? What strategies should be implemented to promote successful social integration of "marginalized" teens?

   d. Do you think Napoleon meets criteria for a diagnosis like Asperger's syndrome? Why or why not?

Homeless Youth/Transgendered Parents

Transamerica (2005; Felicity Huffman, Kevin Zeger): This unusual road movie explores the unfolding relationship between Bree Osbourne, formerly Stanley Chupak (Huffman), a California man undergoing sexual reassignment surgery, and Toby Wilkins (Zeger), a street-hustling teenager who suddenly contacts Bree looking for his father to help him get out of jail for hustling. At the insistence of her therapist, who makes it a condition of her signing the papers for the surgery, Bree goes off to New York City to find her son. After getting him released from jail, she does not reveal her true identity to him. Their relationship unfolds in the course of driving across the country, each searching for a new identity and a new life. (Note: Huffman was nominated for the 2006 Academy Award for Best Performance by an Actress in a Leading Role for this film.)

1 (Ch 3, 0:10:10–0:16:15) Bree picks up Toby from police custody and learns that he has been a street hustler. Bree pretends to be a church worker rather than reveal her identity to him. At a restaurant, she learns about Toby's absence of a family. They go to Toby's crash pad where he reveals his plan to become an actor in Hollywood. Just as she is about to leave him with some money, he shows her a picture of his father and mother, which changes her mind.

   a. How does Toby present himself to Bree? What is his attitude toward this person he believes is a "do-gooder"? What are the daily challenges that street youth face as they try to survive? What are their coping strategies?

   b. What are Bree's reactions to Toby and his plans? What might she be feeling about this young man whom she has never met but who is her biological son?

    c. Why does Bree hide her identity from Toby? Discuss the challenges of transsexuals in society, and how they have to adapt to the attitudes of mainstream Americans.

2 (Ch 5, 0:23:10–0:29:33) Bree and Toby are driving together across country. While he is sleeping, Bree decides to take a detour to visit the boy's hometown in Kentucky. They run into a neighbor who is thrilled to see him, and they go to her home. Thinking she will reunite Toby with his family, she locates his stepfather and brings him to the boy. Their encounter is highly charged and ends in a fistfight. Bree eventually learns that Toby's mother committed suicide and that his stepfather sexually abused him.

    a. What is Bree's fantasy about how to help Toby avoid being a street hustler? What does she discover about the reality of his life? How does that affect her?

    b. What is Toby's view of his hometown? Why did he run away from there? How is he feeling about being back?

    c. Why do homeless youth leave their families? Discuss the issue of "runaway youths." Why are they sometimes referred to as "throwaway youth"?

    d. If Bree brought Toby to your office for counseling, what would be your priorities for treatment?

3 (Ch 11, 1:06:54–1:12:56) Bree and Toby arrive at her parents' home in Phoenix. She has not seen them since beginning hormone treatments, and they are shocked by the transformation. Bree insists that her parents not tell Toby the truth about her being his father.

    a. What are Bree's parents' immediate reactions to her? What are Bree's reactions to them?

    b. How does Bree explain her decision to go through sexual reassignment surgery?

    c. How does Bree's sister react to Stanley/Bree?

    d. What types of feelings can be triggered in parents when they learn of a child's decision to pursue gender reassignment? How might these feelings affect family relationships?

    e. How does the family react when they realize that Toby is Bree's son? What hopes/fantasies are triggered by this revelation?

4 (Ch 12, 1:17:31–1:22:33) Bree's family goes out to a restaurant and a variety of family dynamics are revealed during the dinner conversation. Recall that Toby does not yet know that Bree is his father.

    a. Comment on how Bree's mother treats others. How would you characterize her personality?

    b. Comment on the conversation in the restaurant between Bree and her mother. What is revealed about their relationship? How does this scene help to clarify the sources of Bree's diffidence and insecurities?

    c. How might parents of a person going through sexual reassignment surgery feel about this issue? How might the siblings?

d. What do you make of Bree's mother's offer to Toby? How would you explain Bree's response?

e. What are some of the challenges facing families in which one member has gender dysphoria and is going through sexual reassignment? How might these issues be addressed in family therapy?

5 (Ch 15, 1:35:35–1:39:15) After running away from her in Phoenix, Toby comes to Bree's place in Los Angeles to see if she's had surgery and to see how she is doing. She tells him of her plans and tells him she's missed him. She learns of his current work as a porn movie star, and gives him a gift.

a. How has Bree changed in her way of interacting with Toby? To what do you attribute this?

b. What is the significance of her asking him to remove his feet off the coffee table?

c. How might the children of a transsexual parent feel about his/her parent's decision to go through with sexual reassignment surgery? What issues are raised for them?

d. How might parents going through sexual reassignment surgery feel about their relationships with their children?

e. If Bree and Toby came to your office for help with their relationship, how would you go about treating them? What are some positive traits in each of them that you could identify to help them feel better about themselves and each other? What are some important themes they will need to face?

Immigrant Families/Masturbation/Bullying

The Motel (2005; Jeffrey Chyau, Jade Wu, Samantha Futerman): This touching and funny film focuses on the "coming of age" of a Chinese-American boy faced with the challenges of adolescence in a single-parent family in a nontraditional setting. Thirteen-year-old Ernest (Chyau) lives with his mother, sister, and grandfather in an hourly rental motel where he learns about the intimate details of human relationships.

1 (Ch 1, 0:03:45–0:08:24) This segment includes several confrontations between Ernest and his mother, and scenes of Ernest cleaning up the motel including vacuuming, stripping semen-covered sheets off beds, flushing away condoms, and finding pornographic material. It establishes the context in which Ernest and his sister are growing up and introduces one important theme of the film: Ernest's efforts to gain independence from his overbearing mother.

a. Comment on how Ernest and his mother get along. How would you describe Ahma's (Wu) parenting style? Is this consistent with what is known about the parenting styles of immigrants from China?

b. What is Ernest's reaction to her accusation that he lied about the half day at school? Why do you think he didn't let her know about it? How do most 13-year-old boys try to assert their independence?

   c. What is Ernest's reaction to finding a pornographic magazine in the empty room? How do boys his age approach sexuality?

   d. What is his mother's reaction to finding out that he entered the contest? Why does she tell him that "Honorable Mention" isn't winning? What motivates her to tell him the story of the man in her village back in China who told too many stories?

   e. Why do you think Ernest hid the fact that he entered a writing contest from his mother? Discuss the parent–child relationship from the standpoint of early adolescent development. What are the major conflicts that emerge in this time period? How would you counsel Ernest's mother about handling her son's growing need/desire for independence?

   f. To what extent is the parent-child relationship as depicted here made more complex by (i) the immigrant experience and (ii) the fact that Ernest's father is not in the picture?

2 (Ch 3, 0:8:25–0:11:52) Ernest waits for his friend Christine (Futerman) who works at her parents' Chinese restaurant. He brings her a pornographic magazine from the motel and shares it with her.

   a. The scene begins with Ernest sitting on a dumpster playing with a sharp can, using it to cut light scratches on himself and then play-acting a karate fight scene. How does adolescent play enable them to prepare for adulthood? How do young teens explore their bodies? In your opinion, is this behavior healthy or not? Explain your views about this issue.

   b. Christine sits outside and smokes a cigarette with a bottle of wine nearby. Why do teenagers smoke and drink? What would you say to Christine about these behaviors? How do you address the risks of smoking and drinking with adolescent patients?

   c. What is Christine's reaction to the pornographic material Ernest shows her? Why does she say it's "so gross" and then continues looking at it? Christine challenges Ernest by saying "you like it, don't you?" He agrees. Do girls and boys view explicit sexual displays similarly or differently? How so?

   d. The porn magazine markets "oriental girls" as sexual objects. What are your views about pornography? Is it healthy or unhealthy for young adolescents to look at pornographic magazines? How does pornography on the Internet differ from that which is published in "girly magazines"?

   e. Why does Ernest paraphrase his mother's words when telling Christine that he won "Honorable Mention" in the writing contest? What is her reaction to the news and how does she respond to his statement that it's nothing to be proud of? What makes it hard for Ernest to feel proud of his accomplishment? What do you think this signifies about him?

3 (Ch 5, 0:16:07–0:19:55) Ernest stays up late watching over the motel office. This segment shows him keeping himself entertained and eventually masturbating while looking at the porn magazine. He takes his sister's fur bunny

to clean himself off and accidentally wakes her up. Following this, Ernest witnesses an angry confrontation between lovers outside the motel.

a. Comment on the role of masturbation in adolescent sexual development. What are your views about masturbation? How might your views differ from parents like Ernest's mother? How do you introduce masturbation in a clinical setting? What are your criteria for assessing an adolescent's sexual health status?

b. Contrast the childlike quality of Ernest's play with his growing preoccupations about sex. How do early adolescents manage the transition signaled by the onset of puberty? What would you say to Ernest about sexual development? How would you bring up the conversation?

c. What does Ernest witness? What does he make of it? How do you think living in a motel where people rent rooms for sexual encounters is affecting Ernest? What might it be doing to his sense of intimate relationships?

4 (Ch 8, 0:29:52–0:35:02) A boy staying at the motel challenges Ernest to kiss his sister, threatening to fight him if he doesn't. As he complies with this, his mother finds him and slaps him across the face. Sam, a flamboyant motel guest, calls Ernest over and invites him to have a game of catch.

a. Comment on the bullying episode. Why does bullying occur? How common is this phenomenon in your community? How does bullying affect children and adolescents? What should be done about it? Comment on the racial/ethnic aspects of bullying.

b. How do you imagine Ernest feels about kissing the girl? What do you make of her response to him? How would you characterize their behavior? Is this healthy or not? Explain your view.

c. Why does Ernest's mother slap him? What do you imagine he's feeling as she does this? What is the impact of parental discovery of teen sexual experimentation on parent-child relationships? How would you advice Ernest's mother to handle this delicate issue?

d. As Sam and Ernest play catch, they talk about his family. What do you make of Ernest's physical abilities and how he feels about them? How does Ernest react to Sam's questions about his father? Comment on the feelings that might be going on in Ernest as he is developing a friendship with Sam. What are the developmental challenges of boys growing up in homes with single mothers? How does the absence of a steady male role model affect them? How would you approach this issue if Ernest was brought to your office for counseling?

5 (Ch 15, 0:57:10–1:01:35) Ernest secretly takes his mother's car and drives over to pick up Christine. They go on a drive, where Ernest unsuccessfully attempts to seduce Christine.

a. How does Ernest try to impress Christine? What is her response to him? What "mistakes" does Ernest make in his attempts to seduce Christine?

b. What is going on for each of them in this scene? Which character do you identify with most? In what ways do you identify with him/her?

    c. How do Ernest and Christine each construe their relationship? What happens when they realize that they are not seeing it in the same way? Have you ever been in a relationship with someone in which a similar problem emerged? How did it unfold and what eventually happened?

    d. What do you imagine will happen to their relationship in the future?

    e. How might adults help young people when they encounter disappointment in their early romantic encounters? What would you say to Ernest if he came to you and recounted this painful episode?

Reference

1 Levin HW, Schlozman S. Napoleon Dynamite: Asperger's disorder or Geek NOS? *Acad Psychiatry*. 2006; **30**(5): 430–5.

Acknowledgments

The author wishes to acknowledge Emily Ets-Hokin, PhD (Department of Psychiatry, State University of New York at Buffalo), and Robert Racusin, MD (Department of Psychiatry, Dartmouth Medical School), for their ideas regarding interactive teaching of several movies in this chapter, and for their collaboration on several workshops presented at annual meetings of the American Association of Directors of Psychiatry Residency Training.

6

Blood is Thicker than Water: Family Celebrations and Holidays

Anna Pavlov & Patricia Lenahan

FAMILY CELEBRATIONS, HOLIDAY TRADITIONS, AND RITUALS ARE markers in our lives: for the special occasions that they are intended to be and for the unexpected occurrences and parallel life events that color them. As personal, family, and social expectations regarding these occasions mount with corresponding stress, particularly with respect to the annual events, the holidays can take on an unwelcome and negative light. Factor in strained or difficult family dynamics and additional tensions and stresses shape holidays and family celebrations into unique events.

This chapter incorporates a sampling of traditions from various cultures and religions. Obviously, this selection could not possibly cover all the rich and diverse rituals, celebrations, and holidays that exist.

Spiritual Milestones in Adolescence: The Quinceañera and the Bar/Bat Mitzvah

Quinceañera (2006; Emily Rios, Jesse Garcia): Set in Los Angeles' Echo Park region, this film is centered on a Latino family preparing for their daughter's quinceañera, a significant cultural and religious event occurring when a girl turns 15. The typical dress and aspects of the ceremony are reminiscent of a wedding. Amidst the preparation is Magdalena's unexpected, surprising, and rare pregnancy (secondary to noncoital ejaculation). She leaves her home as her father lashes out at her and understandably refuses to believe that she has not had sexual intercourse. Magdalena goes to live with a gentle and accepting great-granduncle. We see the various struggles of the community she now inhabits and personal redemption on many levels. The scenes offered do not focus on the teen pregnancy per se but on the cultural tradition itself.

1   (Chs 1–2, 0:00:25–0:4:35) The film starts with a whirlwind composite of the quinceañera experience, starting with the opening of the church service for Eileen Garcia. The occasion is described as a spiritual milestone in the life of a young girl when she turns 15. We see images of the intense preparation, the teens that will also be a part of the festivities, the couples walking down the church aisle and forming a bridge for the girl to walk under, picture taking afterwards, and the big party.

   a. What is your reaction to this scene?
   b. If you are not familiar with quinceañeras, what impressions do you have viewing this clip?

2   (Ch 28, 1:24:28–1:26:11) In spite of her pregnancy, Magadalena, after reconciling with her father, has her quinceañera. A stretch limousine approaches and parks. The quinceañera court files out of the vehicle and organizes for the ceremony. Magdalena's cousin Carlos walks her down the aisle as her father looks on with pride.

   a. While a significant tradition, what pressures do such events place on individuals and families?
   b. How might other life events collide with the festivity expected for such milestone occasions? How are they integrated and made sense of?
   c. How would knowing of this Latina tradition affect your interactions with a Latina client or patient at this age?
   d. What traditions from other cultures occur during the adolescent period and mark entrance into spiritual adulthood?

Keeping the Faith (2000; Ben Stiller, Edward Norton, Jenna Elfman): Jake, a rabbi, has a childhood friend who is a priest. They want to bring their religions into the modern world. They are as close as ever as a third friend (Anna) comes back onto the scene.

1   (Ch 9, 27:58–29:21) Rabbi Jake is with a discouraged bar mitzvah boy whose voice is cracking as he is practicing the Haftorah. Rabbi Jake responds by telling him that this is not a talent contest but a rite of passage. "This happens in all cultures. God knew your voice would change at 13." The rabbi encourages the boy to embrace his awkwardness.

   a. What strikes you as you watch this scene?
   b. What is different about how the rabbi addresses the boy's developmental stage? How would you address his frustration?

Sixty Six (2006; Helena Bonham Carter, Eddie Marsan, Gregg Sulkin, Matt Bardock, Alex Black): The story of an English boy named Bernie Rubens (Sulkin) who feels second best in his life and hopes that his bar mitzvah will put him centerstage, only to learn that the English national football team is in the final playoff of the 1966 World Cup Final on his big day.

1 (0:05:52–0:07:38) At their first bar mitzvah class, a rabbi (who is blind) explains the significance of this milestone to the boys. As the scene shifts, Bernie begins meticulous plans for his bar mitzvah. We see scenes from his older brother's bar mitzvah, which Bernie hopes to outdo.
   a. For those who are not Jewish, have you ever been to a bar mitzvah? Is there a tradition/ceremony for an adolescent in your culture?
   b. What "coming of age" traditions exist in other cultures.

2 (0:17:30–0:18:09) Bernie is energized as he plans every detail of his bar mitzvah, from the seating arrangement to the cocktails. This clip can be combined with the previous clip or shown separately.

3 (0:18:32–0:19:30) Fathers attend this bar mitzvah class. One father with his son outlines a rigorous Torah study schedule. He tells the others that his son worked on it 2 hours every night. Other fathers share their experiences and memories.
   a. How are bar/bat mitzvahs different from other "coming of age" milestones?

4 (0:26:10–0:28:26) Bernie is sad that his bar mitzvah reception plans are scaled back because of unfortunate family circumstances. He talks to his rabbi about it, who reframes the situation by telling him smaller receptions are more "exclusive." After this, Bernie now imagines what his reception will be like in a smaller venue.
   a. Discuss the peer pressure to have a big costly party.
   b. How can family expectations add to this pressure (e.g. "keeping up with the Joneses")?

5 (0:54:50–0:56:46) Bernie is studying with his rabbi, who follows along in a Braille text. The rabbi tells Bernie that he has always been his best student and asks him what is wrong. The rabbi talks to him about overcoming obstacles.
   a. Why might these difficult lessons be hard for adolescents to accept?

6 (1:06:10–1:08:11) It's Bernie's bar mitzvah day. He is walking up to the bema and reciting the Torah. Initially he is distracted by the outside noise of soccer fans, but then he remembers the significance of the day and reads brilliantly. His mother and aunt look on very proudly.
   a. What do you imagine Bernie's mother is thinking and feeling?

Marriage and Cultural Traditions

The Family Wedding (2010; America Ferrera, Lance Gross, Forest Whitaker, Carlos Mencia): Two families are forced to set aside their culture clash differences to plan their children's wedding in a few weeks. Unbeknownst to her parents, Lucia (America Ferrera) has dropped out of law school. She and her medical resident fiancé Marcus (Lance Gross), plan to go on a medical mission to Laos and want to get married before they leave.

1 (Chs 10–11, 0:32:48–0:37:33) Marcus and Lucia are getting married in

2 weeks. Their idea for a small and intimate wedding is quickly overtaken by family expectations and Mexican-American and African-American cultural traditions. Lucia strives to blend traditions. In order to aggravate Marcus's father, her father tells him that a Mexican tradition is for the godparents to pay for the wedding but, since Lucia does not have any godparents, the father of the groom foots the bill. The young couple is told that the four words to remember are: "Our marriage, their wedding." The scene changes as we see the bride and her family tasting various foods and picking out flowers.

   a. What is your interpretation of "Our marriage, their wedding"?

   b. How might a couple be able to retain their original vision for their wedding day?

   c. How do couples tackle the issue of who pays for what? How could that be a source of conflict? How does that vary between cultures? How did or do you think your family would participate?

2 (Chs 11–12, 0:38:26–0:41:06) The family is planning the seating arrangements for the reception. The mother of the bride has brought a "seating schematic," a three-dimensional aide to assist with decisions of where to place the guests so that everyone gets along. They imagine various pairings and the social gaffes and conflicts that would arise.

   a. The seating arrangement can be one of the more carefully crafted plans. We see a view of the craziness involved in anticipating how guests will behave if misplaced. How could this add to the stress of the couple and their families?

   b. Despite the best-laid plans, mishaps occur at special occasions such as weddings. How would you respond to a client or patient who told you about something that went very wrong at their wedding (short of the bride or groom not showing up)? How might you help him, her, or them reframe the situation?

3 (Ch 12, 0:41:04–0:41:52) In this scene, Lucia is with her mother and sister at the bridal dress shop.

4 (Ch 17, 0:58:25–0:59:41) Marcus's father and the woman who helped raise Marcus (who is romantically interested in Marcus's father) try out various wedding cakes. Their discussion about why brides and grooms "shove cake in each other's faces" leads to their own cake fight.

   a. Where did the cake tradition originate?

   b. What is your opinion of it? Does it seem like an unkind gesture on such a special day?

5 (Chs 25–26, 1:27:26–1:30:47) This scene can be divided in two: as Lucia is dressing for the wedding, her mother gives her some earrings to wear and has her take a good look at herself in the mirror; meanwhile, in a parallel scene, Marcus's father is helping him with his tie and sharing some deep feelings, apologizing for unkind things he has said about Marcus's mother and marriage in general. After this the wedding procession begins. When Lucia and her father arrive at the front, Marcus pauses to get down on his knees to

ask Lucia's father for permission to marry her (a sore point with him when they first announced their intentions). Mr. Ramirez welcomes Marcus to the family.

    a. Depicted are tender moments between the bride and her mother and between the groom and his father. What strikes you as you view these exchanges?

    b. What is the origin of the tradition for a man to ask his love's father for "her hand in marriage"?

    c. How would you respond to a patient/client who did not want to do this despite it being highly valued by the fiancé's family?

6 (Ch 26, 1:31:12–1:32:29) Three unique Mexican-American symbols are part of the wedding ceremony. The first is the arras, which is a coin that the groom is given to hold and then drops into the open hands of his bride symbolizing mutual protection (that money will never be an issue between them). The second is the veil, which brings them together into one. The final item is the lasso, which symbolizes eternal love.

    a. What impact did the symbolic gestures have on the ceremony?

    b. What are wedding rituals from other cultures? What rituals/symbols would you want at your wedding/commitment ceremony?

    c. What rituals have you seen at weddings/commitment ceremonies?

7 (Chs 26–7, 1:32:30–1:35:02) This is a scene from the reception, opening with a view of the wedding cake. The mariachis are playing and the bride and groom dance, as do the guests. Traditional and contemporary music is heard. Lucia throws her bouquet, which is caught by her sister, and the couple feed each other cake.

    a. To what extent have Lucia and Marcus succeeded in integrating their cultural customs into their wedding ceremony and reception?

    b. Were the planning struggles with family necessary to achieve this outcome? Discuss.

Group Weddings

The Milk of Sorrow (2009): This is the story of Fausta (Magaly Solier), a young woman stricken with a pathological fear that she has contracted the "milk of sorrow" from her mother's breast milk. Women who were raped during the Peruvian civil war and the years of the Shining Path suffer this condition. Fausta's mother would recount for her the full nature and experience of the violence and would even sing her a song about the events.

1 (1:07:59–1:09:58) A group wedding is being held on a dusty plain in the barrio of Lima. All the brides stand and say, "I do" followed by all the grooms. The scene shifts to a procession of friends and families of the grooms. The announcer tells the wedding-goers that the families have saved all year to give the couples a great gift. Music plays in the background as families carry various gifts down the red carpet while the announcer describes each gift.

a. Why are group weddings held in some cultures?

b. What are some of the benefits of them? What are some disadvantages of them?

2 (1:09:06–1:21:20) A procession of trucks and cars carrying the wedding party and guests travels down the dusty road to the reception site, an arid plain overlooking the city. The wedding party is in front of a picture of a beautiful waterfall to have the official wedding photos taken.

a. Western culture is highly individualistic, right down to its ceremonies. What reactions do you have to the idea of such a special occasion occurring at the same time and place for multiple couples?

The Arranged Union

Arranged (2007): This film focuses on the developing friendship between two first-year teachers in a Brooklyn school. Rochel (Zoe Lister Jones), an Orthodox Jew, and Nasira (Francis Benhamou), a Syrian-born Muslim, are confronted by bias and bigotry from both their students and their principal. As a result, they form an alliance and begin to share their feelings and experiences, as both are engaging in their cultural practices of arranged marriages.

1 (0:11:15–0:13:45) Rochel's aunt, Nina (Sondra James), comes to take Rochel to meet the marriage broker. Her aunt notices Rochel's nervousness and acknowledges that although some people may frown on arranged marriages, these marriages succeed in the long run. She adds: "isn't it better to let those who have known you for a lifetime find you a partner?"

a. What do you think about this view?

b. How would you counsel someone who is ambivalent about being in an arranged marriage?

2 (0:34:13–0:36:17) In this scene, Nasira and her family are sitting at dinner. An older gentleman, her father's friend and a prospective mate for Nasira, joins them. Nasira appears uncomfortable and eventually asks to be excused. She runs into the bathroom and her mother, Elona (Doris Belack), joins her. Nasira shares her fears and feelings with her mother about this man.

a. What is your reaction to this process?

b. What must it be like to meet a prospective spouse and not have "sparks fly"?

3 (0:37:06–0:38:21) Nasira and Rochel are sitting at lunch and sharing their experiences with the matchmaking process and the men they have met. They discuss having children and how many they hope to have.

a. Do you know of anyone who had a traditionally arranged union?

b. What do you know about that process?

c. How has the process of an arranged marriage changed over time?

4 (0:41:45–0:43:15) Nasira is talking with her father, Abdul-Halim (Laith Nakli), about his friend. She has many concerns about this suitor, stating that he is 20 years older than her and has never lived in the United States. Abdul asks Nasira if she thinks "Mom and I are a good match." Nasira nods

her assent and Abdul reassures her that he wants the best for her, ending by agreeing that his friend is not a match for her.

  a. Are you surprised that Nasira's father considered his friend as a possible match for his daughter?

  b. Why does Nasira's father ask her if she thinks her mother and he are a "good match"?

  c. What if Nasira's father had not listened to her feelings?

  d. How do arranged marriages fare compared with contemporary marriages?

5 (0:43:40–0:45:13; 0:48:08–0:49:40) In the first scene, Rochel is seen on dates with four men. Her dismay is evident. The second scene finds Rochel and her mother, Sheli (Mimi Lieber) meeting with the matchmaker, Miriam (Peggy Gormley). Rochel shares with them her feelings, stating, "This isn't working. If this is the best there is, I don't want to date." Her mother and Miriam tell her that isn't an option. Rochel responds that she isn't willing to settle.

  a. Discuss the modern version of matchmaking.

  b. Why have matchmaking services such as eHarmony.com and Match.com become so popular? What does this say about our society and culture?

6 (0:50:45–0:51:42) In this scene, Nasira and Rochel are talking. Rochel asks Nasira if she ever thinks the process of an arranged marriage won't work. Nasira says it will work, adding that it worked for their parents.

  a. Discuss what roles Nasira and Rochel serve for each other.

  b. How does the fact that they are from different cultural and religious traditions affect this?

Thanksgiving – Loss and Loneliness

Home for the Holidays (1995): It is Thanksgiving week and 40-year-old Claudia (Helen Hunt) was just fired from her job at a museum. Her teenage daughter is spending the holidays with the daughter's boyfriend and his family, so Claudia must face her parents, siblings and extended family alone.

1 (Ch 7, 0:039:28–0:0:40:40) Adele (Ann Bancroft) tries to set Claudia up with an old high school acquaintance by calling him out to work on their furnace on Thanksgiving Day. Adele pushes Claudia out on the porch to talk with Russell (David Strathairn). Claudia expresses surprise that Russell is working on Thanksgiving Day. He tells her that he is giving his employees the day off because they have family. He goes on to tell her that his brother and sister left town after they lost their jobs and that his parents were killed last summer by a drunk driver. Russell says that he doesn't have anybody anymore and he has no place to go. He adds that his girlfriend married his best friend.

  a. What is your reaction to Russell's account?

  b. How does Russell present to Claudia and what are his expectations?

  c. How might Russell's attitude assist Claudia in coping with her job firing and her attitudes toward her family?

    d. Russell decides to work on Thanksgiving Day. How does this help him cope with the holidays and his personal sense of isolation?

    e. What risks do isolated individuals face at holidays?

Family and Personal Expectations for the Holidays – Christmas

Christmas Vacation (1989; Chevy Chase, Beverly D'Angelo): This film focuses on the Griswolds and their extended family who descend upon their home for Christmas. Clark is striving to achieve the perfect Christmas, yet seems thwarted at every turn.

1 (Ch 4, 0:08:04–0:08:59) Clark (Chase) has taken the family for a drive to find the family Christmas tree. Clark finds one of the largest trees in the field. He ignores his family when they tell him the tree is too big. Although his family seems to be less impressed, Clark embraces them all and says: "The most enduring traditions of the season are best enjoyed in the warm embrace of kith and kin. This tree is the symbol of the spirit of the Griswold family Christmas."

    a. What are Clark's expectations for the holidays?

    b. How do other family members respond?

    c. Are his expectations reasonable?

    d. How might expectations for a "perfect holiday" set people up for disappointment?

2 (Ch 6, 0:15:00–0:15:18) Clark is seen entering a large department store. Christmas music is playing and decorations are blazing brightly. The store is full of shoppers and the scene shifts to piles of money being counted and credit cards being swiped.

    a. How does the commercialization of the holidays contribute to individual and familial stress?

    b. What factors contribute to overspending during the holidays?

    c. What other ways can families celebrate the holidays without increasing their debt or financial worries?

3 (Ch 7, 0:17:50–0:19:35) The doorbell rings and the Griswold family freezes in place. Eventually the door is opened to both Clark's and Ellen's parents. All four parents are talking at the same time and sharing their health problems with one another and with Clark, who says, "This is what Christmas is all about."

    a. What does Clark mean when he says, "This is what Christmas is all about"?

    b. How can the arrival of extended family affect the overall family dynamics?

    c. What childhood memories can their arrival evoke?

    d. What aspects of "family" and tradition do Clark's children learn from these holiday visits?

e. How will this color their expectations and experiences of the holidays as they age?

Holiday Cultural Traditions

Nothing Like the Holidays (2008): The film focuses on the Rodriguez family living in Chicago. Family secrets and dysfunctions are revealed as they make their preparations for celebrating Christmas and for the arrival of all their children returning for Christmas, including their son who is home from Iraq. The family celebrates parranda, a Puerto Rican Christmas holiday tradition in which neighbors go door to door caroling. When they knock on someone's door, the family living in that house is then ready to join in the parranda and the group moves on to the next house. The festivity can end at church or at a big party or both.

1   (Ch 4, 0:14:33–0:15:30) The family is sitting in the living room having drinks. Eddy (Albert Molina) talks excitedly about the upcoming parranda. His son Mauricio (John Leguizamo) is sitting with his wife, Sarah (Debra Messing), a Wall Street attorney. Eddy explains the parranda to her.
    a. What role do cultural traditions play in the lives of the Rodriguez family?
    b. How do you introduce these traditions to someone who has not experienced them before?
    c. What aspects of family and culture are evident in this scene?

2   (Ch 11, 0:1:07:52–0:1:10:38) La Parranda begins as the neighbors come caroling. The family is already dressed in their coats and readily joins in the caroling and in gathering more neighbors. The group grows and the music continues. The scene ends at a community party in the evening.
    a. What cultural and family traditions are important to you?
    b. What is the significance of these traditions?
    c. What losses may immigrant families face in a new country?

Home for the Holidays (see earlier description)

1   (Ch 9, 0:46:00–0:47:20) Gladys (Geraldine Chaplin), Adele's sister, sings a hymn as the family sits down to Thanksgiving dinner. Adele says grace to start the meal and Henry adds his thoughts: "Give me those old pain-in-the-ass traditions like Thanksgiving which really mean something to us, but we can't tell you what that is."
    a. What are the origins of family traditions?
    b. What factors compel families to continue these traditions?
    c. How do families transmit the significance of traditions to younger generations?

Family Dynamics, Relationships, and Crisis Events

Passover, Thanksgiving, and Christmas

When Do We Eat? (2005; Lesley Ann Warren, Michael Lerner, Jack Klugman): This film is an extreme Indie comedy about the Stuckman family as they prepare for and celebrate Passover at their family Seder meal. With a little psychedelic inspiration, the once-gruff and critical patriarch, Ira, embraces the spirit of the holiday, vowing to guide his contentious clan toward forgiveness and harmony.

1 (0:23:00–0:30:10) The family gathers for the Passover Seder, which is held outdoors under a brightly decorated tent – in part to honor the request of one of their now much more religiously observant sons, Ethan. As the family settles in, the Passover symbols on the plate are shown and are described as the foods that tell the story of Passover. The matriarch (Warren) says the prayer while Ethan wants to chant. Ira asserts "no melody." Ethan does the prayers in Hebrew. Ira and Ethan argue over the proper way to have the service. Ira just wants to get through the service. Ethan states, "the Seder is about us escaping from our own impatience and anger."

   a. How do families negotiate differing perspectives on how to carry out religious holidays?
   b. What is Ethan saying in his perspective on the Seder?
   c. While extreme in this film scene, why do families "lose it" on such important occasions? What's really going on?
   d. If you were a family therapist working with the Stuckman family, how would you begin to work with this family?
   e. Is the family's name apt?

Surviving Christmas (2004): Drew Latham (Ben Affleck) is a rich executive who is tired of being alone for the holidays and who thinks that money can buy him everything.

1 (Ch 1, 0:04:15–0:05:20) Drew (Affleck) gives his girlfriend a Christmas gift: a first-class ticket to Fiji, leaving on Christmas Day. She responds that Christmas is a family holiday. She then questions where the relationship is going and states that she has never met his family. She states: "You can't be serious about the relationship if you're not serious about your family."

   a. What are Drew's girlfriend's expectations for the holidays?
   b. How do differences in expectations and experiences regarding holidays and celebrations affect couples and their relationships?
   c. How can these childhood memories and expectations affect adult traditions and relationships?
   d. What potential conflicts may occur when couples do not share similar holiday traditions or expectations?
   e. What suggestions might you give clients/patients regarding coping with the holidays and relationships?

f. What psychological factors contribute to increased depression and anxiety during the holidays?
g. How comfortable are you when clients/patients ask about your holiday plans? How do you frame your response? What about questions about how you spent the holiday?
h. What do you imagine to be the experience of people who do not celebrate Christmas? If you have that background, what was it like growing up and as an adult now?
i. What anticipatory guidance might a couple therapist provide regarding their first holiday together? How should couples navigate dividing their time with family?

Nothing Like the Holidays (see earlier description)

1 (Ch 5, 0:23:30–0:28:09) At the family dinner, Eddy says that he's happy that everyone is together. Anna, his wife, sits sullenly at the other end of the table and announces that she is divorcing him. Mauricio tells them they can't do that, adding "you've been married 36 years." He then asks his father if he has cheated again. Jesse, another son, responds that it is their lives. Dad yells and everyone but Anna and Sarah leave the table.
a. What prompts Anna to make this announcement now?
b. How important is it to Anna to have her children present when she says she is getting a divorce?
c. What reaction does Anna expect from her family?
d. What is the significance of Sarah remaining at the table with Anna?
e. Do individuals sometimes postpone announcing decisions until after the holiday? Why?

Home for the Holidays (see earlier description)

1 (Ch 2, 0:06:53–0:07:25) Claudia's (Holly Hunter) daughter, Kitty (Claire Daines), is driving her to the airport for a trip home for Thanksgiving. Kitty asks her what's wrong. She reminds Claudia what she's got to look forward to: cigarettes, junk food, and Gram's famous stuffing. Claudia cringes and says, "I can't do it." Kitty tells her: "You're going."
a. What role is Kitty assuming in this family?
b. How does Kitty's statement, "you're going," impact Claudia?
c. What are Claudia's misgivings about returning to her parental home for Thanksgiving?
d. What feelings might Claudia have about her daughter's decision not to join the family for the holiday?
2 (Ch 3, 0:12:02–0:13:55) Claudia reluctantly gets off the plane and as she is walking down the corridor, she sees her parents waiting, with her dad filming her arrival. During the drive home, her parents talk about their friends, their

illnesses and each other. Her mother, Adele (Ann Bancroft), comments on Claudia's hair.

    a. How does Claudia react to her parents' conversation? Does it strike you as unusual? Why?

    b. What do you make of Adele's critical comment about Claudia's hair?

3   (Ch 3, 0:16:04–0:16:40) Claudia and Adele are talking. Adele says that Claudia's sister, Joanne (Cynthia Stevenson), is a pain. Adele goes on to say that Joanne will come barging in here tomorrow with her turkey. Claudia says, "we aren't doing a turkey." Adele responds that Joanne is doing hers and we are doing ours.

    a. What family relationships are being displayed?

    b. What is Joanne's role in the family?

    c. What is Claudia's role within the family?

4   (Ch 5, 0:25:05–0:27:30) Tommy (Robert Downey, Jr.) arrives unexpectedly early in the morning with his friend Leo (Dylan McDermott). Claudia wants to know who Leo is and asks why Tommy's lover, Jack, isn't coming. Tommy asks Claudia if she is losing her mind yet. He also asks her how long she has been home. Claudia responds: "14 hours and 14 minutes."

    a. How would you assess Claudia's relationship with her brother?

    b. What role does Tommy play in the family?

    c. What expectations do the siblings have regarding the holiday with their parents?

5   (Ch 8, 0:42:04–0:43:40) Referring to his sister and brother-in-law, Tommy yells "battle stations, battle stations, the wonderful Whitmans are here." Joanne (Cynthia Stevenson) and her husband, Walter (Steve Guttenberg), groan as they recognize Tommy's car. Walter says he was told that Tommy wasn't coming, stating, "I'm not prepared for this. I need time."

    a. How would a family therapist interpret Tommy's reaction ("battle stations") to the arrival of his sister and brother-in-law?

    b. How would you interpret Walter's response that he wasn't prepared to see Tommy?

    c. How would you assess the family dynamics?

6   (Ch 8, 0:44:06–0:45:48) All the men, Gladys and the children are sitting crammed in the living room, while Adele, Claudia and Joanne are preparing Thanksgiving dinner in the kitchen. Leo asks, on behalf of the men, if they should help them. Henry (Charles Durning) responds that the women don't want us in there. As the women continue to work, Joanne says that she can't do everything. Claudia retorts that no one is asking her to.

    a. What is Joanne's perceived role within the family?

    b. How would you interpret Claudia's response?

    c. What gender role assumptions are made?

7   (Ch 9, 0:1:00:04–0:1:01:06) Adele and Claudia are talking. Adele says that nobody means what they say on Thanksgiving. She says, "That's what the day is all about: torture … and giving thanks that we don't have to go through this

for another year, except that we do because they went and put Christmas right in the middle to punish us." Adele reassures Claudia that it all will be OK if they go and stuff themselves so we can't think anymore.

  a. Do you agree with Adele's cynical view on Thanksgiving? Why?
  b. Do holidays become dreaded? If yes, is that a healthy view? If they are viewed this way, what can help so that they become more meaningful and pleasant?
  c. What function do holidays serve?

8   (Ch 13, 0:1:28:02–0:1:45) Claudia finds her Dad dozing and watching old family movies in the basement. He is reminiscing about when the children were growing up.

  a. What is the role of reminiscence in aging populations? How do the holidays provide markers for remembrance?
  b. What feelings and memories is Henry trying to recapture?

Nothing Like the Holidays (see earlier description)

1   (Ch 9, 0:54:16–0:55:24) Eddy (Sarah's father) is driving Sarah to a friend's bar when he suddenly appears to be gripped by pain. Sarah grabs the wheel and narrowly averts an accident. Sarah calls for an ambulance and her father tells her that his medication is in the glove compartment. Sarah looks at it and seems stunned. She asks him if Anna knows. He begs Sarah not to tell anyone. "I just want to enjoy Christmas. Not that they make it easy."

  a. How should Sarah respond to her father's request to not to tell anyone? Discuss family secrets and their consequences.
  b. What are the implications of such a decision on the family and familial relationships?
  c. What are the potential psychological consequences for Eddy of not sharing the fact of his illness?

Holidays and Aging Populations

Lovely, Still (2008): Robert Malone (Martin Landau) is an aging man who lives alone and works in a grocery store. It is days before Christmas when he finds Mary (Ellen Burstyn), a new neighbor sitting in his living room. The film follows Robert and Mary as their relationship develops and as they prepare for a Christmas together.

1   (Ch 10, 1:0201–1:07:04) Robert awakens with Mary lying next to him. She wishes him a Merry Christmas. They proceed to the living room and begin opening presents. Robert leaves to make coffee and tells Mary to continue opening the presents: all of them are for her. Mary suddenly looks terrified as she unwraps the one present Robert had placed under the tree that was for him. Mary holds up a handgun and asks Robert why he gave himself a gun.

He replied that he was tired, tired of being alone, so he was going to end it. Robert is fearful of Mary's response and asks her not to leave him and tells her that he loves her.

a. What factors contribute to suicidality in older adults?

b. What impact do the holidays have for isolated older adults?

c. What can family members and friends do in order to reduce depressive symptoms around the holidays?

d. How do accumulated losses impact mental health and functioning around the holidays?

e. What protective factors may exist to help an aging individual cope with feelings of loneliness?

How About You (2007; Hayley Atwell, Orla Brady, Imelda Staunton, Joss Ackland, Vanessa Redgrave): Based on a story by Maeve Binchy, this Irish film is the story of Ellie (Atwell), the younger sister of Kate (Brady), who owns a residential living facility. When their mother has a stroke, Ellie is left in charge of the facility and the "hardcore four" (known as the "hardcore four" because they have been banned from other facilities). While most of the residents have gone to join their families for the holidays, these four residents have nowhere to go. The behavior of the "hardcore four" is so disruptive that many other residents have moved out, causing Kate to worry that she may lose the home.

1 (0:50:38–0:53:20) Music is playing in the background ("Oh Santa, don't come to my house") as Ellie speaks with Kate on the phone. When Kate tells her that she won't be back for Christmas because of their mother's health, Ellie hangs up on her. She mutters: "I hate Christmas." Minutes later Ellie talks with the "hardcore four" and suggests they have Christmas dinner together. Ellie says: "We can be a family; a dysfunctional one." Noting their reaction, Ellie adds: "You checked out of life and checked into here."

a. What factors affect an individual's feelings about the holidays? Why do people say that they "hate the holidays"?

b. What contributes to increased stress and depression around the holidays?

c. How can a health professional provide anticipatory guidance to individuals regarding coping with the holidays?

2 (0:1:09:46–0:1:13:40) Hazel (Staunton) enters the dining room and informs Ellie that the "committee" (the residents) has decided to share Christmas dinner together. They have made up a shopping list. Hazel tells Ellie that they all will go shopping with her. Donald (Ackland) brings three bottles of wine with him to the Christmas dinner and Georgia (Redgrave) brings an armful of wine and liquor.

a. How might Ellie's confrontation with the "hardcore four," telling them they "checked out of life," have affected their decision to share Christmas dinner?

b. How can families assist their relatives living in residential care facilities during the holidays?

c. The residents have brought bottles of alcohol to the dinner. How should alcohol use be addressed in relation to their age, medical conditions and health facility requirements?

Loss and Loneliness

1 (0:1:20:00–0:1:21:34) The health inspector, Mr. Evans (Darragh Kelly), showed up unexpectedly on Christmas Day and threatened to shut the facility down because of lack of staff and the overall conditions. He now returns and says that he didn't mean to upset them, and that it's Christmas and he had no place to go. Georgia, who answered the door, explains that his wife just left him and tells the group to set another place for dinner.
   a. How can loss or separation and divorce affect individuals during the holidays?
   b. What expectations do people have regarding holidays and celebrations?

Death and the Funeral Rite

Dim Sum Funeral (2008; Bai Ling, Steph Song, Talia Shire, Julia Nickson, Lisa Lu, Kelly Hu, Russell Wong): The Xiao family, a Westernized Chinese-American family, reunite to carry out their mother's last wish for a traditional Chinese funeral. In the process they learn about many other sides to their mother, who they have long experienced as the "Dragon Lady." Talia Shire portrays Viola, the devoted and longtime house manager and former nanny of the children, now all adults.

1 (Ch 1, 0:02:21–0:05:22) Viola (Shire) is in Mrs. Chow's bedroom as she lies deceased in her bed. Viola telephones the family members to notify them and we see their reactions upon hearing the news that their mother, aka the "Dragon Lady," has died. A hearse takes the body away. A shrine with a candle and incense is set up in her memory.
   a. What range of reactions can occur in response to the news of a death?
   b. What burden may be placed on the person doing the notifying?
2 (Ch 1, 0:06:12–0:07:43) Jason (young boy) asks his mother why she is crying so much at the news of her mother's death saying, "Grandma was a total bitch." She tells him grandma was not always that bad. "She was just Chinese." In the next scene, Mrs. Chow's son asks his wife if she is going to take time off to go to the funeral with him. She tells him that she will not be leaving for the funeral tomorrow, as their daughter has a dance recital. Then she asks the piercing question, "Will your mistress be joining you?"
   a. How does it feel to have a now deceased mother spoken about in disparaging terms? Would this be tolerated in some families?
   b. What does the mother's reaction teach her son about family and grief?

3   (Ch 2, 0:07:45–0:12:08) Viola, the longtime house manager and former nanny of the children, tells the family that their mother had one last request for a traditional Chinese funeral that takes 7 days. As Americans, they wonder how they will do this – they do not even speak Chinese. They are told their mother had cancer. Three of the adult children are kneeling at the home shrine.
   a. The family is asked to take on something new to them in order to fulfill their mother's last wish. What opportunities for growth are present?

4   (Ch 2, 0:11:56–0:14:00) While the family is kneeling at their mother's shrine, their youngest sister, who is an actress, and her girlfriend, Dee Dee, walk in with sarcastic remarks. They make fun of the shrine. Then we see the sister in a dramatic emotional display that is not genuine. The next scene is of the family gathered for a meal. No conversation ensues. Alex tells Dee Dee that she is not family and is not welcome here.
   a. Why might uncivil behavior surface during grief and mourning?
   b. Death often brings disconnected and fractious family members together. How might these times be an opportunity for healing and growth?
   c. How is Alex defining "family"? How would you interpret his remarks? Since they are directed to the lesbian partner of his sister, could they refer to nonacceptance of his sister's same-sex partner?

5   (Ch 2, 0:14:22–0:15:58) Two sisters are outside, catching up on what is clearly a strained relationship. A subplot is that Liz's son, Sammy, died about a year ago.

6   (Ch 2, 0:15:59–0:16:41) A sister tells Liz that she and Dee Dee are planning on having a baby through in vitro fertilization. Dee Dee walks up and is reminded that Liz lost her son.
   a. How does her sister's news impact Liz? What do you notice about her body language?

7   (Ch 2; 0:16:42–0:17:22) Liz is inside, looking at a picture of her son; she holds it close to her.
   a. What is compounded grief? How can a current death trigger unresolved grief with past losses. Discuss.

8   (Ch 3, 0:19:52–0:22:07) The family arrives at the cemetery. Viola invites them to find the feng shui. An elderman talks about the plans Mrs. Chow made for the plots. Alex protests that he and his wife will not be buried there. The elder says funerals are for respect. You are grieving for your mother; that is why you are not thinking clearly. Alex stands quietly, thinking.
   a. Why may such outbursts occur during funeral planning and services? How can they be interpreted?

9   (Ch 3, 0:22:08–0:23:20) Dee Dee points out how many years Viola has devoted herself to this family. Viola replies that "there are all kinds of families." Dee Dee looks up at Mrs. Chow's room and thinks she saw the curtain move. Dee Dee asks Viola if she believes in ghosts.
   a. How would you respond to someone who reported feeling the presence or seeing the image of a deceased loved one?

    b. How would you respond to a client/patient who expressed the idea or a desire to join a deceased loved one?

    c. What screening precautions would you want to take with this client/patient?

10 (Ch 5, 0:34:47–0:37:57) Three of the siblings are going through their mother's personal effects. They find out things they did not know about their mother, including a tragedy with her first love and how she met their father in Hong Kong. Liz reflects on having to write a eulogy for a woman "we clearly did not know."

    a. What function do eulogies serve?

    b. How challenging would it be to write a eulogy for someone you felt conflicted about?

    c. In your experience, do eulogies tend to focus only on positive or glorified memories of an individual? If so, why is that?

11 (Ch 5, 0:44:15–0:45:30) The family meets with a funeral planner to select a tombstone. The planner is ostentatious, suggesting a marble altar for their mother. He prefaces his suggestions with: "if it were my mother." He is not listening to the family or even allowing them to talk. The brother steps up and selects something simple and tasteful.

    a. Discuss the funeral rites and burial practices in the Christian, Jewish, Muslim, Buddhist and Hindu religions.

12 (Ch 6, 0:48:19–0:50:19) The family is visiting their mother's dressmaker to request that she make their mother's final dress. They are informed that it is custom in China for the daughters to make the last dress for their mother. The family thinks they knew what their mother thought of them but find out that she was very proud of them each in their own way and continually talked about them. They wonder how she could present this way to others but act so differently toward them. The son's answer is that their mother was "saving face."

    a. Discuss care of the deceased body in various cultural and religious traditions.

    b. What do you know about the tradition of "sitting with the body"?

    c. What are the purposes of scheduled time to "view the body"?

Reading of the Will

1 (Ch 7, 0:54:07–0:55:25) The family is gathered to discuss their mother's estate. Viola announces that their mother made her the executor of her estate. The son protests briefly. They review the contents of her will. Viola announces that they will get nothing but the house coming from their father's will. Their mother gave everything to the Pacific Coast Community Center. They are surprised to learn that their mother believed in charity.

    a. New information and insights into their mother's vested interests and activities is revealed. How does the family reconcile discrepant views of their mother? What does it say about them that they did not know much of what mattered to their mother?

b. How can these insights be a source of distress now that their mother is deceased?

2   (Ch 7, 0:58:54–0:1:00:45) In this scene, the family is gathered by a pyre attended by monks. They are burning items including an old car, a replica of a house, and touching mementos for their mother for her to take with her into the afterlife.

a. What other symbolic rituals have you seen people perform after a loved one's death?

3   (Ch 9, 1:12:30–1:15:12) On the fifth day of mourning, friends pay their respects to the family at the home. Again the family learns about different, kinder sides to their mother. The grandchildren are making different conclusions about their grandmother than what was presented to them by their parents.

a. How do offers of condolence (visits and cards) comfort and assist loved ones?

b. What lessons are the grandchildren taking away from this experience?

Further Reading

- Biziou, B. *The Joy of Family Rituals: Recipes for Everyday Living*. NY: St. Martin's Press; 2000.
- Doherty W, McDaniel S. *Family Therapy*. Washington, DC: APA Press; 2010.
- Frumkin R, Baver M, Mustakas C. Advancing cultural understanding through a "celebrate diversity!" event: perspectives from three voices [personal perspective]. *Multicultural Education*. 2009; **16**(4): [HTML].
- Goldenberg H, Goldenberg I, editors. *Family Therapy: an overview*. 7th ed. Belmont, CA: Thomson Brooks/Cole; 2008.
- Hardy K, editors. *Re-Visioning Family Therapy, Second Edition: race, culture, and gender in clinical practice*. New York, NY: The Guilford Press; 2008.
- Jordan J. *Relational-Cultural Therapy*. Washington, DC: APA Press; 2010.
- McGoldrick M, Carter B, Garcia-Preto N, editors. *The Expanded Family Life Cycle: individual, family and social perspectives*. 4th ed. Upper Saddle River, NJ: Prentice Hall; 2010.
- Ring J, Nyquist J, Mitchell S, *et al*. *Curriculum for Culturally Responsive Health Care: the step-by-step guide for cultural competence training*. Oxford: Radcliffe Publishing; 2008.

7

Aging Progressions: From Independence to Frailty

Roger Y. Wong, Corisande Baldwin,
Patricia Lenahan & Suzanne Classen

THE WELL-KNOWN POPULATION PYRAMID HAS SHIFTED DRAMATICALLY as global aging has occurred. The term "successful aging" is frequently used by baby boomers and may be "synonymous with global cultural norms that emphasize the importance of maintaining independent functioning, continued physical mobility and a sense of well-being."[1] The reality, however, is that many older adults may not be able to "age well" because of myriad factors: chronic illness, poverty, educational deficits, economics, losses and lack of access to health-care services.[1]

Minority elders may face additional challenges when accessing health-care services related to financial constraints, language barriers, cultural norms and traditions and health literacy. In addition, the older LGBTQI (lesbian, gay, bisexual, transgender, queer, questioning, and intersex) community is currently estimated at three million people and is expected to double by 2030. The current age cohort is one that has experienced discrimination, growing up in an era when being homosexual was considered immoral or sinful. This stigma may result in marginalization from the health-care and mental health-care systems and a sense of disenfranchisement from community aging organizations.

This chapter will focus on issues related to "successful" aging, as well as frailty and decline. Gambling-related issues will be addressed in this chapter, but some specific aging-related topics such as substance abuse will be addressed, instead, in Chapter 8 (Chemicals and Processes: Abuse and Addiction).

Intimate Relationships and Aging Adults
. . . .

Lovely, Still (2008): Robert Malone (Martin Landau) is an aging man who works in a grocery store and often appears confused. His world changes when he meets Mary (Ellen Burstyn), who moves in across the street from him.
1 (Ch 3, 0:14:30–0:16:25) Robert's doorbell rings and Mary is standing there. She asks him if they can have dinner the next evening. Flabbergasted, Robert finally agrees. Mary tells him that he should pick a place for them to go on their date. Robert replies, "date?"
   a. Why does Robert seem so surprised?
   b. What attitudes and beliefs does he have about himself? About dating?
   c. How do you feel about dating among older adults?
2 (Ch 5, 0:29:00–0:29:50) Mary and Robert are sitting at dinner, sharing child-hood dreams. Robert is reminiscing about a life not lived. Mary tells him there is no chance to fail if you don't give up. They promise each other that they won't give up.
   a. What does Mary mean when she says there is no chance to fail if you don't give up?
   b. What purpose does Robert's reminiscence serve? Is it a positive or nega-tive activity for him?
3 (Ch 6, 0:38:45–0:40:30) After sledding, Mary asks Robert to be her date for Christmas Eve. Robert looks pensive and replies, "I may have wasted my whole life." Mary reassures him by saying "the past is just something we cannot do anything about; let's just be happy now."
   a. What factors contribute to the development of intimate relationships in aging adults?
   b. What role do societal, cultural, and familial beliefs play?

Boynton Beach Club (2005; Dyan Cannon, Sally Kellerman, Brenda Vaccaro, Joseph Bologna, Michael Nouri, Len Cariou): This film is a some-what stereotypical and clichéd look at a group of recently widowed and single seniors living in an active retirement community, looking for new relationships.
1 (Ch 3, 0:17:10–0:18:40) The bereavement support group is meeting. The leader says that today is a "rap session," which means "nothing is off limits." She asks: "What's on your mind?" A woman raises her hand and looks around. She says: "What do you say to a fellow who is impotent?" A woman sitting behind her shouts out: "Find yourself a boy toy!"
   a. How would you respond to an older patient who is concerned about begin-ning a new sexual relationship?
   b. What advice would you give a patient about sexual dysfunction in older adults?
   c. How would you counsel an older patient about safe sexual practices?
2 (Ch 2, 0:15:10–0:16:37; ch 7, 0:42:06–0:43:07) In the first scene, Harry (Bologna) is on the computer looking at a website, Seniors Seeking Seniors.

He replies to a post from a woman named Florence who describes herself as "55 years young and sexy." Harry is interested. In the second scene, Harry is again chatting with Florence. They make arrangements to meet.

   a. What are the risks and benefits to Internet dating sites? What are the risks of becoming a victim of fiduciary abuse? How would you advise your patients regarding safe Internet usage?

   b. What is the impact of social media on seniors?

   c. How can the Internet be used to facilitate communication, education and services for seniors?

3 (Ch 5, 0:34:19–0:35:11) This scene begins with a look at a water aerobics class attended mostly by women; the scene shifts to a group of men playing cards at the senior center. They are talking about dating and online dating websites. Harry shares his posts with Florence, who wants to see a photo of him. The men advise Harry to send her a photo that's 20 years old, adding "everyone does it."

   a. What are your impressions about the aqua aerobics class? Would you recommend this as a form of exercise for your older patients?

   b. What stereotypic views of a senior retirement community are displayed in this scene?

   c. What advice would you give Harry?

   d. Is "honesty the best policy" or do people exaggerate online?

Driving and Letting Go of the License

1 (Ch 3, 0:23:40–0:24:17) Marilyn (Vaccaro) is in line at the Department of Motor Vehicles. Her license expired more than 20 years ago. The clerk at the counter tells her that she is in the wrong line, tells her which line she needs to go to for her new license and adds that she will need to take the test over because she is 65. He adds: "Do you understand what I'm saying," to which Marilyn angrily replies: "I may be 65, but I am not an idiot."

   a. What is ageism? Are the clerk's assumptions about Marilyn an example of ageism and ageist thinking?

   b. How would you counsel a patient about driving safety?

   c. At what point would you counsel a patient and/or family to discontinue driving? What are your legal obligations in this regard?

That Evening Sun (2009; Hal Holbrook, Barry Corbin, Walter Goggins): Abner Meecham is an aging farmer in rural Tennessee whose disengaged son, an attorney, facilitates Abner's admission to a nursing home. However, Abner has other ideas. He walks out of the facility and back to his farm but he encounters a family living on his farm.

1 (0:27:10–0:28:07) Thurl (Corbin) is talking with Abner (Holbrook) who wants Thurl to take him to town. Thurl shares that he can't do that because

"they took my license away because I hit some folks." Abner asks him how he gets around and Thurl replies: "My daughter comes on Tuesdays and takes me shopping." He adds: "You know what's amazing? After they raise their own kids they come back to raise you."

    a. How would you interpret Barry's remarks about his daughter coming back to "raise" him?

    b. What are the autonomy issues here?

    c. How can the lack of driving affect rural older adults? What can be done to reduce isolation?

Loss and Grief in Aging

Goodbye, Solo (2008): This is the story of Solo (Souleymane Sysavane), a Senegalese cab driver who forges an unlikely friendship with one of his regular passengers, William (Red West), whom Solo calls "Big Dog."

1   (1:13:00–1:14:28) Solo sees a notebook on William's bed. It contains stubs of movie tickets and diary entries. Solo was taken by one entry: "When he laughed, his lip twitched. He looked just like his mother." Solo recalled William talking with the same young man at the ticket office every time he dropped William off at the theater.

    a. How would you interpret this diary entry?

    b. How would you address this issue with William?

    c. What is the role of diaries and reminiscence in aging?

Boynton Beach Club (see earlier description)

1   (Ch 1, 0:5:00–0:6:30) Marilyn (Brenda Vaccaro) greets her daughter and son-in-law at the airport after her husband died after being run over by a woman in the retirement community. Her son-in-law is carrying a dog, saying they brought it for Marilyn as company. She replies that she hates dogs. At home, her daughter is trying to convince her to move up North with them, pointing out that "Daddy did everything for you. You don't know how to balance a check book and you haven't driven in years." Marilyn replies that she will learn.

    a. Marilyn's daughter is clearly concerned about how her mother will cope. Was this an appropriate time for Marilyn's daughter to pose this discussion? What are the stressors for adult children who live in other parts of the country?

    b. Would a pet be an appropriate gift for a bereaved person?

2   (Ch 1, 0:6:50–0:7:350) The scene occurs at the Boynton Beach Senior Center bereavement group. Marilyn attends her first group and seems uncomfortable. Another attendee, Lois (Dyan Cannon), sees her discomfort and says she knows it's difficult, adding, "we've all been there."

    a. Was Lois's comment helpful?

    b. What is the likelihood that Marilyn will return to the group?

    c. What are some of the advantages of support groups? Are there any potential negative consequences?

3 (Ch 2, 0:8:26–0:11:04) Jack Gudson (Len Cariou) attends his first group. Another man, Harry (Joseph Bologna), says it's nice to have another man, stating there are "eight women to every man" here. Jack is asked to introduce himself and he shares that his wife and companion of 45 years died recently. The group leader says: "Grief is a normal process. We have to go through the stages in order to come out the other side."

    a. What symptoms might Jack present in a clinical setting?

    b. Were the group leader's comments helpful? Was Jack ready to hear those words?

    c. How do you counsel patients about grief?

    d. What are the diagnostic criteria for bereavement?

    e. What is "complicated bereavement"?

4 (Ch 3, 0:19:03–0:21:13) Marilyn (Vaccaro) returns to the support group. She stands up and shares that she would like to learn how to deal with her anger. She shares how her husband died (as the result of a woman backing out of a driveway while on her cell phone). When she is finished, Marilyn says: "Sorry, I had to get that out." Lois (Dyan Cannon) convinces Marilyn to join her for coffee after the meeting. Marilyn says: "Two things I don't like: doctors and support groups."

    a. Was Marilyn's anger justified? Is this an example of a grief reaction?

    b. How would you approach a patient who shares with you that she doesn't like doctors? What experiences, attitudes, or beliefs may have contributed to her feelings about physicians?

That Evening Sun (see earlier description)

1 (0:55:40–0:59:34) Abner (Holbrook) and his son, Paul (Goggins) are sitting in a diner having lunch. Paul is trying to convince him to return to the nursing home. Abner says that he lived on the farm alone for 8 years after his wife died. He adds: "I deserve to do with it (life) as I please. I am an 80-year-old man with a bum hip and a weak heart. The road ain't long and winding, it's short and straight. I know that."

    a. What are the ethical dilemmas in this situation?

    b. Is it feasible for Abner to stay on the farm alone? What other options might exist other than a nursing home?

    c. What does the loss of autonomy mean to Abner? How would you counsel a patient regarding moving into an aggregate living situation? What would you say to aid the family in its decision making?

    d. How do these types of dilemmas impact family relationships?

Away from Her (2005; Gordon Pinset, Julie Christie): A touching glimpse into the experience of a couple as one partner moves into a care facility because of a diagnosis of Alzheimer's disease. This movie portrays the heartbreaking moments the spouse of a patient with Alzheimer's experiences, including when the one they love no longer recognizes them.

1 (0:09:56–0:11:15; 0:13:22–0:14:30) The first scene shows Fiona and Grant sitting together in a doctor's office after Fiona had been unable to recall the word "wine." Fiona undergoes an assessment for her memory issues. When she is unable to answer questions, she tries to change the subject. The second scene occurs after Fiona has been diagnosed. Grant and Fiona read and learn what a caregiver must endure as Alzheimer's disease progresses in their loved one.

   a. What type of resources would benefit a spouse whose partner has been diagnosed with Alzheimer's disease?

   b. When thinking about Elizabeth Kübler-Ross's stages of grieving, what reactions might be expected from a spouse after their partner has been diagnosed with Alzheimer's disease?

   c. When a spouse or partner has been diagnosed with Alzheimer's disease, a couple experiences many losses. What losses can you identify that a couple may experience in order to provide them with anticipatory guidance?

   d. What are some ways the expression of grief and loss differs between cultures?

Addictive Behaviors and Older Adults

Vegas Vacation (1989; Chevy Chase, Beverly D'Angelo): Chase and D'Angelo reprise their roles as Ellen and Clark Griswold. This time they take a family vacation to Las Vegas.

1 (Ch 30, 1:21:07–1:25:48) (This scene is also described in Chapter 9 [Betting On Your Life: Pathological Gambling], with a different focus.) The Griswolds have lost all their money except $2, which they bet on keno. They sit next to an older man, Mr. Ellis (Milt Kamen), who strikes up a conversation with Clark (Chase). Mr. Ellis tells Clark that he has a nice family. He shares that he never got married because he was too scared. He adds: "money isn't everything. I sit here alone; nobody cares. If I win, there's nobody to share it with." Clark tells him that at least he has his health and a hobby. Mr. Ellis responds: "A hobby, I've got – health?" Clark tells Mr. Ellis to consider himself part of their family. At that point, Mr. Ellis's numbers come up and he wins keno: "All the years I've waited for this; all the years I've been coming here…" He then appears to die of shock or have a myocardial infarction. When the paramedics arrive, one paramedic says: "He's gone … he was the loneliest guy I ever saw. He'd give anything to have somebody sit with him and say a few nice words."

a. What factors are associated with problem gambling in older adults?
b. What are the risks of addiction developing in older adults?
c. Many senior centers and assisted living facilities organize social outings and day trips to casinos. Does this type of activity contribute to the development of addictive behaviors?

From Successful Aging to Frailty

While many older persons will age successfully, a small number of them will develop multiple complex chronic illnesses that predispose them to functional and/or cognitive decline.[2] These frail older people may have different clinical presentations. Many are "frequent flyers" to many health-care services, as they make multiple visits to the ambulatory clinics, acute care hospitals, and are eventually at increased risk of requiring long-term care facility (nursing home) placement.[3] Frailty is a complex concept, and although various hypotheses exist to explain it,[4] it is an abstract concept to convey to many health-care learners. Cinemeducation can be helpful to put a few faces to frailty. We are certainly not promoting stereotyping all older people as frail, but at the same time we recognize a picture (or movie film in this case) can be worth a thousand words in conveying an abstract concept such as frailty to the novice learner.

This part of the chapter describes several examples of how aging individuals, and frail older adults, are portrayed in films. As always it is important to allow time for reflection and facilitated discussion following each selected scene. Of note, one of the examples uses animated film, which can hopefully inspire a wide variety of film genres to be used in cinemeducation.

Physical Illness as a Basis for Declining Health

The Stone Angel (2007; Ellen Burstyn, Christine Horne, Ellen Page): This film tells the story of an older woman, Hagar, who is physically declining as a result of a cancer diagnosis that has not been revealed to her. Throughout the course of her decline she reflects on her youth, her marriage, and raising her family. This film presents a vivid drama of contrasting the younger person with the older person and personal autonomy.

1 (Scene 1, ch 1, 00:07:23–00:08:19) In this scene, Hagar is at the family physician's office with her son for an assessment for syncope.
   a. How would you assess the family physician's approach to communicating with Hagar? What works well and what does not?
   b. What do you think of the environmental set-up of the office where Hagar is interviewed?
   c. Why do you think Hagar's son behaves in the way he does in this scene?
   d. What about patient autonomy?

2 (Scene 2, ch 2, 00:15:07–00:16:50) In this scene, Hagar's son, who is losing his home and business because of financial difficulties, approaches his
   mother about going into a nursing home. Hagar and her daughter-in-law, who
   is caring for her, become quite upset with each other, and her son is left in
   the middle.
   a. How would you assess Hagar's son's way of breaking the news to Hagar
       that she may wish to relocate to a nursing home? What works well and
       what does not?
   b. What are some possible factors that lead to caregiver stress as portrayed
       in this scene?
   c. What do you think of the financial issues as brought up in this scene? Why
       is Hagar vulnerable to elder mistreatment in terms of finances?

Falls in the Elderly

That Evening Sun (see earlier description)

1 (0:43:00–0:45:00) Abner (Holbrook) is cleaning his gun and talking to his
   dog. He says that he fell down the porch steps last year on a patch of ice. "It
   was December, I broke my hip, no one was around. I thought 'my time has
   come.' All I could do was lie there and ache. A friend of mine came by the
   next day 'on a whim.'" He adds that he spent a few weeks in the hospital and
   knew pretty quickly that he couldn't tend the farm.
   a. What are the potential consequences of falls in the elderly? What can be
       done to reduce their occurrence?
   b. How would you interpret Abner's statement that he thought his time had
       come?
   c. What concerns might you have about guns and older adults?
   d. What might Abner's cleaning his gun signify?

Suicidality and Older Adults

Lovely, Still (see earlier description)

1 (Ch 10; 0:1:02:01–0:1:07:04) Robert and Mary wake up together on
   Christmas morning and begin to open Christmas presents. Robert goes
   into the kitchen to make coffee and tells Mary to open up all the remaining
   presents since they are for her. Mary looks terrified after opening one gift
   that Robert had wrapped and addressed to himself: a gun. Robert returns to
   the living room and Mary asks him why he gave himself a gun for Christmas.
   Robert says that he was tired, tired of being alone, and he planned to "end it."
   a. What are the risks for suicidality in older adults?

    b. How does cognitive decline and/or depression affect suicidality?

    c. What is the impact of loneliness and isolation as people age?

Goodbye, Solo (see earlier description)

1 (Ch 1, 0:02:08–0:0:2:47) William, aka Big Dog, has been one of Solo's regular fares, with Solo taking him to the movies regularly. On this occasion, William offers Solo $1000 to take him to the top of Blowin' Rock on October 20. Solo asks him if he is going camping there. When William doesn't respond, Solo jokingly asks him if he is going to fly away. He then becomes serious and asks, "you're not going to jump are you?"

    a. What sparks Solo's concern and fear that William is going to jump?

    b. What actions should Solo take if he believes William has suicidal thoughts?

    c. What is the significance of October 20?

    d. Do special occasions such as anniversaries and holidays increase suicidal ideation among older adults?

2 (Ch 2, 0:08:37–0:09:40) Solo arrives to pick up William, who has his luggage with him. Solo seems surprised and says that he thought William was going to the movies. William replies that he sold his home and is moving into a motel. At this point, Solo tries to give William the $1000 back.

    a. What prompted Solo to try to give the money back?

    b. What do you think Solo suspected was behind William's motivation to make such a drastic change?

3 (Multiple chs, 0:16:00–17:00; 0:47:50–0:48:40; 1:15:41–1:15:55) In these three scenes, William is getting drunk at a bar, goes to the bank and closes his account, and gives his clothes away.

    a. What do these behaviors represent?

    b. What is the impact of the S.A.D. (suicide-alcohol-depression) triangle in older adults?

    c. Would this constellation of behaviors be significant enough to warrant a psychiatric evaluation or involuntary hospitalization?

4 (01:19:00–01:21:34) William, and Solo arrive at Blowin' Rock. Solo leaves William and walks away. William stares at Solo as he walks away and then William continues climbing to the rock.

    a. Did Solo have any responsibility to stop William?

    b. Do you think William jumped from Blowin' Rock?

    c. What interventions might have helped William cope with his apparent depression?

    d. What types of therapeutic interventions are most appropriate to consider with depressed older adults?

Suicidality in Assisted Living Facilities

Assisted Living (2003; Michael Bonsignore, Maggie Riley, Malerie Boone, Jose Albovias): This faux documentary highlights the experience of Todd, a janitor at an assisted living facility. Through watching Todd at work, the viewer is able to gain an understanding about the experiences of the residents in the facility.

1 (0:33:41–0:35:16) Mrs. Pearlman (Maggie Riley) tells Todd (Michael Bonsignore) a story about her son. She looks at Todd and asks him if she had already told him that story, and he nods affirmatively. Mrs. Pearlman acknowledges her Alzheimer's disease and discusses suicide with Todd.
   a. How can you include a depression screening in your assessment when working with a patient who is in the early stages of Alzheimer's disease?
   b. What are some of the potential indicators for suicidality in a patient diagnosed with Alzheimer's disease?
   c. What would you tell a patient who disclosed they wanted to die? What are your feelings related to a patient's decision or desire to end their life?

Challenges Associated with Living in an Assisted Living Facility

1 (0:00:31–0:00:58; 0:01:00–0:01:32) In the first scene, an unidentified member of the assisted living facility staff explains that the seating in the dining room is assigned because of the number of restricted diets among the residents. In the second scene, Jose (Albovias), the chaplin, speaks about his style of sermon and how he wants to reach the residents.
   a. What challenges would a single adult with no children face when choosing a care facility?
   b. How might religious or cultural factors impact a person's choice of residential facilities?
   c. What are some of the issues a family with limited resources faces when making decisions regarding the residential placement of their loved one?
   d. What are some of the freedoms a person gives up when they move into an assisted living facility?

Therapy Animals

1 (0:06:54–0:07:07) Todd is shown walking down a hallway with a golden retriever. A number of residents are shown petting and showing affection to the dog. Later in the film (1:12:01–1:13:21) the dog's owner, whose name is never identified, reveals the dog died and discusses the positive impact the dog had on the other residents in the assisted living.
   a. What are some of the benefits to having a therapy animal in assisted living?

   b. What are some religious or cultural beliefs that may impact a patient's decision to participate in animal therapy?

   c. How might the dog's death affect a patient who had grown close to it?

   d. What requirements are needed for animals to participate in therapy work?

The Savages (2007; Philip Bosco, Laura Linney, Philip Seymour Hoffman): This film is the story of a disengaged family. Lenny (Bosco) is living with his longtime girlfriend in a retirement community in Sun City, Arizona. When she dies, Lenny's two children, Wendy (Linney), an unsuccessful writer, and her brother, Jon (Philip Seymour Hoffman), a drama professor, are called upon to make living arrangements for Lenny who is suffering from some type of dementing illness.

1   (Ch 11, 0:37:06–0:39:30) Wendy and Jon are accompanying Lenny into the skilled nursing facility. He is being shown to his room when a cat crosses their path. The nurse's aide explains that he is "Winston … we call him the mayor."

   a. How might family members react to seeing a cat walking the halls of a skilled facility?

   b. What are the advantages and disadvantages of having resident pets?

2   (Ch 21, 01:19:04–0:1:20:00) Wendy is bringing her cat into the nursing home. Jon asks her what she is doing. Wendy explains that the cat is going to stay with their father. Jon seems skeptical, but Wendy assures him that it was OK with the staff as long as the cat was vaccinated. She continues by saying: "Apparently it is good for the residents' well-being. They reduce stress."

   a. How would you respond to a family who wanted to bring in a resident pet into a skilled facility?

   b. What potential issues might occur when the facility already has a resident pet(s)?

Social Isolation

Up (2009; Edward Asner, Jordan Nagai, John Ratzenberger): This is an animated film relaying the story of a retired balloon salesman and widower, Carl Fredricksen, who embarks on an adventure sought by his late wife to go to Paradise Falls in South America. The themes addressed in this animated film include identifying the determinants of health and overcoming social isolation. This example illustrates how a different genre of film (animation) can offer a different tool for and experience of cinemeducation.

1   (Scene 1, ch 5, 0:13:25–0:15:14) In this scene Carl is shown struggling to protect his little house, which, although once on a quiet road, is now dwarfed by major construction and skyscrapers.

   a. What are the biological, psychological, and social determinants of health that play a role in Carl's aging as illustrated by this scene?

    b. Why do you think Carl attempts to protect his house in the scene?

    c. Why does Carl behave the way shown in the scene? How would you approach Carl differently if you were the construction staff in the scene?

    d. What factors contribute to frail older adults who are facing change and loss?

2 (Scene 2, ch 7, 0:17:40–0:19:18) In this scene Carl becomes enraged when a construction vehicle damages his mailbox and he acts out violently.

    a. What do you think are the factors that provoke Carl to act out violently? Which of these factors are potentially avoidable?

    b. What role does social isolation play in influencing the way Carl reacts as portrayed in the scene?

    c. If you were the health-care professional providing care to Carl, how might you communicate with him in an attempt to reach out to him?

Cognitive Impairment

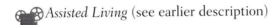 *Assisted Living* (see earlier description)

1 (0:46:05–0:53:25) While in a state of confusion, Mrs. Pearlman repeatedly asks Malerie (Boone), the nurse on duty, to call her son in Australia. Malerie tells Mrs. Pearlman no outside calls can be made from the phone at the front desk and Malerie offers to look up the phone number for her. The nurse discovers there is no number on file for Mrs. Pearlman's son. After hearing her confusion and distress, Todd pretends to be Mrs. Pearlman's son Jeremy on the phone. Initially the conversation was going well; however, when the conversation took a negative turn, Mrs. Pearlman became upset, fell to the floor, and was sedated by Malerie.

    a. Many times when a patient with Alzheimer's disease has delusions, individuals will play along with the delusions. Is there a point where playing into their delusions becomes abusive?

    b. How would you assess a patient for symptoms of elder or dependent adult abuse? How would you assess for abuse in a patient who has dementia or psychosis? When would you be required to make a mandated report?

    c. What steps can you take as part of the treatment team for a patient with little social support, to reduce their risk for potential abuse?

Dementing Illnesses

Intoxicating (2003): William (John Savage), a former boxer, is the father of the busy heart surgeon Dorian Shanley (Kirk Harris). William has dementia and lives at home with an in-home caregiver.

1 (Ch 5, 0:19:26–0:22:40) The caregiver (Allan Rich) has been calling Dorian

for 3 days before Dorian came to his father's house. The caregiver acknowledges that he knows how terrible it is to see your father go through this. Dorian's father, William, is shadowboxing in the living room. Dorian calls to him and William asks him if he could help him find his son. William adds: "It's been so long since I've seen him. I can't remember." Dorian walks outside, sits, and cries. The caregiver emerges from the house and says: "He didn't recognize you? Dorian, at this stage he's doing better than most."

a. How would you counsel an adult child or spouse of a patient experiencing memory loss?
b. What impact does memory loss have on parent-child relationships?
c. What suggestions would you offer Dorian in terms of trying to help William remember him?

2 (Ch 8, 0:37:57–0:40:24; 0:40:36–0:41:30) The caregiver is seen with William who is shadowboxing again. The caregiver is trying to get William to take a shower. When Dorian arrives, William hits him. The caregiver warns Dorian to be careful because William doesn't know him. William turns to the caregiver and tells him he is supposed to help him. Then he says: "Do me a favor and let my son know where I am." In the second scene the caregiver asks Dorian if William has Alzheimer's disease. Dorian replies that it is "pugilistic dementia," the boxer's disease. Dorian adds: "You should have seen him when I was young. He just stayed in the game too long."

a. What are catastrophic reactions in patients with dementia?
b. How would you counsel caregivers and family members in coping with these behaviors?
c. What does Dorian mean when he says his father stayed in the game too long?
d. Are there any differences in working with adult children who are also physicians or other health-care providers?

The Savages (see earlier description)

1 (Ch 1, 0:1:00–0:4:53) The home health aide caring for Lenny's girlfriend, Doris, calls to Lenny, telling him "somebody forgot something in the bathroom. Lenny, you forgot to flush." Lenny ignores him, until the aide comes into the living room and takes his cereal away. Lenny returns to the bathroom and later, when the aide knocks on the door, he sees that Lenny has written a derogatory word on the bathroom wall with his feces.

a. How would you interpret Lenny's behavior?
b. Is fecal smearing a symptom of an underlying disorder or merely a response to being told what to do?
c. How would you explain this type of behavior to family members?

Advanced Directives
•••••••••••••••••••••••••••

1   (Ch 13; 0:45:15–0:49:30) The scene opens with Lenny sitting in an exercise class and shifts to Wendy and Jon talking with the facility administrator who is explaining Medicaid, advanced directives, health proxy and funeral arrangements. Wendy and Jon don't know how to respond. The administrator advises them to talk with their father. The scene shifts again to Jon, Wendy and Lenny sitting in a diner. Jon gives Lenny a hearing aid and tells him how to turn up the volume. The children are reluctant to discuss the advance directives, but state there are some things we need to know. As Jon tries to explain advance directives, Lenny yells "pull the plug" and "unplug me." Jon then asks Lenny "what do we do with you?" Lenny looks disbelieving and says: "you bury me ... are you a bunch of idiots ... you bury me."
   a. How can you facilitate a discussion of advance directives with a patient and family?
   b. When would you advise patients to consider advance directives?
   c. What are some of the commonly held misperceptions about advance directives?

Choosing a Facility
••••••••••••••••••••••••••

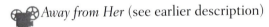 *Away from Her* (see earlier description)

1   (0:14:32–18:06; 0:20:20–25:12) In the first scene, Fiona went skiing by herself. When Fiona was nowhere to be found, Grant went searching for her and found her wandering alongside the road. Once they returned home and Fiona was coherent, she told Grant they have reached that stage, referring to her need to go to an assisted living facility. Grant stated that it must not be a permanent move. The second scene shows Grant on a tour of the assisted living facility. During this time he is informed that new residents are prohibited from having visitors for the first 30 days in order to facilitate their settling in.
   a. What are some of the challenges a couple faces when deciding whether to place their partner in an assisted living or care facility?
   b. Would home-based care be appropriate for a couple when one partner has been diagnosed with Alzheimer's disease?
   c. If Grant and Fiona did not have the resources to cover the cost of a care facility, what would be some of their options? As a member of their treatment team, how would you help a patient discover and access potential resources?
   d. How do you feel about the facility's policy to prohibit visitors during the first 30 days? Would you recommend a facility that adhered to such a policy?

The Savages (see earlier description)

1 (Ch 8, 0:24:00–0:25:30) After meeting with their father's physician, Jon and Wendy are seen sitting in a bar reading pamphlets on Parkinson's disease. While Jon is talking about skilled nursing home placements, Wendy wonders aloud: "Maybe he didn't abandon us; maybe he forgot us."
   a. What is the role of patient education materials when addressing a difficult diagnosis?
   b. What factors must be considered when providing patients and families with these resources?
   c. What other sources of information do patients and families use in order to obtain more information and to clarify issues?
   d. How would you assess Wendy's comment?
2 (Ch 9, 0:30:55–0:31:55) Wendy has remained behind in Arizona while Jon returned to New York to find a place for Lenny. He calls Wendy and says he has found a facility that has an opening. Wendy questions what kind of place it is and Jon replies: "a facility for older people – in this country they are called nursing homes." Wendy asks if it smells. Jon replies: "yes, they all smell." Wendy wants Jon to find an assisted living facility for their father. Jon replies that they won't take him because he has dementia.
   a. What factors contribute to Wendy's reluctance to consider this move?
   b. Is Jon being realistic or is he merely trying to get things resolved for their father?
   c. How would you assist a family in making arrangements for an out-of-home placement?
3 (Ch 10, 0:32:30–0:35:40) Wendy is checking Lenny out of the hospital. She signs him out, gets his medications, and gets a pile of diapers. The nurse says she shouldn't be giving the diapers to Wendy, but she thinks Wendy will need them. The scene then shifts to Lenny being lifted onto the airplane. Suddenly, Lenny appears to become angry, tosses his food in the box, and yells "bathroom." Wendy tries to calm him down, but he is adamant. She assists him to walk down the aisle of the plane. He stops suddenly and looks down at his feet. His trousers have fallen around his ankles, exposing his diapers.
   a. What are the risks of flying with a demented individual? What advice would you give them? Would you medicate an older individual for the flight? How do you alert airline personnel?
   b. Do you think Lenny is embarrassed? What about Wendy? The other passengers?
   c. How can families cope with catastrophic reactions among demented individuals?

Adult Children and Aging Parents
· ·

1 (Ch 4, 0:11:22–0:13:42) Wendy (Linney) has picked up a phone message about her father's behavior and calls her brother Jon, (Hoffman), telling him: "Dad's writing on the walls with his shit." She ends with: "Don't leave me alone with this. You don't even know where he is. This is a crisis." Jon replies that it isn't a crisis.
   a. How would you assess the family relationships based on this interchange?
   b. What factors contribute to family dysfunction?
   c. Who appears to be the primary care provider? Who usually assumes this role in families? Why?

2 (Ch 6, 0:18:00–0:20:15) Jon and Wendy arrive at Doris's home after her death. Doris's daughter explains that Lenny is in the hospital. She continues that while Lenny has been like family for over 20 years, he is their family and they will need to find him a place to stay.
   a. How do Jon and Wendy respond to this?
   b. Are they ready and able to assume responsibility for their father's care?
   c. Do Wendy and Jon "know" their father? What factors may have contributed to their estrangement?

3 (Ch 7, 0:20:29–0:22:40) Jon and Wendy arrive at the hospital. They hesitate before entering the room. Lenny is lying in bed with a nasal cannula, a foley urinary catheter, and he is in restraints. He appears to be asleep, but wakes up and says to them: "Where the hell have you been? You're the late ones." Lenny is agitated by the restraints and Jon goes for a nurse who returns and releases them.
   a. What factors contribute to restraining an older patient?
   b. Are chemical restraints or physical restraints used more frequently? Why?
   c. What is the impact on families in seeing their relatives restrained?
   d. How would you interpret Lenny's remark about Jon and Wendy being the "late ones"? Is Lenny coherent when he makes this comment? What might it tell you about their family relationships?

4 (Ch 11, 0:40:00–0:40:39; ch 12, 0:43:57–0:45:00) Jon and Wendy are standing outside after placing Lenny in the facility. Jon says that their father doesn't know where he is, but Wendy tearfully repeats: "we're horrible, horrible, horrible people." In the second scene, Jon tries to assure Wendy that they are doing the right thing, adding, "we're taking better care of the old man than he ever did of us." Wendy responds that she knows. The scene shifts to Wendy viewing a brochure and video of another facility.
   a. How would you counsel adult children who have been disengaged from their parent and each other? How does this impact their decision-making abilities?
   b. What function does guilt play here?
   c. Is Wendy's search for a more idyllic facility an attempt to assuage her guilt? Is it based on the reality of Lenny's situation and capabilities?

5 (Ch 18, 1:07:00–1:09:58) The scene begins with Jon, Wendy, and Lenny meeting an administrator of admissions at a new facility. She is asking Lenny some mental status questions and admonishes Wendy for trying to help. Jon reminds Wendy that Lenny becomes reactive. The scene ends with Jon and Wendy standing outside. Jon says: "It's not about Dad, it's about your guilt … the nice landscaping is there to obscure the fact that people are dying."
   a. How to you address family members who are trying to prompt their relatives during a mental status exam?
   b. How would you assess Jon's statement?
   c. Is Wendy being realistic about her father's capabilities?

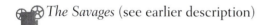 *Goodbye, Solo* (see earlier description)

1 (Ch 2, 0:10:23–0:11:04) They are riding in the cab and Solo asks William if he has a family. Solo wonders why families don't stay together in America. He adds that in his country, families take care of old people: "even if they have no teeth; we put food in their mouths." Solo ends by saying that he's sure that William's family wants to see him.
   a. What cultural and ethnic issue may present in addressing the needs of aging adults?
   b. What is the impact of geographic isolation?
   c. How are older adults viewed in other cultures?

Explaining a Diagnosis

The Savages (see earlier description)

1 (Ch 7; 0:22:49–0:23:27) Wendy and Jon are at the hospital and meeting with the physician. He is showing them a MRI scan. The doctor discusses vascular dementia and why he doesn't see any radiographic indications that vascular dementia is the source of Lenny's problems. The doctor discusses Lenny's symptoms (disinhibition, aggression, masked faces with a blank stare) and says they are characteristic of Parkinson's dementia.
   a. How would you assess this exchange with Lenny's children?
   b. Do you think they understand what the physician is saying?
   c. How would you evaluate this explanation in terms of health literacy issues?
   d. Was it useful to show them the MRI scan?

Sexuality, Dementia, and the Nursing Home

Away from Her (see earlier description)

1   (0:35:40–0:37:45) Once Fiona gets checked in to the facility, she and Grant go to her room to get her settled in. Fiona tells Grant that she would like to make love then for him to leave. Once Fiona is ready for Grant to leave, he walks out of her room while buttoning his pants and receives an admonishing look from a passing nurse.

    a. How does a couple maintain their sexual relationship when one partner resides in a care facility?

    b. Many individuals diagnosed with Alzheimer's disease may act in sexually aggressive or inappropriate manners. What are some interventions that could help a spouse cope with these changes?

    c. Spouses of patients with Alzheimer's disease often end their sexual relationship with their partner for a variety of reasons and some choose to date. What are some of the feelings that a spouse of a person diagnosed with Alzheimer's disease may experience if they choose to date while their partner is in a facility? What are some of the cultural or religious factors that may influence a spouse's decision whether they should (not) pursue a relationship?

    d. At what point is a patient with Alzheimer's disease unable to give consent to engage in sexual activities? How would you counsel the spouse regarding sexuality issues?

Spouses of Patients with Alzheimer's Disease

1   (0:30:38–0:34:50) During the car ride to take Fiona to the assisted living facility, the couple reflects on their troubled past. Grant asks Fiona not to go; however, she persists. Once inside, Grant again pleads with her not to go. Fiona comments to Grant that he could have left her and she appreciates that he stayed with her.

    a. How might you help a spouse cope when their partner no longer recognizes them?

    b. What would be the benefits of a spouse joining a support group?

    c. What are some challenges an LGBTQI (lesbian, gay, bisexual, transgender, queer, questioning, and intersex) couple may face when one partner receives a diagnosis of Alzheimer's disease? What are some of your feelings associated working with LGBTQI couples?

References

1 Lenahan PM. Issues in aging. In: Sahler OJ, Carr JE, editors. *The Behavioral Sciences and Health Care*. 2nd ed. Cambridge, MA: Hogrefe & Huber; 2007. p. 230–4.
2 Ravaglia G, Forti P, Lucicesare A, *et al*. Development of an easy prognostic score for frailty outcomes in the aged. *Age Ageing*. 2008; **37**(2): 161–6.
3 Song X, Mitnitski A, Rockwood K. Prevalence and 10-year outcomes of frailty in older adults in relation to deficit accumulation. *J Am Geriatr Soc*. 2010; **58**(4): 681–7.
4 Abellan van Kan G, Rolland Y, Houles M, *et al*. The assessment of frailty in older adults. *Clin Geriatr Med*. 2010; **26**(2): 275–86.

Further Reading

● Ball M, Perkins M, Hollingsworth C, *et al*. Pathways to assisted living: the influence of race and class. *J Appl Gerontol*. 2009; **28**(1): 81–108.
● Chodosh J, Kado DM, Seeman TE, *et al*. Depressive symptoms as a predictor of cognitive decline: McArthur Studies of successful aging. *Am J Geriatr Psychiatry*. 2007; **15**(5): 406–15.
● Erickson L, Molina CA, Ladd G, *et al*. Problem and pathological gambling are associated with poorer mental and physical health in older adults. *Int Rev Geriatr Psychiatry*. 2005; **20**(8): 756–9.
● Fowler C, Fisher CL. Attitudes toward decision-making and aging and preparation for future care needs. *Health Commun*. 2009; **24**(7): 619–30.
● Gillick MR. *The Denial of Aging: perpetual youth, eternal life, and other dangerous fantasies*. Boston, MA: Harvard University Press; 2006.
● Paulson D, Bowmen ME, Lichtenberg PA. Successful aging and longevity in older women: the role of depression and cognition. *J Aging Res*. 2011; Epub 2011 Jul
● Pinquart M, Sörensen S. Spouses, adult children, and children-in-law as caregivers of older adults: a meta-analytic comparison. *Psychol Aging*. 2011; **26**(1): 1–14.
● Strober L, Arnett PA. Assessment of depression in three medically ill, elderly populations: Alzheimer's disease, Parkinson's disease, and stroke. *Clin Neuropsychol*. 2009; **23**(2): 205–30.
● www.alz.org
● www.aoa.gov
● www.ltcombudsman.org

PART III

Specific Disease States

8

Chemicals and Processes:
Abuse and Addiction

James Tysinger, Patricia Lenahan & Layne Prest

A BROAD DEFINITION OF SUBSTANCE ABUSE IS "THE PROBLEMATIC USE of alcohol, tobacco, or illicit drugs."[1] Substance abuse is so prevalent that it has been called America's number-one health problem.[2] The estimated costs of substance abuse in the United States, including its related effects (e.g., lost work productivity) have been estimated to exceed US$600 billion a year.[3]

Substance abuse has impacted most families in one way or another. Consider, for example, the people you know who have abused one or more substances. Think of the ways substance abuse has damaged these specific individuals, their relatives, and random others (e.g. people who have been injured or killed in accidents caused by people driving under the influence of one or more substances).

Movie clips can be useful in teaching medical learners about substance abuse and its effects.[4] Some films with strong messages about substance abuse (e.g. *Crazy Heart*, 2009) can be viewed in their entirety, or teachers can use selected clips to focus on specific teaching points. Questions to stimulate learner thought and discussion can be obtained from sources like this book, or teachers can devise questions based on the particular objectives they want to attain by showing certain films or film clips.

Films or film clips can also broaden learners' cultural perspectives about substance abuse. For example, clips that show substance abuse among particular cultural groups (e.g. adolescents, college students, the elderly) or depict how people from particular cultural groups (e.g. physicians) respond to people who suffer from substance abuse can give learners specific insights they may otherwise have overlooked. These insights can spur discussions that go beyond medical knowledge.

Likewise, teachers must consider how films or film clips could help learners form or reinforce preexisting negative stereotypes about particular groups. Thus, educators are encouraged to specify their objectives for showing a film or clip and select the appropriate film or clips needed to attain those objectives. Before

the film or clips to learners, clips should be viewed from a fresh perspect-
his regard, cinemeducators would be wise to ask themselves the following
question: "Besides what I want my learners to see in this clip, what *unintended*
messages might the clip send?"

Many of the films cited in this chapter offer examples of polysubstance abuse,
but they may be used for the specific disease states referenced here.

Alcoholism

Crazy Heart (2009; Jeff Bridges, Maggie Gyllenhaal, Jack Nation, Robert
Duvall): This is an excellent film to use to teach people about alcoholism,
its impact on the problem drinker, the nature of his or her relationships with
others, and the recovery process. "Bad Blake" (Bridges) is a 57-year-old country
music singer whose career, personal life, and health are in "bad" shape largely due
to his problem drinking. His out-of-shape body and inappropriate behavior are
the outcome of years of problem drinking, the stress of multiple marriages, the
demands of a life on the road with its requisite budget hotels, and an estranged
relationship with his adult son. At first it appears that Bad's personal life is on the
upswing after meeting Jean Craddock (Gyllenhaal), a newspaper reporter, and
Buddy, her 4-year-old son, but Bad's problem drinking sabotages any happiness
he might find.

1 (0:09:20–0:14:50) Bad is performing in a small-town bowling alley. He was
   drinking before he arrives for the show and then he continues drinking. Bad
   starts singing, but he leaves the stage to throw up. After throwing up, he
   returns to the stage.
   a. What aspects of alcoholism are portrayed in this clip?
   b. How does Bad's problem drinking impact his fans?
2 (0:18:10–0:22:55) Introduced by her piano-playing uncle, Bad meets Jean
   Craddock, a single parent, who works as a newspaper reporter in Santa Fe,
   New Mexico.
   a. What aspects of alcoholism are portrayed in this clip?
   b. Besides alcohol, what other substance does Bad abuse?
   c. What do you learn about Bad in this clip?
3 (0:36:35–0:38:26) After Bad and Jean awaken in bed, Bad talks Jean into
   letting him go to her home so he can cook breakfast for her and Buddy, her
   4-year-old son. Bad and Buddy form a bond. Bad then heads to Phoenix to
   open a concert headlined by Tommy Sweet, one of Bad's highly successful
   protégés.
   a. How does Bad behave toward Jean and Buddy in this clip?
   b. What signs of alcoholism, if any, does Bad demonstrate in this clip?
   c. What would you predict will happen to Bad's and Jean's relationship based
      on the last part of this clip?
4 (0:52:00–0:56:33) After opening for Tommy Sweet in Phoenix, Bad is

returning to Santa Fe to see Jean and Buddy. Bad falls asleep and sustains a broken ankle and concussion when he rolls his SUV in the desert. The latter part of this scene shows a physician interacting with Bad while Bad is confined to a hospital bed.

  a. What does the physician have to say about Bad's health?

  b. What is the physician's diagnosis?

  c. What does the physician's recommend?

  d. Analyze the physician's interaction with Bad. If you had been the physician, how would you approach Bad? Would your approach be the same? Be different? In what ways?

  e. How does Bad respond to the physician?

  f. In your professional practice, how do you screen your patients for alcohol abuse?

  g. What are effective means of screening male and female patients for alcohol use and abuse?

5 (1:06:25–1:07:25) Bad recuperates at Jean's after being released from the hospital. He enjoys spending time with Buddy. In this scene, Buddy and Bad return from a fun-filled outing at a park. Jean arrives home to find an empty house.

  a. Why does Bad rush to his bedroom when he returns to the house? What does Bad do in there?

  b. What is Bad experiencing? How do you explain his behavior?

  c. What does Bad do while talking to Jean? Why does Jean initially refuse to kiss him?

  d. Bad is leaving for Houston. What concern does Jean express to Bad? Is her concern justified?

  e. What dilemma is Jean experiencing in this clip?

  f. Jean says: "It's like living with a rattlesnake." What is she referring to when she says this?

Methamphetamine Abuse/Dependence

Spun (2002; Jason Schwartzman, Brittany Murphy, Mickey Rourke, Mena Suvari, John Leguizamo, Patrick Fugit, Debbie Harry): This movie gives a graphic portrayal of a methamphetamine drug ring. The title refers to a slang term for the aftereffects of a long methamphetamine binge. From the opening scene, this film almost assaults the viewer with a realistic glimpse into the psychosocial and physical havoc caused by meth use.

1 (0:0:00–0:03:45) Ross (Schwartzman) tries to score some meth from Spider (Leguizamo), his local dealer. Also present in the house are Nicki (Suvari), whose boyfriend is Spider's meth "cook" (Rourke), and several other neighborhood characters who are also part of the meth network of dealers and users.

    a. What are the differences among drug use, abuse, and dependence? What signs do you see in these characters of varying levels of meth involvement?

    b. What are the risk factors that contribute to (young) people considering using illicit drugs such as methamphetamine? Which do you see portrayed in this clip?

    c. Choose a character portrayed here and discuss your hypotheses about the interaction of social location, personality, and effects of psychostimulants such as methamphetamine on this person's behavior.

    d. What do you think of the "disease model" of addiction? Are there competing philosophical-theoretical explanatory models?

    e. What kinds of treatment interventions may be most effective with methamphetamine abusers?

2 (0:26:36–0:30:45) Failing to score with Spider for some methamphetamine, Ross makes a deal with the cook – he will be the cook's driver in exchange for a supply of the drug (keep in mind the larger contextual issue in this clip, which is significant).

    a. What are the systemic issues that influence the availability and social acceptability of drug use? How do these intersect with the national and local efforts to combat drug abuse (e.g. the "War On Drugs" and "Just Say No" campaigns)?

    b. What national and regional measures have been undertaken to address drug and alcohol abuse/dependence? What is your perception/understanding of their effectiveness?

    c. Professionals who attempt to intervene with abusers of methamphetamine and other drugs often encounter many barriers to engaging people in effective treatment. What are some of the barriers of which you are aware? Which of these barriers do you see portrayed in this clip?

    d. What changes should be made in order to improve the coordinated efforts of various agencies, professionals and judicial systems to reduce drug abuse and dependence?

3 (0:53:40–0:56:00) This clip illustrates the different methods of ingesting methamphetamine.

    a. Why would people choose to administer a drug by different means?

    b. What are the various effects and unintended side effects of different means of administering a drug?

    c. How might such choices be influenced by the use of other drugs in combination with methamphetamine?

    d. Reflecting on the characters you see portrayed in this clip, what might motivate each to make the choice s/he does?

    e. What are the implications of these choices in determining the most effective methods for treatment?

Substances and Suicidality

El Cantante (2006): This film is based on the true story of Puerto Rican salsa singer Hector Lavoe (Marc Anthony), known as El Cantante. The story of Hector's rise to stardom and ultimate fall due to alcohol, drugs, and depression is told through the eyes of his wife, Puchi (Jennifer Lopez). The film alternates between watching Hector's rise and Puchi's soliloquies about their life together.

1 (Ch 9, 0:59:28–1:01:24) The scene begins with Puchi's reverie to the camera: "12 albums, drugs, a wife, a kid, everything for a breakdown." The scene then shifts to Puchi in bed, waking up to see Hector sitting in a chair with a gun in his hand. Quietly, Puchi reaches for the phone. Hector is next seen in the hospital, as Puchi continues her reverie: "He's not the kind of guy to go to A.A. Private lives stay private." The scene ends with Puchi doing a line of cocaine as her son Tito calls from the other room, asking if they are going to the hospital this week. Puchi replies, "not this week, next week." Tito responds: "That's what you said last week."

   a. How would you interpret Puchi's comments about Hector's "breakdown"?
   b. How would you respond to Puchi's statement that Hector isn't the kind of guy to go to A.A.?
   c. What misconceptions do individuals have about 12-step programs and their attendees?
   d. What is the impact of parental substance abuse on Tito? What interventions would be helpful for him?

2 (Ch 14, 0:1:34:05–0:1:36:26) The scene begins with Hector talking with a friend in Central Park and ends back in his apartment. Hector is talking with a friend about death. Hector says that he can't sleep and that he should have quit (drugs), given that now he can't smile the same and that he can't sing the same.

   a. How would you describe Hector's symptoms?
   b. What type of treatment would be beneficial for Hector?
   c. What risks may be indicated here? How would you intervene?

3 (Ch 14, 0:1:41:14–0:1:42:08) Hector returns to the hotel after an unsuccessful concert and sees Puchi at the bar talking with another man. He enters his hotel room, opens the balcony door, climbs over the railing, and jumps. Puchi is next seen telling the emergency medical technicians to "hurry up." The scene ends with Puchi waiting in the hospital.

   a. What factors contributed to Hector's suicide attempt?
   b. What is the impact of a family member witnessing or being the first on the scene of an attempted suicide?

4 (Ch 15, 0:1:42:18–0:1:43:22) Puchi is talking to the camera and asking: "How do you go through that? Multiple fractures and broken bones including being all messed up inside due to drugs." She adds: "He hit the air-conditioning shaft over a room and bounced. If he had hit the concrete, he would have been dead. He lived 5 more years, but it wasn't real life."

a. How would you interpret Puchi's remark that the aftermath of his suicide attempt "wasn't real life"?

b. What is the impact of suicidality on family and friends?

Family and Relationship Issues

1 (Ch 8, 0:50:25–0:53:15) Puchi enters the apartment and calls for Hector. She finds him in the bathroom injecting himself. Puchi is upset because their son had been left alone to eat at 10 p.m. The couple begins fighting and slapping each other. Hector calls Puchi a whore and leaves, while Puchi calls the doorman, telling him not to give Hector the car keys because he has been drinking. All the while, their son, Tito, sits at the kitchen table, visibly shrinking back.

   a. What is the impact on children who witness parental violence?

   b. What are the A.C.E.s (adverse childhood exposures) for Tito?

2 (Ch 13, 0:1:31:30–0:1:33:56) Their teenage son is accidentally shot and killed by his best friend, and after this Hector becomes pensive. He says to Puchi: "You know, we haven't been straight for 3 hours for 20 years, not since we met, and we go on with life like this. I love you, but it's impossible." Puchi retorts angrily: "Now that our son is dead it all comes clear to you? We're going to break things up to fix things up. Now?"

   a. What is the significance of Hector's statement? How would you respond to a patient who shared this perspective?

   b. How would you counsel a couple at this point in their relationship?

   c. From where does Puchi's anger stem?

On The Outs (2004): This film follows three teenage girls who meet at a juvenile detention facility. Suzette (Anny Marino) is a pregnant pre-teen who is arrested for carrying her boyfriend's gun, which was used in a shooting, while Marisol (Paola Mendoza) is a single mother and a crack addict, and Oz (Judy Marte) is a 17-year-old drug dealer.

1 (0:23:02–0:26:46) Evelyn (Ana Garcia), Oz's mother, is in the kitchen with her son, Chuey (Dominic Colon). She is telling him that she is making a special dinner because the rehab program called and they will have a bed next week. Oz arrives as her grandmother (Gloria Zelaya) sits down to dinner and begins complaining about the burned food. She insisted on praying to get rid of the evil in the house. When Evelyn offers to buy Chuey the new goldfish that he wants, the grandmother taunts Evelyn and asks her if she is going to steal to buy him the fish. She brings up Evelyn's drug use and what it has done to the family: "Your mommy stuck Disney up her arm [referring to a planned trip to Disney World when Evelyn used the money for drugs instead]. Your mommy shot drugs when she was pregnant with you and that's why you are funny in the head." Chuey immediately leaves the table and is

followed by Oz. As Chuey is lying on his bed he says, "Grandma says I'm funny in the head." Oz tries to reassure him. Chuey then confesses that he has smoked weed. She angrily replies, "You don't see me doing that." Chuey responds, "Your mind goes away when you smoke."

a. How would you describe the interpersonal dynamics of this family?
b. What is the impact of intravenous drug use on pregnancy?
c. How has Evelyn's drug use affected her children? Her mother?
d. What are the risks for developing substance use disorders in children of addicted parents?
e. How would you interpret Chuey's remark that "your mind goes away when you smoke"?

2   (0:57:40–0:59:10) Marisol's (Mendoza) daughter was taken into temporary custody after her great-aunt and primary caretaker had a stroke. In this scene, Marisol is meeting with the therapist for a psychiatric evaluation. The therapist asks her how long she has used crack cocaine and what steps she has taken to assist her recovery. Marisol appears anxious and possibly under the influence. She is evasive when answering the question about her drug use, but does not seem to understand the question about what she has done to assist her recovery. The therapist explains that he means a 12-step program. Marisol says she hasn't begun a program yet. While Marisol had hoped for a quick reunification with her daughter, her hopes are dashed when the therapist tells her that he needs to see long-term progress (i.e. 10–12 months of being clean) before they can re-evaluate getting her daughter back.

a. How would you assess Marisol's understanding of what the therapist is saying?
b. What factors may have contributed to Marisol's difficulty hearing what the therapist says?
c. How would you respond to a patient in your office who you suspected was under the influence?
d. What is the impact of Marisol's drug use on her parenting abilities?
e. How would you counsel children separated from their parents because of drug use?

3   (1:02:53–1:05:26) Marisol is meeting with her caseworker. Marisol shares what was discussed during the psychiatric evaluation. The caseworker laughs at the idea that long-term meant a year. She tells Marisol that it could take 4 or 5 years to get her daughter back. Marisol becomes quite upset. The scene ends with Marisol visiting her daughter in foster care.

a. What impact could this delay in reunification have on Marisol's sobriety?
b. How would you interpret the caseworker's laughing?
c. Does Marisol have realistic expectations of treatment and sobriety?
d. How would you instill hope yet remain realistic in treating Marisol?

4   (1:11:51–1:12:56) Oz sees her mother sitting on the curb sometime after Chuey's death. Evelyn asks Oz for drugs. Oz angrily confronts her mother and tells her she should have been on that bus (to treatment). Evelyn says

she couldn't do it. Oz remains on the attack: "No, the dope fiend couldn't make it. I can't believe you're my mother. I shouldn't be going through this. I'm 17." As she walks away from her mother, Oz says that she is done.

   a. What factors contributed to Evelyn's inability to accept treatment?

   b. How would you motivate a patient to engage in treatment?

   c. Oz is dealing drugs. In light of this fact, how would you interpret Oz's remark: "I shouldn't be going through this. I'm 17."

   d. What treatment services would be helpful for Oz?

   e. What type of prevention/early intervention programs would have been helpful for Oz?

   f. What is the role of harm reduction strategies versus abstinence for Oz?

Life Support (2007): Made for HBO, this film is based on the true story of an HIV-postive African-American woman, Ana (Queen Latifah), and three generations of her family in Brooklyn. Ana tries to put her life back together and repair relationships with her mother and teenage daughter while working for Life Support, a community outreach group focusing on HIV/AIDS awareness, prevention, and support for women.

1 (Ch 5, 0:34:25–0:35:26) Ana (Queen Latifah) finds Amare's sister, Tanya (Tracee Ellis Rosa), and confronts her about turning her brother away. Tanya responds angrily, reminding Ana of her past, telling her she may be all righteous now, but she remembers when "all you crackheads were up in my apartment with my parents." Tanya tells Ana that she was the one who had to raise Amare and that she was only 13 at the time: "I had to be out there stealing – diapers, wipes, Similac …"

   a. What is the impact of parental substance abuse on childhood development? What about the parentified child? How did Tanya avoid succumbing to substance use herself?

   b. How did Tanya's sense of responsibility for her brother ultimately impact their relationship?

2 (Ch 7, 0:54:51–0:55:20) Lucille (Anna Deavere Smith), Ana's mother, is sitting in the kitchen talking with Kelly (Rachel Nicks), Ana's teenage daughter. Lucille tells her that Ana has hurt her and that it has taken a long time to forgive her. She adds: "Sometimes I still can't. I try to remember everything she's done since she's stopped messing with those drugs. She does try."

   a. What are the long-term effects of substance abuse on the family and extended family?

   b. How have Lucille's feelings about Ana affected Ana's relationship with Kelly?

   c. How would you counsel a family member regarding the following three choices: (i) forgiveness, (ii) forgetting, and (iii) letting go?

3 (Ch 8, 1:01:10–1:03:35) Ana (Queen Latifah) is seen sharing her story at the support group. She talks about losing custody of her eldest daughter. Ana says: "I was 25 and I signed her over to my mother because of drugs." Her

daughter is now 17 years old and plans to move south with her grandmother. Ana says she is "missing" her daughter and talks about what she has missed as Kelly has grown up. Ana adds: "I feel like I am running out of time. Kelly is almost grown."

a. What reparative efforts might help Ana's relationship with Kelly?
b. What types of therapeutic interventions might be helpful to both Ana and Kelly?
c. What are the risks for Kelly in developing substance abuse issues of her own?

Animal Kingdom (2010): This gritty Australian film focuses on Josh, a quiet 17-year-old boy whose world changes when his mother overdoses in front of him. He is forced to live with his estranged family, including his grandmother who is the head of a dangerous crime family engaged in drug sales and violent crimes.

1 (Ch 1, 0:030–0:2:15) Jay, aka Josh (James Frecheville), and his mother are sitting on the couch watching a gameshow on TV. His mother appears to be asleep. The viewer learns this is not the case when the paramedics arrive and ask Josh what she has taken. Josh replies: "Heroin." He stands alternately watching the paramedics and the TV show. Ultimately, despite their attempts to revive her, the paramedics declare that Josh's mother has died. Left alone in the apartment, Josh calls his grandmother, asking her if she remembers him.

a. How would you interpret Josh's response to his mother's death?
b. Josh appears dispassionate when the paramedics arrive. What impact does exposure to parental drug abuse have on their children?

16 Years of Alcohol (2003; Iain De Caestecker, Lisa May Cooper, Lewis MacLeod, Kevin McKidd, Susan Lynch): This gritty UK film, told in a series of flashbacks, focuses on the life of Frankie (De Caestecker, as a child; McKidd, as an adult) as he observes his father's infidelities, intimate partner violence and alcohol abuse. Frankie begins experimenting with alcohol as a child and demonstrates a propensity for violence.

1 (0:14:41–0:17:48) Frankie (De Caestecker) is seen sitting in the kitchen with a glass of scotch in his hand. He tastes it, makes a face, and slides down the wall. The scene shifts to Frankie in bed, awakened by the sounds of his parents arguing. He goes to the top of the stairs and asks what they are doing. Frankie announces that he is coming down. Frankie sees that the living room has been trashed and things have been broken. He picks up one of the unfinished glasses of scotch, sits, and drinks. The adult Frankie, as narrator, says: "This is not the stuff dreams are made of. Each second here is another education in the art of destruction, the wonder of hate."

a. What is the impact of substance abuse and parental violence on children?
b. How would you intervene with Frankie as a child? As an adult?
c. To what A.C.E (adverse childhood experiences) has Frankie been exposed?
d. What are the potential long-term effects of multiple A.C.E.s?

2 (0:18:00–0:19:30) Frankie's mother has left the family. Frankie walks into a bar where his dad (MacLeod) is sitting. Frankie sits down and his dad sets a drink in front of him. Frankie finishes it.
   a. What message is his father giving Frankie?
   b. Would you consider this a form of child maltreatment?

Crazy Heart (see earlier description)

1 (1:15:44–1:19:50) Just before this scene, Bad starts drinking after his 37-year-old son tells him that he wants no further contact with him. A phone call from Jean and Buddy awakens Bad. Bad tells Jean about his conversation with his son.
   a. Why does Bad abruptly tell Jean that he has to call her back?
   b. What happens to Bad next?
   c. In what condition does Wayne, Bad's longtime friend, find Bad?
   d. What exciting news does Bad share with Wayne while they are fishing. Predict how this news may affect Bad's career.
   e. Consider the advice Wayne gives Bad. How would you have advised Bad?
2 (1:19:51–1:20:45) In this clip Jean tells Bad that she has 4 days off, and she and Buddy want to visit Bad in Houston. However, Jean has some concerns.
   a. What reservation does Jean express to Bad?
   b. How does Bad respond?
3 (1:22:34–1:29:55) Bad and Buddy are throwing coins into a fountain. (Bad sends Jean to a park to rest while Buddy and he go for a walk. The three plan to meet later for lunch.) Bad and Buddy go into a mall.
   a. Describe the atmosphere when Bad and Buddy are in front of the fountain.
   b. Where do Bad and Buddy go after entering the mall?
   c. Describe what happens soon after Bad and Buddy enter the mall. What leads to the choice to go into the restaurant bar?
   d. How does the security guard react to Bad?
   e. How does Jean react when she discovers Buddy is missing?
   f. How does this incident affect Jean and Bad's relationship?
   g. What does Jean do after returning to Bad's home? Why?
4 (1:30:02–1:31:32) This clip depicts Bad's actions after Jean and Buddy leave his home.
   a. What does Bad initially do?
   b. What does Bad say when he phones Wayne? Why does he say it?

Entering Treatment Programs

1 (0:1:31:03–1:34:05) This scene opens with Bad in a recovery program. At first he's shown speaking before a group of men in the recovery program. After that he appears to be thinking and reflecting while walking around the program's

grounds. The scene ends with Wayne picking Bad up from the program.

a. What does Bad tell the others in the recovery plan? What does his story tell you about Bad's personal and professional struggles?

b. What is Bad thinking about when he is walking around the program's grounds?

c. What does Bad tell Wayne? Is Wayne overconfident? What are the struggles Bad is likely to experience as he tries to change?

d. What does Wayne tell Bad? Why does Wayne have special insight into Bad's potential struggles with alcohol?

e. Explain what Wayne means when he says: "One day at a time."

Twelve-Step Programs

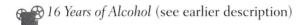 *16 Years of Alcohol* (see earlier description)

1. (0:1:02:04–0:1:07:41) Frankie is attending an A.A. meeting. Jennifer opens the meeting, sharing that it has been quite a good week for her. She talks about trigger events and her desire to drink, but she says, "I held on." Frankie (McKidd) stands up next and introduces himself, saying, "I am a violent man." He continues to share various experiences of his violent behavior.

a. What are trigger events? How can you help a person identify and respond to these events without drinking (or using drugs)?

b. How would you interpret Frankie's statement that he is a violent man?

c. What role does anger management have in an A.A. meeting?

d. Should Frankie be attending another meeting instead? What is the impact of his sharing on other members of the group?

Confessions of a Shopaholic (2009; Isla Fisher, Hugh Dancy, Krysten Ritter, Joan Cusack, John Goodman): Rebecca (Fisher) is obsessed with shopping and finds herself in trouble with her credit cards and a need for a new job. Her friend Suze (Ritter) tries through various means to help her overcome her urge to shop.

1. (Ch 5, 0:23:20–0:25:00) Rebecca and Suze are in a bookstore when Rebecca's credit card is declined because it has reached its limit. Suze finds a DVD that she thinks will help Rebecca, entitled *Control Your Urge to Shop*. The scene shifts to Rebecca and Suze watching the disk at home and responding to the questions posed by the man on the DVD. Rebecca answers "no" to all the questions. He tells his audience to "de-clutter your life," adding that "simplicity and order are your new watchwords." Rebecca is seen shrink-wrapping her clothes and stuffing them into the closet as a response to the concept of de-cluttering.

a. What is the role of self-help books or videos in helping people change problem behaviors?

    b. How would you respond to a patient who brings self-help materials into your office?

    c. Is excessive shopping an addictive process or an impulse control disorder? Define the difference between process and substance addictions.

    d. How would you treat these types of problems?

2 (Ch 11, 0:55:20–058:30) Rebecca is attending a 12-step meeting for compulsive shoppers. Ryuichi (Yoshiro Kono) shares that it has been 6 months, 3 weeks, and 4 days since he has used a credit card. Everyone applauds Ryuichi. D. Freak (John Salley), a former NBA player, says that he "cracked today at Cartier." The meeting leader asked him how many items he bought. D. Freak responds that he bought seven – one for each day of the week. It was then Rebecca's turn. She introduced herself and said she was there as a favor to a friend. She continued by saying she didn't think there was anything wrong with shopping or else "why would there be stores?" Rebecca continues to describe how shopping makes her feel. This triggers responses in several of the group who get up to leave with her, but are brought back by the group leader. The scene ends with Rebecca thawing out her freezer until she finds a credit card.

    a. How would you describe Rebecca's interactions in the group?

    b. Does she believe she has a problem?

    c. What impact does her sharing have on the other group members?

    d. Rebecca has frozen her credit card in an attempt to not use it. What types of behaviors do individuals with addictions (or impulse control disorders) engage in to avoid succumbing to the negative behaviors?

    e. What type of treatment would be helpful for Rebecca?

Recovery and Forgiveness

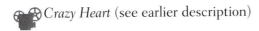

Crazy Heart (see earlier description)

1 (1:34:10–1:36:11) This clip shows Bad singing a song in Wayne's bar. Note Bad's tone and demeanor.

    a. Compare Bad's performance in Wayne's bar with his performance in the bowling alley at the beginning of the movie. What's different?

    b. What does Bad mean when he says: "It's so good to be home"?

2 (1:36:22–1:38:51) Bad is visiting Jean and Buddy's home. He apologizes to Jean, tells her he is sober, and asks her to forgive him. He wants to be a part of Jean's and Buddy's lives again.

    a. Compare Bad's appearance in this scene with his appearance in earlier parts of the movie?

    b. What is Bad's given name? Why is he going to stop using the name "Bad"?

    c. How does Jean respond to Bad's request to "start over"?

Alcohol and Aging

How About You (2007): This Irish film is based on a short story by Maeve Binchy. *How About You* is the story of Ellie (Hayley Atwell) and her older sister, Kate (Orla Brady), who owns a residential care facility. Ellie is visiting over the Christmas holidays when Kate is called away to care for their mother who has had a stroke. Although most of the residents and staff have left to join family for the holidays, Ellie is left in charge of the remaining residents. These residents are known as the "hardcore four" because they have been banned from other facilities. Their behavior is so disruptive that many other residents have left the facility, causing Kate to worry that she may have to close the home.

1 (0:1:01:30–0:1:02:00) Hazel (Imelda Staunton) and Donald (Joss Ackland) are sitting in the pub. Hazel offers Donald some of her drink. Donald, a retired judge, says that the trouble is once he starts to drink, he can't stop. He continues: "I drank my way through two family fortunes." Donald is pensive as he shares: "One day I was sitting in my chambers and three of my colleagues came in and suggested that I retire. I had a few years to go, but no, they insisted I retire that day. And I hope nobody knew."
   a. How would you describe Donald's sense of self?
   b. What is the impact of shame on people?
   c. What are the potential relapse triggers for Donald?
   d. Does aging contribute to his sense of loss?

2 (0:1:09:46–0:1:13:40) The "hardcore four" refer to themselves as "the committee" and say they have decided to have Christmas dinner together. As they are getting ready for dinner, Donald arrives with three bottles of wine that he had been saving, and Georgia (Vanessa Redgrave) enters the dining room with an armful of various types of wine and liquors.
   a. What are the risk factors associated with substance use among an aging population living in an assisted care environment?
   b. Are there legal or ethical issues to consider in such circumstances?
   c. How would you interpret the fact that Donald has "saved" three bottles of wine?
   d. How would you intervene with Donald if you knew of his history of alcoholism?

Relapse Triggers

Life Support (see earlier description)

1 (Ch 9, 01:07:02–01:08:24) Ana (Queen Latifah) and her husband, Slick (Wendell Pierce), have had a fight. Slick arrives home late from work. Ana says she was afraid that he wouldn't come home. Slick replies that he thought about it, adding that he even went by "the old spot" and saw lots of folks there

getting high. The scene ends with Slick saying: "Things aren't perfect, but they are better than when we were getting high."

    a. What factors and stressors contribute to relapse triggers?

    b. How can recovering addicts be counseled regarding coping with relapse triggers?

    c. How would you interpret Slick's comment?

Polysubstance Abuse

Intoxicating (2003): Dorian Shanley (Kirk Harris) is an up-and-coming cardiac surgeon who works long hours, doing countless procedures. He also attends to the needs of his father, William (John Savage), a retired boxer suffering from dementia. Dorian copes with the demands on him by using alcohol and cocaine, trading pharmaceutical drugs he steals from the hospital to pay for his cocaine.

1   (Ch 15, 1:26:30–01:27:51) Dorian is driving to his dealer's home. He grabs a beer, does two lines of cocaine and asks for more. His dealer, Teddy (Eric Roberts), tells him he's had enough. Dorian replies that he will know when he's had enough. He grabs Teddy and shoves him, driving off to a bar where he is seen downing drinks.

    a. Do addicted individuals "know" when they've had enough?

    b. How do individuals under the influence react when someone tells them they have had enough?

    c. What responsibilities would a health-care professional have when seeing a patient under the influence who has driven to the office?

Prescription Drug Misuse

The Savages (2007; Philip Bosco, Laura Linney, Philip Seymour Hoffman): This film is the story of a disengaged family. Lenny (Bosco) is living with his longtime girlfriend in a retirement community in Sun City, Arizona. When she dies, Lenny's two children, Wendy (Linney), an unsuccessful writer, and her brother, Jon (Hoffman), a drama professor, are called upon to make living arrangements for Lenny, who is suffering from some type of dementia.

1   (Ch 9, 0:29:00–0:29:30) Wendy (Linney) is clearing out her father's medications from the medicine cabinet he shared with his now deceased girl friend, Doris. Wendy sees Doris's prescription for Percocet and initially leaves it there. Then, Wendy decides to take the medication with her, popping a pill as she goes.

2   (Ch 16, 0:58:15–0:59:10) Wendy's brother, Jon, has strained his neck. He is leaving for work when he sees an envelope taped to the door, telling him the medications inside will help his pain. Jon looks at the prescription bottle

and returns to speak to Wendy. Jon says: "You stole painkillers from a dead woman?" Then he asks her if they work. Wendy says yes, and they both take Percocet.

3   (Ch 18, 1:05:50–1:06:51) Jon, Wendy, and their father, Lenny, are waiting for their interview at a new nursing home. Wendy tells Lenny that he has to concentrate. She gives him a ginkgo biloba capsule, then reaches for a medication for herself. Jon asks her what she is taking and she responds "an antidepressant … you could use one yourself." Jon replies that it's like a pharmacy in her purse.

   a. Are siblings more likely than unrelated individuals to share proclivities for substance abuse?
   b. Have you encountered polysubstance abuse in your practice? Is it more the norm or the exception?
   c. How does polysubstance abuse complicate recovery treatment?
   d. Can individuals "abuse" antidepressants?
   e. Is prescription drug abuse on the rise? What complicates the treatment of prescription drug abuse? How is it best managed in professional practice?

References

1 Mersy DJ. Recognition of alcohol and substance abuse. *Am Fam Physician* 2003; **67**(7): 1529.
2 Horgan CM. *Substance abuse: the national number one health problem: key indicators for policy update.* Princeton, NJ: Robert Wood Johnson Foundation; 2001: 6.
3 Rehm J., Mathers C., Popova S., *et al.* Global burden of disease and injury and economic cost attributable to alcohol use and alcohol-use disorders. *Lancet.* 2009; **373**(9682): 2223–33.
4 Welsh, CJ. OD's and DT's: using movies to teach intoxication and withdrawal syndromes to medical students. *Acad Psychiatry.* 2003; **27**(3): 183–6.

Further Reading

● Taylor-Seehafer M, Jacobvitz D, Steiker LH. Patterns of attachment organization, social connectedness, and substance use in a sample of older homeless adolescents: preliminary finds. *Fam Community Health.* 2008; **31**(Suppl. 1): S81–8.
● Tolan P, Szapocznik J, Sambrano S, editors. *Preventing Youth Substance Abuse: science-based programs for children and adolescents.* Washington, DC: American Psychological Association; 2007.

9

Betting on Your Life: Pathological Gambling

Nigel E. Turner

GAMBLING CAN BE DEFINED AS RISKING SOMETHING OF VALUE (usually money) for the possibility of gain with an uncertain outcome. Although gambling has existed for thousands of years,[1] the past 30 years have witnessed an unprecedented level of commercial exploitation of gambling. The majority of people in North America engage in some form of gambling and view it as a form of entertainment.[2–5] However, some people are unable to control their gambling and become problem or even pathological gamblers. Pathological gambling is determined by the endorsement of five or more symptoms on the pathological gambling symptom checklist.[6] Problem gambling is a more general term often used to describe excessive gambling regardless of whether or not individuals reach the clinical criteria of five symptoms. The characters in the films discussed in this chapter often do not carry a formal diagnosis, so the term problem gambler will be used instead of pathological gambler.

Problem gambling is similar to alcoholism in that most people who drink or gamble are not addicted to the behavior. Individuals who engage in problem gambling have an addiction-like disorder characterized by excessive gambling, an inability to quit, chasing losses, lying about gambling losses, jeopardizing career opportunities in order to gamble, enormous debt, marital discord, and in some cases criminal activity. In North America approximately 4% of the general public are problem or pathological gamblers.[2,4,5]

Gambling has consistently been a popular topic for myths, books, songs, poems, operas, and more recently films.[7,8] This chapter examines three films that depict different aspects of problem gambling: (1) *Lost in America* (1985)[9] reveals some features of the initiation of a gambling disorder, (2) *Vegas Vacation* (1997)[10] illustrates chasing and youth gambling, and (3) *Owning Mahowny* (2003)[11] illustrates how some problem gamblers turn to crime in order to deal with their financial problems. In addition, these three films also illustrate relationship problems, the marketing and promotion of gambling, and the resolution of the disorder.

Films that illustrate problem gambling

Initiation of a gambling problem

Of the three films discussed, only one, *Lost in America*, deals with the initiation of a gambling problem.

Lost in America (1985; Albert Brooks, Julie Hagerty):[9] This is a comedy about a couple who experience a midlife crisis. An advertising executive, David (Brooks) is passed over for a promotion and is instead asked to move to New York City. He overreacts, becomes hostile, and is fired. He and his wife, Linda (Hagerty), decide to give up their workaday lives and hit the road in a recreational vehicle (RV). Their first stop is Las Vegas, where they plan to renew their wedding vows. Instead of camping in their RV, Linda persuades David to stay in a casino. She loses nearly all their money at the hotel's casino. The couple fight but they reconcile and try to get back on their feet by working. At the end of the film they drive to New York so David can try to get his job back.

1   (Ch 11, 0:31:15–0:33:42) In this clip, the couple arrives in Las Vegas. They see the spectacle of all the bright lights of the Las Vegas strip. They had planned to renew their vows immediately in a little chapel. Linda suggests instead that they wait until the morning and stay in a hotel instead of in their RV.

2   (Chs 13–14, 0:37:56–0:43:08) In this clip, David wakes up to find Linda missing. He finds her at the roulette table obsessively saying "22, 22, 22." She has a small win, which instantly changes David's mood from anxiety to excitement. A moment later he discovers that she has lost nearly all of their money. She tells him that earlier she was up a hundred thousand dollars and that there were people around cheering. She says, "I didn't feel like I had any problems." She says she has only ever gambled once before. Notice also her attempt to get a keno card.

   a. What hints are there in these two clips about the appeal of gambling and the early stages of a gambling problem? (Answer: Availability of gambling, the bright lights, being impulsive, having gambled previously, an early big win, an enthusiastic audience, stressful life experiences.)

   b. In what ways does this film illustrates the difficulty people have in understanding problem gamblers? (Answer: David cannot understand Linda's behavior. People that do not have an addiction often do not understand why the addicted person simply can't stop.)

   c. Linda does not appear to have any psychiatric problem other than gambling. What special challenges and opportunities are there in a case like hers? (Answer: The lack of other psychiatric problems means that it is more difficult to spot her as a "vulnerable" person. On the other hand her case would be fairly easy to deal with therapeutically.)

Chasing Losses and Erroneous Beliefs

One of the key symptoms of problem gambling is chasing losses. Chasing is often associated with erroneous beliefs about random chance. Many problem gamblers believe that the only way they can make good on their losses is to get more money and increase their bets.

Vegas Vacation (1997; Chevy Chase, Ethan Embry, Randy Quaid, Wallace Shawn, Beverly D'Angelo, Sid Caesar, Marisol Nichols):[10] This is a comedy about gambling. Clark Griswold (Chase) earns a large bonus and takes his family to Las Vegas for a vacation. Clark immediately becomes hooked on gambling, and proceeds to gamble away all of the family's money. At the end of the film, they meet an old man who dies after winning a large keno jackpot. The Griswold family takes the old man's ticket, which covers all of Clark's losses, giving the film a happy ending.

1   (Ch 6, 0:14:46–0:17:12) In this clip, Clark starts gambling. Cousin Eddie (Quaid) comes up behind him. Clark makes another bet upon which Eddie says to Clark "that's right, show them who's boss." When the dealer wins, Eddie says, "he's good." Eddie warns Clark that it is people who come to Las Vegas and break the family nest egg that built the town.

2   (Ch 15, 0:41:00–0:42:05) Clark is winning at craps. Eddie comes to watch him play. Clark loses and suggests that Eddie is "bad luck." Clark goes to the cashier to cash a check for a large sum of money. The amount is not specified but Eddie asks if he's buying a Cadillac. Clark says that he is just trying to "get even."

3   (Ch 16, 0:42:38–0:43:38) In this clip, Clark is at a blackjack table and is winning. The dealer is replaced by Clark's nemesis, Marty (Wallace Shawn) and Clark starts losing again.

4   (Ch 21, 0:55:35–0:56:32) Clark is shown taking a large cash advance out of an automatic teller machine. The amount is not clear, but the bills are all $100 bills. He says "payback time." The dealer says to him "you don't know when to quit." This is not given as friendly advice, but as a taunt.

5   (Ch 29, 1:19:17–1:26:15) Clark's losses are finally revealed to the family.
a. Is Clark's behavior rational? (Answer: No.)
b. Many gamblers hold erroneous beliefs about gambling. List some of the erroneous beliefs mentioned in the film. List any accurate statements about gambling made in the film. (Erroneous: the dealer is "good," "shows them who is boss," and the idea that Eddie is bad luck. Accurate: people who break the family nest egg built the town and that Clark doesn't know when to quit.)

Underaged Gambling

Although there are cautionary elements in the depiction of Clark's descent into problem gambling, the social message of his story is completely undermined by the adventures of his son, Rusty (Ethan Embry.) When they arrive at the casino, Rusty is very disappointed to discover that the minimum age for gambling is 21.

1 (Ch 16, 0:42:12–0:42:37) In this clip, the son tries to obtain a false ID so that he can gamble.

2 (Ch 16, 0:44:01–0:45:09) The ID is rejected because the picture is of a black man. He complains to the fake ID dealer and obtains a new one with his picture on it.

3 (Ch 17, 0:46:40–0:47:34) Rusty goes gambling for the first time. Rusty puts a dollar in a slot machine (0:46:50), pulls the lever and wins a car. His new ID is checked and passes inspection.

4 (Ch 19, 0:50:26–0:51:55) Rusty plays craps and has a great run of luck.

5 (Ch 20, 0:53:40–0:54:00) A security officer checks his ID and lets him keep playing.

6 (Ch 21, 0:59:25) Rusty wins another car.

7 (Ch 32, 1:28:50–1:29:31) Rusty tells Clark about the four new cars that he has won. "I put a dollar in and I got a car. I put a dollar in and I got a car." Clark says nothing about Rusty's false ID or his gambling. Instead, Clark hands his wife, daughter, and son keys and the four of them drive off in the four vehicles towards Chicago.

   a. What social problems could be caused by the depiction of Rusty's underage gambling? (Answer: The film may encourage youth to gamble, especially given Rusty's success. The film suggests that it is easy to fraudulently obtain a fake ID.)

   b. *Vegas Vacation* includes a mix of accurate and inaccurate depictions about gambling. Considering the stories of both Rusty and Clark, list some of the unrealistic aspects of *Vegas Vacation*. (Accurate: the glamour of gambling, the cheering of the winners, Clark's obsessive and irrational chasing, erroneous beliefs and deception. Inaccurate: Rusty wins far too often, while Clark's losing streak is equally unlikely. Clark develops a problem too quickly, too few hints to explain it (e.g. no early win) and Clark keeps going back to the same dealer to lose again. The film mostly depicts table games (e.g. craps and blackjack), but gaming machines now make up about 70% of casino revenues. Only the males in the film gamble. All of the scenes in which a gaming machine is played result in a win.)

Turning to Crime

Owning Mahowny (2003; Philip Hoffman, Minnie Driver, John Hurt, Vincent Corazza, Chris Collins):[11] This is a true story about a bank account manager in Toronto, Canada, who embezzled over 10 million dollars from his employer and lost it gambling. Initially he "borrows" money in order to pay off his bookie. He then borrows large sums of money in the hope of winning enough to pay back what he had borrowed. However, each time he loses money he has to borrow more. Eventually he is caught by the police and serves time in prison for embezzlement. This is a very rich film in terms of the depiction of problem gambling. Unlike *Vegas Vacation*, it is a very accurate depiction of the disorder but it focuses more on the consequences of gambling rather than the gambling itself.

1   (Ch 2, 0:05:57–0:07:32) Dan Mahowny's bosses are discussing the new responsibility they have placed on Dan and one of them mentions that he has an impeccable reputation and excellent judgment. A few seconds later, the clip shows two unsavory individuals waiting for Dan in his office. Dan is clearly upset. As the scene unfolds we are gradually made aware that Dan owes money to these individuals – $10,300. In addition, they tell Dan that he is cut off from gambling until he pays them. As the scene ends, Dan arranges to meet his bookies in the parking garage in 1 hour.

2   (Ch 2, 0:07:53–0:08:54) The first of several quiet moments in the film; no background music, only his breathing. Dan is then shown briefly filling out a loan application and the sounds of a street car can be heard in the background.

3   (Ch 3, 0:08:55–0:09:36) Dan is shown giving a check to his bookies. His bookie is not happy about the bank draft. The scene ends with a dispute because his bookies still do not want to let him bet anymore.

4   (Ch 3, 0:09:38–0:10:08) Dan is shown filling out a second loan application. Another quiet moment with him thinking as he puts on his jacket – this time there is music. Dan picks up the second check and tells the teller his client is waiting in his office.

5   (Ch 3, 0:10:19–0:10:53) A third quiet moment where Dan is shown sitting in his car in a parking garage. There is no music, but some ambient noise that hints at the location (the airport). He gets out of his car, saying, "let's do it." Next, he is shown on a plane as the captain announces that they are landing in Philadelphia. Finally his destination is revealed as an express bus passes under a "Welcome to Atlantic City" sign.

6   (Ch 4, 0:16:03–0:16:25) Another quiet moment in his car in the parking garage. He has obviously returned from Atlantic City. The music of a saxophone is heard as well as ambient air traffic noise in the background. He has a single $500 chip in his hand that he is turning over in his fingers.

   a. In what way is the depiction of the bookie different from the stereotype of a loan shark? (Answer: The film does not follow typical stereotypes of loan sharks. They are not threatening him physically; they are threatening to cut him off from further "action.")

   b. What does Dan's reaction to the "threat" from his bookies say about the strength of the addiction? (Answer: The fact that the threat of cutting him off from gambling is sufficient to trigger risking his career and freedom to keep gambling suggests that his addiction is very strong.)

   c. What do the quiet moments in film imply? Is this an effective technique?

(Answer: The film uses these quiet moments to show that stealing money is a difficult decision.)
d. After returning from Atlantic City, Dan is sitting in his car holding a single casino chip in his hands. What does this single $500 casino chip indicate about his weekend in Atlantic City? (Answer: Given the music and his mood, most likely that he has lost the $15 000 except for one last chip.)
e. In the film, Dan keeps embezzling larger and larger sums of money and making increasingly large bets. What is Dan trying to accomplish? (Answer: Dan is hoping to win enough money in order to pay off his debts and put back the money he has stolen. Doubling one's money will work in the short term, but there is an advantage of the house edge so that eventually the player ends up with even larger losses.[12,13])

Relationship Problems

In addition to debt, one of the most harmful consequences of problem gambling is related to relationship problems. All three films depict relationship issues resulting from problem gambling.

Lost in America When Linda's losses are discovered, David is upset but emotionally in control. The couple continues along on their journey.
1 (Ch 17, 0:49:39–0:52:30) This clip shows Linda getting the "silent treatment" as David stews over the conflict.
2 (Chs 18–19, 0:52:30–0:58:32) Linda and David arrive arrive at the Hoover Dam, whereupon they finally erupt into a full argument. Eventually, she leaves him and gets into the car of a complete stranger.
a. What does this scene illustrate about conflicts that can arise between a problem gambler and his or her spouse?(Answer: This scene illustrates how quickly financial losses can lead to marital conflicts. This is particularly problematic given that many women gamble to escape from an oppressive life, including spousal abuse. David is actually remarkably well controlled.)

Vegas Vacation In a number of scenes Clark neglects his wife, leaving her alone while he is off gambling. He also lies to her about the extent of his losses until near the end of the film.
1 (Ch 9; 20:58–22:24) The Griswold family is having breakfast together. When Clark's wife Ellen (D'Angelo) asks Clark how he did the night before, Clark tells her he broke even. His son Rusty then expresses an interest in gambling but Clark sternly tells Rusty that gambling is a serious business. He then sneaks off to bet on roulette and loses $50. He is upset about the loss, but when he returns to the breakfast table, he doesn't mention the gambling.
2 (Ch 19, 0:51:5–0:53:09) Clark ignores Ellen's sexual advances because he is too busy trying to learn gambling games and thinking about gambling.
a. How typical is Clark's willingness to lie? (Answer: Many gamblers do lie

about their gambling, and will indeed say they broke even when they have in fact lost.)

    b. How realistic is it when Clark ignores his wife's sexual advances because of his preoccupation with gambling? (Answer: Clark's reaction to his wife, as well as being very funny, is actually quite believable. At some stage in a gambler's career, some problem gamblers do in fact come to find gambling more satisfying than sex.)

Vegas Vacation. Another important relationship issue is illustrated by Clark's treatment of cousin Eddie (Quaid).

1 (Ch 25, 1:07:18–1:10:00) In this clip Clark admits to cousin Eddie that he has gambled all his money away. Eddie is shocked to find out how much he has lost, but offers to help bail him out by giving him any money that they can find buried in his yard.

2 (Ch 26, 1:10:23–1:12:16) Eddie and Clark go to a bizarre casino that offers games such as guess the number, rock-paper-scissors, war, and guess which hand; once again, Clark loses the money.

    a. Was Eddie's offer to lend Clark his money a good idea or a bad idea? (Answer: In the movie, Eddie is not well off and is amazed by the size of Clark's losses. Problem gamblers often cannot stop gambling until they run out of people who are willing to bail them out.)

    b. What else could Eddie have done? (Answer: A better approach might have been to encourage Clark to talk to Ellen and to seek treatment. The money buried in the yard could have been given to Ellen to help get the Griswolds home.)

Owning Mahowny Dan often lies about his losses or about his activities.

1 (Ch 4, 0:13:36–0:14:22) In this clip, Dan is washing his face in the bathroom. We hear a voice over of a telephone conversation in which he is apologizing to his girlfriend, Belinda (Minnie Driver), for missing their date. He tells her he got tied up. She tells him to have a good weekend. He says that all he needs is "one good weekend."

2 (Ch 4, 0:16:34–0:17:47) Dan and Belinda are relaxing on a mattress in a barren room. She asks him if he won during the weekend and he replies, "sort of." She asks how much he won. He says he came home with $500 (see ch 4, 10:6:03–0:16:25, mentioned earlier.) She says, "cool."

3 (Ch 5, 0:19:05–0:20:22) Dan and his girlfriend and another couple are socializing. Dan's attention is on the basketball game on the TV, rather than on the social get-together.

4 (Ch 6, 0:29:15–0:29:35) Two girls are talking about Dan and his gambling. Belinda defends the time he spends at the track. She says that anyone who works as hard as he does deserves the right to do whatever he wants with his money.

a. With Belinda, Dan sometimes manages to be honest and yet deceptive at the same time. Give an example. (Answer: Dan tells her that he brought home $500 leading her to think he had won. He actually lost all the other money except for the $500 he brought home.)

b. What did Dan mean when he said, "one good weekend"? (Answer: Winning enough to pay off his embezzlement would be all that he would need to get his life back in order. Not only is one good weekend unlikely to accomplish this, it is probable that if it did occur, he would soon gamble himself into another hole.)

c. Throughout the film, Belinda shows a remarkable degree of tolerance over Dan's gambling obsession. Why does Belinda defend Dan's gambling? (Answer: Belinda's relationship to Dan appears to be one characterized by codependency. It may be that Belinda defends Dan's gambling in part because she could be insecure about their relationship.)

Owning Mahowny Dan suggests to Belinda that they get away and spend a weekend in Las Vegas. The scene is a complex one that switches back and forth between several story lines including Dan's gambling, Belinda's disappointment, and the casino managers in Atlantic City and Las Vegas virtually fighting over who owes Dan.

1 (Chs 8–9, 0:40:15–0:49:05) Dan and Belinda travel to Las Vegas for a weekend. Belinda is in the bathroom, Dan tells her he is going for a walk to look around. (0:42:21) Belinda is shown looking bored and lonely. (0:42:52) Dan is shown at the craps table and he is winning.

2 (Ch 9, 0:43:33–0:44:01) Belinda is shown lying down, possibly sleeping. No music. She gets up looking puzzled and concerned. She then goes down to the casino floor looking for Dan. She sees a happy couple in wedding attire going up the escalator as she goes down into the casino looking for Dan.

3 (Ch 9, 0:44:55–0:46:18) Belinda finds Dan at the craps table still winning. A security officer tries to keep Belinda away from Dan. Dan tells her to give him a "couple more minutes." He goes on to say "I'm on a roll," "a few more minutes." He says all of this without even looking at her. She is stunned. After Belinda leaves, you hear someone at the table telling Dan to stay hot now.

4 (Ch 9, 0:46:19–0:46:54) Belinda is shown packing, and then on a plane flying home. A man beside her on the plane says that everyone loses in Vegas.

5 (Ch 10, 0:49:27–0:53:37) Back in their Toronto apartment, Dan says he's really sorry about leaving her alone. Belinda says it's OK and that she understands. She tells him he has a gambling problem. He responds that he doesn't have a gambling problem but, rather, a financial problem. Belinda offers him $2000 and offers to cash in her retirement for another $3000. She asks if that will it make them into a normal couple. He tells her not to worry.

a. List some of the complications of being in a relationship with individuals who are addicted that are illustrated in these scenes? (Answer: Belinda allows Dan his space, which enables his behavior. Her offer to bail him out with her savings would also have enabled continued gambling. On the other hand, her steadfast loyalty to him through his arrest and trial may in part explain his continued abstinence. Her continued love, however, was in part because he had not stolen from her. Oftentimes, marital conflict can trigger relapses.)

b. To what extent is Dan being honest when he says he doesn't have a gambling problem but a financial one? To what extent is he being dishonest? (Answer: Dan's financial problems stem entirely from his gambling problem.)

c. How would you intervene with Belinda if she were your psychotherapy client or your medical patient? (Answer: Belinda could be encouraged to read a book on codependency, go to a Co-Dependents Anonymous meeting or engage in psychotherapy designed to explore self-esteem and family of origin issues.)

Role-Play

After viewing the video clips from these three films, choose one of the interactions between the characters illustrated in one of these films and role-play the scene. Using one of the scenarios portrayed in the movie, the role-play should attempt to show the positive ways the situation could have been resolved. The other learners should be asked to observe the role-play and provide feedback on such processes as nonverbal.

Marketing, Design, and Incentives

A number of scenes in each of the three movies illustrate some of the methods that the casino engages in to encourage gambling.

Lost in America

1 (Ch 11, 0:31:15–0:33:42) As previously described, the couple drives through the sights of the Las Vegas strip.
2 (Chs 15–16, 0:43:32–0:49:39) After David finds out how bad the situation really is, he talks to the casino manager about getting his money back. David suggests that the casino could create an effective marketing strategy centered on returning the money to Linda and David (e.g. "The Desert Inn has Heart.") The manager is polite and patiently explains why he can't give them their money back.
   a. What effect do the sights of the Vegas strip have on the couple? (Answer: Linda appears to be particularly entranced by the sights of Las Vegas and this may in part have triggered her gambling.)
   b. Is David's idea about getting their money back realistic? Is the manager's response reasonable? (Answer: David's idea about giving them back their money is not a realistic idea because the gambling industry relies on losses from gamblers to pay their staff, the infrastructure of the hotel, and profit for the corporation.)

🎥 Vegas Vacation

1   (Ch 4, 0:07:08–0:09:00) The Griswold family sees the sights and sounds of Las Vegas.
2   (Ch 5, 0:09:05–0:10:25) The family is instructed on how to find their room through the maze of the casino.
   a. What do the reactions by the characters in these two films to the sights and sounds of Las Vegas tell you about the marketing of gambling? (Answer: In both *Lost in America* and *Vegas Vacation* the characters are entranced by the sights of Las Vegas and this may in part have triggered their gambling.)
   b. The description of how to get to the elevator is actually a fairly accurate description of the layout of many Las Vegas casinos. Why do casinos make finding one's way around so difficult? (Answer: The confusing layout of casinos forces the hotel guest to see all the sights and sounds of the games and, as with sights and sounds outside, entices players to start playing.)

🎥 Owning Mahowny

1   (Ch 3, 0:11:00–0:14:35) This series of short scenes brilliantly introduces us to the world of casino gambling. As Dan enters the Atlantic City casino for the first time, he is stopped by security to allow Mr. N. and his entourage to walk through the door, past the gaming tables and the gaming floor in general. The casino manager greets Mr. N. Dan is then shown at the craps table. Everyone is smiling and well dressed. A beautiful woman is seen at the table with Dan, winning and jumping up and down in joy. Mr. N is shown winning a throw at craps. Dan is in the background watching Mr. N.
2   (Ch 5, 0:21:31–0:27:00) In this series of short clips, Dan cashes in for $100 000. His friend Doug (Corazza) is taken to a new room because the large deposit has triggered an upgrade. Victor Foss (Hurt) introduces himself to Dan and tells him, "my casino is your casino." He asks Dan if he wants anything. Dan says he'd like ribs with no sauce. Dan's ribs are ready, but the casino doesn't want to interrupt him. A casino manager orders them to have fresh ribs on permanent standby. After running out of money, they offer Dan the ribs but he refuses. He wanders into a stairwell where he finds Bernie (Collins), a busboy who offers him some ribs (with no sauce). Dan laughs when he realizes those were the ribs he had ordered.
3   (Ch 15; 1:18:57–1:18:57) This scene is nearly an exact repetition of the aforementioned VIP scene with Mr. N., but this time it is Dan entering the casino in a limo with an entourage. The manager calls him Dan, not Mr. M., but otherwise says the exact same thing: "an honor and a pleasure."
   a. What do these scenes tell us about the allure of gambling? (Answer: These scenes illustrate the glamour of gambling and, in particular, the manner in which a big gambler is turned into the center of attention.)

b. What do the scenes about the room and the ribs tell us about the casino's business practices. (Answer: Gamblers often want to be the center of attention. People who risk large sums of money are rewarded with attention, free food, free drinks, show tickets, and other complimentary benefits.)

Consumer Protection/Duty of Care Exercise

Manufacturers of products can be sued or even charged if they knowingly manufacture unsafe products. In recent years some public health advocates have argued casinos also have a duty of care to their customers.[14] In *Lost in America*, David asks the casino for his money back. He proposes a marketing campaign centered on the idea that "The Desert Inn has Heart." His idea was probably unrealistic, but it may be possible to come up with a consumer protection policy that prevents financial disasters like the one shown in these films. Come up with a series of rules that could be implemented that protects people from excessive gambling, but does not interfere with those gamblers who do not gamble excessively. Is it possible to balance casino profits, the fun of gambling, and consumer protection?

Resolution of the Problem

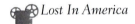 *Lost In America*

1 (Ch 28, 1:23:20–1:28:08) The couple get back together, end up in a small town in Arizona, and struggle to get back on their feet. In this clip, they decide to go to New York so that David can try to get his job back. Throughout the last half of the film there is no additional depiction of gambling and Linda does not talk about wanting to get back into the "action."
a. In the film the resolution focuses entirely on the couples' return to the "rat race." Is this a realistic depiction of a solution to a gambling problem? (Answer: Linda does not seem to crave gambling after leaving the casino, which is somewhat unrealistic. However, the couple does not have any money to gamble. In addition, at the time (1985) legal casinos in the United States were restricted to Nevada and New Jersey. It is possible that simply being away from temptation would help her abstain.)

Vegas Vacation

1 (Ch 29, 1:19:17–1:26:15) In this clip, Clark's losses are finally revealed to the family. Ellen gathers together the two remaining dollars that they have and tells Clark to get their money back. To do this they march through the mouth of the MGM lion and into the keno lounge, where they bet their last $2. While waiting for the outcome, they befriend a lonely old man, Mr. Ellis (Sid Caesar), who is sitting beside them. The Griswolds lose their bet, but Mr. Ellis wins and dies from the shock. The Griswolds take Mr. Ellis's ticket and recoup all their losses.

2 (Ch 29, 1:26:15–1:26:23) The camera opens on a huge sign spelling out "Fun." As the camera pans down, Ellen tells Clark that she hopes he now understands the "dangers of gambling." Clark then responds that gambling is what made America great, suggesting that he learned nothing from his experiences.

   a. At the end of the film the Griswolds' problems are solved by a miracle win. What message does this win give players about gambling? (Answer: Hollywood happy endings may encourage people to chase their losses in the false belief that they can win back the money if they just keep gambling.)

   b. Clark appears to be able to walk away from the casino with his winnings. How realistic is his recovery? (Answer: Clark's ability to walk away from the casino with his winnings without any lingering cravings is not realistic.)

   c. In his 1999 book, Dement[7] describes several films about gambling as having irresponsibly happy endings. Is *Vegas Vacation* an irresponsible film? (Answer: *Vegas Vacation* is an odd mix of cautionary tale (Clark's story), an unlikely success story (Rusty), and an irresponsibly happy ending.)

Owning Mahowny

1 (Ch 17–18, 1:29:11–1:35:20) In this series of short scenes, Dan's crimes are revealed. Dan has lost again and is returning to Toronto. The police have finally figured out that he is engaged in criminal activity and are waiting for him. He calls his girlfriend, and suggests they go to Niagara Falls, but she hangs up on him (1:30:20). Dan drives away from the airport. The police follow him. Dan's old car breaks down on him. Dan is arrested for theft over $200. During questioning, he tells the police that he does not have a gambling problem but that he has a "financial problem." The bank finds out about their losses and asks if anyone else was in on it.

2 (Ch 19, 1:36:12–1:37:30) Dan and Belinda find out that eleven employees including Belinda have been suspended and that one of the managers has taken an early retirement. Dan shows remorse.

   a. Discuss the idea of "hitting bottom" as it relates to *Owning Mahowny*. Contrast this with the other two films.(Answer: Hitting bottom occurs when an addict reaches a point where they can no longer deny their addiction. The bottom is different for each individual. Dan hits bottom when he is arrested.)

Treatment

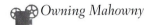*Owning Mahowny*

1   (Ch 19, 1:39:29–1:40:31) In this final scene, Dan is in therapy. When his
    therapist asks him to rate the thrill of gambling from 0 to 100, he says "100."
    He then is asked to rate the greatest thrill of his life other than from gambling,
    to which he says "20." The therapist asks if he can live with a maximum of
    20. He says he can.

    a. Does his response make any sense to you? (Answer: Dan's response may
        seem bizarre, but is consistent with his refusal of most of the compliment-
        ary benefits offered by the casino, including free drinks, show tickets, and
        a prostitute. The addiction has basically taken over his reward system.)

    b. Of the three films, this is the only one that depicts treatment. Why do
        you think the films are reluctant to show therapy? (Answer: Films typic-
        ally focus on the glamour and intrigue of gambling. The only other film
        that we know of that depicts treatment is *Fever Pitch*[15] but this film is not
        currently available.)

    c. What are the most effective therapeutic approaches to treatment of
        problem and pathological gambling? (Answer: Treatment for gambling
        problems is modelled on treatment for substance abuse and may con-
        sist of individual, couple, and family therapy. Therapy often begins with
        motivational interviewing and may also include learning alternative leis-
        ure activities, coping skills, dealing with past traumatic events, or relapse
        prevention.[16] Problem gambling treatment also includes education about
        erroneous beliefs about random chance and a greater emphasis on money
        management. Gamblers Anonymous may also be an effective treatment
        strategy, either alone or in conjunction with formal therapy. Clients should
        also be screened for comorbid conditions such as substance abuse, sex
        addiction, depression, anxiety, or attention deficit hyperactivity disorder.)

Discussion
. . . .

All three films have scenes in which a winning gambler is depicted as the center
of attention. *Lost in America* has only a relatively short segment about gambling itself, but the crisis caused by the casino dominates the second half of the
film and forces the rebellious couple to return to the "rat race." Although *Vegas
Vacation* has an irresponsibly happy ending,[7,8] this film is actually a rich source
of information on the disorder (especially in terms of chasing) that can be used
for education, as long as the inaccuracies are pointed out. *Owning Mahowny* is
a very rich source of information on one particular consequence of gambling –
crime. It also is one of the few films about gambling that shows a gambler in
therapy (albeit very briefly). None of these films provides a comprehensive view
of the disorder, but taking into account all three, most of the major aspects of

problem gambling are covered, including: (1) initial development of the disorder, (2) chasing losses and erroneous beliefs, (3) youth gambling, (4) crossing the line into criminal behavior, (5) problems with relationships, (6) the marketing and promotion of gambling, and (7) the resolution of the disorder.

Limitations

These films do not show a full spectrum of gambling games. Most films about gambling focus on table games (e.g., blackjack, poker) and very few show problems associated with slot machines.[8] However, most problem gamblers seek treatment for problems associated with gaming machines.[16]

References

1 Schwartz DG. *Roll the Bones*. New York, NY: Gotham Books; 2006.

2 National Opinion Research Center. *Gambling Impact and Behavior Study*. Report to the National Gambling Impact Study Commission; 1999. Available at: www3.norc.org/projects/Gambling+Impact+Behavior+Study.htm

3 Turner NE, Wiebe J, Falkowski-Ham A, *et al*. Public awareness of responsible gambling and gambling behaviours in Ontario. *Int Gambling Stud*. 2005; **5**(1): 95–112.

4 Wiebe J, Mun P, Kauffman N. *Gambling and Problem Gambling in Ontario 2005*. Guelph, ON: Ontario Problem Gambling Research Centre; 2006.

5 Shaffer HJ, Hall MN, Vander Bilt J. Estimating the prevalence of disordered gambling behavior in the United States and Canada: a research synthesis. *Am J Pub Health*. 1999; **89**: 1369–76.

6 American Psychiatric Association. *Diagnostic and statistical manual of mental disorders: fourth edition, text revision (DSM-IV-TR)*. Washington, DC: American Psychiatric Association; 2000.

7 Dement JW. *Going for Broke: the depiction of compulsive gambling in film*. Lanham, MD: The Scarecrow Press; 1999.

8 Turner NE, Fritz B, Zangeneh M. Images of gambling in film. *J Gambling Issues*. 2007; **20**: 117–44.

9 Katz M (producer), Brooks A (director). *Lost in America* [motion picture]. United States: Geffen Film Company, Warner Brothers; 1985.

10 Weintraub J (producer), Kessler S (director) *Vegas Vacation* [motion picture]. United States: Warner Bros; 1997

11 Camon A, Hamori A, McLean A (producers), Kwietniowski R (director). *Owning Mahowny* [motion picture]. Canada: Alliance Atlantis; 2003.

12 Turner NE. Doubling vs. constant bets as strategies for gambling. *J Gambling Stud*. 1998; **14**: 413–29.

13 Turner NE, Horbay R. Doubling revisited: the mathematical and psychological effect of betting strategy. *Gambling Res*. 2003; **15**: 16–34.

14 Sasso WV, Kalajdzic J. Do Ontario and its gaming venues owe a duty of care to problem gamblers? *Gaming Law Rev*. 2006; **10**: 552–70.

15 Fields F (producer), Brooks R (director). *Fever Pitch* [motion picture]. United States: MGM; 1985.

16 Problem Gambling Project Staff. *Problem Gambling: a guide for helping professionals*. Toronto, ON: Centre for Addiction and Mental Health; 2008.

10

Tragedy and Transcendence: Cancer

Kim Goodman, Suzanne Classen & Patricia Lenahan

"CANCER IS A TERM USED FOR DISEASES IN WHICH ABNORMAL CELLS divide without control and are able to invade other tissues."[1] The mere mention of the word "cancer" elicits a myriad of emotions both from the health-care professional and from the patients and families who receive the diagnosis. The medical terminology associated with disease is difficult for many patients who may, for example, equate the word "tumor" with "cancer." Clearly, the diagnosis of cancer elevates the importance of the health-care provider-patient relationship. The importance of prevention (e.g. avoidance of tobacco, engaging in healthy and active lifestyles), risk reduction and routine screenings also require a healthy provider-patient relationship.

Based on rates from 2005 to 2007, the National Cancer Institute states that more than 40% of men and women born today will be diagnosed with cancer during their lifetimes.[1] The lifetime risk of developing cancer is nearing one in two adult males and females.

Minority and underserved communities often experience an unequal cancer burden[1] due to a variety of factors. Therefore it is important to develop culturally and linguistically appropriate community interventions that are evidence based, in order to increase routine screenings and to modify risk behaviors to enhance prevention efforts and to improve early detection.

One example of the impact of cancers in underserved populations is the rise of AIDS-related cancers in Africa. According to a recent study, "Africans infected with AIDS have a 30–90% times higher risk of acquiring Kaposi sarcoma, a five times higher risk of developing lymphoma and at least double the risk for cervical cancer."[2]

Delivering and Receiving Bad News

Bloom (2005): This is the story of the intersecting lives of the youngest daughter of an upwardly mobile Latino family in Chicago and her court-ordered therapist, Dr. Sharon Greene (Mara Monserrat), who is coping with problems of her own: infertility and concern for her terminally ill mother. Letty (Jessi Perez) barely graduated from high school and, much to the dismay of her mother, soon became pregnant with Lisa, now aged 5. Letty's second child, Beto, was born with cerebral palsy. Letty alternately lives with her parents and her new boyfriend, Ernesto, an abusive drug dealer.

1 (Ch 7, 0:57:15–0:59:45) Ruthie (Greta DeBofsky), Sharon's mother, has just had a biopsy and is in recovery. Her physician daughter and son-in-law are sitting with her as Dr. Agrawal (Ken Mines) enters the room. David (Bill Ferris) the son-in-law stands up immediately and asks if those are the results. Dr. Agrawal looks at Ruthie who just woke up and suggests that they step outside. Despite the physician's efforts to delay the discussion, Ruthie says that she's on pins and needles. She adds: "You're beginning to scare me." Dr. Agrawal says there is no easy way to say this and tells them that the tumor was malignant. David immediately wants to know the next step, while Dr. Agrawal wants to give Ruthie time to digest the information.
    a. How would you assess Dr. Agrawal's delivery of bad news? Was there anything he could have done to make sharing the diagnosis easier?
    b. What is the impact of having to share bad news with both the daughter and the son-in-law who also are physicians?
    c. What is the focus of Sharon and David?
2 (Ch 8, 1:05:40–1:08:00) Ruthie and Sharon (Mara Monserrat) are seeing the specialist, Dr. Harris (Winston Evans). He shares with Ruthie that she has an aggressive pancreatic cancer. Ruthie asks what would happen if she did nothing. She presses the physician to give her specifics about how much time she has left. He replies 3–6 months without chemotherapy. Sharon, her daughter, is beside herself and insisting that Ruthie has to have chemotherapy.
    a. How might a patient interpret the word "aggressive"?
    b. What is the potential impact of literacy and health literacy when sharing a diagnosis and a prognosis?
    c. The physician is matter-of-fact in sharing the information. How might the patient and the family view this dispassionate approach?
    d. Was the physician's approach to sharing information impacted by being a colleague of the patient's daughter?
    e. What role did Sharon's insistence that Ruthie have chemotherapy play? Could Sharon force Ruthie to have chemotherapy?

The Bucket List (2007; Jack Nicholson, Morgan Freeman): A movie about Edward Cole (Nicholson) and Carter Chambers (Freeman), two men from very different worlds who meet in a hospital and discover that they have one thing in common: a terminal cancer diagnosis. Together, they survive treatment and develop a plan for coping with the end-of-life process.

1 (Ch 6, 0:26:30–0:27:46; 0:28:40–0:29:27) Dr. Hollis (Rob Morrow) enters the room to give Edward the results of his tests. He asks Edward how it is going, quickly adding, "dumb question." He tells Edward that he has "6 months, a year if we're lucky." Dr. Hollis says there are experimental protocols that they can try. Edward, who had been watching TV when the doctor came in, says: "Hey, Doc, you're blocking my view." When the doctor asks Edward if there is anything he can do for him he says, "get familiar with Carter's case." In the second scene, Dr. Hollis returns to talk with Carter. Although the viewer doesn't hear what is said, it is clear that the prognosis is not good. Edward and Carter share a glance that speaks volumes.

   a. How would you assess the quality of the doctor-patient relationship?
   b. Dr. Hollis tries to offer hope that appears to be rejected by the patient. How should a health-care professional respond?
   c. Edward asks his doctor to look at the chart of another patient and to speak with him. What are the ethical issues involved?
   d. The disparities between those who are well insured and can secure a different level of care are demonstrated here. How might this affect the confidence Carter has in his own doctor and treatment?

Clinical Trials and Cancer

The Big C, Season 1 (2010; Laura Linney, Oliver Platt, Reid Scott, Idris Elba, Gabriel Basso): This Showtime television series depicts the life of Cathy Jamison (Linney), who has been newly diagnosed with stage IV melanoma, and her experiences coming to terms with her diagnosis. Cathy played by society's rules her entire life, but upon receiving her diagnosis she defies society's expectations and lives life her way. The entire first season is available on most standard television streaming and downloading providers.

1 (S1E13, 0:08:46–0:10:08) Cathy, her husband Paul (Platt), and her oncologist, Todd (Scott), discuss the potential of her participation in a clinical trial. Her oncologist informs them that he has registered her for a spot in a clinical trial. Todd explains to them that it will be 6 months before she is able to participate, if at all. Cathy, Paul, and her oncologist discuss what the remaining treatment options are while weighing the risks and benefits. Cathy opts to wait for the clinical trial.

   a. What are some of the potential risks for a patient involved in a clinical trial?
   b. If a patient lacks the resources to investigate information about clinical trials on their own, is it ethical for their doctor or other members of their treatment team to discuss the option with them?
   c. In certain cultures, doctors are not questioned by patients and are often

seen as authority figures. What cultural values may impact a patient's decision to participate in a clinical trial if (not) recommended by their physician?

Pediatric Cancer

My Sister's Keeper (2009; Cameron Diaz, Jason Patric, Sofia Vassilieva, Thomas Dekker): A film about the emotional, physical, and ethical challenges a family faces when a child is diagnosed with a chronic and life-threatening form of cancer.

1 (Ch 4, 0:10:10–0:10:51) In this scene, the Fitzgerald family is informed that their young daughter, Kate (Vassilieva), has leukemia.
   a. What minor steps does the doctor take in this scene to comfort the family?
   b. What, do you imagine, are some of the initial thoughts/feelings the parents might be experiencing in this scene?
   c. What other members of the multidisciplinary team might have been helpful to have present when informing the Fitzgeralds of their daughter's diagnosis? Why?

2 (Ch 7, 0:23:30–0:24:28; 0:25:27–0:26:21) In the first scene, Kate expresses her frustrations with feeling sick, tired, and "looking different" from other people her age. According to Erik Erikson's developmental theory, Kate is in the adolescent stage of development, known as identity versus role confusion. At this time in development, feeling accepted by and connected to one's peers is particularly important.[3] This scene also reinforces a mother's love for her child when Sarah Fitzgerald (Diaz) shaves her head in an effort to normalize her daughter's appearance and provide support. In the second scene, Kate begins to express some of the challenges her cancer diagnosis has had on the entire family system. It is important to recognize that cancer does not just affect the individual, but the entire family.
   a. What are some of the common activities, cares, and concerns of teenagers?
   b. How might having a cancer diagnosis and/or receiving cancer treatment (e.g. chemotherapy) impact a teenager?
   c. What psychosocial resources could you offer to help Kate and her family cope with the cancer diagnosis?
   d. How might Kate's cancer diagnosis and treatment impact her parents and siblings?

3 (Ch 10, 0:38:42–0:41:51) This scene helps illuminate two different phases of the grief and loss process constructed by Elizabeth Kübler-Ross. Upon receiving news of Kate's rapidly declining health status, Kate appears to be in acceptance of the information. Sarah Fitzgerald (Diaz), Kate's mother, seems to remain in denial. In order to cope with her daughter's illness, Sarah seems to deny the need for additional resources. This is seen when Sarah refuses services from the Make A Wish Foundation and hospice.

    a. What are your beliefs regarding death and dying? What are your values regarding quality of life versus quantity of life?

    b. How might Sarah's and Kate's views on quantity versus quality of life differ?

    c. What is your understanding of hospice care? Who qualifies? What services are provided?

    d. How might a therapist help a parent cope with the impending loss of a child?

4   (Chs 13–14, 0:50:45–0:58:19) In these scenes Kate interacts with another cancer patient whom she meets in the hospital. Taylor (Dekker) quickly becomes her boyfriend. These scenes highlight the importance of peer relationships, peer acceptance, self-image, and sexuality during the adolescent stages of development.

    a. How would you explain these aspects of adolescent development to parents and hospital staff?

    b. What is the importance of peer relationships and sexuality at the end of life?

    c. How does having a cancer diagnosis impact her self-image?

    d. How does Kate's relationship with Taylor impact her sense of self?

5   (Ch 24, 1:33:32–1:36:41) In this scene the viewer witnesses a pivotal moment between a mother and a child. It is during this conversation that Sarah Fitzgerald begins to process and face the inevitable death of her child. Kate is finally able to communicate with her mom through art. Kate comforts her mom and together they face her impending death.

    a. How might expressive therapies (e.g. art, movement, music, and so forth) be used to help cancer patients and their families communicate and cope with a cancer diagnosis and/or loss? In what other situations would these adjunctive therapies be useful?

    b. How might the loss of Kate impact Sarah? How will Sarah's identity, roles, and family dynamics change?

    c. What resources might be available to Sarah and her family? What interventions might you use to help Sarah cope with the loss of her child?

    d. What is the role of cultural beliefs, spirituality, and religion in coping with loss?

Children of Cancer Patients

The Big C, Season 1 (see earlier description)

1   (S1E13, 0:23:42–0:26:29) Adam (Basso), Cathy's son, discovers a storage room filled with presents from Cathy for future events, such as his high school graduation and his 26th birthday. After he finds these presents, he begins to cry as he faces the reality of his mother's probable death. This is this first

time Adam has shown any emotion regarding Cathy's diagnosis. This can be compared with earlier in the episode (0:18:45–0:20:10) when Cathy and Paul tell Adam that she has cancer and that she will be receiving treatment – at that time his reaction was ambivalent and unemotional.

a. What type of support and interventions would benefit an adolescent whose parent has been given a terminal diagnosis?

b. What are some behavioral changes that might be expected from an adolescent during the grieving process?

c. What are some of the ambiguous losses experienced by an adolescent when their parent is diagnosed with a terminal illness or advanced cancer?

Cancer and Sexual Minorities: Telling His Story

Southern Comfort (2001): This documentary, a Sundance Film Festival award winner, is the story of Robert Eads, a terminally ill 52-year-old female-to-male transgendered man living in rural Georgia. The film follows Robert with his "chosen family" of friends and family of origin during the last year of his life.

1 (Ch 3, 0:13:21–0:15:31) In this scene Robert talks about his diagnosis and his attempts to obtain treatment. Robert says that he was diagnosed a year ago after waking up in a pool of blood. He learned that he had cancer of the cervix, uterus, and ovaries. He shares that he spent 3 weeks calling doctors asking for appointments. His friends, Tom and Debbie, also share their attempts to get help for Robert. They state that Robert was refused care by more than 20 doctors and by "countless" hospitals. Robert adds: "the last part of me that is female is killing me."

a. What resources exist for individuals who are transgendered?

b. How would you respond to Robert's statement that the last part of him that is female is killing him?

c. Robert shares that he had asked for a hysterectomy but was told he didn't need it since he was perimenopausal at the time of transition. What role does hormonal treatment (testosterone) have on the potential to develop cancer?

2 (Ch 10, 1:11:40–1:12:15; 1:14:40–1:15:01) Robert says that he made a bargain with God to be able to attend one more Southern Comfort meeting. He adds that he has terminal cancer and that he was "supposed to be gone months ago." Robert is smoking and sees the irony in this. He says that his bones and lymph nodes are full of cancer, but not his lungs. Robert has been smoking since he was 5 years old and isn't going to quit. He adds: "as long as I keep my lungs full of smoke, they'll be fine."

a. How does an important goal, meeting, or date influence a patient with a terminal condition to "hang on"?

b. What can health-care providers do to help patients identify the important things in life for them?

c. How would you respond to Robert's statement that as long as he keeps his lungs full of smoke, they'll (lungs) be fine?

d. In view of the prevalence of lung cancer, and this patient's overall health, would you have encouraged him to stop smoking? Why/why not?

Coming to Terms with the Diagnosis

1 (Ch 11, 1:17:15–1:18:09) Robert is talking about his cancer: "Do I want to die? No. Am I afraid of dying? No." He goes on to share that he wants to live long enough to see his grandson grow up, to walk Lola down the aisle and to make her his wife. He adds: "Sometimes you don't get what you want."

a. How would you respond to a patient who expresses similar emotions and feelings?

b. What solace can you offer him? Would this be helpful?

c. How would you assess his understanding of his condition and his coping skills?

The Decision to Discontinue Treatment

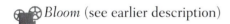 *Bloom* (see earlier description)

1 (Ch 11, 1:21:16–1:25:45) Ruthie and Sharon are having coffee. Ruthie seems uneasy. She tells Sharon that she called Dr. Harris and told him that she wouldn't have any more treatment. Sharon becomes angry and tells her mother not to be "childish" and that she doesn't understand what she's saying. Ruthie tries to reassure Sharon, telling her that it's OK. Sharon replies: "it may be OK for you, but it's not OK for me." Ruthie tells Sharon that she has no energy and that she wants to die with dignity. Sharon retorts: "there's no dignity in death." Ruthie continues that she's had a great life and a great husband and daughter. Sharon persists and says: "Don't you want to live to see your grandchildren someday?" Sharon asks her mother how she can be so calm and so optimistic.

a. What factors contribute to Ruthie's decision to end treatment?

b. What is the impact on Sharon both as a daughter and a physician?

c. How might Ruthie's physician intervene to help this family?

d. Is Sharon being selfish in wanting her mother to continue treatment? How would you counsel her?

The Bucket List (see earlier description)

1 (Chs 7–8, 0:35:25–0:38:00) Carter's wife, Virginia (Beverly Todd), arrives at the hospital and enters the room. Edward says hello and says that he will

give them some time. Virginia is upset, asking, "What kind of hospital is this? There's not a doctor within a mile of here." She says she regrets that they didn't go to a university hospital. She gets on the phone, calling another doctor. Carter tells her to stop. He shares with her that he and Edward are going away. She becomes even more upset, demanding to know how he can give up and quit fighting. She adds: "Why don't you tell our children that you've given up on them."

    a. How would you respond to the spouse of a terminally ill patient who questions the care he has received?

    b. What services may be helpful to the spouse and adult children in processing the information?

    c. How would you evaluate Carter's decision to discontinue treatment?

Alternative Therapies

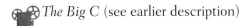

The Big C (see earlier description)

1 (S1E11, 0:05:02–0:06:48) In this scene, Cathy and her oncologist discuss her decision to pursue alternative treatment. Upon receiving her diagnosis Cathy decided not to start traditional treatment because of the low success rate and fear of the negative side effects. On this visit, she discusses with her oncologist the different types of alternative therapies for cancer, including one she has just begun without his knowledge. She is met with resistance by her oncologist to treatments that are not used as supplements to traditional treatment but, instead, as curative modalities.

    a. If a patient chooses to receive treatment from a curandero, sangoma, medicine man, or other healer, what are some of the challenges they may face from their oncologist and other individuals within their treatment team?

    b. What steps can a health professional take to enhance their sensitivity to their patients' cultural beliefs regarding folk and alternative therapies?

    c. How can physicians inquire about a patient's interest in or use of alternative therapies? How might this affect the quality of the doctor-patient relationship?

The Impact of Surgery and Coping with Multiple Medical Problems

All of Us (2008): This documentary focuses on Mehret Mandefro, an Ethiopian-American internal medicine resident at Montefiore Medical Center who treats many HIV-postive African-American women. Dr. Mandefro wants to understand why so many women of color are affected and decides to develop a research project on HIV and minority women. The movie focuses on two of Dr. Mandefro's patients.

1 (0:17:04–0:18:25) Tara explains that she had surgery to remove her vulva because cancer had invaded the skin. She says she is "not just fighting one disease, I'm fighting two." The scene shifts to the obstetrics and gynecology office, where the physician tells her that she will need another surgery. Tara responds: "I just hope my numbers don't drop."

   a. How does Tara's status as HIV positive affect her ability to "fight" both diseases?

   b. Tara expresses concern about her "numbers dropping." How does her focus on HIV affect her coping with cancer?

   c. Tara acknowledges that she is fighting not one but two diseases. How would you respond to this statement?

   d. What is Tara's understanding of her cervical cancer and its impact on her relationship with her partner?

Companion Animals and Social Supports

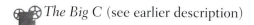 *The Big C* (see earlier description)

1 (SO1EO1, 0:05:47–28:56) For the first time, Cathy begins to talk about her cancer with someone other than her oncologist. She discusses her treatment options and her reasons for not pursuing chemotherapy. The viewer finally sees Cathy cry and process her emotions regarding her diagnosis and prognosis. Initially, the viewer perceives she is talking to a friend or possibly a therapist. As the camera angle changes, the viewer learns Cathy is talking to the neighbor's dog.

   a. Many patients have a strong emotional bond with an animal. How does this bond help them cope with their diagnosis and treatment?

   b. What are the physical and mental health benefits for patients who participate in animal assisted therapy?

   c. What are some of the challenges a patient with a terminal diagnosis may face when caring for their pet?

Intimate Relationships, Sexuality, and Cancer

All of Us (see earlier description)

1 (0:24:20–0:26:00) Dr. Mandefro visits Tara at home after her surgery. There are pills all around the nightstand and the room is in disarray. Tara rests on her side, the only position that doesn't make her hurt. She says she feels like

giving up with the pain. Tara shares that after the surgery she "feels funny as a woman" adding: "I don't recognize myself down there."

   a. What anticipatory guidance/patient education might have prepared Tara for the surgery and the postoperative period? How would you involve her partner in this discussion? Would you want him to see the surgical site?

   b. How would you respond to Tara's statement "I don't recognize myself down there"? In what way has the surgery affected Tara's self-image, both as a woman and as a sexual being?

   c. What are the potential sexual consequences of this surgery? What are the possible psychological sequelae? How would you counsel Tara and her partner regarding resuming sexual relations?

The Big C (see earlier description)

1 (S1E06, 01:34–02:12) At various times in the series, Cathy engages in intercourse. In this scene, when Cathy's partner Lenny (Elba) discovers a metastasis, she becomes visibly uncomfortable and evasive. Later in the episode (0:14:07–0:14:30), Cathy is engaged in an intimate moment with Paul, who is also unaware of her cancer. He expresses his desire to change positions during intercourse, which would expose her metastasis to him. Again, she becomes uncomfortable and avoids discussing her diagnosis.

   a. What are some issues that concern many cancer patients regarding their sexuality?

   b. In addition to married individuals or those in long-term relationships, single adults are also diagnosed with cancer. What are some of the obstacles that single adults face when dating and being intimate with partners?

   c. How might patients cope with body image changes when their bodies show visible signs of a previously internal problem?

   d. How might a doctor or other member of a patient's treatment team be more aware about their LGBTQI (lesbian, gay, bisexual, transgender, queer, questioning, and intersex) patients' needs?

Southern Comfort (see earlier description)

1 (Ch 10, 0:15:40–0:16:32) Lola Cola, Robert's lover, shares her feelings: "For the first time last night … in a long time … we got back to that space that we shared when there's no cancer, no medications to worry about. There's just 'us' connected so thoroughly … it was beautiful, it was a gift." The scene shifts to Robert sitting in his wheelchair with Lola in front of him. Robert states: "The main thing she [Lola] tells me is don't hold on for me. I can't help but hold on for her."

Cancer in Later Life

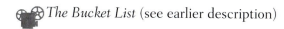 *The Bucket List* (see earlier description)

1 (Ch 4, 0:14:23–0:15:00; ch 5, 0:17:12–0:23:06) These two scenes introduce the viewers to some of the physical side effects of chemotherapy (e.g. nausea, vomiting, weakness, chills, and so forth). The connection between the physical challenges faced in cancer treatment and the overall spirit, mental health, and well-being of a person is highlighted when Edward (Nicholson) states, "Somewhere, some lucky guy is having a heart attack." Viewers are also exposed to the benefits/challenges of caregiving and psychosocial support networks.

   a. How might a cancer diagnosis, cancer treatment, pain, and/or discomfort impact the psychological, social, and spiritual well-being of a person and/or his or her support system?

   b. What are some of the positive and potentially challenging aspects of having a strong support system? What are some of the potential benefits/challenges of being alone while coping with a cancer diagnosis? If a natural support system does not exist, what other options are available to a client/patient?

   c. What are some of the differences between Edward and Carter (Freeman) highlighted in this scene? How might their life choices influence their ability to cope with a cancer diagnosis and the life review process?

2 (Ch 6, 0:24:09–0:29:24; ch 7, 0:29:45–0:35:26) In Chapter 6, Edward and Carter discuss Elizabeth Kübler-Ross's stages of grief. Edward had asked Carter if he had considered suicide. When he said no, Edward said, "you are in the first stage, denial." While both scenes illustrate issues related to grief and loss, they also highlight issues related to coping with a terminal cancer diagnosis. Both Edward and Carter demonstrate what is thought of as a need to maintain normalcy and control. The scenes also provide an example of male coping styles.

   a. What are Elizabeth Kübler-Ross's five stages of grief and loss and what occurs at each stage?

   b. What coping mechanisms do Edward and Carter utilize when learning of their prognosis?

3 (Ch 11, 0:47:15–0:49:33; ch 19, 1:17:50–1:19:21; ch 22, 1:17:50–1:29:12) In these scenes, we are introduced to the concepts of spirituality and prayer, commonly used forms of complementary and alternative medicine, especially among African-American families. Prayer and spirituality are often used to provide comfort and hope during times of grief and loss. Engaging in a life review, wondering about God, and questioning spirituality are often part of the grief process. We are also reminded in Chapters 19 and 22 of our earlier discussion regarding the benefits/challenges of psychosocial support when Edward and Carter return home from their travels.

a. How is the presence of psychosocial support depicted in these scenes?

b. What might you say to a patient/client coping with end-of-life issues and spirituality? Whose role is it to introduce issues of religion and/or spirituality? How do you assess if addressing spirituality is a beneficial intervention?

c. How might you help someone reflect back on their life and plan for their death?

d. What topics might be important to introduce to a client/patient living with a terminal cancer diagnosis (e.g. advanced directives, wills, funeral planning, and so forth)?

e. How might you support caregivers, friends, and family members coping with loss?

Saying Goodbye

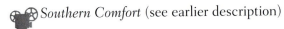 *Southern Comfort* (see earlier description)

1   (Ch 11, 0:1:22:10–0:1:25:12) It's Christmas time and Robert has entered the hospice. Everyone has gathered in his room. Robert talks about going fishing with Cas before it snows. The scene shifts to photos of everyone, Robert's "chosen family," at "SoCo" (Southern Comfort, an annual meeting of trans-gendered persons in Atlanta). Lola is lying in the bed with Robert. She shares: "As the end drew near, I noticed a change in his breathing. I gathered him in my arms and told him how much I loved him and he left." Lola's final words in the film are: "Nature delights in diversity, why don't people?"

a. Everyone knows that Robert will not survive and have an opportunity to go fishing again. How would you evaluate this statement? What is the purpose of Robert's saying this?

b. How would you respond to Lola's final words? What message is she trying to convey?

References

1   Howlader N, Noone AM, Krapcho M, *et al.*, editors. SEER *Cancer Statistics Review, 1975–2008.* Bethesda, MD: National Cancer Institute. Available at: http://seer.cancer. gov/csr/1975_2008 (last accessed 12/01/11)

2   Brower V. AIDS-related cancers increase in Africa. *J Natl Cancer Inst.* 2011; **103**(12): 918–19.

3   Abrams AN, Hazen EP, Penson RT. Psychosocial issues in adolescents with cancer. *Cancer Treat Rev.* 2007; **33**(7): 622–30.

Further Reading
●●●●●●●●●●●●●●●●●●●●●●

- Chang KH, Brodie R, Choong MA, *et al.* (2011). Complementary and alternative medicine use in oncology: a questionnaire survey of patients and health care professionals. *BMC Cancer*. 2011; **11**: 196.
- Engler M, Brock T, Lehman M, *et al.*, directors. *The Big C* [television series]. United States: Perkins Street Productions; 2010.
- Houtzager BA, Grootenhuis MA, Hoekstra-Weebers JE, *et al.* Psychosocial functioning in siblings of pediatric cancer patients one to six months after diagnosis. *Eur J Cancer*. 2003; **39**(10): 1423–32.
- Hurwitz CA, Duncan J, Wolfe J. Caring for the child with cancer at the close of life: "there are people who make it, and I'm hoping I'm one of them." *JAMA*. 2004; **292**(17): 2141–9.
- Koenig HG, Larson DB, Larson SS. Religion and coping with serious medical illness. *Ann Pharmacother*. 2001; **35**(3): 352–9.
- Kübler-Ross E. *On Death and Dying*. New York, NY: Macmillan; 1969.
- Kutner JS, Steiner JF, Corbett KK, *et al.* Information needs in terminal illness. *Soc Sci Med*. 1999; **48**(10): 1341–52.
- Meropol NJ, Egleston BL, Buzagl JS, *et al.* Cancer patient preferences for quality and length of life. *Cancer*. 2008; **113**(12): 3459–66.
- Roesch SC, Adams L, Hines A, *et al.* Coping with prostate cancer: a meta-analytic review. *J Behav Med*. 2005; **28**: 281–93.
- Visser A, van der Graaf W, Hoekstra H, *et al.* Stress response symptoms in adolescents during the first year after a parent's cancer diagnosis. *Support Care Cancer*. 2010; **18**(11): 1421–8.
- Young B, Dixon-Woods M, Findlay M, *et al.* Parenting in a crisis: conceptualizing mothers of children with cancer. *Soc Sci Med*. 2002; **55**(10): 1835–47.

11

Your Sugar is High, M'am:
Diabetes

John D. Stokes

DIABETES IS BECOMING ONE OF THE MAJOR MEDICAL PROBLEMS facing this country and the world. An estimated 260 million people worldwide have diabetes, including over 25 million in the United States. It is estimated that 7 million people worldwide develop diabetes annually. The rate of new diagnoses of diabetes is rapidly accelerating. Having diabetes can shorten one's life expectancy by 5 to 10 years and diabetic complications can have a dramatic effect on quality of life. Diabetes places an extreme financial burden on the medical care system. It has been estimated that 1 of every 4 dollars spent by Medicare is somehow related to diabetes. In 2010 it was estimated that most countries spent up to 10% of their medical care dollars on diabetes.

Preventing diabetes is now thought to represent a major savings in the medical care area. Studies have shown that delaying the onset of diabetes by even 5 to 10 years can result in significant savings over the lifetime. Unfortunately movies generally do not portray diabetes in a realistic light. There seems to be a concentration on type 1 diabetes with the focus on the attention-grabbing complications. However, in reality 90% of the individuals with diabetes have type 2 diabetes; where complications have a tendency to occur after years of hyperglycemia. The complications seen for type 1 are typically hypoglycemia (which can be very dramatic) and renal failure. The complications seen with type 2 diabetes in the movies can again include hypoglycemia and cardiovascular events. Unfortunately, day-to-day life with diabetes is rarely portrayed.

Editor's note: *Soul Food* (1997) is an excellent movie that portrays diabetes in a minority population, a group particularly at risk for the development of diabetes. Scenes from this film were included in volume one of *Cinemeducation* in the chapter addressing chronic health problems. Jason Statham's "Diabetes" on YouTube provides yet another *unrealistic* look at diabetes. However, this 2-minute clip may be useful in sharing with patients in a group medical visit to encourage an exploration of their feelings about having been diagnosed with this illness.

Steel Magnolias (1989; Sally Field, Julia Roberts, Shirley MacLaine, Dolly Parton, Dylan McDermott): *Steel Magnolias* seems to be either the most loved or most hated movie with diabetes as a major theme. In way of background, the story is based on the author, Robert Hartling's, younger sister. He had trouble dealing with her death and it was suggested that he write about it. The story was originally staged as an off-Broadway production in 1987, but based in the late 1950s. It then was staged on Broadway in 2005, in addition to the movie release in 1989. Shelby Eatenton (Julia Roberts) and her mother M'Lynn (Sally Field) are two of the main characters. The movie begins with the preparations for Shelby's wedding at the Eatenton home.

1   (0:17:44–0:28:20) The women have gathered at Truvy's (Dolly Parton) beauty parlor to have their hair done for the wedding. Shelby mentions that she would like to grow old with someone. She also states that she plans to keep her job at the hospital because she loves being around the babies. M'Lynn states that she shouldn't be on her feet all day and she should be "nicer to her circulatory system." Earlier in the film, Jackson Latcherie (Dylan McDermott), Shelby's prospective husband, raised the question of whether Shelby would be able to have children. Now Shelby is talking about adoption.

   a. What does M'Lynn mean when she says that Shelby should be nicer to her circulatory system?

   b. What impact does her hypoglycemic episode have regarding her future planning?

   c. What advice would you give to prospective couples about childbearing when the woman has diabetes? Would your advice differ if the patient had been diagnosed with type 1 or type 2 diabetes?

2   (0:24:20–0:26:00) Shelby begins to realize that something is wrong; she is becoming hypoglycemic. There is a close-up of the look of terror on her face and she begins sweating. She becomes combative and gradually recovers after being forced to drink juice. There is talk of adopting children.

   a. What was the personal impact of this hypoglycemic episode for Shelby?

   b. How would you counsel a patient who presents with these symptoms and a desire to become pregnant?

3   (0:46:00–0:59:20) After her wedding, Shelby returns to the Eatonton home for Christmas. Shelby tells M'Lynn that she is pregnant (0:53:20). Shelby says that she wants a child of her own and that she wouldn't be able to adopt. M'Lynn says "Your body has been through so much. You're special." Shelby replies that diabetics have babies "all the time."

   a. How would you interpret M'Lynn's remark that Shelby's body has been through so much?

   b. Does M'Lynn seem pleased at the prospect of being a grandmother?

   c. What advice would you give to this family?

4   (1:13:06–1:15:30) Shelby has had her baby. She is back at Truvy's beauty shop. Truvy notices Shelby's dialysis fistula while she is getting a manicure. Shelby has her long hair cut short to be "easier to manage." She states that her

kidneys failed during the pregnancy and that she is going to have a transplant and M'Lynn is going to be the donor.

    a. How can the contemporary monitoring and treatment technology allow women with diabetes to live normal reproductive lives?

    b. What is the impact of dialysis on a young mother?

5 (1:22:14–1:23:03; 1:27:00–1:32:30) During the first scene, Shelby has the transplant. In the second scene, Shelby is with her son. She collapses and is taken to the hospital. She is seen in the hospital on a ventilator. The family gathers. Apparently days go by. Shelby doesn't respond and the ventilator is discontinued resulting in Shelby's death (1:32:12).

    a. This was a time of difficult management filled with myth and superstition about the illness.

    b. How has the results of the Diabetes Control and Complications Trial changed our attitudes about type 1 diabetes treatment?

    c. What are the various stages of development of hypoglycemia?

    d. How does hypoglycemia unawareness hinder the treatment of hypoglycemia?

    e. What are appropriate methods to treat hypoglycemia?

    f. How is diabetes treated differently in pregnancy?

    g. How do codependency and controlling behavior interfere with effective diabetes treatment?

(Author's note: It helps in looking at this chain of events to realize that this occurred in the 1950s and 1960s, even though we were spared the sight of sharpening needles and boiling of glass syringes. Tools now commonplace for good control did not exist then. Control was difficult for type 1 patients. Even into the 1970s women with type 1 diabetes were commonly hospitalized and placed on bed rest for a large portion of their pregnancies. Dialysis was difficult and transplantation was highly experimental and dangerous.)

This Old Cub (2004): This movie is a documentary that reviews the playing career and postcareer events in the life of Ron Santo. Unfortunately, diabetes steals the spotlight. Ron was diagnosed with diabetes at age 18, soon after signing a Major League Baseball contract. He decides to hide his diabetes. In the extra material included on the DVD, he relates that he spent a month in the hospital learning how to deal with diabetes and how to adjust to the way he was feeling related to his blood sugar level. He states he was able to get through his first season off insulin. However, before starting spring training for his second season, he had lost 35 lb in a 3-month period and was started on insulin. Ron Santo shares how he had to spend a month in the hospital again to learn how insulin affected him.

Ron was always keeping orange juice and candy in the dugout. He was judging what his blood sugar was by how he felt. He states that one of the reasons that he signed with the Cubs was that there were no night games at Wrigley Field, which would have caused further disruption in his routine. This was at a time when there were no good monitoring tools available, just urine testing. Only the old animal insulins were available then. He relates in an anecdote how he managed to hit a game-winning grand slam home run with two outs while he was having a severe hypoglycemic episode.

The movie spends a lot of time on how Ron Santo dealt with his severe peripheral vascular disease and neuropathy resulting in the below the knee amputation of both legs. The movie frequently jumps from baseball to diabetes-related problems. Sometimes there is even a narrative about diabetes while a baseball scene is being shown. Sometimes the opposite occurs.

1 (0:1:50–0:13:00) Much time is spent with Ron in rehabilitation. He gets out of bed after his amputation and is seen using a walker. His blood sugar is checked while he is sitting in a wheelchair. Ron rationalizes the result and gives himself an insulin injection.
   a. How do patients with diabetes cope with their disease?
   b. What factors contribute to his rationalization? Is this a common response of patients with diabetes?

2 (0:22:00–0:23:18) The scene goes from showing Ron walking on crutches to clicking his heels after a cub victory. This was characteristic after a Cub win on their race for the 1969 championship.
   a. How would you interpret this scene?
   b. What is the impact of diabetes on a professional athlete? Does it differ from other individuals?

3 (0:27:00–0:36:50) Ron talks about his upcoming surgery on a radio show. He has the surgery and is seen in a rehabilitation facility. This scene shows the rehabilitation process. Ron finally is discharged from the facility to his home in Arizona.
   a. What is the impact of a sports figure – or a well-known individual – sharing their health-related problems?
   b. How can Ron's family be prepared to address his needs at home?
   c. What is the impact of an amputation on an athlete?

4 (0:53:11–0:54:24) Ron shares his experiences working with the Juvenile Diabetes Research Foundation. He talks about starting the Ron Santo Diabetes Walk and how over the years he has raised $50 million for the Juvenile Diabetes Research Foundation.
   a. What is the impact of a celebrity or sports figure as a champion for disease research?
   b. How does this use of his celebrity affect Ron personally in his own fight against the disease?

5 (1:14:00–1:17:50) Ron gets up, puts on his prostheses and then the protective devices, and takes a shower. Afterwards, he goes about his daily routine, driving to Wrigley Field to broadcast a Cubs game.
   a. How would you assess Ron's coping skills?
   b. How has he been able to adapt to his illness? What supports contribute to this?

6 (1:21:00–1:21:30) Finally, Ron shares that he has had diabetes for 45 years. He had to have a coronary bypass surgery in 1999, one leg amputated in 2001, and the other in 2002. He states that he feels that he has beaten it.
   a. What new developments are there for diagnosing and treating diabetes?
   b. What are reasons that people "hide" diabetes?
   c. What interventions can help vascular disease in diabetes?
   d. How can a positive outlook and acceptance help in diabetes treatment?

Memento (2000; Guy Pearce, Carrie-Anne Moss, Joe Pantoliano, Jorja Fox, Steve Tobolowsky): This film centers on Lennie (Guy Pearce), who has a significant injury during an attack. As a result, he cannot remember any new information for more than a few minutes. The movie is filled with flashbacks. There are scenes where apparently he attributes what happened to him to other people. He is seen going around the Los Angeles area looking for the man who killed his wife. (Actually, it was the man who attacked him and his wife.) We learn that he is the one who really "killed" his wife by repeatedly injecting her with insulin, since she was testing his memory, and he did not remember doing it.

1 (0:26:50–28:30; 1:27:00–1:30:00) In the first scene we see Lennie, an insurance company investigator. He has the memory of a "case he investigated" where Sammy (Tobolowsky) had a head injury and couldn't remember anything new for more than a few minutes. Sammy can give his wife (Harriet Sanson Harris) an insulin injection without any difficulty. In the second scene, Lennie remembers Sammy giving his wife repeated insulin injections although he didn't remember giving them to her. This results in her death. Later, Lennie is talking with a rogue cop, Teddy (Pantoliano) after killing a guy he thought previously killed his wife but didn't. At this point, Lennie remembers injecting his wife (Fox) with insulin repeatedly. He says that she wasn't diabetic.
   a. What are potential problems of improper insulin injections?
   b. Discuss the frequency of the lethal complications of hypoglycemia and who is at risk for this?
   c. How can potentially hazardous medications be used safely in patients with psychiatric illnesses?
   d. Are there potential uses for insulin-induced hypoglycemia outside of diabetes?

The Godfather Part III (1990; Al Pacino, Andy Garcia, Sofia Coppola, Talia Shire, Diane Keaton): In the final instalment of the Godfather trilogy, Michael Corleone (Al Pacino) struggles with a heavy heart to make the family business legitimate, but he's pulled into more bloodshed after he makes a lucrative business deal with the Vatican. Meanwhile, Sonny's son, Vincent (Andy Garcia) works hard to become Michael's protégé. Michael Corleone has diabetes and in several scenes is shown indulging in pastries.

1 (1:06:00–1:24:50) At a family meeting in his kitchen, Michael is discussing business issues. He has a "diabetic" stroke and is taken to the hospital. His family is present. Michael gradually recovers and is able to run the family business from the hospital.

   a. What is the impact of stress on chronic health conditions?

   b. How would you advise patients about coping with stress?

   c. Would you encourage patients to work from the hospital?

2 (1:39:07–1:44:30; 1:44:55–1:47:13) In the first scene, Michael is in Italy and is trying to influence a cardinal (who later becomes pope). Michael has a hypoglycemic episode and ravenously drinks juice and eats candy. In the second scene, he is discussing his confession with Connie (Talia Shire) as she prepares his insulin for him.

   a. How can patients be prepared to cope with variations in blood glucose?

   b. Is this scene realistic? How can patients minimize hypoglycemic episodes?

   c. What is the role of family in coping with diabetes? How can they be helpful or unhelpful?

3 (1:56:30–1:56:55) After walking around in the village, Michael asks Kay (Diane Keaton) to drive back, stating that his eyesight bothers him and his eyes are weak.

   a. How can diabetes affect vision, both acutely and chronically?

   b. How do codependency and denial interfere with diabetes treatment?

   c. How is stroke related to diabetes?

Derailed (2005; Clive Owen, Jennifer Aniston, Vincent Cassel, Melissa George, Addison Timlin): Advertising executive Charles Schine (Owen) is set up for a one-night stand with Lucinda Harris (Aniston), whom he meets on a train. When they are in their hotel room, LaRoche (Cassel) breaks into the room. Things really progress after that. The story is complicated by Charles's being married to Deanna (George) and having a daughter with type 1 diabetes. Their daughter has had three renal transplants fail and is on home dialysis, causing financial problems for the family.

1 (0:3:10–0:5:10) At breakfast Deanna checks Amy's (Timlin) blood sugar and draws up insulin in the syringe. Amy gives herself the injection. The hospital calls wanting a fax of her blood sugar results.

   a. Why is Amy not using an insulin pump and a continuous glucose monitoring device?

   b. How might such monitoring devices potentially affect her overall health and psychological well-being?

2 (0:11:50–0:13:30) Charles is seen at work and having an argument with his boss. Charles faxes the blood sugar results. Charles has just lost a big client. After work while at home, Deanna reviews the blood sugar results. She leaves to go to a Parent Teacher Association meeting.

   a. What role do family members play in caring for a child with diabetes?

   b. How does this impact the family as a whole and the parents as a couple?

3   (0:23:00–0:24:40) Amy has a seizure in the middle of the night and Deanna gives her a glucagon injection. Amy gradually recovers. The dialysis machine is seen in the background. Later that day Charles discusses Amy's situation while he is at lunch with Lucinda.

   a. What is the impact of this scene on the patient and her parents?

   b. What sources of support are utilized?

   c. Why is Charles discussing this with Lucinda instead of his wife?

   d. How might a chronic illness affect the marital relationship?

4   (0:42:30–0:45:15) After being mugged while trying to have an affair with Lucinda, Charles is home in the bathtub trying to recover from the mugging. Deanna hooks up Amy to the dialysis machine. At the same time, Charles answers a call from LaRoche. He tells his wife it is a business call.

   a. How does renal failure occur in diabetes?

   b. Would control be better using different methods of insulin administration (pens, pumps) and monitoring (continuous monitoring)?

   c. How does the financial cost of chronic illness affect families?

   d. How does diabetes affect families?

Black Book (2006; Carice Van Houten, Sebastian Koch): Rachel Stein (Van Houten) is a Jewish singer in Holland during World War II. She witnesses her family being gunned down trying to escape the Nazis. She goes into hiding and joins the underground in an attempt to survive. There she infiltrates a Nazi command post, but unfortunately the underground also has been infiltrated. After several near misses, Rachel finally escapes to Israel and joins a kibbutz as a teacher. There are just two main scenes dealing with diabetes.

1   (0:38:25–0:40:00) Rachel is preparing for an assignment to infiltrate a Nazi staff office. She learns that insulin had been included in an airdrop of supplies to the resistance. Rachel remarked that she worked in the past with a comedian who had diabetes and that he would have to eat a large amount of candy if he overdosed himself with insulin.

2   (2:00:00–2:06:50) After the Allied liberation, Rachel is captured as a collaborator. Eventually she is able to break away with the resistance officer (Koch) who was the Nazi spy. He injects her with a large amount of insulin to help "calm her." She survives by eating a large amount of chocolate and escapes.

   a. What treatments were available for the treatment of diabetes in the 1940s?

   b. What misconceptions about diabetes are shown in these scenes?

   c. How can people living in war-torn areas have their medical needs met?

   d. How can patients and families be prepared to cope with the effects of natural disasters when access to care and medications may be limited for a period of time?

Chocolat (2000; Juliette Binoche, Judi Dench, Carrie-Anne Moss, Leslie Caron, Alfred Molina): This movie deals with what happens in a small puritanical village when a young mother (Binoche) and her daughter, Anouk (Victorie

Thivisol), are blown in by the North Wind and establish a chocolate shop there. This occurs during the height of Lent and their shop is directly across the street from the church. At first the shop and the rich sensuous chocolate scandalizes the town but the residents of the town later accept and learn to savor the sweetness.

1   (1:15:09–1:24:00; 1:31:30–1:32:00) Armande Voizin (Dench) has a fight with her daughter, Caroline Claimant (Moss), when Armande is found having a cup of chocolate. She shows the bruises on her legs from insulin injections. Caroline wants her mother to live a healthier lifestyle. Later there is a party for Armande. She indulges freely in all the rich foods and drinks. In the second scene, Armande does not feel well. She leaves the party and goes home with her grandson, Luc (Aurelien Parent-Koenig). Later he finds her in her chair, dead.

  a. What are potential adverse effects of insulin injections?
  b. How does alcohol ingestion result in delayed hypoglycemia in diabetes?
  c. How does ignoring appropriate lifestyle changes affect diabetes complications and mortality?
  d. How does labeling patient behaviors or food intake as "good versus bad" interfere with achieving good control?

Panic Room (2002; Jodi Foster, Kristin Stewart, Forest Whitaker): Meg Altman (Foster) and her daughter, Sarah (Stewart), move into an old brownstone building in New York City. Their unit contains a panic room. Shortly after moving in, three burglars break in with the objective of recovering something left in a safe in, of all places, the panic room. There is a chase in and out of the panic room, with Sarah's diabetes becoming a major side plot. What appears to be a GlucoWatch is seen. (This is not a GlucoWatch but a fabrication – at the time the movie was filmed, the GlucoWatch was unavailable.)

1   (0:9:35–0:12:19) Shortly after moving in, Meg and Sarah are eating pizza. Meg is drinking wine and Sarah is drinking coke. They are talking about school. There is a brief glance at the GlucoWatch reading of 87. There is a glimpse of insulin bottles in the refrigerator.

  a. How would you counsel this parent about dietary adherence?
  b. What developmental factors should health-care providers be aware of in addressing chronic illness in adolescent/pre-adolescent patients?

2   (0:31:00–0:39:32) Meg and Sarah lock themselves in the panic room during the burglary. Meg questions Sarah about hypoglycemic symptoms. Sarah says she is OK and won't let her mother see her GlucoWatch reading. Sarah checks for emergency supplies in the panic room. Meg tells Sarah to calm down and not get herself upset.

  a. Who appears to be more "upset"?

3   (1:04:55–1:07:15) After a while Sarah becomes hypoglycemic. Her GlucoWatch reading is 42. Meg tells Sarah to stay calm. Sarah and Meg both look for glucose sources in the panic room, without success.

4   (1:13:21–1:27:15) Sarah's condition deteriorates further. The GlucoWatch

sounds an alarm. Sarah has a seizure. Meg opens the panic room door and gets the glucagon kit from the refrigerator. The thieves realize something has happened and go to the panic room and find Sarah alone. Meg returns and throws the glucagon kit into the panic room before the thieves can close the door. One of the thieves (Whitaker) finally draws up the glucagon and gives Sarah the injection. Sarah gradually recovers.

    a. What other behaviors can be seen with hypoglycemia other than seizures?

    b. What should people with diabetes have in their disaster preparedness kits?

    c. How do "diet rewards," such as coke and pizza, interfere with diabetes control?

Further Reading

- Ben-Ami H, Nagachandran P, Mendelson A, *et al*. Drug-induced hypoglycemic coma in 102 diabetic patients. *Arch Intern Med*. 1999; **159**(3): 281–4.
- Cherrington A. 2005 Presidential Address: Diabetes; past, present, and future. *Diabetes Care*. 2006; **29**(9): 2158–64.
- DECODE Study Group. Glucose tolerance and mortality: comparison of WHO and American Diabetes Association diagnostic criteria. *Lancet*. 1999; **354**(9179): 617–21.
- Diabetes Control and Complications Trial Research Group. The effect of intensive diabetes treatment on the development and progression of long-term complications in insulin-dependent diabetes mellitus: the Diabetes Control and Complications Trial. *N Engl J Med*. 1993; **329**(14): 977–86.
- Hadley-Brown M. Issues concerning optimal diabetes care. *Diabetes Prim Care*. 2007; **9**(3): 213–5.
- Hanssen KF, Dahl-Jorgensen K, Lauritzen T, Feldt-Rasmussen C. Diabetic control and microvascular complications: the near-normoglycemia experience. *Diabetologia*. 1986; **29**(10): 677–84.
- Hepburn DA, Deary IJ, Frier BM, *et al*. Symptoms of acute insulin-induced hypoglycemia in humans with and without IDDM: factor-analysis approach. *Diabetes Care*. 1991; **14**(11): 949–57.
- International Diabetes Federation (IDF). *IDF Diabetes Atlas*. 4th ed. Brussels: IDF; 2009. Available at: www.diabetesatlas.org/ (last accessed 12/01/11)
- Koivikko ML, Salmela PI, Airadsinen KEJ, *et al*. Effects of sustained insulin-induced hypoglycemia on cardiovascular regulation in type 1 diabetes. *J Clin Endo Metab*. 2006; **91**(3): 851–9.
- Kroc Collaborative Study Group. Blood glucose control and the evolution of diabetic retinopathy and albuminuria: a preliminary multicenter trial. *N Engl J Med*. 1984; **311**(6): 365–72.
- Nathan D, Cleary P, Jye-Yu M, *et al*. Intensive diabetes treatment and cardiovascular disease in patients with type 1 diabetes. *N Engl J Med*. 2005; **353**(25): 2643–53.
- Powers AC. Diabetes mellitus. In: Braunwald E, Fauci AS, Kasper DL, *et al*., editors. *Harrison's Principles of Internal Medicine*. 15th ed. New York, NY: McGraw-Hill; 2001. pp. 2109–37.
- Rivera N, Ramnanan CJ, An Z, *et al*. Insulin-induced hypoglycemia increases hepatic sensitivity to glucagon in dogs. *J Clin Invest*. 2010; **120**(12): 4425–35.

- Schmittdiel JA, Uratsu CS, Karter AJ, *et al.* Why don't diabetes patients achieve recommended risk factor targets? Poor adherence versus lack of treatment intensification. *J Gen Intern Med.* 2008; **23**(5): 588–94.
- Solli O, Stavem K, Kristiansen I. Health-related quality of life in diabetes: the associations of complications with EQ-5D scores. *Health Qual Life Outcomes.* 2010; **8**: 18.
- UK Prospective Diabetes Study (UKPDS) Group. Effect of intensive blood-glucose control with metformin on complications in overweight patients with type 2 diabetes (UKPDS 34). *Lancet.* 1998; **352**(9131): 854–65.
- UK Prospective Diabetes Study (UKPDS) Group. Intensive blood-glucose control with sulphonylureas or insulin compared with conventional treatment and risk of complications in patients with type 2 diabetes (UKPDS 33). *Lancet.* 1998; **352**(9131): 837–53.
- University Group Diabetes Program. A study of the effects of hypoglycemic agents on vascular complications in patients with adult-onset diabetes. *Diabetes.* 1970: **19**(Suppl. 2): 747–830.

12

The Heart of the Matter: Cardiac Disease

Jonathan Alexander, Matthew Alexander, Anna Pavlov &
Patricia Lenahan

CARDIAC DISEASE REMAINS THE NUMBER-ONE KILLER IN THE UNITED States. Despite major improvements in prevention, early detection, and prompt treatment with a vast array of pharmacologic, device, and surgical treatments, the impact of cardiac disease on the elderly patient population remains significant. A large number of patients in primary care settings will have cardiac risk factors for disease. Many will be on medications and counseled about healthy lifestyles. The importance of counseling, behavior management, and motivational interviewing in cardiology, as well as family and internal medicine, practices cannot be stressed enough.

The following films have elements in them that address several aspects of treating cardiac disease: the significance of stress in precipitating cardiac events, importance of risk factors in causing heart disease, and the role of lifestyle modification after a cardiac event. In addition, this chapter will deal with sexuality and heart disease, noncompliance, complications from substance abuse, and biopsychosocial-spiritual issues relevant to heart transplant.

Stress/Coronary Artery Disease

Dr. Zhivago (1965; Omar Sharif and Julie Christie): An all-time classic film, this movie tells the story of Dr. Yuri Zhivago (Sharif), a romantic Russian doctor/poet who finds his life changed by the Russian Revolution of 1917 and the chaos that subsequently ensues. Zhivago is witness to the tremendous upheaval brought about by the Revolution and we are shown his struggles between his loyalty to his wife, Tonya (Geraldine Chaplin), and his passionate love for his mistress, Lara (Christie).

1   (Ch 58, side 2, 1:12:41–1:15:57) Yuri returns to Moscow several years after

the war. While traveling on a tram on his way to work, he sees a woman walking the street and he believes her to be Lara, his mistress, from whom he has been separated for many years. As he rushes to get off the tram, he suffers a fatal heart attack before he is able to catch up to this woman (who turns out not to be Lara). We witness his intense emotional longing in this scene.

a. This scene illustrates the importance of stress in precipitating a cardiac event, in this case Yuri's strong emotional longing for Lara. This particular phenomenon has recently been referred to as the "broken heart syndrome" (Takatsubo's cardiomyopathy). Do people indeed die from broken hearts?

b. What is the interplay between intense emotion and cardiac events?

c. How can we best counsel patients with heart disease (or with risk factors for heart disease) to modify their exposure to intense emotional stress whether that stress is financial, job related, intrapersonal, or interpersonal in nature?

In Good Company (2004; Dennis Quaid, Topher Grace, Scarlett Johannson, Marg Helgenberger): Ad salesman, Dan (Dennis Quaid), must take a junior position after a corporate shakedown. Even worse, he now reports to a much younger boss, Carter (Topher Grace), a business school graduate who espouses a sales approach branded Synergy that is at odds with Dan's sales style.

1   (Ch 5, 0:24:04–0:25:08) Dan and his wife are at an obstetrics visit. They are listening to the baby's heart beat. Dan becomes overwhelmed and has an arrhythmia, thus becoming the patient. The doctor then examines Dan and asks if he has been under a lot of stress. Dan announces that he is getting demoted at work.

a. How big a cardiac risk factor is work stress?

b. How would you, as a cardiologist, attempt to help Dan deal with his stress (i.e. referral, short-term counseling, bibliotherapy, and so forth)?

c. What do you think of how the physician interacted with Dan? Would you have responded any differently?

d. Have you ever been in a situation when you are seeing one patient and the person accompanying them becomes the "patient"? How did you respond? How would you respond in the future?

e. What issues regarding documentation and liability exist when a "companion" becomes the patient? How would you resolve these issues?

f. What would be your primary concerns for Dan's heart? How would you address these in the office?

The Noncompliant Cardiac Patient

The Wrestler (2008; Mickey Rourke, Marisa Tomei): Rourke plays an aging professional wrestler, Randy "The Ram" Robinson, who was a sensation in the 1980s but who is now way past his prime. Randy works part-time in a supermarket. After winning a local match, he is invited to wrestle in a 20th anniversary rematch in Wilmington, Delaware, against his former foe, The Ayatollah (Ernest Miller). To prepare for this fight, Randy increases his training, which includes the use of steroid injections.

1 (Ch 9, 0:34:10–0:37:04) In a preparatory match, Randy suffers a heart attack. He is taken to the hospital where he has coronary bypass surgery. A hospital-based cardiologist tells Randy that he has had a heart attack and that he can't wrestle or use steroids any more. Despite this warning, which is echoed by Cassidy, his stripper girlfriend (Tomei), Randy decides to wrestle in the anniversary match, with deadly consequences. In the movie's final scene, Randy suffers a fatal heart attack while performing his classic move.

   a. How realistic is the scene showing the interaction between the physician and Randy?

   b. Would Randy have been more compliant with the doctor's recommendations if he had been his primary care provider rather than a hospitalist?

   c. Comment on the general lack of eye contact between the physician and the patient? Comment on the issue of names? The physician's tone?

   d. How can we motivate patients to take better care of themselves after a cardiac event? What is the role of motivational interviewing in this regard?

   e. Would Randy have been more compliant if the hospitalist had taken more time or asked to speak with a loved one? Is this realistic?

   f. What is the role of cardiac rehabilitation following a heart attack and/or coronary artery bypass graft surgery?

   g. How can we counsel patients about strenuous activity following heart attacks?

   h. How can the use of steroids facilitate the development of coronary artery disease?

Solitary Man (2009; Michael Douglas, Susan Sarandon, Mary-Louise Parker, Imogen Poots, Bruce Altman): Ben Kalman (Douglas) is a "60ish" car salesman in New York whose life is falling apart – professionally, personally, and physically. He has difficulty controlling his impulses and denies both aging and his potential heart disease through compulsive drinking and womanizing.

1 (0:1:00–0:2:50) Ben is at his physician's office for his annual physical. He's ready to leave and says, "see you next year" when Dr. Steinberg (Altman) tells him, "It will probably be sooner. I don't love your EKG." Ben questions him and Dr. Steinberg says there is an irregularity that could be serious. He tells Ben he will set him up with a CAT scan.

   a. How would you assess Ben's response to the information provided him by Dr. Steinberg?

   b. What aspects of a patient's personality impact their willingness and ability to participate in further needed treatment?

   c. Is Dr. Steinberg aware of Ben's problem drinking? If not, why do physicians and other health-care professionals often miss this diagnosis? If he is aware, why does he not provide counseling to Ben about the harmful impact of alcohol abuse on heart disease?

2 (01:18:00–0:1:19:20) Ben is in the hospital after a physical assault. The nurse (Simone Levin) enters the room and tells Ben that the doctor will be in soon to review the results of his tests, which, she informs him, were run while he was sedated. Ben appears anxious and asks what kinds of tests were ordered, to which the nurse replies (obliquely) "heart tests." Ben immediately stands up, takes off one monitor, and asks what else he is attached to. He announces that he is leaving. The final part of the scene shows Ben's cell phone with a message from Massachusetts General Hospital, which he ignores.

a. How do you understand Ben's reaction?

b. How might the nurse have interacted differently with Ben (i.e. perhaps by naming Ben's anxiety; by being more specific about the types of tests that had been run; by verbalizing how Ben might still be in a stressful state because of the physical assault, and so forth)?

3 (0:1:21:56–01:25:15) This scene begins with Ben in Dr. Steinberg's office. The doctor says that he had ordered the CAT scan 6½ weeks ago. He asks Ben about his cheating behavior, attempting to link that with Ben's not showing up for the test. Ben shares that he had planned to have the test, but got scared. He went into a bar for a couple of drinks to relax and "picked up the first girl who would go home with him." The scene ends with Ben sitting on a park bench as his ex-wife, Nancy (Susan Sarandon), approaches and sits down. They begin talking about his life in general and his health. Ben says that he isn't going to go to the doctor and "give him that kind of power." He adds that he is not going to get those "beta-blockers that slow you down and stuff."

a. What do Ben's comments to Nancy say about patient nonadherence in general?

b. Why does Dr. Steinberg not pursue more information about Ben's drinking behavior? What is the relationship between alcohol abuse and impulsivity? What would have been the best way for Dr. Steinberg to counsel Ben about alcohol abuse?

c. Are there ways that Dr. Steinberg might have diminished the imbalance of power between him and Ben?

d. Where is Ben in terms of his readiness to change? What might have to happen for him to take greater responsibility for his health?

e. How can physicians manage difficult patients who are in denial about their condition? How can health-care providers practice self-care so that they don't bring these patients "home with them"?

Sexuality and Heart Disease

Something's Gotta Give (2003; Jack Nicholson, Dianne Keaton): Harry Sandborn (Nicholson) is a wealthy 63-year-old New York music mogul who has a fondness for younger women. Early in the film, while having foreplay with Marin, a woman in her 20s, he suffers a heart attack. Dr. Julian Mercer (Keanu Reeves) treats him, giving him the diagnosis and discussing guidelines regarding future activity. Jack subsequently develops a relationship with Erica Barry (Keaton), Marin's mother. During an argument that develops after Erica sees him with another woman, Harry suffers chest pain and is rushed to the hospital fearing another heart attack. Another physician sees him and diagnoses him as having had a panic attack. He advises Harry to relax.

1 (Ch 6, 0:18:25–0:19:48) Dr. Mercer discusses the use of Viagra and nitroglycerin.
    a. Is it appropriate to discuss sexual activity in older male patients, especially those with cardiac disease? Do you feel comfortable initiating a discussion about erectile dysfunction, especially with the spouse present? If so, how would you lead such a discussion? Educators should consider a role-play using the characters in the film to practice engaging in such a dialogue with a patient.
    b. Are erectile dysfunction drugs such as Viagra, Levitra, and Cialis contraindicated in patients with coronary artery disease, following heart attacks, coronary intervention, or bypass surgery? What guidelines are appropriate in cardiac patients? What are the contraindications to their use?
2 (Ch 21, 1:25:48–1:27:23) Jack suffers recurrent chest pain.
    a. What guidelines do you discuss with patients with documented coronary artery disease concerning the issue of when to come to the hospital or seek medical attention with recurrent chest discomfort? What is the role of nitroglycerin in patient care?
    b. Do you discuss the importance of reporting cardiac symptoms to medical personnel in those patients with cardiac disease? How do you prescribe nitroglycerin, discussing side effects and interactions with other medications?
    c. How can you educate patients to tell the difference between panic attacks and heart attacks?

Heart Transplant

Return to Me (2000; Minnie Driver, David Duchovny, Carroll O'Connor, Robert Loggia, Joely Richardson): A building contractor donates his wife's heart after she's tragically killed in an accident. A year later, he falls in love with a waitress, only to discover she had received a heart transplant at the same time and place.

1 (T5C5, 0:08:01–0:09:38) Grace is in a hospital bed appearing to have

difficulty breathing. Her friend Megan is at her side, asking her items from a questionnaire, when she notices that Grace appears to be struggling more. However, Grace is fooling her friend, who becomes alarmed and asks what she needs. When the joke is over, Megan quips, "you almost gave me a heart attack, if you'll excuse the expression." Grace asks Megan to promise to take care of her grandfather because she may never get a heart transplant. Megan tries to be hopeful and instill hope in Grace.

    a. In life-threatening situations, how do patients, families, and health-care professionals balance hope, humor, and reality?

    b. What is your reaction to Grace's brand of humor? Discuss patient and family use of humor to cope with challenging and life-threatening illness.

    c. Discuss the use of "gallow's humor" by health-care professionals.

    d. Where does the expression "you almost gave me a heart attack" originate?

2 (T5C8, 0:16:09–0:18:02) Two older men are working in a restaurant when the phone rings. They seem to know that it could be word about a heart for Gracie. Grace's grandfather says he will be at the hospital. Grace is being wheeled into the operating room with her grandfather and Megan at her side. Grace thanks her grandfather for always taking care of her and says if she does not make it, she wants him to know she loves him. She is wheeled through the operating room doors as Megan and her grandfather look on.

    a. How can physicians best help patients cope with the tremendous sense of vulnerability experienced prior to surgery?

    b. How can family members be best cared for while waiting for the outcome of a loved one's surgery?

3 (T5C9, 0:18:03–0:20:25) Meanwhile following the death of his wife, Bob returns to his home with his friend, Charlie. Bob sees a note left by his wife earlier in the day. Their dog is looking to the door and Bob tells him, "she is not coming home." Charlie leaves and Bob envisions the last hours he had with his wife at a fundraiser. He weeps deeply.

    a. One person's tragedy (death) becomes another's opportunity (transplant) and chance for life. Discuss this ironic fact of life.

4 (T5 C10, 0:23:33–0:23:38) We see in this very short scene an operating room monitor a heart beat that registers for the first time from the transplanted organ. (If you continue until 0:24:00, the scene changes to Bob having an image of his wife with the sound of the beating heart.]

    a. How do you feel when you see this scene?

    b. How does this scene impact your sense of life's wonder?

5 (T5C12, 0:28:21–0:29:24) Grace is seeing her doctor and talking about how she and her grandfather only have each other. The physician has his head down writing notes and making perfunctory comments. He tells her to "add these to your morning medications." Grace reflects that she should be happy just to be alive. The doctor leaves the room and Grace makes a flip remark to the nurse that the doctor is a good listener.

    a. What does the doctor do well? What could he do better?

    b. How might the physician have expressed empathy and understanding rather than becoming preoccupied with his notes?

    c. In what ways are empathy and understanding vital to successful doctor-patient interactions?

Post-Transplant Surgery

1 (T5C13, 0:29:58–0:31:17) Grace and Megan are walking around at the zoo. Grace debates whether to mail an anonymous letter she has been carrying around thanking the family who donated their loved one's heart, which she received in the transplant.

    a. What do you think about Megan's comment that she is sure that, 1 year past, the donor's family has moved on?

    b. What is a realistic time line for grieving the loss of a loved one?

2 (T5C19, 1:02:24–1:03:00) Grace is sitting at a mirror looking at her midline chest scar in the mirror.

    a. What thoughts might Grace be having?

    b. How could heart transplant (and other major) surgery(ies) and their resulting scars affect a patients desire and ability to find a love relationship and engage in sexual intimacy?

    c. What advice would you give a woman in a similar position as Grace or one who has a scar from a surgery such as a mastectomy?

3 (T5C21, 1:10:03–1:10:27) Grace is out on a first date with Bob, who asked her about her parents. She tells him that her mother died of heart disease when Grace was 5 years old and her father took off when her mother's illness interfered with his plans.

    a. What are the rates of heart disease in women? How do these compare with men?

    b. Contrast the stressors that contribute to heart disease in men and women.

Paris (2008; Romain Duris, Juliette Binoche, Fabrice Luchini, Albert Dupontel, François Cluzet [with French subtitles]): Pierre (Duris) is a young cabaret dancer sidelined by a heart condition, and awaiting a risky transplant surgery. His sister, Élise (Binoche), gives up her work as a social worker to help care for him. She and her children move in with him. Pierre confides to her that one of his distractions is watching the people in the streets of Paris from his apartment window, their lives gradually intersecting with a diverse array of strangers.

1 (0:04:28–0:04:56) In this scene, we see an echocardiogram of a beating heart. A doctor is explaining what is going on to Pierre who is looking on. The doctor points to the center of the heart, noting that the heart beat is irregular, that the treatment seems to be helping but … and the scene cuts off at this point.

    a. What are the advantages of taking time to educate patients about bodily organs germane to their diseases?

   b. How do cardiologists determine who is a candidate for heart transplant (i.e. age, diagnosis, history of other conditions, history of addictive behavior, and so forth)?

   c. How can a cardiologist best bring up the issue of a heart transplant with a patient (i.e. leave time to fully explore the issue; balance realism (what will happen if the transplant does not occur) with optimism (80% 1- to 2-year survival rate post transplant with favorable long-term survival, as well; review details of why, where, by whom, and so forth).

2 (0:07:12–0:07:32) Pierre is out of breath and rests after climbing stairs in his apartment building. An older woman following tells him that he is "like an old geezer and needs to exercise," unaware of his heart condition.

   a. What impact might this interaction have on Pierre's compliance with his medical regimen?

   b. How can patients' social networks either help or hinder their motivation to follow their medical regimen?

Communication with Family Members

1 (0:09:36–0:12:56) Pierre sits down with his sister, Élise, and tells her that he is sick and that his days are numbered. He says that he may need a heart transplant. She yells at him for not telling her sooner and then apologizes, asking if he has told their parents, which he has not done (and wishes not to). Out his window, Pierre watches other people live their lives and tells Élise that they become the heroes of little stories that he imagines.

   a. Why do patients sometimes choose to not tell close family members about their serious medical conditions?

   b. How would you advise a patient who asked you to keep their medical condition a secret from his or her loved ones?

2 (0:33:20–0:35:35) Élise comes from behind Pierre as he is looking out the window. They debate how to disclose his situation to her children. She wants to make up a less harsh reality for them – namely, that he is weak and not working – while he opts for being straight with the children. In the end, Pierre answers the children's questions.

   a. How would you advise a patient in a situation like this? What factors might you take into account (i.e. age of children; others stressors in the children's lives; preferences of the spouse, aunt, uncle, and so forth) when advising a patient to either tell or fudge the truth with their offspring?

3 (0:48:35–0:49:47) Pierre is seen at his cardiologist's office after feeling sick. He tells his doctor that he just had one beer because of intense cravings. The doctor reminds him that, "with beta-blockers and the other medications, one drop of alcohol and you vomit." His physician tells him that the whole team will need to see him more regularly (including an endocrinologist and psychiatrist) and that they all recommend a transplant. The scene concludes

as they walk out into the hallway and we hear the doctor telling Pierre that he is doubling his dose of digoxin.

    a. What do you make of this physician's response to the patient's having had a drink? How would you have handled the situation?

    b. What is the interaction of alcohol with beta-blockers and other heart medicines?

    c. What are the interpersonal and legal problems posed by concluding a patient interview in a hallway? How could this interchange have been handled differently?

4 (1:59:00–2:02:19) Pierre is in a taxi headed to the hospital for transplant surgery. In the days and months before this time, he has become a keen observer of the human condition. As he is driven through the streets of Paris, he reflects on the people doing everyday things and not realizing how lucky they are – walking, breathing, running late. We see images of various people while the background music slows down and then stops.

    a. What do members of the transplant team do to help prepare patients for heart transplant surgery?

    b. Is there a role for the referring cardiologist in helping their patients (and patients' families) prepare emotionally for heart transplant surgery?

Disclosure Following Heart Transplant

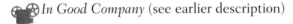*In Good Company* (see earlier description)

1 (T5C27, 1:34:45–1:36:27) Grace tells Bob that she is going away and that over a year ago she had surgery … a heart transplant. She tells him that she did not know, referring to the fact that Bob's deceased wife was her donor.

    a. What barriers might people have to revealing that they are the recipient of an organ donation?

    b. Reflect on the feelings that Bob might have upon hearing the news that his deceased wife was Grace's donor?

Further Reading

- Prasad A, Lerman A, Rihal CS. Apical ballooning syndrome (Tako-Tsubo or stress cardiomyopathy): a mimic of acute myocardial infarction. *Am Heart J*. 2008; **155**(3): 408–17.
- Sharkey SW, Lesser JR, Zenovich AG, *et al*. Acute and reversible cardiomyopathy provoked by stress in women from the United States. *Circulation*. 2005; **111**(4): 472–9.
- Wittstein IS, Thiemann DR, Lima JA, *et al*. Neurohumoral features of myocardial stunning due to sudden emotional stress. *N Engl J Med*. 2005; **352**(6): 539–48.

The Emergence of a Chronic Illness: HIV

Patricia Lenahan & Hans House

THE TERMS HIV AND AIDS HAVE INSPIRED MANY EMOTIONS AMONG health-care providers, patients and communities. Stigma, shame, isolation, and abandonment have accompanied this diagnosis. Randy Shilts's 1987 book *And the Band Played On* (subsequently made into a TV docudrama in 1993) offers one of the better-known histories of the early HIV epidemic. Initially, HIV/AIDS was viewed as a terminal illness. However, as more scientific information and newer classifications of drugs and treatments have become available, HIV/AIDS has become a chronic illness for those who have access to the medications and who adhere to the treatment regimen.

Despite treatment advances, HIV remains an ongoing health crisis that disproportionately affects racial and ethnic minorities. Women and minority group members comprise a significant percentage of new infections and are considered vulnerable populations who are at high risk for developing HIV. These communities already face innumerable disparities and challenges including: poverty, substance abuse, homelessness, unequal access to health care, and low levels of literacy and health literacy. Multiple studies cite a link between sexually transmitted disease, intimate partner violence, lack of personal empowerment, and other factors, with increased risks of developing HIV for minority women. Minority women may also have significant comorbidities including substance abuse, depression, posttraumatic stress disorder, and intimate partner violence.

Recent data from the World Health Organization and Centers for Disease Control and Prevention provide a startling reality of this complex disease. HIV/ AIDS has become a global pandemic, with populations in sub-Saharan Africa at high risk. Cultural myths also have contributed to increasing rates of infection in children, while many other children are left as orphans.

HIV and AIDS: Then and Now
• •

Angels in America (2003; Ben Shenkman, Justin Kirk, Jeffrey Wright, Al Pacino, Emma Thompson, Patrick Wilson, James Cromwell): Made for HBO, *Angels in America* is an adaptation of Tony Kushner's Pulitzer Prize–winning play about AIDS in New York in 1985. At this time, AIDS is a new disease and little if any treatment is available. The story centers on four gay men and their friends and family as they struggle to deal with their homosexuality and their mortality. The six-part miniseries is available on two discs.

1 (Disk 1, track 1, 0:17:40–0:19:44) Prior (Justin Kirk) shows his partner, Louis (Ben Shenkman), his first Kaposi's sarcoma lesion, shocking and horrifying Louis. Prior deals with the news differently, cracking puns about the cancer's name.
   a. What are the Kübler-Ross stages of grief? Where stage is Prior at on this continuum from denial to acceptance? How about Louis?
   b. What would you do to help Louis in hearing the news of his partner's illness?

2 (Disk 1, track 1, 0:49:30–0:51:47) Prior and Louis talk in bed. Prior describes the symptoms of his disease including proteinuria, chronic diarrhea, and hematochezia. Louis does not think he can cope with Prior's illness.
   a. What are some of HIV's effects on the kidneys? What effect do antiretroviral medications have on the body?
   b. How is Prior's illness affecting their relationship?
   c. Does Louis have an ethical duty to Prior? Is he justified in focusing his concern on his own health?

3 (Disk 1, track 1, 0:53:50–1:01:40) Ray Cohn (Al Pacino) is being examined by his physician, Henry (James Cromwell). Henry describes the course and pathology of HIV to Ray, and informs him that he likely has the disease.
   a. Henry lists a number of conditions from which Ray is suffering. Which of these are AIDS-defining illnesses?
   b. Ray explodes at his doctor for stating that he acquired HIV from homosexual contact. How does Ray view his own sexuality? How has he convinced himself of this view?
   c. Ray insists that he has liver cancer, not AIDS. If you were Ray's health-care provider, how would address his denial?

4 (Disk 1, track 2, 1:01:48–1:03:39) Prior's condition worsens, as he awakens with dyspnea, fever, and bloody diarrhea. Yet he begs Louis not to call an ambulance.
   a. Why doesn't Prior want to go to the hospital? What does he fear?
   b. Louis' horror at Prior's condition grows stronger. What does Louis fear?
   c. If you were to see Prior as a patient in his depicted condition, what would be your treatment priorities? How would you approach his stabilization?

5 (Disk 1, track 3, 2:02:20–2:06:00) Prior is being examined by Nurse Emily (Emma Thompson) and describes his symptoms, including nausea, diarrhea,

and a "fuzzy tongue." His dentist says "yuck" when looking in Prior's mouth and has taken to wearing condoms on his fingers. Prior then describes the funeral of a friend who died of "bird TB" and that he was afraid to go to the funeral because he might catch "bird TB." We then see Prior manifest religious hallucinations.

   a. How do the actions of Louis and Prior's dentist contribute to Prior's sense of isolation and shame?

   b. What are some of the many causes of diarrhea in patients with AIDS?

   c. What does Prior mean by "bird TB"? Can he catch it from a corpse? How is it acquired?

   d. How do hallucinations relate to AIDS?

   e. How can you put patients more at ease when conducting a history and physical?

Coping with the Initial Diagnosis and Partner Notification

El Cantante (2006): This film is based on the true story of Puerto Rican salsa singer Hector Lavoe (Marc Anthony), known as El Cantante. The story of Hector's rise to stardom and ultimate fall due to alcohol, drugs, and depression is told through the eyes of his wife, Puchi (Jennifer Lopez). The film alternates between watching Hector's rise and Puchi's soliloquies about their life together.

1 (0:1:23:27–0:1:24:28) Hector is in the doctor's office. The physician tells him that he is HIV positive and that it doesn't matter how he got it. He suggests that Puchi should be tested, "just in case." Hector returns home and shares the information with Puchi. He tries to reassure her by saying that the disease may not show symptoms for years.

   a. What approaches might be helpful in delivering bad news?

   b. What advice might be helpful for an HIV-positive patient to share his status with his partner?

Yesterday (2005): This film is set in the KwaZulu-Natal province of South Africa, an area that has been disproportionately affected by HIV/AIDS. The story focuses on one family coping with HIV: Yesterday (Leleti Khumalo), her daughter, Beauty (Lihle Mvelase), and her husband, John (Kenneth Kambule).

1 (0:38:01–0:40:38) Yesterday (Leleti Khumalo) learns that she is HIV positive. The physician tells her that her husband should be tested. Yesterday embarks on a long journey to Johannesburg where her husband works in a mine. Yesterday waits for her husband to emerge from the mines after his shift. She shares her diagnosis with him and he beats her. The mine supervisor looks out his window and observes the violence but does nothing.

   a. What are the potential risks in sharing a diagnosis of HIV with a partner?

   b. How might the physician have helped Yesterday in addressing this issue?

c. What is the prevalence of intimate partner violence associated with HIV?

One Week (2000): This film follows Varon Thomas (Kenny Young), his fiancée Kiya (Saadiqa Muhammed), and Varon's friend, Tyco (Eric Lane), in the week prior to Varon's wedding when he is informed that one of his former sexual partners has tested positive for HIV.

1 (1:22:52–1:27:06) Varon is sitting on the bed, again trying to reach Kiya on the phone. He picks up the gun and cocks the trigger, putting it to his head. The screen goes black as the gun goes off. In a flash back, the scene shifts to the health center where Varon is waiting to be seen. Kiya joins him unexpectedly. They walk in to the office hand in hand to hear the results of the HIV test. The scene shifts again to a montage of photos of their wedding, of Varon attending classes at Chicago State and pictures of their baby. It ends with a billboard for the health center. It shows Varon and Kiya with the caption: "Living with HIV."
   a. What factors contribute to Varon's resiliency?
   b. What is the role of family, community and spiritual supports? How can they be mobilized to assist HIV-positive individuals?
   c. How can resiliency be identified and used therapeutically?
   d. What was the impact of Kiya's demonstration of support?

2 (0:23:16–0:27:25) Varon and his fiancée Kiya are sitting in the health center waiting for him to be called in to see the worker. Stacy Watts (Pam Mack), the worker, explains why she needed to see him, says she cannot reveal the name of the person who named him, and explains partner notification. Bryon responds, "I ain't burnin'." Stacy reports that one of his former sexual partners has tested positive for HIV. She urges him to get tested and explains the privacy aspects of the testing. The results will be available in 1 week … after his scheduled wedding. Byron reluctantly agrees to the test. He lies to his fiancée about the reason for the visit.
   a. Varon says that he isn't "burning." What type of sexually transmitted infection does Varon assume Stacy will test for?
   b. How does Varon react when Stacy tells him that one of his partners is HIV positive?
   c. What would have been a better way to deliver this news to a patient?

3 (0:32:00–0:33:00) Varon stands in front of the bathroom mirror, examines his face, his sclera, and feels his genitals.
   a. What signs and symptoms is Varon looking for?
   b. What knowledge does he have about HIV and its symptoms?
   c. How can patients be better prepared to understand this disease?

4 (0:43:00–0:46:30) Tyco, Varon's friend who has been sleeping on his couch, comes to Varon's work and begs him to leave work. While they are driving, Tyco tells him that he is HIV positive.
   a. What feelings and initial reactions can be evoked when learning a friend is HIV positive?

b. Varon is still awaiting for his own test results. How does Tyco's admission of his HIV status affect him?

5 (0:48:00–0:48:56) Varon and Tyco are talking about his former sexual partner who tested positive for HIV. While they are talking, Varon learns that he has had sex with the same woman as Tyco.
   a. What reactions might be expected?
   b. How does Varon respond to this information?

6 (0:54:17–0:55:53) Varon wants to tell Kiya about the HIV test, but before he has a chance to do so, she tells him that she is pregnant.
   a. What are the risks of transmitting HIV to a partner?
   b. What are the risks of transmitting HIV to an unborn child?
   c. What anticipatory advice would have been helpful for Varon to have received from his health-care provider or clinic?
   d. How might the health-care provider have assisted Varon in preparing to discuss his HIV test and possible results with his fiancée?

7 (1:09:56–1:11:35) Varon arrives late for his wedding rehearsal. He tells Kiya that they need to talk. He tells her that he was fired and about the HIV test. Kiya hits him and announces to everyone that the wedding is off.
   a. What is the potential impact of both losses (job and health status)?
   b. How would you evaluate Kiya's response?
   c. How might this discussion have been handled better?

Suicide and Suicidality

1 (1:17:21–18:56) Varon returns home to find that Tyco committed suicide in the bathroom. The gun is still in his hand and the walls are covered with blood. The scene ends when the police arrive and the coroner removes the body.
   a. What interventions might have helped Tyco?
   b. What is the impact of Tyco's suicide on Varon since he fears that he is also HIV positive?
   c. What type of trauma therapy might be helpful to Varon?

2 (1:19:01–1:19:23) Varon scrubs the bathroom walls to remove the blood. The water in the sink turns red.
   a. What is the impact of a completed suicide on the person who finds the victim?
   b. What types of trauma services would be useful to assist Varon in coping with the death of his friend in his home?

Life Support (2007; Queen Latifah): Made for HBO, this film is based on the true-life story of an HIV-positive African-American woman, Ana (Queen Latifah), and three generations of her family in Brooklyn. Ana lost custody of her daughter because of her drug use. Years later, she is trying to get her life back together and to repair relationships with her mother and teenage daughter. At the same time, she is working for Life Support, a community outreach group focusing on HIV/AIDS awareness, prevention, and support for women.

1   (1:10:25–1:16:30) Ana (Queen Latifah) receives a phone call in the middle of the night. Someone has spotted Amare (Evan Ross), a friend of her teenage daughter who is HIV positive because of drug use and has stopped taking his antiretroviral medications. Ana and her husband, Slick (Wendell Pierce), find Amare sitting on a park bench, looking at his sister's apartment window. Amare is coughing, sweating, and breathing with difficulty. Amare reminisces about observing Ana and his parents using drugs when he was a child and his subsequent rejection by his sister. Ana unsuccessfully tries to reach Amare's sister and calls 911 for Amare's attempted suicide. The scene shifts to the hospital, with Ana telling her daughter that Amare might not make it.
   a. What is the role of the family in the life of the HIV-positive individual?
   b. What are the effects of childhood exposures to drugs?
   c. How might a health-care provider have intervened with Amare?
   d. What might have motivated Amare to adhere to his treatment regimen? What factors are associated with decreased adherence in adolescents who are HIV positive?
   e. What are the risk factors for suicide? What factors might mediate these risks?

HIV and Intravenous Drug Use

1   (0:00:07–0:02:14) Various women meet at a support group and discuss how they acquired HIV. One woman shares that she was with a man whom she knew was "shooting drugs." "I told him to get a test before we did anything, but then I threw it all out the closet … $10000 in this arm and $5000 in this arm … he talks about being tested … I'm ready to kill him, kill myself." Another woman shares that she told herself "it was all BS." He was with another woman and shot drugs. I was young, he was older … I asked him and he said no … a basket of condoms sat there."
   a. How can a prospective sexual partner initiate a discussion about HIV testing?
   b. What are the risks associated with HIV transmission and intravenous drug use? What precautions should prospective sexual partners take?
   c. How would you interpret the second woman's statement about the basket of condoms sitting there? How can health-care providers empower women to assume greater responsibility for their sexual health?
2   (0:28:03–0:29:35) Ana leads a group. She tells the women: "if your man just came out of prison, get him tested." She then goes on to share her story of living with the virus for 10 years, telling the group that she and her husband are both HIV positive and shot cocaine. Ana ends the group saying, "If you'll

stop dying, I'll stop talking about it." One woman stays behind and asks Ana, "how would you suggest that I talk to my man about taking the test?"

a. What are the risks of acquiring HIV among incarcerated males?
b. How would you interpret Ana's statement: "if you'll stop dying, I'll stop talking about it"?
c. How would you counsel a woman who was reticent to ask her partner to be tested?

Women and HIV

All of Us (2008): This documentary film focuses on Mehret Mandefro, an Ethiopian-American internal medicine resident at Montefiore Medical Center who treats many HIV-positive African-American women. Dr. Mandefro wants to understand why so many women of color are affected and decides to develop a research project on HIV and minority women. The movie focuses on two of Dr. Mandefro's patients.

1 (0:5:12–0:6:26) Viewers are introduced to Chevelle Wilson, a 37-year-old HIV-positive woman. Chevelle shares that she used to have sex for drugs. Chevelle takes Dr. Mandefro to the area where she traded sex for drugs and says she doesn't like to go there because it's a "relapse trigger." As they are walking in the area, Chevelle hugs a man, a janitor from a local school. Afterwards, Chevelle shares that he used to be one of her "tricks." Chevelle says: "Men was a drug for me."
   a. How would you respond to Chevelle's statement that men were a drug for her?
   b. What is a relapse trigger?
   c. Chevelle says that her old hangouts are relapse triggers for her. What advice would you give a patient regarding coping with relapse triggers?

2 (0:7:06–0:10:12) Tara Stanley, aged 36, is also HIV positive and has early stage cervical cancer. Dr. Mandefro makes a home visit and Tara talks about her family, telling the doctor that she grew up in a family of heroin addicts, that she was physically abused by her mother, and sexually abused by a man in her mother's life. Tara says: "my mother pimped me out until I was 25" and that she had been abused and raped. She also shares that she had been in an abusive relationship. When questioned about her HIV status, Tara says: "I didn't have any self-esteem" and that she was promiscuous and didn't use condoms.
   a. How does childhood sexual abuse impact women?
   b. What is the incidence of HIV-positive status in women who have been sexually abused as children?
   c. What additional risk factors are associated with HIV in women?
   d. What is the prevalence of HIV-positive status in minority women?

3 (0:17:04–0:18:25) Tara explains that she had surgery to remove her vulva

because cancer had invaded the skin. She says she is "not just fighting one disease, I'm fighting two." The scene shifts to the obstetrics and gynecology office, where the physician tells her that she will need another surgery. Tara responds: "I just hope my numbers don't drop."

a. How would you assess Tara's health literacy?

b. Tara acknowledges that she is fighting not one, but two diseases. How would you respond to this statement?

c. What is Tara's understanding of her cervical cancer (in light of her stated concern about her "numbers dropping")?

4 (0:24:20–0:26:00) Dr. Mandefro visits Tara at home after her surgery. There are pills all around the nightstand and the room is in disarray. Tara rests on her side, the only position that doesn't make her hurt. She says she feels like giving up with the pain. Tara shares that after the surgery she "feels funny as a woman," adding: "I don't recognize myself down there."

a. What anticipatory guidance/patient education might have prepared Tara for the surgery and the postoperative period? How would you involve her partner in this discussion?

b. How would you respond to Tara's statement "I don't recognize myself down there"?

c. What are the sexual aspects of this surgery? What are the possible psychological sequelae?

HIV and Pregnancy

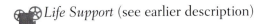

Life Support (see earlier description)

1 (0:11:25–0:13:25) Deyah (Chyna Layne) walks into the center and talks with Ana. Deyah is pregnant and HIV positive. She isn't taking her medications and hasn't told her husband of her HIV status. She tells Ana that she was HIV positive when she had her daughter 9 years ago. Deyah says she wants a healthy baby and wants to go back to Jamaica to see the "Obeah Man." Ana advises her to take her medications and to tell her husband about her HIV status.

a. What is the role of culture in disease management?

b. How might Ana have responded in a more culturally sensitive way?

c. What are the risks of HIV transmission in pregnancy?

d. What precautions should Deyah take?

e. How would you advise Deyah to initiate the discussion about being HIV positive with her husband? What are the potential risks of such disclosures?

The Role of Education and Support Groups

Rent (2005; Anthony Rapp, Adam Pascal, Rosario Dawson, Jesse L. Martin, Wilson Jermaine Heredia, Taye Diggs): Rent is a film adaptation of the Broadway musical by Jonathan Larson. Based on the opera *La Bohème*, the musical tells the story of a group of artists in New York's East Village, struggling with life, relationships, finding money to pay the rent, and with HIV infection. The film is set in the early 1990s, before the advent of highly active antiretroviral therapy. Despite this, the messages about grief and a sense of isolation still ring true for patients with HIV today.

1   (0:38:10–0:41:50) Mark (Anthony Rapp) arrives at a community HIV support group and stumbles when introducing himself. One of the members shares his concerns and the group sings their support.

   a. When Roger introduces himself to the group, his verbal stumble creates a separation between him and the support group members. When meeting a patient with HIV, what can you do to put that patient at ease?

   b. What are the concerns faced by the members of the support group?

   c. How can you help a patient with these same fears?

   d. What support services are available in your hospital or community?

All of Us (see earlier description)

1   (0:35:40–0:38:30) Dr. Mandefro joins Chevelle at her HIV women's group. One of the women says that she only had sex with one man and that he was on the "down low." She says she will remain a spinster.

   a. What is the impact of HIV-positive status on sexuality and dating?

   b. How would you respond to this woman's statement?

   c. What does the "down low" refer to?

   d. What are the risks of being on the "down low" on other relationships?

2   (0:41:56–0:44:30) Mehret (Dr. Mandefro) decides to hold a "truth circle" with her friends before she has one with patients. Her goal is to learn more about the sexual behaviors of women. Mehret describes her friends as "successful, educated, and multicultural," a contrast with her patients. During the truth circle, several of the women share that they didn't use condoms consistently or at all, despite what they know about disease transmission.

   a. What are the ethical issues involved here?

   b. How do the comments of her self-described "educated and successful" friends contribute to her understanding of the complexities of HIV prevention?

   c. What is the impact of sexual knowledge versus personal empowerment? How generalizable is this information? How could this type of group knowledge affect prevention programs?

Life Support (see earlier description)

1   (0:22:11–0:23:52) Sandra (Gloria Reuben) shares at the support group. She tells the group that she has met someone, but that she hasn't told him yet that she is HIV positive. Sandra says she plans to tell him this weekend. Another woman in the group responds by saying that rejection is hard. She adds: "Some say to give him the condom, others say just come straight out with it."

   a. What are social and emotional consequences of revealing one's status as HIV positive?
   b. How can an individual's HIV status affect decisions about sexual activity?
   c. What are the effects of rejection when HIV status is revealed?
   d. How can a therapist help an HIV-positive individual explore possible responses of key people in that person's life?

2   (0:9:45–0:11:17) Ana meets at the center with other peer counselors. She holds a female condom. She tells them that a younger woman asked her what it was. Ana adds: "older women don't know about it." She discusses the advantages of the female condom with the women, i.e. that women can wear it for a while, that they can be prepared. Ana tells the peer educators that they can order the vagina demonstrator to use as a teaching aid.

   a. What does Ana mean when she says, "older women don't know about it"?
   b. How would you counsel a woman on condom use? Female condoms? What are the advantages and disadvantages of female versus male condoms?

HIV in Incarcerated Populations

Carandiru (2003): This film is based on the book *Estação Carandiru* (*Carandiru Station*), a true story of the work of Dr. Dráuzio Varella, a Brazilian physician who served as an unpaid doctor at the overcrowded Carandiru Prison in São Paulo from 1989 to 2001. In the movie, Dr. Varella (Luis Carlos Vasconcelos) is seen caring for the more than 8000 inmates, listening to their stories and learning more about the transmission of HIV/AIDS, a disease that affected many of the prisoners. (Carandiru prison was the site of the "Carandiru massacre" in 1992. This incident ultimately led to the closure of the facility.)

1   (0:12:51–0:15:30) Dr. Varella (Luis Carlos Vasconcelos) interviews and examines various HIV-positive patients. Some of the patients/prisoners also are intravenous drug users and dealers while others contracted the disease through unprotected sexual contact with male and female partners. The patients share their stories with the doctor. One prisoner tells the doctor: "You come in here sick and they treat you with respect."

   a. What are the challenges in caring for an HIV-positive population who are incarcerated?
   b. What types of prevention efforts would be effective in working with this patient population?

    c. How would you interpret the prisoner's statement that one is treated with respect if ill?

2 (0:27:34–0:29:12) Dr. Varella interviews "Lady Di" (Rodrigo Santoro), a transvestite. Lady Di states that she doesn't do drugs but smokes pot. The doctor asks Lady Di how many sexual partners she has had and she replies, "about 2000."

    a. How would you respond to this patient?

    b. What prevention techniques might be effective with this patient?

3 (1:28:30–1:30:45) Lady Di and her partner, Dr. Varella's assistant, get their HIV test results. Lady Di opens hers and begins to cry, "I'm clean!" Her partner responds: "You've had over 2000 men and you're clean? We're both clean!"

    a. What are the risks of HIV infection among sex workers?

    b. How can the health-care community provide preventive services to sex workers?

    c. What are the risks for developing HIV in incarcerated populations? What factors can contribute to this risk? How can this risk be mitigated?

HIV-Related Disorders

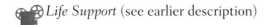

Life Support (see earlier description)

1 (0:48:21–0:49:21) Ana sees her physician who asks her to describe how the sensations in her feet have changed and if the Neurontin helps. Ana admits that she stopped taking the medication because she "couldn't get past the bathroom." The doctor can replace it with Vicodin, but advises Ana to slow down or she could lose the use of her feet. The doctor continues to talk about HIV and its effects. Ana responds: "What do you want me to do? Lie in bed and think about dying?"

    a. How would you characterize this interchange between the doctor and Ana?

    b. How can health-care providers minimize the likelihood of nonadherence to medical regimens?

    c. What are the risks of prescribing Vicodin to a recovering drug addict?

All of Us (see earlier description)

1 (0:51:50–0:53:41) Chevelle and Mehret are talking about Chevelle's fiancé, Robert, who also is HIV positive, and the plans for their wedding. Chevelle says that she loves Robert with "all my heart" but also acknowledges that he gets on her nerves. Chevelle shares with Mehret that Robert has HIV-dementia. The scene shifts to Chevelle picking up Robert at the hospital, a discussion of the upcoming wedding and greeting their son, Robert Jr., when they get home.

a. What are the effects on a caregiver who is also HIV positive?

b. What kinds of stressors does the caregiver experience as the disease progresses? How does this decline affect the HIV-positive caregiver?

c. What are some guidelines on when and how to talk with children about a parent's HIV status?

Loss/Death

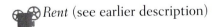*Rent* (see earlier description)

1 (0:50:30–0:54:17) Roger copes with the loss of his girlfriend from AIDS and struggles to acknowledge his own HIV-positive status. After Mark encourages Roger (Adam Pascal) to go out with the group that night, he makes his way to the community support group, joining Tom (Jesse L. Martin) and Angel (Wilson Jermaine Heredia). The group sings their fear of dying alone and without dignity.

2 (1:40:30–1:45:21) Roger is frustrated with Mimi (Rosario Dawson), who used her past relationship with the landlord Benny (Taye Diggs) to secure the group's rent problem and then re-starts using heroin. As the song, "Without You" plays, a montage of the support group gets smaller and smaller. Finally, Angel takes ill and succumbs to an opportunistic infection.

a. Describe the context of the musical. How has therapy for HIV changed since it was written?

b. Do you believe patients today are any less fearful of the diagnosis?

c. Review the use of viral load and CD4 count in tracking disease severity.

d. Opportunistic infections have become less common since the development of highly active antiretroviral therapy, but they still occur. Which infections have you experienced as a clinician?

e. Angel develops lesions on his chest before he dies. What are these lesions and have you seen a patient with this condition?

Life Support (see earlier description)

1 (1:19:58–1:22:30) The peer counselors of the outreach group, Life Support, organize a monthly rooftop memorial where they release balloons for those who have died. Family, friends, and supporters attend the memorial. As the group gathers and begins to release their balloons, Ana reminds everyone in attendance what this ceremony is about: "for those who struggle with the virus, the fears, those who fear us, those who judge us, ignore us, for those we love and who love us, and for those who stand with us: the doctors, nurses, friends and family."

a. How would you interpret these comments?

b. What impact does this ceremony have on the survivors and family?

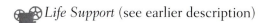*Yesterday* (see earlier description)

1   (0:1:22:40–0:1:24:26) The teacher joins Yesterday at John's grave outside the village. She says she has seen her visiting the gravesite every day throughout the winter. Yesterday now has multiple lesions on her face and neck and seems more fragile. The teacher reminds Yesterday that school will be starting next week and talks about how much she is looking forward to teaching Beauty. Reluctantly, the teacher adds that, when the time comes, she will love Beauty as if she were her own daughter.
    a.   At what point should an HIV-positive parent discuss his or her status with his or her children?
    b.   Beauty has lost one parent to HIV. What social and emotional effects occur in children who grieve the loss of a parent?
    c.   Beauty is getting ready to begin school. In view of the villagers' concerns about the virus, how might this affect Beauty's ability to make friends?
    d.   What anticipatory guidance should health-care providers offer to HIV-positive parents?

Impact on Health-Care Providers

Life Support (see earlier description)

1   (0:44:36–0:45:14) Ness (Tony Rock) is attends a support group. He tells the group that he contracted HIV during the 2 years he spent "shooting up." Ness is now taking azidothymidine (AZT) and talks about his experience getting his AZT prescription filled. Ness states "the guy behind the counter was all cool until he saw what it was … he put the paper up on the counter like he'd catch it."
    a.   In what ways do the reactions of health-care providers affect the patient's potential adherence to a medical regimen or their motivation for treatment?
    b.   How can an experience like this affect a patient's emotional well-being?
    c.   What is the role of shame and stigma in individuals with HIV? How can health-care providers reduce such feelings?

Angels in America (see earlier description)

1   (Disk 2, track 2, 1:18:00–1:20:50) In the hospital room, Joe (Patrick Wilson) tells Roy that he is gay. Roy stands and rips out his intravenous line, dripping blood on the floor and on Joe.
    a.   How would you respond to this scene? What concerns would you have?
    b.   How do you utilize universal precautions in the hospital?
    c.   Would you touch the skin of a patient with HIV without gloves? Would

you shake their hand? What if you knew they didn't have HIV? What if their status is unknown?

2   (Disk 2, track 1, 0:09:30–0:16:00) Roy is a patient in the hospital under the care of Belize (Jeffery Wright). He is very abusive toward Belize, even demanding to be treated by a white nurse.

   a. How does Belize remain professional in the face of such abuse? How would you react?

   b. Explain the concept of transference.

   c. How would you respond to a patient with a terminal disease who says, "Am I going to die?"

   d. Describe the risks and benefits of a double blind trial. When is it ethically acceptable to offer patients a 50/50 chance of getting only a placebo? What benefits does a placebo demonstrate?

3   (Disk 2, track 1, 0:46:45–0:51:20) Roy uses his political connections and acquires his own supply of AZT. Continuing to abuse Belize, he relents to part with some of his supply only when Belize plays his game of insults.

   a. In general, patients with greater resources have access to more specialized care. Does this result in better outcomes? How does society determine what health-care resources are essential?

   b. Belize exceeds his scope of practice by taking Roy's medication. Does the end justify the means in this case?

   c. How effective is AZT monotherapy for HIV infection?

   d. How do you respond to a patient asking, "Am I going to die?"

   e. Describe the risks and benefits of a double-blind trial. When is it ethically acceptable to offer patients a 50/50 chance of getting only a placebo? What benefits do a placebo demonstrate?

Carandiru (see earlier description)

1   (0:2:18:00–0:2:18:27) Dr. Varella is on the train leaving Carandiru after the massacre. He says that AIDS prevention work in jail took him to Carandiru in the 1980s (he volunteered as an unpaid physician at Carandiru from 1989 to 2001). His reverie continues: "I heard stories, made real friends, learned medicine and penetrated a few of the mysteries of life in jail which would have remained inaccessible if I were not a doctor."

   a. What prompts a physician to engage in volunteer service?

   b. What expectations might a health-care provider have in working in a prison?

   c. Dr. Varella says he has made real friends and learned medicine at Carandiru. How would you interpret this statement?

HIV/AIDS in the Global Arena: The Impact of Culture

3 *Needles* (2005): This film was released on World AIDS Day to bring attention to the global AIDS crisis. The movie takes place in three different geographic regions: an ethnic minority community in rural China, where a black market blood procurer (Lucy Liu) unwittingly causes all but one member of the community to become infected with HIV; the pornography industry in Montreal, where a porn star substitutes his father's blood for his own in order to pass the mandatory monthly tests; and a missionary clinic in South Africa, where children are raped in order to "cure" the plantation workers of their disease.

1 (0:24:00–0:25:00) The black market blood seller (Lucy Liu) goes to the hospital with contractions. The doctor asks her how she knows she is sick. She responds that her father is sick. When the doctor inquires about the father's illness, she replies that he is "like a skeleton." The doctor says that he can't give her any medications without a test. He asks her where she is going to deliver her baby. Her only response is "I'm having contractions 4-to-6 hours apart." The doctor tells her: "you know you can't breast feed the baby?" She later delivers the baby alone in a field.
   a. Why did Liu's character choose not to tell the doctor directly about the HIV?
   b. How did the doctor convey that he understood what she didn't say?
   c. What aspects of doctor-patient communication are evident here?

Yesterday (see earlier description)

1 (1:36:00–1:38:18) A young child is taken to the clinic in South Africa. The nurse states: "this child has been raped." When the child returns home, her older brother is asked how it happened. He explained that it was one of the plantation workers with the virus and the only way to be cured was to pass it on to a virgin.
   a. What is the prevalence of HIV infection in children in sub-Saharan Africa?
   b. What public health approaches are most likely to effect a change in light of prevailing beliefs about causation and cure?
2 (1:05:35–1:07:49) The village teacher arrives at Yesterday's home and asks to talk with her outside. She relates that all the villagers are talking about John, saying that he has "the virus." Yesterday confirms this and adds that she has it, too. Yesterday also shares her fears about everyone knowing, relating a story about a young woman in another village who was stoned to death when her HIV status became known.
   a. What is the impact of these fears on Yesterday?
   b. How can health-care providers inform communities about the realities of this disease?
   c. What are some cultural myths about disease causation?
3 (1:08:00–1:09:47) The villagers talk, saying that John should not be allowed

to live there, fearing that he would infect all of them. The teacher tries to assuage their fears by conducting an educational session in her classroom. She tells the women how HIV is transmitted. She says: "your husbands are bringing it to you." The women react angrily.

   a. What educational programs might be helpful to address the villagers' fears?

   b. How is knowledge about HIV communicated in rural and disadvantaged communities?

   c. How would you characterize the women's responses when the teacher tells them that their husbands are bringing the disease home to them?

Complementary and Alternative Medicine

1 (0:23:08–0:25:54) Yesterday collapses in her doorway and Beauty goes for help. The next day, Yesterday visits the Sangoma (Nandi Nyembe), the village medicine woman. The Sangoma asks her how long she has had the "falling illness." She also questions why Yesterday went to the medical clinic first and not to see her. The Sangoma says she will examine Yesterday and has her breathe into a bag before she throws the shells and stones. The Sangoma tells Yesterday that she has lots of anger and that she must let it go. Yesterday replies that she isn't angry. The Sangoma agrees to treat Yesterday (she inhales vapors from a teapot), but says that the treatment may not help if Yesterday doesn't let go of the anger.

   a. What percentage of HIV-positive individuals utilize complementary and alternative therapies?

   b. What expectations did Yesterday have in seeking help from the Sangoma?

   c. What role do culture-bound syndromes and cultural healers play in HIV treatment?

2 (0:26:45–0:27:50) Yesterday drinks tea with the new teacher in the village whom she befriended. The teacher says she heard about Yesterday's collapse and asked what the Sangoma said. The teacher suggests that maybe Yesterday has diabetes, adding that diabetics can collapse when their sugars are too low. She urges Yesterday to go back to the clinic to see the doctor.

   a. What is the impact of the teacher's concerns?

   b. What does Yesterday think is wrong with her?

3 (1:09:51–1:10:56) Yesterday travels to a hospital in another village where AIDS patients are treated. She is told there isn't any room and that John can be added to the waiting list. Yesterday observes the Sangoma sweeping an empty bed and inquires about it. She's told that the bed will be filled by the evening and that the waiting list is the only recourse for John.

   a. What is the impact of advanced HIV on the caregiver?

   b. What services would have been helpful to Yesterday?

   c. What was the purpose of the Sangoma's sweeping of the bed?

Cultural Barriers to Safe Sex Practices and Partner Notification
· · · · · · · · · · · · · · · ·

1 (0:38:01–0:40:38) Yesterday arrives at the clinic. The doctor asks her if she uses a condom. Yesterday appears stunned and offended, telling the doctor that she is a married woman. The doctor asks her if her husband has any other wives and where he is. Yesterday explains that her husband works in the mines in Johannesburg. The doctor clearly has shared the diagnosis (not seen by viewers) and explains that her husband needs to be tested as soon as possible. Yesterday asks the doctor if she is going to "stop living." The physician has a pained look on her face as she searches for a way to respond to this question.
   a. How might a physician best answer this question?
   b. How can a health-care provider balance reality and preserve a sense of hope?
   c. What other personal information would be helpful for the physician to know about Yesterday in order to respond to this question?

2 (0:56:20–0:59:09) Yesterday's husband, John (Kenneth Kambule), has returned to the village. He sits at the table wrapped in a blanket, sweats, and appears to have chills. His face is covered with lesions. He shares with Yesterday that he used to run to the toilet every 5 minutes at the men's hostel, but that there were no toilets in the mines underground. He adds that he "stunk like an animal" and that no one would come near him. John tells Yesterday that he didn't want to believe what she told him about HIV, until the shift boss made him go see a doctor and the doctor said, "like you," referring to his having the same disease as his wife.
   a. Why did John wait so long to seek medical care? What fears might he have had?
   b. What is the potential impact on employment if someone is HIV positive?
   c. John could not say that he was HIV positive or that he had the virus. He says, "The doctor said like you." Why was he unable to say that he had the virus?

3 (1:00:05–1:01:35) Yesterday is at the clinic. The physician tells her that she is doing very well, that her body is strong and is keeping the disease in check. Yesterday smiles and replies that it isn't her body, pointing to her head. Yesterday says that she's made up her mind to live until her daughter starts school the next year. The doctor seems surprised to learn that Yesterday has a daughter and seems to struggle with this information. Yesterday tells the doctor that John is very ill and in pain. She asks if there is anything the doctor can do for him. The physician replies that she'll see what medications she might have for him.
   a. Why is the doctor seemingly so concerned that Yesterday has a daughter?
   b. Should the doctor suggest that Beauty be tested for HIV?
   c. What are the risks of HIV transmission to children of HIV-positive parents?

Further Reading

- Acevedo V. Cultural competence in a group intervention designed for Latino patients living with HIV/AIDS. *Health Soc Work.* 2008; **33**(2): 111–20.
- Cargill VA, Stone VE. HIV/AIDS: a minority health issue. *Med Clin North Am.* 2005; **89**(4): 895–912.
- Eshel A, Moore A, Mishra M, *et al.* Community stakeholders' perspectives on the impact of the minority AIDS initiative in strengthening HIV prevention capacity in four communities. *Ethn Health.* 2008; **13**(1): 39–54.
- Kurth AE, Celum C, Baeten JM, *et al.* Combination HIV prevention: significance, challenges, and opportunities. *Curr HIV/AIDS Rep.* 2011; **8**(1): 62–72.
- Littlewood RA, Vanable PA. Complementary and alternative medicine use among HIV-positive people: research synthesis and implications for HIV care. *AIDS Care.* 2008; **20**(8): 1002–18.
- Rao D, Pryor JB, Gaddist BW, *et al.* Stigma, secrecy, and discrimination: ethnic/racial differences in the concerns of people living with HIV/AIDS. *AIDS Behav.* 2008; **12**(2): 265–71.

14

The Stakes are Very High: High-Risk Obstetrics

Jo Marie Reilly, Patricia Lenahan & Snezana Begovic

PREGNANCY IS OFTEN ONE OF THE HAPPIEST TIMES IN THE LIFE CYCLE of the family. However, several factors may be present that contribute to potential problems, thus designating the pregnancy "high risk." Factors associated with high-risk pregnancies include the following: (1) age, either young (under 15) or advanced maternal age (over 35); (2) being underweight or obese; (3) a history of difficulties in previous pregnancies; (4) violence during pregnancy; (5) and pre-existing health conditions such as hypertension, diabetes, and being HIV positive. Other health conditions may develop during pregnancy itself: pre-eclampsia, gestational diabetes, and preterm labor. Lifestyle issues such as smoking and alcohol consumption can contribute to potential problems with the fetus. Illicit substance use and abuse also add to risk factors.

Adolescent Pregnancy

The United States has the highest rate of teenage pregnancies in the developed world and the highest teenage abortion rate. Teenage pregnancy is formally defined as a pregnancy in a young woman who has not reached the age of 20 years when the pregnancy ends. It also usually refers to unmarried minors who become pregnant unintentionally.

Teen pregnancy is one of the most difficult experiences a young woman may ever face. In addition, there are significant health risks for both the baby and the mother. Teenagers usually don't receive timely prenatal care, and they have a higher-risk pregnancy because of complications related to pregnancy-induced high blood pressure, preterm labor, and infections. Risks for the baby include low birthweight, intrauterine growth retardation, and premature birth. Both the mother and the baby are also at risk socioeconomically. Teen pregnancy creates an emotional crisis resulting in feelings of shame and fear, as well as stress of how to break the news to parents. Obtaining additional support for teen moms can be challenging.

Education of both medical professionals and teenagers is crucial in the prevention and treatment of teenage pregnancy. Film clips can help demonstrate some of the emotional trauma young women experience and assist medical staff to reflect on how to better manage and support teenage moms.

Juno (2007; Ellen Page, Michael Cera, Jennifer Garner): This movie addresses the impact of a teen's unplanned pregnancy, her emotional changes, and her courageous decision regarding her unborn child. It also depicts health-care professionals who can improve their care of teen moms.

1   (0:05:34–0:06:40) After a positive pregnancy test and on her way home, Juno (Page) plays with a rope and imitates hanging herself. She feels desperate and scared about what to do next. She is also confused about how she could become pregnant after having sexual intercourse only once.
   a. (0:07:06–0:08:22) Juno talks to her friend about her pregnancy and discusses plans with her. She is looking for support from a friend.
2   (0:22:51–0:27:00) After some time, Juno decides to talk to her father and stepmother. When she sits them down, they expect other "bad news" but not that she is pregnant. Juno makes the decision to give the baby up for adoption and receives full parental support and understanding.
   a. What do you think about Juno's reaction?
   b. What do you think of her girlfriend's reaction? How would you assess the level of education Juno and her friend have about sexuality and pregnancy?
   c. What do you think of her parents' response? How typical is this response? How else could they have reacted?
   d. How do you think the parents' prior life experience and behavior affected the way they respond to Juno?
3   (0:17:55–0:19:19) Juno goes to an abortion clinic called Women Now. She is greeted by a receptionist and runs away. Juno decides she is not having an abortion.
   a. What prompted Juno's response?
   b. How would you counsel an adolescent who is considering an abortion?
   c. What legal issues should be considered?
4   (1:23:50–1:25:50) This is the labor scene. Juno delivers a healthy baby boy with support from her stepmother and her friend.
   a. What do you think about how the doctor addressed Juno's labor pain? Should she get pain medications if an epidural was not an option yet?
   b. What is the best way to manage teen labor? How is it usually handled? Do teens experience more pain during labor?
   c. How can a health-care provider counsel and prepare an adolescent patient for labor and delivery?

Difficult Decisions during Pregnancy

Challenges in Facing an Unplanned Pregnancy

Waitress (2007; Keri Russell, Nathan Fillion, Cheryl Hines): This film chronicles a small-town waitress's journey in a troubled marriage with an unplanned and unwanted pregnancy. Her pie-baking gives her an opportunity to start her life again.

1 (Scene 1, 0:2:22–0:3:35) Jenna discovers she is pregnant and the pregnancy is unplanned. She feels it will trap her into staying in an unhappy marriage and she shares this with her friends.
   a. How do you respond to a woman with an unplanned and unwanted pregnancy who feels very alone?
   b. How would you respond if a patient stated, referencing her pregnancy, "Now I'll never get away from Earl"?
   c. How would you screen for abuse during pregnancy?

Knocked Up (2007; Seth Rogen, Katherine Heigl): This is the story of Alison, who gets pregnant after an intoxicated evening with Ben, a man she just met, and their journey through her pregnancy.

1 (Scene 5, 0:3:40–0:5:40) Alison confirms her pregnancy at the doctor's office with Ben present. They are shocked and upset.
   a. How do you respond to a couple who struggles with an unplanned pregnancy and are emotionally upset?
   b. What counseling strategies would you employ to offer pregnancy options to a couple?

Ambivalent Feelings about Pregnancy

Waitress (see earlier description)

1 (0:1:18–0:4:45) Jenna describes the letter she would write to her baby about how she feels about her pregnancy. She describes how unfit and unworthy she feels to be a mother.
   a. How do you respond to a woman who is ambivalent about her pregnancy and has no connection to her infant?
   b. What questions would you ask to assess the severity of her disassociation with her pregnancy?
   c. How helpful would you find the approach depicted by Jenna's friends, of using a journal to help a pregnant woman through a difficult journey?

Cultural/Spiritual Issues Surrounding Pregnancy Decisions

Saved! (2004; Jena Malone, Mandy Moore, Macaulay Culkin, Patrick Fugit): The movie is about the hypocrisy and hype of a religious high school and a teenager's journey growing up, discovering her boyfriend is gay, and in becoming sexually active with him to "cure" him, she becomes pregnant.

1 (0:0:00–0:3:40) Mary discovers she's pregnant. She has a very religious family, friends, and school and she doesn't know how to handle being pregnant.
   a. What counseling strategies would you employ to help a teenage girl who discovers that she is pregnant and all alone?
   b. How would you respond to a family in which cultural and religious factors may cause conflict as they consider options for an unplanned teenage pregnancy?

Tentative Hopes: Pregnancy after Miscarriage

Bloom (2005): This is the intersecting story of the youngest daughter of an upwardly mobile Latino family in Chicago and her court-ordered therapist, Dr. Sharon Greene (Mara Monserrat), who is coping with problems of her own: infertility and concern for her terminally ill mother. Letty (Jessi Perez) barely graduated from high school and, much to the dismay of her mother, soon became pregnant with Lisa, now aged five. Letty's second child, Beto, was born with cerebral palsy. Letty alternately lives with her parents and her new boyfriend, Ernesto, an abusive drug dealer.

1 (0:54:53–0:55:36) Sharon is sitting on the exam table in Dr. Sabbagha's office after having labs drawn. The doctor enters the room smiling and says, "it looks like a go, you're definitely pregnant." Dr. Sabbagha tries to caution Sharon that it is early and that anything can happen, especially with her previous miscarriage. He encourages her to slow down.
   a. How would you assess Dr. Sabbagha's approach?
   b. Do you think Sharon heard his words of caution?
2 (0:55:55–0:57:11) Sharon is sitting looking at an old photo album and smiling when David comes home. She hints that she is very hungry and wants to go out to eat. David is distracted with his phone. Sharon says she is really hungry, now that she's eating for two. She asks David if he heard what she said … that she was pregnant. David embraces Sharon and says how happy he is.
   a. How can health professionals support the "tentative hope" that is present in couples as they discover "they are pregnant"?
   b. What may be the best counsel for very early expectant parents after a very difficult journey to conception, particularly as they are eager to "share their news" with family and friends?

Multiple Miscarriages

1 (1:10:25–1:10:34; 1:13:04–1:15:37) Sharon is in session with a patient when she suddenly grabs her abdomen. The patient asks if she's OK. She tells the patient he will have to leave and as she stands up, she passes out. The scene shifts to the hospital where David sits holding Sharon's hand. When she awakens, Sharon asks what's going on. She says she doesn't remember

anything other than the ambulance ride. David reluctantly tells her that she had to have surgery for a tubal pregnancy. Sharon tearfully asks why this keeps happening to her and why God hates her so much. She adds that she hates God, too, and tells David that she wants to be alone.

a. What are some of the best resources for women who have just lost a pregnancy in the hospital and are grieving? How can her partner best be supported?

b. How can health-care professionals best support a grieving woman who has spiritual needs and is hurt and angry with "her God"?

c. How can the health-care team provide a supportive physical environment for a woman who has lost a child when she is often on the labor and delivery ward and other women are delivering healthy term babies?

Fears about Physician's Care during Pregnancy

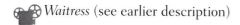*Waitress* (see earlier description)

1 (Scene 3, 0:0:00–0:02:07) Jenna goes for her first prenatal visit and the doctor that she knows and trusts and who delivered her first baby has retired. She is shocked and upset and is distrustful of her new physician.

a. How do you feel when you are with patients who have disappointment and expectations in your care and may not have given you a chance?

b. How do you respond to patients who express disappointments in their pregnancy that may be a manifestation of fear and hurt?

c. How do you "cover for a colleague's" obstetrical patient "on call" when they already have a strong established relationship with another provider?

Labor and Delivery

A Father's Role during Labor and Delivery

Knocked Up (see earlier description)

1 (0:3:10–0:4:36) Jenna is in early labor at home and Ben is trying to support and comfort her as she prepares to go to the hospital.

a. What is the expectation about the role of a father during labor and delivery?

b. How can the health-care provider counsel a couple so that they are best prepared for labor and delivery?

c. How can a physician best include a father in the birth process?

Complications during Delivery

1 (0:2:26–0:5:04) Jenna's baby is having decelerations and she, Ben, and the doctor are stressed in responding to the potential crisis.
   a. How can physicians best prepare patients for potential problems in labor and delivery?
   b. How can physicians help patients develop realistic birth plans as they prepare for childbirth?
   c. How do we best respond to a potential birth crisis and communicate a plan of action to a concerned patient and family?
2 (0:05:45–0:06:50) Jenna's baby is crowning and Jenna is trying to push and breathe through the process.
   a. How can physicians help both comfort and respond to a woman in pain as she delivers her baby?
   b. How can physicians best prepare a pregnant woman for her pregnancy pain management options prior to delivery?

Violence in Pregnancy

Nil By Mouth (1997): This is the story of a working-class London couple, Ray (Ray Winstone) and Val (Kathy Burke), and their multigenerational family, which is beset by many problems including a brother's drug addiction.

1 (Ch 16, 1:14:49–1:18:14) Ray has been drinking and is sitting at the table brooding. He wakes up Val and tells her that he wants to talk to her downstairs now. Ray is upset that Val had been playing pool with friends. He wanted to know where she met one of the men and asked if she was having an affair. He accuses her of having an affair. As Ray becomes increasingly angry, Val looks more scared and begins shaking. Ray continues screaming, calling her names, hitting and kicking Val in the stomach and the abdomen. Val is pregnant. Their daughter, Michelle (Leah Fitzgerald), is seen sitting at the top of the stairs.
   a. What is the incidence of intimate partner violence (IPV) in pregnancy?
   b. How may Val physically and emotionally present to a health-care provider as a pregnant IPV victim?
   c. How does this scene illustrate the power and control that is the hallmark of IPV?
   d. What are some of the physical risks to Val's pregnancy and her developing baby as a result of her abuse?
   e. What legal responsibilities do health-care providers have regarding violence during pregnancy?
2 (Ch 18, 1:22:25–1:25:03) Val is lying in the hospital bed as her mother arrives. Janet confronts Val and says, "It's murder really, isn't it?" She adds: "If they only knew," implying that Val has not shared what actually happened to her with the medical staff. Janet asks Val if Ray knows where she is. Janet

tells her how everyone feels and what they would like to do to Ray. Val is upset that so many people know what happened to her, stating that she didn't want anyone to know. The scene ends with Janet asking Val if she still loves Ray.

a. How can health-care providers best encourage family members and friends to help support an IPV victim?

b. What role should family members play in notifying health-care providers and/or law enforcement about known IPV in a family member's home?

Substance Use and Abuse during Pregnancy

On the Outs (2004): This movie follows the lives of three adolescent girls in the inner city who meet in juvenile detention. Suzette (Anny Marino) was found carrying her boyfriend's gun after he killed another teen, while Marisol (Paola Mendoza) is a teen mother who is addicted to crack cocaine, and Oz (Judy Marte) is a 17-year-old drug dealer and daughter of an addicted mother who is in and out of treatment. Oz acts as a surrogate mother to her mentally challenged brother Chuey (Dominic Colon).

1 (0:23:02–28:34) Evelyn (Ana Garcia, aka Rockafella), Oz's mother, is preparing dinner and talking with Chuey. She tells him that she is making dinner in honor of a call that she received from the treatment program and that a bed has opened up for the following week. As Oz comes in and joins the family, Chuey tells his mother that he wants to buy a new goldfish the next day. When she offers to buy it for him, her mother, Abuela (Gloria Zelaya), sits down and begins to confront Evelyn about her drug use, her stealing, and selling things from the house to buy drugs. Abuela tells Chuey "your mommy stuck Disney in her arm." (This was a reference to Evelyn's taking the money the family had saved for a Disney World vacation and using it to buy drugs.) Abuela continues: "your mommy shot drugs when she was pregnant with you and that's why you are funny in the head." Chuey jumps up from the table and runs to his room, followed by Oz who tries to console him as he cries: "grandma says I'm funny in the head."

a. What are some of the physical risks that a pregnant drug-using woman may impose on her developing infant?

b. How is the pregnancy and labor of a woman with a history of substance abuse best handled (e.g. supporting the pregnant mother and, simultaneously, the health needs/rights of the developing infant)?

c. What resources can a health-care provider best mobilize to help a pregnant woman who is currently "using" to stay clean and sober during and after her pregnancy?

d. How can a health-care provider best support the continued health and well-being of an infant that has been born to a mother who was using illicit substances during her pregnancy?

Infertility and In Vitro Fertilization

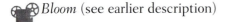

Bloom (see earlier description)

1 (0:20:16–0:22:45) Dr. Sharon Greene (Mara Monserrat) has just finished a session with her patient and calls for the results of her personal pregnancy test. The expectant and hopeful look on her face changes to one of devastation. At home that evening, Sharon paces, bottle of wine in her hand. Her husband, David (Bill Ferris), arrives home and asks what happened today and if she spoke with Dr. Sabbagha. Sharon replies, "it didn't work again." David's attempts to be supportive are met with anger.
   a. What is the impact of failed conception on a marriage?
   b. How would you counsel a spouse/partner in situations like this?

2 (0:23:06–0:25:34) Sharon goes into the kitchen and David follows her. He asks when Dr. Sabbagha said they could try again. Sharon tells him "a few weeks" but adds that she doesn't know how much more she can take. David tries to be supportive and says they need to be patient. Sharon angrily retorts that she is tired of being patient after 2 years and more than 1 year of seeing the specialist, 9 months of shots, and four attempts at in vitro fertilization (IVF). David's further attempts to be supportive produce more anger with Sharon saying he doesn't understand "what happened" when it means that she is unable to conceive a child and that she will be barren and childless for the rest of her life. They each lay blame on the other in terms of their careers and their needs to finish residencies and/or fellowships. David finally adds, "who's to say that you were ever able to conceive a child at 26 or 39?"
   a. How can health professionals support couples who are desperate to conceive a child of their own and struggle with the limitations and challenges of IVF?
   b. What suggestions can a clinician make to a couple, bearing in mind that the divorce rate for couples who are trying to conceive through IVF is higher than the general population, to help them achieve balance and maintain a healthy, honest, and realistic dialogue through their infertility journey?
   c. How can health professionals best advise couples who have elected to delay their childbearing and families secondary to their career aspirations?

3 (0:26:38–0:27:16; 0:27:31–0:28:40) Sharon is having lunch with her mother, Ruthie (Greta DeBofsky), and is very quiet. Ruthie says she's been meaning to ask about the IVF. Sharon says she doesn't want to talk about it and hurries her mother out of the restaurant. Ruthie presses the point in the car, saying, "that last miscarriage almost killed you," adding "sometimes enough is enough," and reintroducing the idea of adoption. Sharon angrily says, "this part of my life is not open for discussion."
   a. How would you interpret Ruthie's comment?
   b. What impact might this type of issue have on a familial relationship?

4 (0:35:00–0:36:15) Sharon and David are having a party. Sharon learns that her best friend is pregnant for the third time "without even trying" and that David has withheld the information from her. Sharon asks, "can't I be happy for them and sorry for me at the same time?" Sharon adds: "I can't be complete without a child of my own."

   a. How can health-care providers best counsel couples who are struggling with unsuccessful attempts in becoming pregnant as well as the staggering costs of IVF?

   b. How should health-care professionals best approach couples who are adamantly opposed to alternative family options when IVF fails?

   c. What are some strategies to help couples and their families deal with the tremendous sense of pain, grief, and loss that occurs during the infertility process?

Making Grace (2004; Ann Krsul, Leslie Sullivan [as themselves]): This film is an intimate portrait of a lesbian couple's efforts to conceive a child. The documentary chronicles their unique emotional journey from sperm donor anxieties to their daughter Grace's first birthday.

1 (0:02:07–0:05:29) The scene begins with Leslie talking about pregnancy cycles. It then shifts to the couple on the Staten Island Ferry discussing how it would have been better psychologically if Leslie were the one to get pregnant. Ann talks about being 37 and wonders why she did not try getting pregnant before. She calculates the number of "tries" she has left. Ann wonders if she has damaged her body by past lifestyle habits. The scene concludes with Ann's statement that "every month is a huge trial."

   a. What are some of the emotional issues a health-care professional may anticipate in counseling a lesbian couple who is trying to decide who should carry the pregnancy?

2 (0:05:50–0:06:47) Leslie talks about how she never felt she needed to give birth to a child. She feels lucky that Ann wants to go through pregnancy. Ann recounts that she got pregnant the first time they tried to conceive, but it was an ectopic pregnancy. After the procedure, she had to wait 3 months before she could try again.

   a. What are some of the challenges unique to a same-sex couple who want to conceive a biological child?

3 (0:0:7:41–0:0:8:26) Leslie discusses the couple's differences in anxiety around being pregnant, getting pregnant, and being a parent – with Ann being the more anxious.

   a. How can a health-care professional help a same-sex couple navigate the challenges and potential biases they may encounter in the health-care system while trying to conceive a biological child?

   b. What resources are available for gay couples as they address issues unique to their pregnancy and birthing experiences?

4 (0:1:05:23–0:1:07:02) Leslie and Ann talk about the intense stress having a

child places on a relationship. "Any problems you had before are only magnified or problems that you have in your own personal self. You're working with incredible sleep deprivation. You end up fighting more." They share that they've probably had the worst fights since becoming parents.

a. What resources may a health-care professional suggest to a gay couple as they anticipate issues unique to parenting a child?

Advanced Maternal (and Paternal) Age

Today in the United States every fifth woman has her first child after the age of 35. This number is even higher in professional women, who usually decide to postpone having children until a later age.

Most of these pregnancies are uneventful, but advanced maternal age can bring some pregnancy risks such as high blood pressure, gestational diabetes, preterm babies, still births, low birthweight, increased C-section rate, and congenital birth defects. It is also not uncommon that these women face different challenges being pregnant at an older age, such as fear of complications, work obligations, and sometimes lack of support and understanding from the family.

Father of the Bride Part II (1995; Steve Martin, Diane Keaton, Martin Short): George Banks (Martin) finds out that both his newlywed daughter and his wife, Nina (Keaton), are pregnant at the same time. Our focus here is on Nina's reactions and emotions when she finds out she is pregnant.

1 (0:34:23–0:36:55) Nina reads about menopause, to explain her symptoms of fatigue and a late period. George is in a midlife crisis and in denial over what is happening.

a. What do you think of Nina's explanation of her symptoms? How would you explain George's denial?

2 (0:37:19–0:41:00) Nina and George are at the doctor's office to hear her test results. They hear the news that Nina is not in menopause but is pregnant. Both of them are in shock. George doesn't believe he is the father.

a. What do you think of Nina's and George's reaction? How you can explain George's behavior?

b. Was the doctor's reaction appropriate? Would you do anything different?

3 (0:43:01–0:43:57) George and Nina are on the way home from the doctor's visit. They see things differently.

a. What do you think of Nina's reaction to the news of her late life pregnancy?

b. How would you explain George's thoughts?

4 (0:45:07–0:48:47) George and Nina are at their daughter's house, breaking the news about the pregnancy. Their daughter is stunned. Nina finally expresses all her feelings about her pregnancy.

a. What was the daughter's reaction? What do you think about her comments? What could she have said instead?

    b. What do you think of Nina's feelings about her pregnancy? Is this an unusual reaction?

    c. As a physician, how do you handle an advanced maternal age pregnancy?

    d. What advice can you give to the family of an older pregnant woman?

In Good Company (2004; Dennis Quaid, Topher Grace, Scarlett Johannson, Marg Helgenberger): Ad salesman Dan (Quaid) must take a junior position after a corporate shakedown. Worse, he now reports to a much younger boss, Carter (Grace). Much to his surprise, Dan's wife (Helgenberger) becomes pregnant.

1 (Ch 2, 0:08:14–0:09:45) Dan returns home from work quite late. He heads to the bedroom. He is privately worried that his college-bound daughter, Alex (Scarlett Johannson), is pregnant. He asks his wife questions about his daughter's romantic life, only to find out that his wife is also pregnant. At first he is confused as to how this is possible. He replies that he thought she was "done with all that." At first he is shocked but then happy. He says, referring to a newborn son, "that means when he is 21, I'll be 72."

    a. What are some of the unique health concerns of the patient with advanced maternal age?

    b. What are the risks associated with pregnancy in older women?

    c. How can a health-care provider best counsel and prepare an older couple for the additional fetal testing that they may consider?

    d. How can a health-care professional provide anticipatory counseling and facilitate planning for any infant health challenges?

    e. What are the potential effects on the marital relationship?

    f. How would you respond to a prospective father regarding his age-related concerns?

2 (Ch 5, 0:24:04–0:25:08) Dan and his wife are at an obstetrics visit. They are listening to the baby's heartbeat. Dan is overwhelmed and has an arrythmia. He becomes the patient. The doctor examines Dan and asks if he has been under a lot of stress. He announces that he is getting demoted at work.

    a. What are the potential compounding effects of an unplanned pregnancy and job difficulties for the father?

    b. What impact might these issues have for the couple? For the pregnant woman?

    c. How should a health-care professional respond to an overwrought family member while trying to care for the primary patient?

    d. What are some of the stressors that an older couple may anticipate as they consider being "older parents"? What resources may be available to help them?

Further Reading

- Devries KM, Kishor S, John son H, *et al*. Intimate partner violence during pregnancy: analysis of prevalence data from 19 countries. *Reprod Health Matters*. 2010; **18**(36): 158–70.
- Hueston WJ, Geesey ME, Diaz V. Prenatal care initiation among pregnant teens in the United States: an analysis over 25 years. *J Adolesc Health*. 2008; **42**(3): 243–8.
- Keeling J, Mason T. Postnatal disclosure of domestic violence: comparison with disclosure in the first trimester of pregnancy. *J Clin Nurs*. 2011; **20**(1–2): 103–10.
- Lutz KF. Abused pregnant women's interactions with health care providers during the childbearing year. *J Obstet Gynecol Neonatal Nurs*. 2005; **34**(2): 151–62.
- Martins MV, Peterson BD, Almeida M, *et al*. Direct and indirect effects of perceived social support in women's infertility related stress. *Hum Reprod*. 2011; **26**(8): 2113–21.
- Stewart M. We just want to be ordinary: lesbian parents talk about their birth experiences. *MIDIRS Midwifery Digest*. 2002; 12: 415–18.
- Toevs K, Brill S. The essential guide to lesbian conception, pregnancy and birth. Los Angeles, CA: Alyson Books; 2002.

Resource List

- Resources for Health Care Providers Caring for Lesbian Patients.
- Gay and Lesbian Medical Association – 459 Fulton Street, Suite 107, San Francisco, CA 94102.

PART IV

Mental Health Issues

15

From Burnout, Harassment, and Job Loss to Despair, Engagement, and Recovery: Workplace Issues

Anna Pavlov

MOST PEOPLE SPEND OVER ONE-THIRD OF THEIR ADULT LIVES AT WORK. Factor in extended commute times and individuals can average more than 10–12 hours away from home. Some workers can leave their job behind at the end of the day or shift while many take work and/or work worries home with them. The technological revolution now allows individuals to be available "24/7." Even vacation time is not necessarily a protected time.

As this book is going to press, the world is ever so slowly emerging from the economic recession of 2008. Although economic indicators have improved, job growth has not.[1] As such, and during other similar periods in history, work takes on a sense of urgency, in terms of both acquiring it for those who have lost their jobs and holding on to it for those still employed. During this recession, pressure to find a job has been intense and with the passage of time, when prospects are poor, can lead to tremendous despair.

Work defines one's identity, life, and access to both the basic necessities of life and the "American Dream." According to the 2008 Annual Stress in America survey conducted by the American Psychological Association,[2] 80% of Americans were stressed about their personal finances and the economy. Half of those surveyed said they were increasingly stressed about their ability to provide for their family's basic needs.

In 2010 the survey[3] found nearly 75% of Americans reported being stressed to the max. For men, unemployment continued at the same time that unemployment benefits ran out. For 3 consecutive years, worries about jobs, mortgage, money, and how to pay the bills have been top stress factors for many Americans. These unhealthy stress levels can put individuals at risk for developing chronic illnesses such as depression, anxiety, diabetes, and heart disease at the same time that health insurance may be gone or threatened by job loss.

The nature of one's work can also contribute to unhealthy stress levels. Long hours, a difficult work environment including unfulfilling and repetitive tasks, and poor management are issues with which many workers cope. Clearly, some jobs are just about "paying the bills" as there is wide variability in job satisfaction. Coping with work stress has been a longtime focus of occupational and health psychology researchers and clinicians.[4,5]

Industrial/occupational psychologists have developed strategies to increase productivity and retain valued employees through many approaches including worker input/autonomy, incentives, recognition/rewards, and flexible scheduling.[6] With greater numbers of women in the workforce, flexible work schedules to accommodate the needs of families and including more women in top managerial positions have become a new mandate.[7]

The progressive decline in US manufacturing and service jobs through technology and outsourcing has been a major contributing factor to job loss and has not been without a human cost.[8] Downsizing has changed work culture and morale. In some cases, it has exacerbated workplace stress, with pressure on the fewer workers remaining to do more.

Workplace issues such as worker safety, equality in pay, gender discrimination, sexual harassment, disability rights, and, more recently, rights for families caring for a loved one while protecting one's job (the Family and Medical Leave Act of 1993) have evolved through various legal challenges and precedents.[9-13] However, their application is not universally and strictly enforced as some individuals and institutions have been slow to recognize evolving views and the law.

As an example, despite the fact that there is equality in pay laws, many women, while now surpassing men with college and advanced degrees, still make 77 cents for every dollar earned by a man. Even though women choosing lower-paying and more portable careers to accommodate family responsibilities, including caring for an elder relative, may account for some of this gap, it can't explain 40% of the difference.[14]

This chapter provides film clips depicting various aspects of the workplace. In addition to the films presented here, the reader can find several excellent documentaries that focus on the impact of globalization such as *American Jobs* (2005) and the Academy Award–winning documentary *Inside Job* (2010), which focuses on the deeply rooted corruption that led to the global economic crisis of 2008.

The Daily Grind

Office Space (1999; Ron Livingston, Stephen Root, Jennifer Aniston): In this comedy about the mundane and demoralizing aspects of the work world, Peter Gibbons (Ron Livingston) highlights the indignities of office life in a cubicle. He conspires with his cubicle cohorts to embezzle money from their soulless employers. While this film was released in 1999, the scenes selected do not appear dated and reflect current realities.

1   (Ch 2, 0:03:50–0:06:49) We see a glimpse into the daily realities of an office worker in a cubicle including the repetitive nature of some tasks and ridiculous rules. Character Peter Gibbons is especially sensitive to the daily onslaught.
    a. What is your reaction to this scene? Can you relate? In what ways?
2   (Chs 3–4, 0:06:49–0:09:16) We see other coworkers frustrated by the technical failures and other indignities of the daily grind.
3   (Ch 5, 0:10:39–0:12:39) Murkowski is running toward a trio of coworkers with a rumor that their company, Initech, is downsizing. He believes this is because the company is bringing in a "consultant."
    a. How might office rumors/gossip be useful?
    b. In what ways can they be counterproductive or harmful?
4   (Ch 6, 0:17:18–0:18:20) The dreaded staff meeting where the manager is telling employees to ask themselves with every decision they have to make, "Is this good for the company?" The consultant is introduced who will help them and find ways to make things run more smoothly.
    a. How might consultants be useful to an organization?
    b. In what ways do employees respond to them?
5   (Ch 7, 0:19:02–0:20:48) Peter Gibbons tries to avoid being asked to work on a Saturday. His plan is to dash out a little early on Friday afternoon. However, he is not successful and, in addition to being told to come in on Saturday, he is also told to work on Sunday too.
    a. Are there industries in which working additional hours is sometimes necessary?
    b. How can companies meet their needs and also respect employees' off duty time?
    c. How can workers set boundaries on extra work without fearing loss of their job?
6   (Ch 8, 0:20:49–0:23:32) Gibbons sees an occupational hypnotherapist so that he can be hypnotized to forget about his dreadful feelings toward his work. The therapist takes him through a relaxation self-hypnosis exercise suggesting that his concerns about his job will melt away. In a comedic twist, the therapist sweats profusely and passes out but Peter feels much better.
    a. Is Peter's attempt to cope by seeing an occupational hypnotherapist a useful strategy?
    b. What advice would you give someone who repeatedly complained about their job?
    c. Have you ever been in a job that became or started out as too difficult to tolerate?
7   (Ch 10, 0:25:45–0:26:11) We view another boring company meeting with additional minutiae.
    a. How can office meetings become more productive and less dreaded?
8   (Ch 18, 0:45:14–0:46:19) The consultant and manager callously talk about

who will be fired and that entry-level people will be hired to replace them and some of the work will be outsourced. They discuss that Friday would be the best day of the week to fire people.

    a. What reactions do you have to viewing this scene?

    b. Why do you think they behave this way?

9 (Ch 20, 0:48:13–0:49:44) Peter and Michael are at a bar talking about the injustices in the work place. They reflect on how human beings spend their workdays.

    a. If Peter Gibbons were your client/patient, how would you respond to his complaints?

    b. What advice would you give someone about coping with work stress? What about coping with repetitive tasks? What do you think an industrial/organizational psychologist or other professional would recommend?

    c. What work injuries are office workers more prone to develop?

    d. What adjustments are available to reduce risk of those injuries (ergonomics and so forth)?

    e. What physical symptoms can surface as a result of job dissatisfaction?

    f. What emotional symptoms can surface as a result of job satisfaction?

    g. How do you get through monotonous or unpleasant aspects of your work?

Job Loss – Downsizing: Methods, Spin, and Emotional Fallout

Up in the Air (2009): Ryan Bingham (George Clooney) flies around the country firing employees on behalf of companies downsizing. Natalie Keener (Anna Kendrick) is Bingham's trainee. Jason Bateman stars as Bingham's boss.

1 (Ch 1, 0:03:06–0:04:02) A variety of individuals share their feelings about losing their jobs. One man stated, "I feel like people I work for are my family and I died."

    a. What reactions do you have to these statements? What surprises you?

    b. Have you known a friend or family member who lost their job?

2 (0:04:03–0:05:48) Ryan Bingham, the bearer of bad news, is shown speaking platitudes, and asks the employee for his key card.

    a. What do you know about how companies handle layoffs/terminations?

3 (0:20:05–0:20:36) Craig (Jason Bateman) summarizes to his group the dismal economic state of businesses and homeowners. He enthusiastically exclaims, "This is our moment." They will change operations to save costs themselves. Instead of traveling to companies to fire employees, they will terminate them via video camera.

    a. What is your reaction to this method?

    b. If you worked for this company, what suggestions would you have about how to manage this without firing employees via videocam?

    c. How can the industrial organizational literature inform this process?

Breaking the Bad News of Job Loss

1 (0:32:33–0:34:27) Bingham and Keener break bad news to a series of employees that they are losing their jobs. There is an extended discussion with one who asks, "what do you suggest I tell them?" (referring to his children).
   a. How would you answer this?
   b. What health issues might you see in an individual and family affected by unemployment?
   c. How might unemployment affect access to medical care/insurance coverage?
   d. Discuss the ripple effects of unemployment?

In Good Company (2004; Dennis Quaid, Topher Grace, Scarlett Johannson, Marg Helgenberger): Advertising salesman, Dan (Dennis Quaid) must take a junior position after a corporate shakedown. Worse, he now reports to a much younger boss, Carter (Topher Grace), a business school grad who espouses a sales approach branded Synergy that's at odds with Dan's style.
1 (Ch 12, 0:54:18–0:54:48) An employee is leaving the company and his coworkers say goodbye to him.
   a. What do you imagine the dismissed coworker is feeling?
   b. How are coworkers affected by seeing colleagues leave?
2 (Ch 13; 1:03:48–1:04:37) Carter fires a succession of three individuals. One woman says, "But I have worked here for 5 years." Office furniture is being piled up as the workforce is reduced.
   a. See questions from first film clip.

Up in the Air (see earlier description)

1 (0:41:09–0:43:00) Ryan Bingham and Natalie Keener are meeting with a female employee who calls on them to be direct. She asks, "I'm here to be fired, right?" When Natalie responds that, "We are here to talk about your future," the employee tells them her future plans are "to jump off a beautiful bridge by her house." Natalie is shown walking away upset. Ryan then tries to comfort and reassure her that people say these things all the time. It's part of the trade. They say crazy things but they do not actually do it.
   a. How would you have handled the employee's response?
   b. What safeguards would you have considered?
2 (1:38:36–1:39:54) News comes that the aforementioned employee has killed herself by jumping off a bridge. Inquiry is made as to whether she gave any signs of depression.
   a. How prevalent is suicide secondary to job loss? What are the risk factors?
   b. What follow-up should the company have made in response to this tragic event?

3 (1:42:08–1:43:04) A variety of individuals reflect back on how they survived unemployment.
   a. Do you know someone who lost their job during the 2008 economic downturn and/or the years that followed?
   b. What is the emotional impact of job loss via downsizing?
   c. How would you respond to a client/patient who lost their job and appeared despondent?
   d. How are remaining workers affected by downsizing?
   e. Discuss the methods used and how they make the bad news even worse.
   f. Is there a way that employees could be notified more humanely? Is there a more humane way to downsize a company?

Outsourcing: Our Work Culture and that of Others

Outsourced (2006; Josh Hamilton, Asif Basra, Ayesha Dharker, Matt Smith):When his department is outsourced to India, customer call center manager Todd Anderson (Josh Hamilton) heads to Mumbai to train his successor (Asif Basra). Amusing culture clashes ensue as Anderson tries to explain American business practices to the befuddled new employees. In the process, he learns important lessons about globalization – and life.

1 (Ch 1, 0:00:58–0:03:38) Todd Anderson, a customer call center manager, is called into his supervisor's office and told that their phone jobs will be sent offshore. There will be a restructuring of order fulfillment. His supervisor says, "Any American job done online or over the phone is going overseas. The savings are incredible (eight heads for one)." Todd is asked to notify employees that their jobs have been outsourced. He is told he is needed in India to train the replacements. He does not have a real choice because he will lose his benefits.
   a. What is your reaction to this inside view of business?
   b. Are there alternatives to outsourcing?
   c. Are there companies that are trying to manage in other ways?

2 (Ch 3, 0:18:09–0:20:39) Tom has arrived in Mumbai, India. The local man hired to be the manager is driving him to the office. He tells Todd that they work from 6 in the morning to 6 in the evening. He also shares that this new position and great pay will allow him to marry his longtime love. They are in a rural area and arrive at a dilapidated, unfinished building, which is the call center with a sign saying "Fulfilment." He is told that because of outsourcing, all the real estate in Bombay and other cities is not available. Todd is shocked as they pull up and he is introduced to his new trainees. The building is incomplete with ongoing bricklaying and a cow in an adjacent area. Todd learns that the average time to resolve a customer call is over 12 minutes. He becomes noticeably ill and leaves the building.

    a. What is your reaction to the Indian manager's description of what this job will mean for him and the hours that his workers expect to put in?

    b. Does this description alter how you view those to whom jobs are outsourced?

3 (Ch 4, 0:21:59–0:24:24) Todd tells the employees that the numbers are not what they should be and that they need to work faster. He requests that they learn American idioms. Todd advises them that if customers want to know where they are from, say "Chicago." In training them, his suggestions highlight deceitful practices.

    a. What is your reaction to this scene?

    b. What is your reaction when you get a customer call representative from another country?

    c. What are the common complaints/frustrations that people voice?

4 (Ch 4, 0:26:41–0:27:36) Todd observes many kindnesses in the Indian culture in contrast to an increasing awareness of some of his own culture's business tactics, which are nonsensical and cruel. We see him telling his employees that they are losing money on every call. They are still taking an average of 12 minutes per call. The supervisor states that progress has been made because they have gotten it down from 15 minutes. We see the supervisor telling his employees to go faster and faster.

    a. What is your reaction to this scene?

    b. What cultural differences do you see with respect to time?

    c. What aspects of your work environment are nonsensical and aggravating?

    d. What are the time issues in your work?

5 (Ch 7, 0:48:07–0:48:45) Todd and the manager are having coffee and talking about their respective cultures. He points out to Todd that he hates his job and hates his boss. "Why not choose something else?" Todd explains, "In my culture, it makes sense to work your ass off and to get into credit card debt so you can have that 50" plasma."

    a. Do you think this is an accurate description of Western work culture? Why or Why not?

    b. Does this description characterize your work life?

    c. How hard is it to resist entrenched aspects/values of one's culture?

6 (Ch 12, 1:23:34–1:24:51) There is a call from an irate American who asks to speak with a supervisor. When she takes the call, the American tells her that he lost his job last month to outsourcing. She is as understanding as she can be and tells him that they have located American-made products similar to theirs as an alternative for customers who feel as he does. She is ready to refer him to a company that makes the same product he has ordered but is stopped when he finds out the other product costs $212 more.

    a. Do Americans want it both ways, having products "Made in America" and at low prices (that are only possible with overseas production/workers)?

    b. Would you be willing to pay more for a product made in the United States to support American business?

7   (Ch 12, 1:25:51–1:26:29) Todd's supervisor has just arrived in India and tells him that the company is pulling out of India and outsourcing to China. There they can get 20 workers for the price of one. They go online in China the next day.

   a. What reactions do you have to this decision?

   b. Are human factors considered at all?

8   (Ch 12, 1:26:38–1:29:23) Todd goes to find the workers at a club after the shift. He announces the bad news that their jobs have been outsourced to China. He talks to people about what this loss means. The manager tells him that the employees are now well trained and are in a good position to find jobs with other companies. However, as manager, his prospects are not as bright and jeopardize his chance to marry his longtime love.

   a. The original recipients of outsourced work are now outsourced themselves. What is your reaction to this scene?

The Older Worker

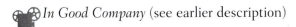 *In Good Company* (see earlier description)

1   (Ch 1, 0:02:59–0:04:19) Dan (Dennis Quaid), who has been head of Ad Sales for *Sports America* magazine for 20 years, is meeting with an ad executive, a prospective client, who has been convinced not to advertise in print. Dan is asked if he is worried about the rumor that his parent company is about to be sold.

   a. Companies must adapt to ever changing trends. How is this especially challenging for older workers?

2   (Ch 3, 0:10:56–0:11:25) We see a newspaper headline that Teddy Kay of GlobeCom is acquiring Waterman Publishing, responsible for *Sports America* magazine. Anxiety fills the office as employees worry that they will be fired.

   a. *See* questions under The Daily Grind, p. 192 (3).

3   (Ch 3, 0:11:32–0:12:30) Dan is told that he is no longer head of ad sales. Carter Deria, a hotshot from GlobeCom will be directing sales. Dan protests that his sales team works very hard. He is reminded that he is not a kid anymore.

   a. How might older workers feel threatened and demoralized by younger "upstarts"?

   b. How might younger, more tech savvy workers devalue or minimize the contributions of more senior workers?

   c. Do you think older workers are valued for their experience and worldview?

   d. What can older workers do to keep their edge and compete with younger workers?

   e. How does compensation work against retaining and hiring older workers?

4   (Chs 3–4, 0:16:34–0:19:25) Carter is meeting the employees at the magazine

and then is shown his new office, which is still Dan Foreman's office. Dan walks in and realizes that this young guy is his replacement. Dan asks Carter his age and then states, "26 years old and you're my new boss." Dan also asks about his experience with ad sales to which Carter replies that he does not have much. Carter then asks Dan his age. When Dan tells him he is 51, Carter exclaims, "You are a year older than my dad."

   a. How might generational differences in work values, technology, and world view create conflict at work?
   b. What is your experience of this in your setting?
   c. How would you imagine an older worker feels to be reporting to a much younger coworker? What about if the younger coworker was not respected by the older one?
   d. Discuss generational cohorts (Gen X, Gen Y, and so forth).

Ethics in the Workplace

1 (Ch 6, 0:25:49–0:29:42) Carter is speaking with the team and is very nervous. He has an agenda and says he has to increase ad sales by 20%. He appears to flounder but eventually gets his confidence back by talking about "synergy," a pep talk he has obviously borrowed from someone else. When Carter presents his ideas, Dan asks if that isn't cheating.

   a. Have you ever had to carry out a plan that made you feel uncomfortable? How did you handle that situation?
   b. Would you handle it any differently today? Why or why not?

2 (Ch 6, 0:29:46–0:31:55) Dan and Carter are at lunch. Carter says he has to cut salaries. He has to cut $300K from the sales team immediately. At first Dan mistakenly thinks he is being fired. Carter tells him he is not letting him go and when Dan asks what benefit is in it for him as Carter's "wingman," he sarcastically states that getting to keep his job is a benefit.

   a. What is your reaction to this scene?
   b. How would you talk with an older employee who needed to consider retirement due to poor job performance? How about for a physical or mental impairment? Would you take any special measures in doing so?
   c. How would you talk with a younger employee about the benefits of respecting the skills and institutional memory that older workers bring to the table?

Balancing Work and Family

Baby Boom (1987; Diane Keaton, Harold Ramis, James Spader): JC Wyatt is a high-powered management consultant in New York who has worked her way up the corporate ladder and stands ready to accept a partner position.

However, fate intervenes when she is given a baby after a distant relative dies. She initially plans to put the baby up for adoption but changes her mind. While this film was released long ago, the scenes selected reflect many ongoing realities.

1   (Ch 1, 02:24–03:37) We get a glimpse into JC's life as she walks and talks, and works at the same time and expects her subordinates to be available for her at all times.

   a. How are men and women with this work style sometimes judged differently?

   b. Would you have a harder time working with a man or a woman with this work style? Why?

2   (Ch 1, 03:54–0:06:38) JC is having lunch with Fritz, her boss. When he asks her how many hours she works now, she casually estimates that she works 70–80 hours per week. Fritz tells her that she is being considered for partner but that the hours will get worse. He adds that normally he does not think of her as a woman but he has to now as she is being considered for this position. He wonders if her partner will expect "a wife" one day or if children are in her future.

   a. Is it legal to ask an employee this question?

   b. Would the same question be asked of a man?

   c. Discuss pro-family work policies.

3   (Ch 2, 0:12:56–0:0:16:12) JC is rushing to a lunch meeting dragging the child in tow. She leaves the baby with the coat check attendant. We hear a baby crying in the background. Her lunch partner is distracted and wonders what is going on. JC presents as distracted. Then the baby is brought to her table and, needless to say, she is not making a good impression.

   a. How could such a scenario create a negative impression? How might someone else interpret this?

   b. How might coworkers respond when a parent stays home with a sick child or leaves the office for childcare responsibilities?

   c. Do you think there are office strains between those workers with and those without children? Discuss.

   d. How might work hour flexibility and telecommuting eliminate some of these problems and result in greater productivity?

4   (Ch 5, 0:34:00–0:36:32) Fritz and a visitor walk into JC's office and see baby Elizabeth in her chair. JC brings Elizabeth to the office, jeopardizing her move to partner. JC looks for someone to take the baby.

   a. What is your reaction to this scene?

   b. Do you have compassion for parents in this situation? Why or why not?

   c. Does your workplace have childcare on site?

   d. What is the worker satisfaction of companies that do?

Gender Discrimination and Sexual Harassment

North Country (2005; Charlize Theron, Jeremy Renner, Frances McDormand, Richard Jenkins, Sissy Spacek): Based on a true story, set in Northern Minnesota, Josey Aimes (Theron) decides to work in the mine industry against the wishes of her father. The extreme taunting, intimidation, and gender discriminatory behavior was grounds for the landmark 1984 class action lawsuit that resulted in the first successful sexual harassment case in the United States (Jenson vs. Eveleth Mines).

Domestic Violence Wrongly Attributed to Job Loss

1 (0:14:05–0:14:30) Josey is talking with her mother about her ex-partner. Her mother appears to excuse his behavior. Josey states back, "Wayne beat me because he was out of work. Is that what you are saying?"
   a. Is the stress of losing a job and financial pressures ever an excuse for domestic violence?
   b. Is an increase in family violence expected during economic downturns?

Unwanted Sexual Advances

1 (Ch 9, 0:44:08–0:45:24) This scene involves veiled threats and intimidation. Bobby Sharp and Josey were involved in high school. Bobby arranges to be alone with Josey and asks her, "Want to kiss and make up? What's the matter with you, Josey?" She rebukes his advances and gets away.
   a. What is your reaction to this scene?
   b. Does the fact that Bobby and Josey had a prior romantic relationship change this from being intimidation and an unwanted sexual advance? Discuss.
2 (Ch 10, 0:48:37–0:49:17) Josey describes the work conditions to her father who does not approve of her working at the mine. She tells him that she goes to work scared and worries that she might get raped. He offers no empathy or concern.
   a. What advice would you give Josey about how to stay safe in her work environment?
   b. What do you think about her father's response?
   c. How would you approach this with her?

Reporting Sexual Harassment in the Workplace

1   (Ch 13, 1:01:55–1:04:33) Josey meets with the head of the mine company. When she started working there, he made it a point of introducing himself and told her to see him if she had any problem. He tells her that he has been "briefed" on her complaint and then asks for her resignation. His tone is patronizing when he discusses how emotional this has been for her.
   a. What recourse do workers typically have when management is not responsive to their needs?
   b. Do you think most workers would stop there? Why or why not?
   c. What forms of gender discrimination continue to exist?
   d. Discuss the WalMart class action suit heard by the Supreme Court in 2011. It is based on the blatant denial of qualified women to managerial positions over men with less experience and performance.
   e. What are your thoughts on the state of sexual harassment?
   f. Why do so many women decide not to pursue complaints?
   g. What can end up happening to their original concerns?
   h. Could they then become victims of other forms of discrimination/retaliation?

Gender Discrimination/Inequity in Pay/Unions

Made in Dagenham (2010; Sally Hawkins, Miranda Richardson, Bob Hoskins): This is a dramatization of the landmark 1968 labor strike initiated by hundreds of women who rebelled against discrimination and demanded the same pay as men for their work in Ford's British automobile manufacturing plants.
1   (Ch 4, 0:19:37–0:23:30) Rita O'Grady and her union representative meet with the company men. They remind her that a formal grievance is in place and the machinist case will be heard. She tells them that the women's work is very important and is semiskilled labor. She brings out leather fabric pieces from her purse to make her point. She asserts that they are entitled to the wages that go with semiskilled labor, not those of unskilled labor.
   a. Why is making change in the workplace so difficult?
   b. What is the effect of Rita's persuasive technique?
2   (Ch 8, 0:42:07–0:43:52) The women have received notices about their "flagrant" behavior and aggressive disregard for the complaint procedure. Mrs. O'Grady gets frustrated and angry over their disregard and inaction and informs the men that there will be an all out work stoppage until their complaint is addressed. She asserts that this strike is about fairness. "Equal pay or nothing."
3   (Ch 6, 0:29:27–0:29:53) Some of the women are on strike with signs to support the machinists.
4   (Ch 8, 0:47:50–0:48:38) Their strike enlarges to equal pay for all women not

just their plant machinists. Rita O'Grady asserts that every single one of them is entitled to the same pay as men.

   a. From a historical perspective, how difficult do you imagine it was to stand up for a cause (such as equal pay for women) in a different era?

   b. Is equal pay for women still an issue today? Discuss.

   c. Access to promotions is another way that gender discrimination may manifest. Discuss.

5 (Ch 14, 1:26:54–1:29:14) Rita O'Grady speaks to the National Union on behalf of the female machinists. She affirms they are not separated by sex but by those willing to accept injustice. Equal pay for women is a right.

   a. What is your reaction to Rita's speech?

   b. Discuss the history of unions and labor.

   c. What issues and controversies have unfolded with unions over time? Discuss the pros and cons.

Health Discrimination: Disability, HIV, and Chronic Health Issues in the Workplace

Philadelphia (1993): Attorney Andrew Beckett (Tom Hanks) launches a wrongful termination suit when his law firm finds out about his HIV-positive status and his homosexuality and fires him. Denzel Washington costars as Joe Miller, the initially homophobic lawyer who takes Andy's case.

1 (Chs 11–13, 0:26:31–0:31:33) Andy Beckett shows up at an attorney's office to find a lawyer who will take on a wrongful termination lawsuit. He explains that he believes he was set up once the partners realized he had AIDS. In flashback sequences, we see how the firm fires him in a meeting of the managing partners. Joe Miller (Washington), who clearly becomes anxious about contagion after hearing that Andy has AIDS, declines the case.

   a. Does fear of contagion still exist for HIV?

   b. How about for cancer and other diseases?

2 (Ch 16, 0:39:59–0:42:31) Miller has a chance meeting with Andy at a law library. He asks if there is a legal precedent to which Andy answers that there is and passes him the legal brief to read. Miller reads out loud the Supreme Court's Vocational Rehabilitation Discrimination Act of 1973, which prohibits discrimination against otherwise qualified persons. AIDS is protected as a handicap under the law.

   a. Discuss the Vocational Rehabilitation Discrimination Act of 1973?

   b. What is the Americans with Disabilities Act of 1990?

   c. What accommodations can typically be made?

3 (Chs 20–22, 0:49:10–0:53:03) Miller is in court outlining the case to the jury. He states that Andy is afflicted with a debilitating disease and made the decision to keep it private. He made a legal choice to keep the illness to himself and then his employer found out. When they fired him because

he had AIDS, they broke the law. The other side says they fired him before they knew he had AIDS. They contend that Andy is lashing out because he is dying and is filled with rage.

a. What is your reaction to this scene?

b. How would you advise a client/patient about disclosing HIV status?

c. What other scenarios can lead to competent workers/professionals being unjustly released from their jobs?

d. How would you advise a client/patient about disclosing another type of chronic illness?

References

1 Zakaria F. A flight plan for the American economy. *Time Magazine*. 2011, May 30.

2 American Psychological Association 2008 Annual Stress in America Survey. Available at: www.phwa.org/media (last accessed 12/01/11).

3 American Psychological Association 2010 Annual Stress in America Survey. Available at: www.phwa.org/media (last accessed 12/01/11).

4 Dewe P, O'Driscoll M, Cooper C. *Coping with Work Stress*. West Sussex, UK: John Wiley & Sons; 2010.

5 Cooper C, editor. *International Handbook of Work and Health Psychology*. West Sussex, UK: John Wiley & Sons; 2009.

6 Zedeck S, editor. *APA Handbook of Industrial and Organizational Psychology*. Washington, DC: APA Publishing; 2010.

7 Barreto M, Ryan M, Schmitt M. *The Glass Ceiling in the 21st Century: understanding barriers to gender equality*. Washington, DC: APA Publishing; 2009.

8 Morgan S, editor. *The Human Side of Outsourcing: psychological theory and management practice*. West Sussex, UK: John Wiley & Sons; 2009.

9 *Equal Pay Made Law*. Directgov. Available at: www.direct.gov.uk/en/Nl1/Newsroom/DG_191258 (last accessed 12/01/11).

10 Jenson vs. Eveleth Mines (Sexual Harassment lawsuit 1984). FindLaw. Available at: caselaw.findlaw.com/us-8th-circuit/1136685.html (last accessed 12/01/11).

11 United States Department of Transportation. *Vocational Rehabilitation Act of 1973*. Available at: www.access-board.gov/enforcement/rehab-act-text/intro.htm (last accessed 03/31/12)

12 US Department of Justice. *Americans with Disabilities Act*. Available at: www.ada.gov (last accessed 12/01/11)

13 US Office of Personnel Management. *Family Medical Leave Act*. Available at: www.opm.gov/oca/leave/HTML/fmlafac2.asp (last accessed 12/01/11).

14 Foroohar R. The 100% solution. *Time Magazine*. 2011, May 23: 22.

Further Reading
∙∙∙∙∙∙∙∙∙∙∙∙∙∙∙∙∙∙∙∙∙∙∙∙∙∙

- Grace M. *What Movies Teach about Workplace Ethics, Harassment and Romance.* Available at: www.myarticlearchive.com/articles/5/034.htm (last accessed 12/01/11).
- Hedge J, Borman W, Lammlein S. *The Aging Workforce: realities, myths, and implications for organizations.* Washington, DC: APA Publishing; 2006.

16

Saying Goodbye:
Loss and Bereavement

Michael Kahn

COPING WITH LOSS IS ONE OF LIFE'S GREATEST CHALLENGES. THIS IS true whether it is an individual coping with loss, the friends and family of that individual, or the medical establishment. Often, extended family members and friends don't know how to react to grieving loved ones. Some individuals choose to avoid the issue, discount it or offer a hurtful or insensitive platitude. Physicians may find that their medical skills and training leave them ill equipped to deal with the emotional and interpersonal terrain of grief and loss.

Though we share common grief reactions, each person's experience, as well as each family's experience, of grief and loss is unique. Having said that, there are universal ways to help grieving individuals feel supported. Cinemeducation is an excellent tool to help health-care professionals learn more about the grief experience and how to best support individuals, their families and their communities in coping with loss and grief.

Effect of Grief on Couples/Families
. . . .

In The Bedroom (2001; Tom Wilkinson, Sissy Spacek, Nick Stahl, Marisa Tomei): This is the story of a New England couple (Tom Wilkinson, Sissy Spacek) whose college-aged son Frank (Nick Stahl) is dating an older woman, Natalie (Marisa Tomei). After Natalie's ex-husband murders Frank, the couple is faced with dealing with their terrible loss and coping with the resultant strain in the relationship.

1 (Ch 14, 1:26:32–1:30:27) In this scene, Ruth (Sissy Spacek) arrives home after seeing her son's murderer, who is out on bail, in the grocery store. Matt (Tom Wilkinson) attempts to start a conversation, which escalates into conflict.
    a. Describe the emotions expressed by Ruth and Matt.

b. The couple argues about the appropriate way to grieve their son's death. Discuss your reactions to their conversation.

c. Is there a right way to grieve?

d. What do Matt and Ruth each do to fuel the conflict? What could each have done differently to avoid the escalation?

e. Do men and women grieve differently? Are there considerable intra-gender differences as well?

f. What percentage of couples stay married after the loss of a child? How do you explain these findings?

In America (2003; Paddy Considine, Samantha Morton, Djimon Hounsou): Based on a true story, *In America* is about an Irish family who emigrates to the United States and attempts to make a life for themselves in New York City.

1 (Ch 2, 0:01:38–0:03:34) This scene begins with the parents and their two daughters at the Canada-US border. The parents appear nervous as the family is asked questions by the border guards, including "How many kids do you have?" The couple has a deceased son, Frankie, who died previously.

a. Do you think deciding how to refer to a deceased child is a typical dilemma faced by grieving parents? Why does each member of this particular couple answer the way they did?

b. If you were in this situation, how would you answer this question from the border guard?

c. How can a marital relationship best survive the death of a child?

d. What resources for grieving parents are available in your community?

Numb (2007; Matthew Perry, Lynn Collins, Kevin Pollack, Bob Gunton): In this "dramedy," Hudson Milbank (Perry) plays an emotionally deadened screenwriter with complicated personal relationships. His attempts at feeling better, including therapy, are not helping until he enters into a relationship with Sara (Collins).

1 (Ch 13; 1:14:21–1:17:15) Hudson receives a phone call informing him that his father has died. After the funeral, family and friends have gathered at the family home. Hudson's interactions with his brother and mother are suboptimal.

a. What emotions have you observed in grieving family members?

b. What is the role of the helping professional when working with grieving family and friends? Discuss an instance when you were faced with grieving family/friends. How did you respond?

c. Consider your own losses and/or those of family/friends. Have any of the losses presented relationship challenges? How so?

Reactions to Loss
· ·

Shadowlands (1993; Anthony Hopkins, Debra Winger, Joseph Mazzello, Edward Hardwicke): This is a touching film about the relationship between the solemn writer and Professor CS "Jack" Lewis (Hopkins) and the vibrant poet, Joy Gresham (Winger).

1   (Ch 22; 1:58:12–1:59:27) Following Joy's death and funeral, Jack is concerned about aspects of his grief and shares those concerns with his brother, Warnie (Edward Hardwicke).
   a. Jack is concerned that he can't "see" Joy anymore or remember her face. Is this a normal reaction to grief?
   b. Critique Jack's brother's response, "I don't know what to tell you."
   c. What would you have said to Jack in this circumstance?
   d. What is your reaction to Jack's theory about suffering?

Mystic River (2003; Sean Penn, Tim Robbins, Kevin Bacon): In this dark tragic film, three childhood friends are reunited subsequent to the death of one of their daughters. Sean Penn plays the grieving father, Jimmy Markum.

1   (Ch 13, 0:43:56–0:45:50) Jimmy's father-in-law, Theo (Kevin Conway), arrives at a post-funeral gathering. He shares a previous experience with loss and then tells Jimmy that Jimmy doesn't have the luxury to grieve because he has "domestic responsibilities" – specifically, Jimmy's wife and children. Jimmy then erupts in anger.
   a. Was Jimmy's anger at Theo appropriate? Explain.
   b. How comfortable are you with your own or another's anger? Have you ever had clients or patients become angry at you for not responding appropriately to them? What has that been like for you?
   c. How would you have responded to Theo?
   d. What societal messages are relayed to men about grief and the expression of vulnerable feelings other than anger?

Truly, Madly, Deeply (1990; Alan Rickman, Juliet Stevenson): Nina (Stevenson) is overwhelmed by the death of her boyfriend, Jamie (Rickman). To her blissful surprise, Jamie reappears to her as a ghost. This leads to complications in her life and in her ability to process her grief.

1   (Ch 3, 0:16:26–0:19:18) Nina is in a session with her psychotherapist. The scene starts with a voiceover of her session while the viewer sees her putting laundry on a line. The therapist is very passive in this scene. (I frequently use this scene in workshops for psychotherapists. Many object to the therapist's inaction. What needs to be emphasized here is that *Truly, Madly, Deeply* is a British film so cultural differences are a factor. Second, the therapist could actually have impeded the client's grief process by saying or doing anything. I do think, however, that the therapist should have checked on the client's safety and said something supportive or validating to her prior to her leaving).

a. How did you feel watching Nina express her grief?

b. What feelings does she express? Are they "normal"?

c. At one point Nina says, "I know I shouldn't do this," seemingly embarrassed to be expressing her grief in this way in front of another person. Remember, this is a British film. How does culture impact processing and expressing grief?

d. How comfortable are you expressing emotions in front of others?

e. Is it appropriate for doctors to express emotions in the presence of patients or their family and friends?

f. Do you find it helpful to discuss with a colleague a particularly difficult interaction with a patient and/or family? Please explain.

The Messenger (2009; Ben Foster, Woody Harrelson, Jena Malone, Samantha Morton): Sgt. Will Montgomery (Foster) is injured in Iraq by an improvised explosive device. Having returned to the United States to recover from injuries to his eye and leg, Sgt. Montgomery is assigned to the casualty notification team. His job is to notify families of killed soldiers. He is partnered with the more experienced Captain Tony Stone (Harrelson). Through "on the job" experience, Will learns about the impact of grief and loss.

1 (Ch 3, 0:15:13–0:18:17) In this scene, Sgt. Montgomery is on his first notification. He and Captain Stone inform a family that their loved one has died.

a. Is the mother's reaction extreme? What is the range of emotional and behavioral reactions that might occur when you give bad news to a client or family?

b. As a health-care provider, have you had to deliver similar types of devastating news to family members whose loved one has died? If so, what was that experience like for you?

c. What is the most professional way to respond to a patient getting angry with you and even possibly attacking you? Are there policies or practices in your workplace that deal with this issue?

d. What is the significance, if any, of the mother being an African-American woman in trying to understand the intensity of her reaction?

A Single Man (2009; Colin Firth, Julianne Moore, Nicholas Hoult, Matthew Goode): This is the story of gay English professor George Falconer (Firth) who is dealing with the sudden death of his partner (Goode) of 16 years.

1 (Ch 2, 0:03:23–0:07:39) It has been 8 months since his partner's death and George is struggling to cope with the loss. He dreams that he walks into the accident scene and kisses his partner's dead body.

a. Describe George's grief experience in emotional, physical, and spiritual terms.

b. What happens to George physically after he says that he feels as if he is "sinking," "drowning," and "can't breathe"?

c. Recall a loss of your own. Can you relate to George's statements "waking up has actually hurt" or "It takes time in the morning for me to become George."?

Friends and Family Reactions to Grieving Individuals

Shadowlands (see earlier description)

1 (Ch 22, 1:59:27–2:00:53) Although ambivalent, Jack (Anthony Hopkins) eventually decides to attend a university gathering. He quickly leaves after hearing his pastor's comments about grief and loss.
   a. What specific comments trigger Jack? Why do many people respond with clichés and platitudes when speaking with someone who is grieving?
   b. Discuss whether you think Jack's anger is appropriate. What did Jack's expression of anger accomplish?
   c. How do you respond to angry patients or family members? If the anger is in response to grief, do you respond differently?
   d. The pastor discusses his beliefs about loss. What role does spirituality/religion play in dealing with loss?

The Namesake (2006; Kal Penn, Tabu, Irrfan Khan): American-born Gogol Ganguli (Penn) is the son of Indian immigrants Ashima and Ashoke Ganguli (Tabu, Khan) and prefers to be called Nick. He is torn between his parents' traditions and his desire to fit in among his friends in New York.
1 (Ch 20, 1:25:09–1:27:01) Nick/Gogol's father has died. His girlfriend, Maxine, attends visitation at the family home.
   a. Critique Maxine's interaction with Nick/Gogol. How supportive is she?
   b. Why does Nick get so angry with Maxine? What could she have done differently in attempting to be helpful to Nick?
   c. How does culture or ethnicity influence how a family grieves?

Smoke (1995; Harvey Keitel, William Hurt, Forest Whitaker): A Brooklyn cigar store and its owner, Auggie Wren (Keitel), are at the center of the vignettes in this film. One of the featured characters is Paul (Hurt), a disheartened and grieving writer.
1 (Ch 3, 0:12:20–0:17:36) Auggie shows Paul photos he has taken from the same street corner and at the same time for 4000 days. While looking at the photos, Paul sees an image of Ellen, his deceased wife. She was murdered in a neighborhood shooting. Paul is overcome with emotion and begins to cry.
   a. Critique Auggie's response to Paul's grief. If you were Paul, would you have felt supported?
   b. Auggie says nothing and simply remains present with Paul's grief. Is there anything Auggie could have said to Paul that would have helped him feel better?

c. How does the fact that Ellen was murdered possibly complicate Paul's grief?
d. How did you feel watching the scene?

Health-Care Provider Interactions with Grieving Families
••••••••••••

Little Miss Sunshine (2006; Abigail Breslin, Greg Kinnear, Paul Dano, Alan Arkin, Toni Collette, Steve Carell): In this poignant and funny film, the Hoover extends family travels by Volkswagen van to California so that Olive (Breslin) can compete in the Little Miss Sunshine beauty contest.

1 (Ch 13, 0:51:10–0:55:17) In this (at times) humorous scene, the paternal grandfather (Arkin) has been rushed to the hospital after not waking up at the motel at which the family was staying. The family is at the hospital waiting to hear about his medical condition. The doctor enters and delivers the news that the grandfather has died. Later, a social worker enters to discuss post-death procedures with the man's son (Kinnear).
    a. Critique the doctor's delivery of the news that the grandfather has died, including his choice of language to describe the death and the body. Was it appropriate to deliver the news to the entire family? What would you have done differently? Suggestion: Role-play an alternative approach.
    b. Have you been in a similar situation with a grieving family? How did you handle it? What impact did the encounter have on you?
    c. What is the role of the physician in caring for a bereaved family?
    d. Critique the social worker's interactions with the son. How do you cope with the day-to-day stress of your job? What do you do to take care of yourself?
    e. Do practice/hospital policies sometimes complicate a family's grieving process? If so, how?
    f. How does a health-care professional deal with the necessary procedures and paperwork required at the workplace and be relational as well?

The Namesake (see earlier description)

1 (Ch 18, 1:12:51–1:18:21) Ashoke (Khan) calls Ashima (Tabu) to tell her that he is at the hospital because he is experiencing stomach discomfort. He assures her that he will call her when he gets home. Having not heard from him for some time, Ashima calls the hospital. After a frustrating wait and being asked to spell her name five times, she is informed by an intern that he has "passed away." After hanging up the phone, she reacts to her grief.
    a. Critique how the intern interacts with Ashima and informs her of the death. Would you have done anything differently?
    b. Are there any policies/practices at your hospital or practice that need to be changed to be more supportive of grieving family and friends?
    c. How would you have responded to Ashima's grief?

     d. Does the fact that the death occurs at Christmas factor into your answer?

     e. How do you cope with your own emotional reactions to the death of a patient?

The Messenger (see earlier description)

1 (Ch 2, 0:07:52–0:10:15) In this scene Sgt. Montgomery learns of his assignment to the casualty notification team. Captain Stone informs him of the rules when engaging with the family. He says never to use terms like "lost or expired or passed away," to be clear by saying "killed or died" and to call each casualty by name, not "the deceased or the body."

     a. What terms are used at your hospital or practice to refer to the fact that someone has died?

     b. What terms do you use? How do you refer to the deceased patient?

     c. Captain Stone said touching the next of kin is forbidden. Do you or your hospital or practice have formal or informal rules when interacting with a grieving loved one, including rules on touching?

     d. Would you ever touch a patient or loved one who is in emotional pain?

     e. What do you see as your "job" when someone is grieving?

2 (Ch 10, 0:54:44–0:57:05) An interpreter joins Sgt. Montgomery and Captain Stone to help them notify a Hispanic father of his daughter's death.

     a. How does the fact that the father does not speak English impact the delivery of the tragic news?

     b. What emotions is the father experiencing? After he hears the news, he looks back at a child in the apartment. What do you think is going through his mind?

     c. Have you had to deliver news of a death to a family whose primary language is not English? If so, what was the experience like for you?

Grief and Loss Issues for Gay, Lesbian, Bisexual, and Transgender Individuals

A Single Man (see earlier description)

1 (Ch 3, 0:07:39–0:11:25) Sometimes, an individual's grief is complicated by society's general lack of acknowledgment of the loss. In this scene, George learns of his partner's death and is told by his partner's cousin that he is not welcome at the funeral because it is "just for family."

     a. Recall a time when you learned of a death. What was it like? How did you react?

     b. Have hospital or practice policies/practices prevented a loved one from being with a patient? Is there anything that can be done to change the policies/practices?

c. George visited his neighbor (Moore) to fully express his grief? Why do you think that was helpful for him? (Hint: Grief shared is halved).

d. How do you think George's exclusion from the funeral impacts his grieving process? Are there other conditions, such as HIV and end-stage alcoholism, when patients and their families feel excluded from society and alone in their grief?

Speaking with Children about Grief and Loss

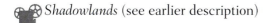

Shadowlands (see earlier description)

1 (Ch 23, 2:01:09–2:04:17) Even though he is unsure what to say, Jack (Anthony Hopkins) speaks with Joy's son (Joseph Mazzello) about his mother's death.

a. Are you wary of speaking with someone who is grieving, particularly children? Why?

b. What did you like about Jack's conversation with the boy?

c. Would you have done anything differently?

d. Is it appropriate for a medical professional to touch or hug a dying or grieving child?

e. How did you feel while watching the scene?

Tender Mercies (1983; Robert Duvall, Tess Harper, Betty Buckley, Wilford Brimley, Ellen Barkin, Allan Hubbard): *Tender Mercies* is about alcoholic drifter and once famous country singer Mac Sledge (Duvall) and his relationship with a widow (Harper) and her young son Sonny (Hubbard). The movie also focuses on Mac's relationship with his ex-wife (Buckley) and their daughter (Barkin).

1 (Ch 5, 0:13:12–0:15:26) In this scene, Sonny gets into a fight with another boy after the boy insults Sonny's father and stepfather. Sonny later asks his mother questions about his father who was killed in Vietnam.

2 (Ch 21, 1:24:17–1:26:25) In this related scene, Sonny asks his mother more questions about his father.

a. It is said that being available to a grieving child's questions is more important than even having the answers to such questions. Despite this observation, critique the mother's responses to Sonny's questions in both scenes.

b. In the first scene, why did Sonny's mother decide to take him to the cemetery? Was it a good idea?

c. How do you respond to a child's illness or death related questions?

Spiritual Questions

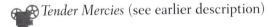 *Tender Mercies* (see earlier description)

1 (Ch 20, 1:20:06–1:24:15) Mac (Duvall) visits his ex-wife Dixie (Buckley) after they discover that their daughter has died in an automobile accident.
   a. What do you think of Harry's (Brimley) physical response to Dixie's anger?
   b. Should the nurse have responded differently? How would you have responded?
   c. In this scene, Dixie was not given medication. What is your opinion of the use of medication for those who are grieving a loss?
   d. The scene depicts Mac and Dixie's spiritual questions related to the loss. How do spirituality and religion impact grief?
   e. How do your spiritual/religious beliefs about death impact your interactions with grieving families?
   f. Rosa Lee (Harper) asks Mac, "You OK?" and says nothing further. Was this effective? If so, how?

Rituals

About Schmidt (2002; Jack Nicholson, Hope Davis, Dermot Mulroney, Kathy Bates): Warren Schmidt (Jack Nicholson) is an insurance actuary whose wife dies shortly after his retirement. He later finds her letters indicating that years ago she had an affair with his close friend. He decides to take a road trip to his daughter's wedding and comes to terms with his life.
1 (Chs 15–16, 1:13:26–1:15:17) Schmidt "speaks" to his wife Helen during a post-death grief ritual on the roof of his camper.
   a. Discuss the importance of rituals in processing grief. How does Schmidt's ritual help him process his grief?
   b. How common is guilt in reaction to a loss?
   c. Have you been asked by family/friends to participate in any rituals for dying or deceased patients? What factors did you consider in your decision on whether or not to participate? If you did participate, what was it like?

Non-Death-Related Grief and Loss

The Messenger (see earlier description)

1 (Ch 5, 0:30:23–0:31:10) Sgt. Montgomery (Ben Foster) injured his eye and leg during active duty. In this scene, a doctor is examining Sgt. Montgomery's eye. Sgt. Montgomery attempts to lighten the mood with some humor.
   a. An individual can experience non-death-related grief, such as when he/

she loses normal body functioning. Discuss further, listing the variety of occurrences that may trigger grief in patients or clients? Would you manage these grief reactions in any way differently from those that occur after a death?

b. What do you think of the doctor's interactions with Sgt. Montgomery? Could he have been more empathic? How?

Up in the Air (2009; George Clooney, Anna Kendrick, Vera Farmiga): Ryan Bingham (Clooney) travels around the country firing people for employers unwilling to do it themselves.

1 (Ch 6, 0:32:20–0:34:22) Natalie Keener (Kendrick), a new colleague of Ryan's, recommends that their company fire people via videoconferencing to save money. She accompanies Ryan on a trip to observe the actual process.

2 (Ch 8, 44:32–44:55) Ryan and Natalie inform more people that they have been fired.

3 (Ch 17, 1:42:01–1:43:05) In this scene, individuals discuss the impact of being fired.

a. The grief experienced by those who lose jobs is similar in nature to that experienced by those who bear the death of a loved one. How do you explain this phenomenon?

b. Describe the emotions expressed by the individuals in these scenes.

c. What mistakes did Natalie Keener make in the first scene (Ch 6)? What was she attempting to do and why do you think her approach was unsuccessful?

d. Describe a time when you said something to a grieving family that was not received in the way you intended. In retrospect, what would you do differently?

e. What differences in the reactions of the fired workers did you notice in the last scene (Ch 17) when compared with the prior scenes? What mechanisms help individuals cope with sudden loss such as job termination?

Further Reading

● Engstrom F. *Movie Clips for Creative Mental Health Education*. Plainview, NY: Wellness Reproductions and Publishing; 2004.
● Humphrey K. *Counseling Strategies for Loss and Grief*. Alexandria, VA: American Counseling Association; 2009.

17

Hard Lives: Trauma from Abuse and Violence

Patricia Lenahan, Jo Marie Reilly,
LaTasha K. Crawford, Peter Cronholm,
Roger Y. Wong, Corisande Baldwin & Michael Metal

VIOLENCE IS A MAJOR PUBLIC HEALTH CONCERN. VIOLENCE EXPOSURES are associated with negative health outcomes at all stages of life. The World Health Organization defines violence as: "The intentional use of physical force or power, threatened or actual, against oneself, another person, or against a group or community, that either results in or has a high likelihood of resulting in injury, death, psychological harm, mal-development or deprivation."[1] Violence can be described in terms of self-directed behaviors (self-abuse or suicidal behavior), interpersonal (community or domestic – i.e. child, partner, or elder abuse), or collective (social, political, or economic). The nature of the violence inflicted may be physical, sexual, psychological, or forms of deprivation or neglect. Violence as a construct can be thought of as occurring within a nested ecological context of the individuals involved with regard to the relationships, communities, and society in which the violence occurs.

Compelling data suggest that exposures to violence correlate strongly and in a dose-response relationship with poorer health and increased mortality. The Adverse Childhood Experiences (ACE) Study[2] continues to explore how exposures to categories of abuse, neglect, and household dysfunction in the first 18 years of life are related to health in later life by comparing health outcomes with patient's ACE-score. ACE-scores are simply the count of adverse childhood experiences reported by patients. As the ACE-scores increases, the risk for the following increase in a strong and graded fashion: alcoholism and alcohol abuse, chronic obstructive pulmonary disease, depression, fetal death, health-related quality of life, illicit drug use, ischemic heart disease, liver disease, risk for intimate partner violence, multiple sexual partners, sexually transmitted diseases, smoking, suicide attempts, unintended pregnancies, early initiation of smoking, early initiation of sexual activity, and adolescent pregnancy.[3]

The mechanisms supporting the connection between poor health and violence exposures are related to social, emotional, and cognitive impairment from the adoption of negative health-risk behaviors which result in disease, disability, and social problems and, ultimately, increased mortality.[4]

Child and elder abuse affect some of the most vulnerable populations. Elder abuse is one of the least studied forms of domestic violence, and includes emotional abuse, physical violence, and neglect, but financial mistreatment can also be a factor. Other forms of violence and abuse that affect individuals and society include bullying in its various forms, gang-related violence, human trafficking, and other forms of gender-based violence.

More than three million reports of child abuse occur annually, one-third of which are substantiated.[5] Cited rates of prevalence are 11.9 per 1000 children, with two-thirds of cases occurring among children aged less than 12 months and four-fifths are less than 3 years of age.[5] Approximately 1500 children die annually as a result of child maltreatment (81% are less than 3 years of age).[5]

With an incidence of approximately 1.5 million women and 834 700 men raped and/or physically assaulted by an intimate partner annually in the United States, intimate partner violence (IPV) is a common form of violence exposure.[6] IPV has a large body of evidence supporting associations with exposure to adverse physical and mental health outcomes.[7–11] Because of disproportionately high rates of female IPV-associated injury, IPV is commonly used to describe female survivors of male perpetrated violence in heterosexual relationships. IPV can be bi-directional, it can affect men as survivors, and it occurs in same-sex relationships. IPV affects both men and women of all demographic and socioeconomic groups.

Impact of Emotional Violence on a Child
∙∙

White Oleander (2002; Robin Wright Penn, Michelle Pfeiffer, Renee Zellweger): This is the story of Astrid's (Alison Lohman) journey to independence as she struggles with the challenge of a manipulative mother and living in a succession of foster homes.

1 (Scene 4: Arrested, 0:00:00–0:01:54) Astrid observes her mother being arrested and sentenced to a jail term after it is discovered that her mother killed her boyfriend.
    a. What is the impact of a parent's violent behavior on a child?
    b. As a health-care professional, what steps can be taken to reach out to a child and identify with their isolation and fear when they have witnessed their parents' violence?
    c. What is the role of law enforcement in identifying and preventing child abuse and intimate violence?
2 (Scene 6, 0:0:01:02–0:01:17) Astrid has flashbacks of her mother's boyfriend breaking into their home.

    a. How do violent flashbacks play a role in a child's ability to heal from the violence they have experienced?

    b. How can a health-care provider best help prepare a child to heal from their experiences?

3 (Scene 8: The Enemy, 0:00:30–0:4:52) Astrid goes to visit her mother in jail for the first time.

    a. What is the impact on a child when they see their parent in jail and handcuffed?

    b. How does a child handle the conflict of living with a foster parent with different viewpoints and values from which they've been raised?

4 (Scene 25: The Price of Belonging, 0:00:1:50–0:4:30) Astrid, now a grown adult, tries to find closure and peace with her mom.

    a. What is the long-term impact of emotional manipulation on a child?

    b. How does a grown woman heal after years of neglect and abuse from her mother?

    c. How can a professional help treat a child who has been neglected and abused by her parents?

Sexual Orientation

Violence Because of Sexual Orientation

Boys Don't Cry (1999; Hillary Swank, Chloe Sevigny, Peter Sarsgaard): This movie tells the true story of Brandon Teena (Swank), a woman who believes that she is a man and struggles with violence and abuse for her sexual orientation, her love for Lana (Sevigny), and tries to be accepted and loved for who she is.

1 (Scene 2: Lincoln 1993, 0:00:00–0:01:14) Brandon (Teena) is being chased by men who are angry when they discover she is not a man and she has been romantic with on of their sisters.

    a. What advice would you give Brandon (Teena) as she divulges her gender orientation to you?

    b. How do we respond to the sexual orientation of others?

    c. How would you support Brandon (Teena) as she struggles with the violence that she incurs while struggling to live her life as a man?

2 (Scene 18: Are You a Girl?, 0:01:06–0:02:52) Lana's friends and family confront Brandon (Teena) about her sexual orientation and they threaten to kill her if she is a lesbian.

    a. How would you approach a mother's horrified reaction that her daughter is involved with a man "with a sickness"?

    b. How would you respond to Lana's friends who want to "kill Brandon" if she is a lesbian and "messing with Lana"?

3 (Scene 19: The Rape, 0:00:00–0:04:32) Brandon (Teena) is recounting her gang rape by two "friends" who discover she is a woman and rape her.

a. How would you respond to the violence and betrayal that Brandon (Teena) suffered as a result of her sexual identity?
b. Could Brandon's rape have been avoided?
c. Could Brandon's murder been avoided?

La Mission (2009; Benjamin Bratt, Max Rosenak): Che Rivera (Bratt) is an ex-con, sober alcoholic and single father to Jess (Jeremy Ray Valdez), a high school senior. His father's pride and joy, Jess enjoyed "cruising" with his father's car club in the San Francisco Mission district and has been accepted to UCLA in the Fall. Jess is also gay and spending more time away from home with his boyfriend. His father becomes violent after discovering photos of his son with Jordan. While his father struggles to deal with his son's sexual orientation, Jess is socially harassed at school and shot. His father must come to terms with his son's identity when Jess rejects his father's denial of his son's sexual orientation and refuses to return home.

1 (Ch 7, 0:34:07–0:35:55) In this scene, Jess walks the hallways at school with students calling him derogatory names and gossiping over the physical beating by his father. His father arrives home after work and finds a derogatory name spray-painted on their garage door.
   a. What resources or actions could a parent take to deal with derogatory names Jess is called at school? In the community?
2 (Ch 14, 1:18:11–1:19:40) In this scene, a gang member harasses Jess and Jordan as they are walking. When Jordan tries to verbally defend them, the gang member shoots Jess.
3 (Ch 19, 1:43:36–1:48:02) Living alone and relapsed, Che encounters an Aztec ceremony on the sidewalk. It is for a grieving family and mother of the deceased young man who shot Jess. Viewing the photo of the deceased boy who'd harassed Jess, Che reflects on his harassment against his son, Jess.

Cultural and Ethnic

Ethnic and Racial Induced Violence

Gran Torino (2008; Clint Eastwood, Bee Vang, Atney Her): This movie tells the story of Walt Kowalsky (Eastwood), a hardened, racist, ex–Korean War vet and his journey with the acculturation challenges and injustices experienced by his Hmong neighbors, particularly the teens, Tou and Gracie.

Racial Violence and Bullying

1 (Scene 3: Chill with Us, 0:00:00–0:01:31) Thao (Vang) is racially bullied by neighborhood Latino gang and "rescued" by some members of a rival Hmong gang.
   a. How would you respond to the racial insults experienced by Thao?

b. How can we advocate for minority youth who are exposed to violence?

c. What are the emotional and physical consequences of racism and prejudice for minorities in this country?

d. How can we intercede with youth who are exposed to violence?

Youth Violence and Gangs

1 (Scene 7: Get off My Lawn, 0:00:00–0:2:30) Thao is pressured by some local Hmong gang members to join their gang and when he resists, they get violent with him.

a. What are the directors portraying about the way youth are pressured into gangs?

b. How did Thao respond to the violence he experienced?

c. How can we advocate for minority youth to resist violence as a way of life?

2 (Scene 9: Crazy Old Man, 0:00:00–0:04:30) Sue (Atney) and her boyfriend are bullied and attacked by some African-American local gang members.

a. How can youth of multiple racial backgrounds live peacefully in their neighborhoods?

b. Did Sue's boyfriend's efforts to "relate" to the African-American gang members help his situation or further incite them?

c. Did Sue's efforts to defend herself improve or antagonize the racial tensions and hostility she experienced?

3 (Scene 20: Making Him Look Bad, 0:00:00–0:01:30) Thao is attacked and bullied by the local Hmong gang for getting a job.

a. Why was Thao penalized by the local Hmong gangs for trying to make a better life for himself?

b. How would you respond to a patient that you recognized was victimized by gang violence?

c. How would you advise a teen or family that was being victimized by gang violence?

Incest

Precious (2009; Mo'Nique, Paula Patton, Mariah Carey, Lenny Kravitz, Gabourey Sidibe): This movie tells the story of Precious Jones (Sidibe), an inner-city high school girl who is illiterate, abused, obese, and pregnant and her journey to redemption and empowerment with the help of an alternative-school teacher.

1 (Scene 2: Principal's Office, 0:02:22–0:03:04) Precious's mother throws an object at the back of her head and her father rapes her.

a. How did Precious respond to her mother's request for cigarettes?

b. What message does Precious's father send to her as he tells her he loves her and then he rapes her?

c. What is the prevalence of incest in families?

Parental Emotional and Physical Abuse

1 (Scene 3: Each One Teach One, 0:03:10–0:05:50) The principal of Precious's school goes to her home and tries to encourage her to go to an alternative school. Her mother is very upset and becomes violent.
   a. What provoked Precious's mom's act of violence?
   b. How does her mother's emotional and physical abuse affect Precious's ability for success?
   c. What can teachers do to become more aware of possible sexual, physical, or emotional abuse of their students?

2 (Scene 11: Eat it Up, 0:00:20–0:03:33) Precious's mother wants her to go to the welfare office instead of going to school and tells her she is too dumb to learn.
   a. How does Precious's mom continue to undermine her self-worth?
   b. How does Precious's mom use food to manipulate her?
   c. What us the impact of the emotional and physical abuse on Precious's ability to improve herself?

3 (Scene 19: Ruined My Life, 0:00:18–0:01:15) Precious brings her newborn baby home from the hospital and her mother throws him on the ground and starts fighting with Precious.
   a. How does Precious's mother now try to use her new grandson as a cause for continued violence?
   b. How can a health-care professional empower a victim of violence?
   c. What is the role of law enforcement in identifying or preventing violence?

Impact of Sexual Abuse on Families

1 (Scene 24: On Her Own, 0:0:05:22–0:07:40) Precious's mother tells the social worker how she let Precious be abused by her husband and wasn't able to intervene.
   a. What was your response to Precious's mother's explanation of how she allowed her daughter to be abused by her husband, Precious's father?
   b. How can a health-care provider respond to a mother who is so disturbed by her own dysfunction that she is unfit to safely parent?
   c. What are the potential long- and short-term emotional sequelae of childhood victims of incest and physical abuse?

Intimate Partner Violence: Physical and Psychological Abuse

Take My Eyes (2005): In this Spanish film, Pilar (Laia Marull) is engaged in a physically and psychologically violent relationship with her husband,

Antonio (Luis Tosar). While she has the support of her sister, Ana (Candela Pena) who takes in Pilar and her young son, Juan, Pilar's mother believes she belongs at home with her husband. Antonio wants his family back, alternately seducing and terrorizing Pilar, forcing her to make an ultimate decision.

1 (0:59:00–1:02:45) The family is coming back from a party at Antonio's brother's home. Antonio is angry about the preferential treatment he believes his brother is receiving. Pilar is quiet and Antonio asks her what she is thinking. She responds "nothing" and Antonio stops the car on the road, begins yelling, gets out, kicking the car and breaking the window. Pilar and Juan are huddled together. Antonio comes home from work the next night with a gift for Pilar, telling her "nobody understands me like you do."

    a. How does Antonio's sense of resentment towards his family of origin affect his relationship with Pilar and Juan?

    b. Antonio brings Pilar a gift and tells her no one understands him like she does. What phase of the cycle of violence does this scene demonstrate?

    c. How would you counsel a patient who shares information regarding an interchange such as this?

2 (1:06:00–1:07:02) Antonio arrives home before Pilar. He demands to know where she went at lunch and who she was with. He also demands to know why she didn't answer her cell phone, especially after he left three messages. He slams her against the wall and Pilar begins to cringe and tremble.

    a. What is the impact of Antonio's violence on Pilar?

    b. What is the impact of jealousy on relationships?

    c. How would you counsel a patient regarding a jealous partner? What are the potential risks?

The Decision to Leave:

1 (0:1:12–0:3:26) It's the middle of the night and Pilar is seen frantically waking up Juan and gathering clothes together. She flees her home, arriving at her sister Ana's house. Pilar's fear is evident. Safely inside Ana's home Pilar notices that she is wearing her bedroom slippers. She says: "I'm still wearing my slippers. How stupid am I?"

    a. Why do people stay in abusive relationships?

    b. What are the risks associated with leaving an abusive relationship?

    c. What is the impact of leaving on the children?

    d. How does Pilar's decision to leave in the middle of the night affect Juan?

    e. How would you interpret Pilar's statement: "How stupid am I?"

2 (0:04:25–0:0:6:35) Ana arrives at Pilar's home to get some of her things. She notices broken dishes and food thrown on the wall. Ana finds copies of hospital records in Pilar's clothing drawer. Before she can look at them thoroughly, Antonio arrives. He tells her to get out and to send Pilar home.

    a. What advice would you offer family and friends regarding going to the victim's home?

    b. How could the situation have been addressed in a safer manner?

3 (1:34:50–1:38:20) Pilar had returned to Antonio, only to be abused again. After the last incident, Pilar visits Ana and asks her to care for Juan until she gets settled. Pilar adds: "I need to see myself. I haven't seen myself for so long." Later, Antonio is home drinking as Pilar and her friends arrive to get her things. Antonio and Pilar only exchange glances.

    a. What factors led to Pilar's decision to leave Antonio?

    b. How can health-care and mental health professionals support a patient like Pilar?

    c. What interventions might a health-care provider have made to help Pilar reach this decision earlier?

    d. What is the impact on Juan? What interventions would be helpful for him?

    e. What recommendations would you make regarding parental (Antonio's) visitation?

Family Violence in the Military

The Great Santini (1979; Robert Duvall, Blythe Danner, Michael O'Keefe): Bull (Duvall) is a Marine Corps fighter pilot and veteran of both the Korean War and World War II. Transitioning from war to a time of peace, he struggles with an identity in flux. Showing symptoms of posttraumatic stress disorder and alcoholism, he becomes both physically and verbally abusive toward his wife and children.

1 (0:09:15–0:011:40) Lillian (Danner), Bull's wife, and their children are at the airport awaiting Bull's return home. The youngest daughter offers to punch her Mom who says that she can't remember what it was like with him home.

    a. The mother downplays the question. What can this be a symptom of?

    b. What are the possible reasons the children are not excited to see their father?

    c. What does the mother's insistence that the children approach their father in a specific order possibly indicate?

2 (0:30:50–0:39:28) Ben (O'Keefe) and Bull are playing basketball and Ben wins. Bull becomes physically aggressive on the court and verbally abusive following the game. Bull practices in the rain, seemingly oblivious to the inclement weather.

    a. Why does Bull become physically aggressive when his son is playing well against him?

    b. What behaviors does Ben mimic following the assault? As a therapist, how would you address this?

    c. The wife indicates an inability by Bull to communicate his feelings effectively. How does this help/hurt the relationship he has with the family?

3 (1:08:00–1:11:18) The rival team foul Ben. Bull comes down from the stands and tells him, "Get him or I'm gonna get you!"
   a. How is Ben's behavior a learned response?
   b. In what ways does Ben display regret following the game?
4 (1:27:30–1:29:00) Bull returns home drunk and begins physically abusing his wife. Hearing the commotion, the children rush in and defend their mother.
   a. What are the potential long-term issues for a child who consistently witnesses spousal abuse in the home?
   b. How does the response of the children indicate protective factors for the children?
   c. What are some of the reasons that Bull believes this to be appropriate behavior?
   d. How does the mother's defense of Bull affect the family's beliefs about right and wrong?

Substance Use and Intimate Partner Violence

Bloom (2005; Mara Monserrat, Jessi Perez): This is the story of the youngest daughter of an upwardly mobile Latino family in Chicago and her court-ordered therapist, Dr. Sharon Greene (Monserrat), who is coping with problems of her own: infertility and concern for her terminally ill mother. Letty (Perez) barely graduated from high school and, much to the dismay of her mother, soon became pregnant with Lisa, now five. Letty's second child, Beto, was born with cerebral palsy. Letty alternately lives with her parents and her new boyfriend, Ernesto, an abusive drug dealer.
1 (1:10:37–1:12:31) Letty and Ernesto are at a bar with friends. Ernesto is playing pool and he says to Letty: "bring us some beers, bitch." Letty tells him to get them himself. Ernesto becomes enraged as his friends laugh at his inability to get Letty to do what he wants. Ernesto grabs Letty, pushes her, hits her, slams her head on the pool table, and kicks her.
   a. What impact can alcohol or drug use have on intimate partner violence perpetration? Does substance abuse cause or exacerbate violent behavior?
   b. How did Letty's refusal to acquiesce to Ernesto in front of his friends impact his reaction?
   c. Why did no one intervene to stop the violence?

Honey and Ashes (*Miel et Cendres*) (1996; Naji Najeh, Amel Hedhili, in French and Arabic): This Tunisian film focuses on the intersecting lives of three women in a North African country who are caught between traditional culture and values and a desire to be independent. One woman, an MD, studied medicine in Russia and fell in love there, but succumbed to family pressure and returned home to enter an arranged marriage. The second woman is a university professor whose husband is also a professor and is jealous of his wife. The third woman is a university student who has fallen in love with a young man the family does not like.

1   (0:41:15–0:44:45) Moha (Najeh) and Amina (Hedhili) have returned from a party. Moha continues to drink and smoke and page through books on the shelf. He becomes visibly more upset when he reads an inscription in one of the books: "to my dear Amina." Moha goes into the bedroom and initiates an argument with Amina about her abortion, stating "you would have given me a son." Amina reminds him that he wanted her to have the abortion so that she could finish her doctorate. An enraged Moha begins choking, hitting, and punching Amina, ultimately knocking her down and stepping on her hand and fingers repeatedly. Moha's neighbors arrive at the door and tell him that it is "enough," adding: "I know what you are capable of. He is just like his father."
    a.   What are ways to prevent intimate partner violence?
    b.   What factors contributed to Moha's behavior?
    c.   Why are men always thought of as the perpetrators?
    d.   Which batterer typology does Moha represent?
    e.   What resources are there for the abuser?
    f.   What effect might alcohol have had on his behavior and mood?

Take My Eyes (see earlier description)

1   (1:24:15–1:28:28) Pilar is ironing her blouse when Antonio comes home and gets a beer. She tells him that she is going to Madrid the next day to guide an exhibition. Antonio isn't happy, but continues to drink and falls asleep on the couch. The next morning Antonio becomes angry when Pilar gets ready to leave. He rips up her art book, tears off her clothes, and locks her nearly naked on the balcony. He later grabs her and pulls her back in when she urinates on the floor. Antonio tells her to go clean herself up.
    a.   How would you interpret Pilar's response?
    b.   What symptoms might a patient present who has experienced what Pilar has experienced?
    c.   What is the impact of humiliation on individuals who have been abused?

Stalking

1   (0:08:10–0:11:20) Pilar goes to a phone booth and calls Antonio, but hangs up before he can answer. Antonio is waiting for her when she arrives back at her sister's home. Pilar is clearly frightened and runs inside. She locks the door, but opens the small grate to talk to Antonio. He hands her a small gift and swears that he is going to change, begging her to come home. Antonio alternately acts seductive and abusive, finally pounding his fists on the door.
    a.   What constitutes stalking?
    b.   What are the risks associated with stalking?

    c. What advice should a health-care provider offer a patient who is the victim of IPV?

    d. What is the impact of technology and social media on stalking and stalking behaviors?

    e. What advice would you give a stalking victim regarding social media, smart phones, and GPS devices?

2 (1:15:40–1:17:00) Antonio tells Pilar that he has homework. He mentions that he was at the museum earlier in the day and saw her there. Antonio adds that she looked quite pretty. Pilar appears surprised and says she didn't see him.

    a. Is it uncommon for stalkers to remain "invisible" to the victim?

    b. What actions might a stalking victim take to decrease the likelihood of further stalking behaviors?

    c. What are the risks associated with being stalked?

    d. How might an adolescent view this type of behavior?

Batterer Threats of Self-Harm

1 (1:30:50–1:33:20) After Juan leaves the dinner table, Pilar tells Antonio that she doesn't love him anymore. He promises that it will never happen again. Pilar doesn't believe him and Antonio senses that he is losing her. He says he'll kill himself if she leaves and he goes to the kitchen and grabs a knife. Pilar tries to get it away from him, but he manages to cut himself several times on the forearm. Later at the hospital, Pilar is told that he has superficial injuries but will be kept overnight for observation.

    a. What aspects of the cycle of violence does this scene portray?

    b. How should a victim of IPV respond to the threats of self-harm by the batterer?

    c. What is the role of the medical provider in identifying the suicidal risks as well as the potential for further IPV?

Violence during Pregnancy

Nil By Mouth (1997): This UK film is the story of a working-class London couple, Ray (Ray Winstone) and Val (Kathy Burke), and their multigenerational family who is beset by many problems including a drug-addicted brother.

1 (Ch 17, 1:18:40–1:20:40) Michelle is playing with her dolls while Val is looking at her bruises in the bathroom when Val's mother Janet (Laila Morse) comes in. Val quickly sends Michelle into the other room and contrives an elaborate story for her mother, telling her about being run over. Janet asks what the hospital said about the baby and Val continues with her story, assuring her mother that the baby is OK.

a. Why do women who are victims of IPV contrive stories to "cover up" the physical signs of their abuse?
b. How does Val's mother respond to Val's elaborate story?
c. How do we respond to victims of violence when we sense their fear and their hesitance at divulging their true stories?
d. What do young children learn from watching their parent's victimization?

Using the Child to Get to the Mother

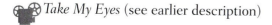 *Take My Eyes* (see earlier description)

1 (0:15:41–0:17:00) Juan and Antonio are playing soccer. Antonio asks Juan lots of questions about Pilar and what she is doing. Initially Juan answers his father's questions, but when Antonio asks him if Pilar's decision to leave was permanent, Juan becomes evasive and says he doesn't know. Antonio starts to kick the ball hard and directly at Juan. Antonio grabs Juan by the shoulder and reminds him of what happens to boys when they don't tell the truth.
  a. What is the incidence and prevalence of child abuse in families where intimate partner violence occurs?
  b. What "message" is Antonio giving Juan?
  c. What is the impact of Juan's being caught between his parents?

Children's Exposure to Intimate Partner Violence

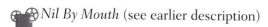 *Nil By Mouth* (see earlier description)

1 (1:14:49–1:18:14) Ray (actor) has been drinking and is sitting at the table brooding. He wakes up Val (actor) and tells her that he wants to talk to her downstairs now. Val had been playing pool with friends and Ray accuses her of having an affair. Things turn violent and Ray begins hitting and kicking Val as their daughter, Michelle, listens in and observes from the top of the stairs.
  a. What behavioral and health symptoms might occur in children who are silent witnesses to parental violence and abuse?
  b. What are the potential long-term sequelae of living in a violent home?
  c. What ACE events are evident in this home?
2 (1:21:23–1:22:15) Val and Michelle are watching TV when Val says she is going to the bathroom. She begins to experience severe abdominal pain and cramping, collapsing on the stairs. Val calls to Michelle and asks her to go get her aunt.
  a. What role do children play in helping protect the violent parental perpetrator?

    b. How do children help/hinder an IPV victim's efforts at stopping the family violence?

    c. What advice/resources should health-care providers give to an IPV victim about how to best protect her children from family violence?

Honey and Ashes (see earlier description)

1 (0:49:45–0:51:00) Said, Moha's brother, comes to the apartment and hugs Amina. She asks him to take her to the hospital. As Amina is getting into the car, she meets Moha, who is with their daughter. The little girl asks what happened to her mother and where she was going. Moha tells his daughter that mommy fell down the stairs when she came to get you at Granny's. He insists on taking Amina to the hospital. At the hospital, the little girl offers the explanation that her mommy fell down the stairs.

    a. Moha associates Amina's injury with coming to get her daughter. What kinds of feelings could this elicit in her daughter?

    b. Describe how people hide abuse?

    c. Batterers often offer plausible explanations for the injuries they have inflicted. Do you think Moha's daughter believed him?

2 (0:55:00–0:56:08) Amina comes home from the hospital with a cast on her arm. She sees all the papers strewn around the bedroom and moves them around with her feet. Her daughter enters the room and asks what she is doing. She says she wants to play "riddles" with her mother. She asks Amina who is the biggest and strongest person in the world. Amina responds, "God," but her daughter says, "no, it's Papa."

    a. How would you interpret the daughter's response?

    b. What is the impact of being exposed to violence in the home?

    c. How can this early exposure affect adult development and relationships?

Bloom (see earlier description)

1 (1:31:50–1:32:47) Letty has returned from a therapy session where she angrily defended herself as being a good mother. She had reassured Dr. Greene that her daughter Lisa did not know about the violence and abuse. Letty walks by Lisa's room where she is playing with her dolls. Letty overhears Lisa talking for her dolls: "I told you to keep your mouth shut. You can't hit me. Yes, I can." Lisa has her dolls hitting one another. It continues with Lisa saying, "You can't hit Lisa … I'll call the cops." Letty enters and asks Lisa what she is doing. Lisa quickly responds that she isn't doing anything wrong. Letty reassures her that she isn't doing anything wrong and attempts to distract her daughter.

    a. What are the adverse childhood effects of witnessing parental violence?

    b. How does "child's play" mimic adult behaviors?

c. What is the impact on Letty of seeing her daughter re-create abusive scenarios in her play?

d. Victims of abuse often think their children aren't aware of what is occurring. How would you counsel them in this regard?

e. What is the incidence and prevalence of child abuse associated with intimate partner violence? Letty's youngest child has cerebral palsy. What is the likelihood of child abuse occurring around disabled children?

Take My Eyes (see earlier description)

1 (1:30:50–1:33:20) Pilar, Antonio, and Juan are sitting quietly at dinner. Antonio comments that it is more like a funeral than a family dinner. Juan asks to be excused and to go visit a friend. Antonio tells him to finish his dinner, but eventually allows him to leave.

a. How would you interpret Juan's response?

b. How are family members affected by intimate partner violence?

Public Health Implications of Violence and Abuse

1 (0:12:16–0:12:58; 0:20:20–0:21:50) Ana confronts Pilar, telling her that she saw the medical records. Pilar's resolve is weakening, especially after her mother says she should work things out with Antonio and go home. Ana becomes infuriated and again confronts Pilar, stating: "mother doesn't want to believe it … all the falls in the hospital records, the tendonitis, torn muscles, loss of vision in one eye … the bastard kicked you in the kidney."

a. What are the costs associated with IPV?

b. What type of injuries might trigger suspiciousness on the part of the physician?

c. How could a physician respond to a patient who has a history of multiple suspicious injuries?

d. How could a physician intervene with a patient who has this type of history?

e. What is the role of the family in the cycle of violence?

f. Other than physical injury, in what other ways to do people affected by abuse or violence present in health-care settings?

Batterers' Treatment

1 (0:21:50–0:24:35) Antonio is seen attending a batterers' treatment group counseling session. The therapist asks one man why he thinks his wife is crazy. He responds that she is "hysterical," going around saying that I beat her. Group members snicker and another man shares that his wife provokes

him so he beats her up, adding that "after a good slap she calms down." The therapist introduces another man, Julian, who had been a member of the group two years earlier. Julian states that he thought he was normal, but "I had erased her personality." Julian continued and shared an incident where he knocked out his wife and thought he had killed her. All the men were attentive and sitting forward.

    a. What impact did Julian's "story" have on the group?

    b. How would you interpret Julian's statement that he "erased his wife's personality"?

    c. How did that affect Antonio?

    d. What purpose did the therapist have in inviting Julian back to the group? Was this approach successful?

2 (0:27:25–0:29:25) The therapist is attempting to elicit what arouses the men's anger. He asks the group how they feel when they get physically violent, how do they recognize it and control it. He discusses time out and distractions. He asks the group to remember a time when they felt peaceful. Some men offer suggestions while Antonio remains quiet and when asked directly, says he can't think of anything. The men were then asked to write out their feelings.

    a. What technique is the therapist demonstrating?

    b. What does Antonio's silence signify?

    c. How could a therapist engage a quiet or nonparticipatory member in the group's discussion?

3 (0:51:40–0:53:20) The therapist attempts to engage the group in role-play, asking one man to be "the husband" who is coming home from work and another man "the wife." He asks them what usually happens. The men are clearly uncomfortable and respond minimally to this approach. Nervous laughter is heard from the rest of the group.

    a. What could the therapist have done in order to create a better role-play situation?

    b. How would you interpret the reactions of the role-play participants, as well as the group members?

    c. What stereotypic behaviors and reactions did the men describe regarding the causes of their violence?

Individual Therapy for the Perpetrator

1 (0:34:42–0:36:30) Antonio is seen in individual treatment. The therapist pushes Antonio to talk about Pilar and what he misses in her. Antonio shares some feelings and the therapist asks him if he has ever apologized to Pilar. Antonio merely frowns.

    a. What techniques was the therapist using?

    b. How could Antonio's reaction to the issue of apologies be interpreted?

    c. What communication issues might exist between the couple?

d. At what point, if any, would you consider couple therapy? What are the risks associated with it?

2 (1:07:17–1:09:30) Antonio returns to individual therapy after an incident in which he became angry because Pilar didn't come home for lunch or answer her cell phone. Pilar cringed and trembled as he slammed her against the wall. However, when he shares the incident with the therapist, he says that he didn't touch her. The therapist asks Antonio to focus on his erroneous thinking and asks him to write out his feelings, step by step, in a journal. The therapist asks Antonio to describe how he felt when Pilar didn't answer the phone, what were his thoughts, and how he could have stopped them sooner. The therapist asks Antonio about "rational thoughts." Antonio responds that he just wants a "normal" relationship.
   a. What technique is the therapist using?
   b. How can a therapist facilitate Antonio's understanding of the abuse?
   c. What aspects of Antonio's social and family history would be relevant to discuss?
   d. How would Antonio describe a "normal" relationship?

3 (1:13:10–1:15:00) The therapist enters, telling Antonio that he was told the situation was urgent. Pilar has returned home, but Antonio is upset and angry because he couldn't reach Pilar on the phone. He tells the therapist that she is changing because she has a job. Antonio is fearful that she will leave again, adding, "why should she stay with a guy like me?"
   a. How should a therapist respond to this statement?
   b. What risk factors should the therapist consider?
   c. What perpetrator behaviors might indicate an escalation of violence?
   d. What are the risks for the victim during this stage of the relationship?

The Role of the Health-Care Provider

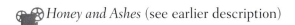 *Honey and Ashes* (see earlier description)

1 (0:51:25–0:53:25) Amina, Moha, and their daughter are at the hospital. The physician emerges and asks why she was called out. Moha wants pain medication for his wife. The physician looks at Amina and pointedly asks, "who did this to you?" She adds: "Tell me, don't be afraid." Moha angrily says, "this isn't the police, she fell." Their daughter adds, "mamma fell down the steps when she came to get me." The doctor doesn't believe them and states: "You tell me this lady fell down the stairs, that's easy. Lies don't heal."
   a. How would you respond to a patient who has suspicious injuries?
   b. What interventions could have been made to offer help?
   c. How could a health-care provider interpret the daughter's response?
   d. What reporting responsibilities do you have in situations like this?

Taking a Violence-Related History

Life Support (2007): This HBO film is based on the true-life story of an HIV-positive African-American woman, Ana (Queen Latifah), and three generations of her family in Brooklyn. Ana lost custody of her daughter because of her drug use. Years later, she is trying to get her life back together and to repair relationships with her mother and teenage daughter. At the same time, she is working for Life Support, a community outreach group focusing on HIV/AIDS awareness, prevention, and support for women.

1   (0:55:25–0:56:23) Ana arrives at the health center as Sandra (Gloria Reuben) is putting up a flyer for a memorial service. Ana expresses surprise, stating that she had seen Deyah the week before and she was "as healthy as can be." Sandra responds that it wasn't the virus that killed her: it was her husband. He shot her. Sandra asks Ana if she had done a domestic violence screen. Ana replies that she had asked Deyah the questions. Sandra tries to be supportive, telling Ana that there wasn't anything else she could have done. Ana is seen standing in front of the flyer saying: "Damn, damn, why didn't you say something?"

   a. When is it appropriate to ask domestic violence screening questions?
   b. How might you assess both the verbal and nonverbal responses of individuals to the questions?
   c. What factors should you consider in conducting a screening interview?

The Role of Law Enforcement: Reporting Intimate Partner Violence

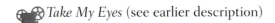

Take My Eyes (see earlier description)

1   (1:28:45–1:30:39) Pilar is seen sitting at the police station after a violent and degrading episode. She states that she wants to report an assault. The officer questions Pilar regarding who assaulted her and the nature of assault. She tells the officer that the perpetrator was her husband and that he insulted her verbally and broke everything. The officer asked about bruises. Pilar tearfully stated that the bruises were inside. After hearing all this, the officer tells her about pressing charges, finding a safe home, and shares that Antonio will be contacted and asked to make a statement. Pilar is visibly upset, says that she's sorry to have bothered him and gets up to leave. The officer follows her, offers her a glass of water, and urges her to stay.

   a. How did Pilar interpret the officer's questions?
   b. What could the officer have done to reassure Pilar?
   c. What constitutes a safety plan?

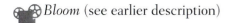*Bloom* (see earlier description)

1 (Ch 9, 1:16:00–1:17:50) Letty has been knocked unconscious by Ernesto and awakens to two concerned police officers kneeling over her. The officer announces that they were here to help her. They tell her not to worry, that Ernesto has been arrested and won't bother her.
   a. What is the impact of the officer's statement?
   b. How did this expression of concern affect Letty?
   c. How realistic is the reassurance of the police officer that Ernesto won't be able to bother her?

Elder Maltreatment: From Neglect to Abuse

Iris (2001; Judi Dench, Jim Broadbent, Kate Winslet): This film is the true story of an English novelist and philosopher, Iris Murdoch, who is diagnosed with Alzheimer's disease while her husband John Bayley struggles to care for her. The film depicts the realities of a devastating disease and raises many important issues pertaining to frail elders with dementia, such as functional decline, wandering, incontinence, and caregiver stress/burnout.

1 In this scene Iris's husband John awakens in the night to hear his wife wandering downstairs and singing. He reflects back to when they were young at a time when they would attend parties together and she would sing. Her singing is interrupted when she becomes incontinent of urine. In this scene it becomes evident that John is having difficulty coping as his home is becoming more cluttered.
   a. What are the biological, psychological, and social determinants of health in someone like Iris who has a dementia?
   b. How would you describe the husband's behavior in dealing with his wife's incontinence? What are some possible reasons for his behavior in this scene?
   c. The husband appears to feel stressed. Thinking back to your past experience, how do you know if a care provider for a frail older person is feeling stressed?
   d. Based on the clutter and deterioration, would this constitute potential elder neglect?

2 (Scene 4, ch 8, 00:45:20–00:46:54; ch 11, 1:10:331:11:50) In these scenes John, Iris' husband, is having more difficulty coping and begins to lash out at Iris.
   a. What are the signs of caregiver burnout as portrayed in the scene?
   b. What can we, as health-care professionals, offer to older people with dementia and their care providers to prevent burnout?
   c. What support services and resources are available to people with dementia in your community?

d. What aspects of neglect and potential elder maltreatment are demonstrated here?

Violence Directed Toward Companion Animals

Amores Perros (2000; Emilio Echevarría, Gael García Bernal, Goya Toledo): Three stories of the complexities of love and life are interconnected by way of a car accident. Octavio starts to use his pet Rottweiler in a dog-fighting ring to raise money to run away with his brother's wife. A couple's rocky relationship is tested after their pet dog gets trapped beneath the floorboards of their apartment. El Chivo is a homeless man who befriends stray dogs and revisits his former trade as a murderer for hire. Viewers should be warned that some scenes contain graphic content and coarse language.

1 (0:03:30–0:04:36) In this scene we see the inner workings of a dog fighting ring as Pancho takes one of his dogs to his next dog fight. A dead dog from the previous fight is dragged away, bets are placed, and the next dog fight starts.

2 (0:54:04–0:56:48) In this scene Octavio brings his dog Cofi to one last fight against another one of Pancho's dogs. Frustrated that Cofi has killed several of Pancho's dogs during previous fights, Pancho shoots Cofi. Octavio and his friend place a bleeding Cofi on the back seat of the car and escape, but not before Octavio stabs Pancho in the abdomen.

3 (1:59:56–2:02:52) Cofi has recovered from his wounds and has become one of El Chivo's faithful canine companions. In this scene, Cofi's past as a vicious dog is brought to light when El Chivo arrives home to find that Cofi has attacked and killed the other dogs that cohabited in El Chivo's makeshift home.

a. If you suspect neglect, animal abuse, or animal cruelty, to whom can you report it?

b. Why do you suppose animal abuse and animal cruelty is linked to other types of crime?

c. What effect might a history of abuse have on a pet, even after he/she has been rescued from an abusive environment?

d. What effect might the behavior of an abused pet have on the new owner?

The Good Son (1993; Macaulay Culkin, Elijah Wood): After his mother passes away, Mark (Wood) goes to stay with his extended family for a few weeks in the winter. His cousin Henry's (Culkin) pleasant façade begins to wear thin as Mark spends more and more time with him. Henry's deception makes everyone suspicious of Mark, especially once he begins to make accusations about Henry. Eventually we learn just how disturbed Henry is, as he attempts to take the life of a neighborhood dog and several members of his own family.

1 (0:24:40–0:26:07) When Henry and Mark are taking a shortcut across a neighbor's pier in their neighborhood, the dog that guards the pier chases

them. After narrowly escaping, Henry turns around and taunts the dog, growling and barking at the dog just beyond its reach.

2   (0:32:32–0:34:44) Henry has made a homemade gun and likes to show it off to Mark. The two boys take it out for target practice. Mark suggests he aim for a sign, but Henry chooses instead to aim for the dog that chased them the day before. His aim is true and the dog dies, forcing them to hide the body of the dead dog in a nearby well. The full extent of Henry's vindictive, homicidal nature emerges as the rest of the movie unfolds.

   a. What behaviors or attitudes might make you more suspicious of Mark's potential for animal abuse or cruelty?
   b. Discuss the connection between animal abuse and domestic violence. What other type of crime has animal abuse been associated with?
   c. What effect might shooting the dog have on Henry? What effect might witnessing this act of cruelty have on Mark?
   d. Why are some people that witness animal cruelty reluctant to report it?
   e. As a veterinarian, what would you tell a client whose pet has presented with injuries that you suspect to be caused by abuse?
   f. What resources are available to pet-owners who suspect their pet is the subject of abuse or cruelty enacted by family members in the home? By strangers in the neighborhood?
   g. Does your state legislation include provisions for pets in domestic violence protection orders?

References

1   Krug EG, Dahlberg LL, Mercy JA, *et al.*, editors. *World Report on Violence and Health*. Geneva: World Health Organization; 2002.

2   Centers for Disease Control and Prevention. *Adverse Childhood Experiences (ACE) Study: data and statistics; prevalence of individual adverse childhood experiences*. Available at: www.cdc.gov/ace/prevalence.htm (accessed April 26, 2011).

3   Centers for Disease Control and Prevention. *Adverse Childhood Experiences (ACE) Study: major findings*. Available at: www.cdc.gov/ace/findings.htm (accessed April 26, 2011).

4   Centers for Disease Control and Prevention. *Adverse Childhood Experiences (ACE) Study: pyramid*. Available at: www.cdc.gov/ace/pyramid.htm (accessed April 26, 2011).

5   *Child Maltreatment 2004*. Washington, DC: U.S. Government Printing Office; U.S. Department of Health and Human Services, Administration on Children, Youth and Families; 2006.

6   Tjaden P, Thoennes N. *Full Report of the Prevalence, Incidence, and Consequences of Violence against Women: findings from the National Violence against Women Survey*. NCJ 183781. Washington, DC: U.S. Department of Justice, Office of Justice Programs, National Institute of Justice; November 2000.

7   Coker AL, Davis KE, Arias I, *et al.* Physical and mental health effects of intimate partner violence for men and women. *Am J Prev Med*. 2002; **23**(4): 260–8.

8   Coker AL, Smith PH, Bethea L, *et al.* Physical health consequences of physical and psychological intimate partner violence. *Arch Fam Med*. 2000; **9**(5): 451–7.

9 Cronholm PF. Intimate partner violence and men's health. *Prim Care*. 2006; **33**(1): 199–209.

10 Campbell JC. Health consequences of intimate partner violence. *Lancet*. 2002; **359**(9314): 1331–6.

11 Cronholm PF, Straton JB, Jaeger J. Intimate partner violence: identification, treatment, and associations with men's health. In: Giardino A, Giardino E, editors. *Intimate Partner Violence, Domestic Violence, and Spousal Abuse: a resource for professionals working with children and families*. St. Louis, MO: STM Learning; 2010. pp. 285–302.

Further Reading

● Wigglesworth A, Mosqueda L, Mulnard R, *et al*. Screening for abuse and neglect of people with dementia. *J Am Geriatr Soc*. 2010; **58**(3): 493–500.

18

Blood Lust:
Suicide and Cutting

Crystal Wilson & Layne Prest

SUICIDE IS THE ELEVENTH-LEADING CAUSE OF DEATH IN THE UNITED States among all ages. It is the second-leading cause among 25- to 34-year-olds and the third-leading cause among 15- to 24-year-olds.[1] It is estimated that one person commits suicide every 15 minutes.[1]

Risk factors include family history of suicide, family discord, medical illness, substance abuse, and mental illness. Psychosocial factors such as personal loss (i.e. losing a job, divorce, death of a loved one), isolation, and difficulty dealing with life transitions also place people at increased risk of suicide. Males are three to five times more likely to die by suicide than females.[2] Elderly white males have the highest incidence of suicide among the general population.[2]

Self-mutilation or self-injury refers to a number of harmful and deliberate behaviors that directly injure the body's tissues. This does not include behaviors such as getting tattoos or body piercing. Common methods of nonsuicidal self-injuring include cutting, burning, punching, or throwing oneself against objects to cause bruising or bleeding. The prevalence of self-injury is estimated to be approximately 1%–4% in the general population, with the younger population being most at risk. Approximately 15% of adolescents and between 17% and 35% of college-age persons have a history of self-injury.[3] It may be assumed that self-injurious behavior is a suicidal gesture when, in general, it has a different function.

Reasons for self-inflicted harm are many and may include exerting punishment on oneself, attention-seeking, attempt to negate feelings of numbness or detachment from reality, and to control intense negative emotions.[4] It is necessary to distinguish whether a behavior is self-harm, a suicidal gesture, or a suicide attempt.

Primary care physicians serve an important role in identifying patients at risk for suicide and self-injury. It is estimated that more than 40% of those who committed suicide had contact with a health professional in the days, weeks, or months, prior to their death.[5] Similarly, it is estimated that nearly 22% of primary care patients have a history of self-injury.[6] It is important to recognize the signs and symptoms of suicidal behavior in order to prevent suicide and to provide treatment for depressive disorders. Health-care professionals must also respond effectively and screen those individuals that engage in nonsuicidal self-injury who need to develop more adaptive coping skills and often be treated for underlying disorders.[7–9]

Adolescent Suicide and Family Dysfunction

The Virgin Suicides (1999; James Wood, Kathleen Turner, Kirsten Dunst, A. J. Cook, Hanna R. Hall, Leslie Hayman, Chesle Swain): This American drama portrays the tragedy of suicide in a "normal" middle-income family. The story is told from the perspective of one of a group of five teenage boys who are fascinated by the mystery surrounding the Lisbon girls, five sisters who all eventually kill themselves.

1   (Ch 2, 0:04:49–0:06:20; 0:07:23–0:08:50) This scene begins the retrospective narration about the theories people had regarding the suicide of five girls from the same family. Everyone has a hypothesis about how life gets as bad as it does for this family.
    a. What are the risk factors which contribute to young people considering suicide?

2   (Ch 4, 0:11:40–0:18:55) After one of the Lisbon girls attempts suicide by cutting her wrists, their parents agree to allow them to have a party to "get things back to normal." They invite the five neighborhood boys for whom they have become the objects of fascination and infatuation.
    a. What are the methods which are more likely to lead to an eventual suicide? Discuss what you know about variability among males and females, people of different ages, and across cultures.
    b. Should this first attempt be considered self-harm, a suicidal gesture, or a suicide attempt? What distinguishes the three?
    c. What are family and peer group members' typical reactions to suicide ideation, attempts, and completions?

3   (Ch 12, 1:06:35–1:25:02) In the face of a parental lockdown of the house, the other four girls commit suicide in this last scene. But they do so only after a protracted period of isolation in their home, broken up only through undercover communication with their friends in the neighborhood.
    a. How do you make sense out of what happened?
    b. As health-care providers, what would you recommend to parents and other family or community members about how to deal with the aftermath of a suicide?
    c. What do you think about the phenomenon of suicide epidemics?

Suicide after Incarceration
. . . .

Shawshank Redemption (1994; Tim Robbins, Morgan Freeman, James Whitmore): A man (Robbins) imprisoned for a murder he claims he did not commit forms a long-lasting friendship with a fellow prisoner who helps him deal with life behind bars.

1   (Ch 17, 0:57:15–1:05:40) Brooks, (Whitmore), a recently released inmate who has spent almost 50 years in prison, has a hard time dealing with life outside of prison.

   a. What risk factors for suicide can you identify in Brooks?

   b. Given Brooks' reaction to being paroled, what steps, if any, should have been taken prior to Brooks' release to help him ease back into life outside of prison?

   c. Recently released prisoners are at a much greater risk of suicide than the general population, especially in the first few weeks after release.[7] What resources should the prison and probation system have in place?

   d. What community resources would you recommend to Brooks if he were your client/patient?

Suicide and Substance Abuse
. . . .

Leaving Las Vegas (1995; Nicholas Cage, Elisabeth Shue, Julian Sands): Ben (Cage), a down-and-out screenwriter who loses his job secondary to alcoholism, moves to Las Vegas to drink himself to death. There he meets a prostitute, Sera (Shue), and forms an odd relationship.

1   (Ch 1, 0:06:00–0:09:05) In this scene, Ben is drinking excessively. When he meets a prostitute, he tells her his wife has left him.

2   (0:13:30–0:15:54) Ben gets fired from his job and receives a severance check from his boss. When asked what he is going to do now, he says he is going to move to Las Vegas.

3   (0:20:48–0:22:38) Ben gets rid of everything in his house prior to leaving for Vegas.

4   (0:31:53–0:34:20) Ben has met a prostitute, Sera, who he almost hit with a car. He pays her to come to his room for sex but changes his mind and just wants her company. Ben admits to Sera that he came to Las Vegas to drink himself to death.

   a. Ben is intent on committing suicide. How may Ben's character present for a medical evaluation? How would you screen for suicidal intent?

   b. What risk factors for suicide can you identify in Ben?

5   (0:46:30–0:54:45) Ben and Sera go on their first date. She attempts to understand why he is killing himself through drinking. In the following clip, Sera falls in love with Ben. She invites him to stay at her place. In a flash-forward scene, she speaks with her psychologist about him. Back at her place, Sera

tells Ben she wants him to move in with her to which he responds that she doesn't know how bad is alcoholism is. When she insists he stay with her, he tells her he will but she can never ask him to stop drinking.

    a. What do you think about Ben and Sera's relationship? What is codependency?

6 (1:40:40–1:47:04) (Warning: this scene has strong sexual content.) Sera visits Ben in his hotel room after they have been apart for several days. She realizes how Ben's drinking has taken its toll on him. In his last moments, they say they love each another.

    a. In what way does Sera enable Ben's drinking?

Suicide Following Death of a Loved One

What Dreams May Come (1998; Robin Williams, Cuba Gooding, Jr., Annabella Sciorra): Chris (Williams) dies in a car accident after losing his children 4 years prior to his death. While he is enjoying what is depicted as heaven, he learns that his wife and soul mate, Annie, has committed suicide and has gone to hell. This movie shows the journey and risk Chris is willing to take in order to find her and bring her to the heaven he inhabits.

1 (Ch 2, 0:04:48–0:07:35) Annie and Chris lose their children in a car accident.

    a. Describe what you imagine Chris and Annie must be going through.

    b. Why is the lost of a child so traumatic?

    c. Discuss the stages of grief.

    d. What resources are available for parents who have lost their children?

2 (Ch 3, 0:07:36–0:14:40) Chris dies after being hit by a car while helping a hurt motorist.

3 (Ch 5, 0:19:52–0:21:20) Annie writes in her journal about her feelings, having lost her husband and her children.

    a. What do we learn about how Annie handled the loss of her children? Who does she credit with helping pull her through it?

    b. How does she feel about her psychiatrist?

    c. What resources would you recommend for her at this point?

4 (Ch 9, 0:51:22–0:52:47) Annie discusses her impending suicide.

    a. What do we notice physically about Annie in this clip?

    b. What does Annie mean by her statement, "I swear that California is the strangest place. They sort of push you into it so that you can get it done before your shrink commits you."

5 (Ch 9, 0:53:25–0:55:50) Chris learns that Annie has killed herself and has gone to hell.

    a. Discuss various religious views on suicide (i.e. Christian, Muslim, Jewish, Hinduism, and so forth). In these religions, what happens to people who kill themselves?

   b. Think about your personal views on suicide. How might your views on suicide influence what you tell a patient who is suicidal?

   c. How would you feel if a client/patient, who endorses suicidal feelings, states that he/she would not act on those feelings because of their religion? Does that serve as a deterrent?

A Single Man (2009; Colin Firth, Julianne Moore, Nicholas Holt, Matthew Goode, Jon Kortajarena): George (Firth), a British college professor, has a difficult time dealing with the loss of his longtime gay lover, making him consider ending his life. However, several small but meaningful interactions with friends, as well as people he meets, make him reconsider.

1   (Ch 1, 0:00:40–0:06:00) George has a dream in which he comes across the dead body of his lover, Jim. When he awakes, he reminisces about waking up in the morning with Jim.

   a. Discuss the symbolism behind George's dream of drowning and his grief over losing Jim.

   b. How would you counsel someone like George about the grief he/she feels from losing a loved one?

   c. How does being a part of a gay/lesbian couple potentially complicate the grief process?

   d. Are gay/questioning youth at greater risk for suicide? What prevention efforts are under way?

2   (Ch 10, 0:29:40–0:35:40) In this scene George cleans his office. Kenny (Holt), the young student who has taken an interest in George from his class, notices and asks George if he is going on vacation. Next George goes to the bank to collect his valuables from the safety deposit box.

   a. Why do you suspect George is gathering his personal belongings?

3   (Ch 14, 0:40:28–0:40:57) George buys bullets for his gun.

4   (Ch 15, 0:44:40–0:47:50) George meets Carlos (Kortajarena), a young drifter outside a convenience store. When Carlos tells George he needs someone to like him, George tells him he is going away.

5   (Ch 17, 0:51:00–0:54:35) George lays out all of his important papers, keys, and a suit with a note. He then tries various positions to determine which is the most appropriate for him to shoot himself.

   a. In the previous scenes, what warning signs does George give regarding his intent to kill himself?

Suicide Following Relationship Loss

The Good Girl (2002; Jennifer Aniston, Jake Gyllenhaal, John C. Reilly): A bored, thirty-something retail worker named Justine (Aniston) brings excitement and drama into her life when she has an affair with a young coworker, Holden (Gyllenhaal), who puts her world at risk.

1   (Ch 20, 1:10:42–1:12:55) Holden tells Justine he has stolen money from the store where they both work. She tells him she is pregnant; he believes it is his baby. He plans for her to meet him at the hotel the next day so they can run away together.

2   (Ch 21, 1:18:00–1:20:00) After Holden realizes Justine is not coming to meet him and has instead given his whereabouts away to the authorities, he kills himself.

   a. What warning signs does Holden give regarding his intentions?

   b. What are other warning signs people give prior to committing suicide?

Suicide Secondary to Mental Illness

The Hours (2002; Nicole Kidman, Julianne Moore, Meryl Streep): This drama intertwines the lives of three women: Virginia Woolf (Kidman), an accomplished author with a history of mental illness; a 1950s housewife (Moore); and a twenty-first-century book editor (Streep).

1   (Ch 1, 0:00:47–0:03:40) Virginia writes a letter to her husband, Leonard, explaining her decision to drown herself.

   a. What does Virginia's letter reveal about her motivation for suicide? What mental disorder do you think Virginia suffered from?

   b. How do you think Virginia perceives her relationship with her husband? What does she think is going to happen to him once she dies?

2   (Ch 10, 0:44:00–0:48:47) Virginia's sister comes to visit. In this scene, Virginia's sister tells her she is sorry she did not invite her to her party but thought she would not come. Virginia states, "even crazy people like to be asked." Next, Virginia's niece and nephew discover a dying bird. Virginia becomes entranced with the bird after talking to her niece about death.

   a. How was mental illness treated during this time period? Did it vary depending on social status?

   b. Discuss Virginia's fascination with the bird.

3   (Ch 12, 1:05:32–1:08:26) Virginia recites lines from her book, *Mrs. Dalloway*, in her head while in a trance.

   a. Based on Virginia's passage in her book, how do you think Virginia views death?

4   (Ch 14, 1:17:03–1:25:43) Virginia's husband frantically tries to find her when he learns she has left the house. He discovers her at the train station where they get into an argument.

   a. What else do we learn about Virginia's mental illness? How does her husband understand her illness? How do Virginia and Leonard's views on her treatment differ?

   b. What is the biggest risk factor for completed suicide?

The Secret Life of Bees (2008; Dakota Fanning, Queen Latifah, Jennifer Hudson, Alicia Keys): This movie, set in the South during the Jim Crow era, is the story of 14-year-old Lily (Fanning), who runs away from home with her nanny (Hudson) to get away from her abusive father and find more information about her deceased mother. She meets the Boatwright sisters who take her and her nanny in and teach Lily the secrets of beekeeping.

1. (Ch 9, 0:31:50–0:33:20) May explains that the Boatwright sisters had another sister named April but she died when she was young.
2. (Ch 10, 0:37:20–0:38:50) August explains why May gets upset easily and is often emotional.
   a. How might the "wailing wall" be therapeutic? What similar technique is suggested to patients during counseling?
   b. What coping strategies does May lack for dealing with death or loss?
   c. Discuss a differential diagnosis for May's condition.
3. (Ch 17, 1:07:38–1:12:10) May drowns herself after learning Zach has "gone missing" after being taken by white men who did not like him sitting beside Lily in the movie theater.
   a. What strategies could the Boatwright sisters have used to prevent May's death?

Suicide Secondary to Extreme Guilt

Seven Pounds (2008; Will Smith, Rosario Dawson, Michael Ealy, Woody Harrelson): A man devastated by an accident decides to dedicate his life to help seven strangers have a new lease on theirs.

1. (Ch 11, 0:46:33–0:47:37) Ben (Smith) has a flashback of a car accident.
2. (Ch 15, 1:01:29–1:04:43) Connie contacts Ben after she decides to leave her abusive boyfriend. Ben leaves his house to Connie and her family so they can stop being victims of domestic violence.
3. (Ch 19, 1:19:10–1:21:21) Ben has another flashback to the car accident that took his wife's life. He then donates bone marrow to a child with cancer. As he is limping back to his motel room, he speaks with the motel owner about how long he plans on staying there.
   a. What warning signs for suicidal intent can you identify in these clips?
4. (Ch 26, 1:45:48–1:51:20) The cause of the accident Ben keeps thinking about is finally revealed. Ben commits suicide by placing a poisonous jellyfish into a tub with himself and ice water to preserve his organs for Emily and the other strangers he intends to help.
5. (Ch 28, 1:52:30–1:53:20) Ben's brother, Tim explains to Emily why he killed himself.
   a. What is survivor's guilt? What medical/mental condition is this phenomenon associated with?

b. What therapy could have been offered after the car accident to help Ben deal with his guilt and possibly prevent his suicide?

Nonsuicidal Self-Injury

Thirteen (2003; Holly Hunter, Evan Rachel Wood, Nikki Reed, Jeremy Sisto): Melanie (Hunter) is the mother of 13-year-old girl Tracy (Wood) who is on the brink of moving from early to middle adolescence. As a divorced single parent of two teenagers, Melanie struggles to find the balance between structure and allowing them to learn through experience. The challenges mount as Tracy is strongly influenced by her new best friend, Evie (Reed), who lives in foster care to escape an abusive home. Tracy's newfound interest in a different style of clothes, a new circle of friends, and older boys escalates to include risk-taking behavior, shoplifting, huffing, and self-mutilation in the form of cutting.

1 (Ch 2, 0:2:38–0:7:35) This scene illustrates the often challenging middle school context of early to middle adolescent development – a changing social fabric and consumer culture, the demands related to changing identity, less supervision and increased independence, peer pressure, and evolving ideas about sexuality and intimacy.
   a. What factors shape adolescent development? Discuss nature versus nurture issues.
   b. How do cultures vary in their perspective on female psychosocial development? Discuss cross-cultural observations, experiences, studies that you have encountered which suggest how to help shape a "healthy" or "normal" development.
   c. How can pressures to "fit in" contribute to overwhelming anxiety and self-harming behavior?
   d. How should parents interact with their daughters to foster healthy development and thus reduce the risk for depression/anxiety/poor coping?

2 (Ch 8, 0:17:25–0:23:45) In this scene, Tracy, pushed by her own need to be seen as cool and pulled by pressure from her new friend Evie, leaves her old friends behind. This clip illustrates the struggles parents can have as they try to foster independence and relationships with peers with their fears about the risks of letting go too quickly. During a trip to the mall, Tracy convinces her mother to leave them relatively unsupervised. In the end, Melanie confronts both her suspicions that she has been manipulated as well as a new perspective on her daughter's blossoming identity as a young woman.
   a. What is the relationship between parental authority/permissiveness and risk-taking behavior?

3 (Ch 15, 0:35:13–0:42:00) In the face of mounting pressure from the increasingly risky behavior she is involved in within her peer group and the escalating conflict within the family involving her mother's relationship with a man who is a negative influence on her sobriety, Tracy's self-harm becomes more serious.

a. What are known to be the factors contributing to self-harming behaviors? Which can you identify in this series of clips from the movie *Thirteen*?

b. What are some other self-harming behaviors and what is their function for the individual?

Manic (2001; Joseph Gordon-Levitt, Don Cheadle, Zooey Deschanel): Lyle (Gordon-Levitt), an emotionally charged teenager, enters the juvenile rehabilitation unit of a psychiatric hospital after severely injuring a baseball teammate. While in the unit, he meets Dr. Monroe (Cheadle) who tries to help him and the other adolescents on the ward deal with their emotional and psychological issues.

1 (Ch 4, 0:14:56–0:16:25) Lyle thinks about the kid he beat up at the baseball game. As he thinks about the incident, he starts hurling himself against his room walls.

a. What is the function of Lyle's hurling himself against the wall? What are other common reasons adolescents self-injure? What is affect regulation?

2 (Ch 4, 0:17:00–0:17:40) Kenny asks a fellow rehabilitation patient why she cuts herself.

a. In this scene, the patient admits to having overdosed before and now cuts herself for relief. What do you think may be this patient's motive for cutting?

b. How would you explore this patient's desire to cut herself? What questions would you ask?

c. What are some techniques primary care physicians can use to motivate self-injurers to stop causing harm to their bodies? What are techniques mental health professionals might employ to help clients decrease self-harming behaviors?

d. What community resources are available?

3 (Ch 17, 1:11:32–1:13:16) Dr. Monroe talks to Lyle about his self-injury and rage.

a. What do you think about Dr. Monroe's speech?

b. How would you counsel Lyle?

Painful Secrets (2001; Sean Young, Kimberlee Peterson, Robert Wisden, Rhea Perlman): Dawn (Peterson) is a shy girl who has trouble fitting in with the other girls at school. She also has a difficult time dealing with her overbearing mother (Young) and her hands-off father (Wisden). In order to deal with her emotions, she turns to cutting. With the help of a psychologist (Perlman), Dawn learns to deal with her emotions in a less destructive manner.

1 (Ch 2, 0:11:29–0:16:06) When Dawn's mom helps her carry in an art project to school, she makes her uncomfortable by insisting Dawn socialize with her "friends." Dawn's mom does not realize these are not her friends but girls who pick on her at school. After the humiliating experience, Dawn runs away to cut herself. Lorraine, another school misfit, catches her.

a. What warning signs for self-injury does Dawn exhibit?

2 (Ch 2, 0:16:14–0:20:45) When Dawn's teacher discovers her bleeding in class, the principal alerts her parents. They come to school to talk to the principal. They were unaware of Dawn's cutting.

3 (Ch 3, 0:22:57–0:24:24) Dawn's parents discuss the idea of having Dawn see a therapist.

   a. Describe Dawn's parents' reactions. What do you think about her father's question prior to leaving the principal's office?

   b. What do you think of the principal's discussion with Dawn's parents? What would you recommend for Dawn and her parents at this point?

4 (Ch 3, 0:20:55–0:22:56) Dawn's mother attempts to understand why Dawn cuts herself while on a shopping trip.

5 (Ch 5, 0:30:13–0:32:53) Dawn's mother attempts to remove all of the sharp objects Dawn has access to in order to prevent further cutting.

   a. In what ways may Dawn's mother's interactions with her influence her cutting behavior?

   b. Comment on Dawn's family's dynamics.

6 (Ch 4, 0:25:48–0:29:43) Dawn talks to Lorraine about her boyfriend and tells her she had sex with him. Dawn is unexpectedly introduced to Lorraine's therapist, Dr. Parella, while out in the mall.

   a. What do you think about Dr. Parella's approach to have Dawn see her? Is validation a good technique?

7 (Ch 6, 0:38:38–0:44:26) Dawn confides in her father how she feels she can never do anything right. After he gives her advice, she goes to the garage to burn herself.

   a. What do you think about Dawn's father's advice? How might his behavior influence her self-injurious behavior?

8 (Ch 7, 0:46:40–0:49:18) Dawn meets with Dr. Parella. She tells her she is not going to stop. Dr. Parella explains to her she is going to teach her how to speak.

9 (Ch 7, 0:51:41–0:53:40) Dawn talks to Dr. Parella about abandonment concerns as well as issues with her mother. Dr. Parella suggests Dawn talk to her mom about how she feels.

10 (Ch 9, 1:02:26–1:04:09) Dr. Parella suggests Dawn's mom come to counseling. She then addresses Dawn's relationship with her father.

11 (Ch 10, 1:07:06–1:09:32) Dawn's parents meet with Dr. Parella and Dawn.

   a. What issues are addressed?

12 (1:13:00–1:15:17) Dawn gets upset after her mother refuses to let her visit Lorraine in the hospital. She cannot stop rocking herself.

   a. What impact can self-injury on family members and loved ones?

Black Swan (2010; Natalie Portman, Mila Kunis, Vincent Cassel, Barbara Hershey): In this psychological thriller, Nina (Portman) is an emotionally dysfunctional and somewhat frigid ballerina who desperately wants to play the lead role in *Swan Lake*. The role requires the lead dancer to portray the White

Swan and the Black Swan. While she masters the role of the sweet, innocent White Swan with ease, she has difficulty portraying the darkly sensual Black Swan. Her struggle to become the perfect White/Black Swan leads her down a path of psychological destruction.

1 (Ch 1, 0:04:20–0:05:06) Nina's mother notices a scar on her back and asks her about it. Nina says it is "nothing."

2 (0:37:34–0:39:09) Nina's mother sees the scars on her back are getting worse and states that she has been "scratching again." She calls it a "disgusting habit" and clips Nina's nails.

   a. What do you think of Nina's mother reaction to Nina's injuries? How might her reaction be counterproductive to helping Nina stop her injurious behaviors?

   b. How have Nina and her Mom treated this behavior before?

28 Days (2000; Sandra Bullock, Viggo Mortensen, Diane Perkins, Steve Buscemi): Sandra Bullock plays Gwen, a newspaper writer whose alcoholism is noticeably out of control when she ruins her sister's wedding then subsequently steals and crashes a limousine. She is forced to go to an inpatient rehabilitation center for treatment. There she meets an interesting group of people who help her realize she can succeed in recovery.

1 (Ch 5, 0:13:36–0:14:50) In this scene, Gwen's roommate Andrea eats chocolate as a way to deal with her heroin craving.

2 (Ch 14, 0:43:03–0:44:10) Andrea talks about her inspiration to stay off of heroin during group therapy. In the following scene, she appears irritated during visitation day.

3 (Ch 15, 0:49:40–0:51:35) Gwen returns to her room at rehab and catches her roommate injuring herself. Andrea admits it was because her mother would not come to visit her.

   a. What psychiatric illnesses are associated with self-injury?

A Thin Line Between Love and Hate (1996; Martin Lawrence, Lynn Whitfield, Regina King, Della Reese): When a womanizer (Lawrence) meets a beautiful stranger, he tries to seduce her but gets more than he bargained for when she turns out to be emotionally disturbed.

1 (Ch 14, 1:12:10–1:14:37) After Darnell stands Brandi up on her birthday to spend time with his childhood sweetheart, he finds her birthday cake with a knife stabbed in it on his sweetheart's front porch. He visits Brandi and tells her he wants to be just friends.

2 (Ch 16, 1:16:38–1:18:03) Brandi breaks into Darnell's house and tries to cook him breakfast.

   a. What do you think of Brandi's affect? Would you be concerned at this point?

   b. Should Darnell have reacted differently?

3 (Ch 16, 1:18:47–1:21:42) Brandi injures herself and goes to the hospital. She

lies about her name and uses Darnell's sweetheart's name to get Darnell to visit her in the hospital.

   a. What was Brandi's motive for hurting herself?

References

1 Centers for Disease Control and Prevention. *Understanding Suicide: fact sheet, 2010.* Available at: www.cdc.gov/violenceprevention/pdf/Suicide-FactSheet-a.pdf (last accessed 12/01/11)

2 American Foundation for Suicide Prevention. www.afsp.org

3 Kerr P, Muehlenkamp J, Turner J. Nonsuicidal self-injury: a review of current research for family medicine and primary care physicians. *J Am Board Fam Med.* 2010; **23**(2): 240–59.

4 Whitlock, J. *The Cutting Edge: non-suicidal self-injury in adolescence.* ACT for Youth Center of Excellence. Available at: www.actforyouth.net/resources/rf/rf_nssi_1209.pdf (accessed May 3, 2011).

5 Pirkis J, Burgess P. Suicide and recency of health care contacts: a systematic review. *Br J Psychiatry.* 1998; **173**: 462–74.

6 Weiderman M, Sansone R, Sansone L. Bodily self-harm and its relationship to childhood abuse among women in a primary care setting. *Violence Against Women.* 1999; **5**: 155–63.

7 Pratt D, Piper M, Appleby L, *et al.* Suicide in recently released prisoners: a population-based cohort study. *Lancet.* 2006; **368**: 119–23.

8 Jobes D, Rudd M, Overholser J, *et al.* Ethical and competent care of suicidal patients: contemporary challenges, new developments, and considerations for clinical practice. *Prof Psychol.* 2008; **39**(4): 405–13.

9 Raue P, Brown E, Meyers B, *et al.* Does every allusion to possible suicide require the same response? A structured method for assessing and managing risk. *J Fam Pract.* 2006; **55**(7): 605–12.

19

Personality Typing, Anyone? The Myers-Briggs Personality Indicator

Matthew Alexander, Kelly Breen Boyce,
Leslie L. Pitt & Kevin Krause

THE MYERS-BRIGGS TYPE INDICATOR (MBTI) HAS BEEN CALLED "THE world's most widely used personality assessment tool,"[1] with estimates of as many as two million annual assessments. Based on the theories of Carl Jung and developed by Katharine Cook Briggs and her daughter Isabel Briggs Myers, the MBTI is routinely used in business, couple therapy, career counseling, leadership training, and education. The MBTI measures personality by typing psychological preferences along four scales: (1) Extrovert-Introvert, (2) Thinking-Feeling, (3) Sensing-Intuition, and (4) Judging-Perceiving. These four dichotomies make 16 possible combinations and these are called "types." Four basic temperaments can be found among the 16 types.[2] Although variations have been observed, studies have shown strong support for construct validity, internal consistency and test-retest reliability of the MBTI.[3–5]

In this chapter, we will provide cinematic examples of each of the four scales of preference followed by examples of each of the four temperaments.

Extroversion/Introversion

Extrovert/Introvert – Introverts tend to get energized by being alone; extroverts get energized by being with others. While introverts tend to think before speaking or acting, extroverts tend to speak/act and then reflect.

The Station Agent (2003; Patricia Clarkson, Peter Dinklage, Bobby Cannavale): Fin McBride (Dinklage), a man with dwarfism, inherits a desolate train station and relocates there after the death of his best friend. A talkative hot dog vendor, Joe Oramas (Cannavale), and Olivia Harris (Clarkson), a woman dealing with her own troubles and losses, befriend him despite his desire to be left alone. Despite their differences, the three become good friends.

1   (Ch 3; 0:10:15–0:12:30) In this scene, McBride (Dinklage) walks outside his train station to find a vendor selling hot dogs. While only wanting coffee, the vendor, Joe Oramas, (Cannavale), attempts to engage him in conversation.

   a. Name five characteristics of McBride which type him as an introvert. Name five characteristics of Oramas that type him as an extrovert.

   b. Despite their differences, these two characters become friends. How do extroverts and introverts complement each other? How do they irritate each other? What are some challenges that extroverts and introverts face when they are romantically involved?

   c. What are common stereotypes about introverts? What are common stereotypes about extroverts?

Amélie (2001; Audrey Tautou, Mathieu Kassovitz): A young Parisian woman, Amélie Poulain (Tautou), decides to spend her free time coming up with imaginative ways to help the people in her life find love and happiness. Though Amélie is able to secretly help those around her, she struggles with shyness to pursue her own love, Nino Quincampoix (Kassovitz).

1   (Ch 2, 0:12:09–0:13:38) In this scene, Amélie describes her favorite activities, from watching movies to skipping stones. She talks about her past relationships with men, which were not very fulfilling.

   a. How are Amélie's favorite pastimes similar to those of other introverts? What might an extrovert need to enjoy similar activities?

   b. To an outsider, how might an introvert's facial expressions and outward emotionality appear?

2   (Ch 15; 1:36:22–1:40:22) After a series of games and strategies, Amélie has told the man with whom she's infatuated, Nino (Kassovitz), to meet her at the café where she works. Nino walks in, hoping to meet her for the first time, but Amélie avoids him. Later, Amélie has a moment of personal reflection in her apartment.

   a. How do Amélie's actions demonstrate the traits of an introvert? Conversely, how do they demonstrate the traits of someone with shyness? How can you distinguish between introversion and shyness?

   b. When Amélie watches TV alone, the man on-screen speaks directly to her, reprimanding her for being "too introverted." Is his assessment correct? What are a few misconceptions about introverts?

   c. Does Amélie experience problems outside of shyness that are typical of introverts?

Rushmore (1998; Jason Schwartzman, Olivia Williams, Bill Murray): The film follows 15-year-old Max Fischer (Schwartzman), a student at Rushmore Academy prep school, who is immersed in numerous extracurricular activities.

Fischer bounces between his many friends, activities, and the budding love-triangle between his adult friend, Herman Blume (Murray), and Rushmore teacher Miss Cross (Williams). Fischer struggles to balance his desires with the pain and problems of those around him.

1   (Ch 8, 0:31:31–0:33:23) Hoping to impress his adult crush, Miss Cross (Williams), Fischer (Schwartzman) somehow manages to head up the construction of a Marine Observatory Center on the baseball diamond of his high school. Fischer jumps between his hired construction worker, assistants, and a news reporter, and is upset to learn that Miss Cross is not attending.

   a. How does Fischer demonstrate the traits of an extrovert? How are extroverts perceived in relation to other people?
   b. What are common stereotypes about extroverts?
   c. From the clip, how do extroverts tend to problem solve?
   d. What kind of problems do extroverts such as Fischer experience as compared to introverts?

Thinking/Feeling

Thinkers/Feelers – Thinkers tend to use objective means to make decisions whereas feelers tend to be more subjective in their decision making. Feelers tend to wear their emotions on their sleeves whereas thinkers are more reserved in showing their emotions.

Frost/Nixon (2008; Frank Langella, Michael Sheen, Rebecca Hall): Set in 1977 after the resignation of President Richard Nixon (Langella), television personality David Frost (Sheen) secures a series of television interviews with Nixon. Hoping to illuminate Nixon's post-Watergate disgrace, Frost underestimates Nixon's cunning while Nixon underestimates Frost's determination.

1   (Ch 2, 0:08:44–0:10:21) In this scene, Frost (Sheen) chats with his friend and producer John Birt (Matthew MacFadyen) about the possibility of securing an interview with Nixon.

   a. How are Frost's interactions with people in this scene reflective of someone with a Feeling (F) preference?
   b. What factors motivate Frost's desire to interview Nixon? Are such motivations typical for people with an F preference?
   c. How would you perceive Frost in a social context? How might other people perceive those with an F preference?

2   (Ch 3, 0:12:02–0:15:02) Here Nixon chats with his literary agent, Swifty Lazar (Toby Jones). Over lunch, the subject of being interviewed by Frost comes up.

   a. Originally, Nixon is reluctant to be interviewed by Frost. How does Nixon make his decision to be interviewed? How do people with a Thinking (T) preference typically arrive at decisions?

      b. Later in the film, Nixon quips that the reason he lost the debate to JFK was because of the sweat on his upper-lip. How would you perceive Nixon in a social context? How might other people perceive those with a T preference?

3 (Ch 5, 0:23:48–0:28:15) In this scene, Frost (Sheen) and his new girlfriend Caroline (Hall), visit Nixon (Langella) in the house where the interview takes place. Nixon entertains his guests with an anecdote about former Soviet president Brezhnev.

      a. How are Frost's reactions to Nixon and the Secret Service typical of someone with an F preference? What are some of the ways that people with an F preference make decisions?

      b. How are Nixon's statements indicative of someone with a T preference?

      c. In the context of the sensitive (and highly pressured) TV interview within the film, what problems might surface on-camera with someone who has a T preference? Similarly, what problems might surface on-camera with someone who has an F preference?

Doubt (2008; Meryl Streep, Philip Seymour Hoffman, Amy Adams): Set in a Catholic middle school in 1964, Father Flynn's (Hoffman) relationship with a young student is questioned by a naïve nun, Sister James (Adams). Though there is no strong evidence of an inappropriate relationship, head nun Sister Aloysius makes it her mission to persecute and intimidate Father Flynn.

1 (Ch 4, 0:15:35–0:18:14) In this scene, all the nuns eat their dinner together in uncomfortable silence. Sister Aloysius (Streep) asks Sister James (Adams) what she thinks the priest's sermon was about.

      a. What is important to Sister Aloysius in this scene? What do people with a T preference tend to prioritize as important in their decision making?

      b. How do people with a T preference feel about ambiguity? How do Ts try to overcome it? When problem solving, how do people with T preference treat the opinions of themselves and others?

2 (Ch 11, 0:57:30–0:1:02:47) In this scene, Father Flynn (Hoffman) approaches Sister James (Adams) while she reads a letter from her sick brother. Adams asks Father Flynn if his relationship with a student was inappropriate.

      a. How does the conversation between Father Flynn and Sister Adams demonstrate an F preference?

      b. How does Father Flynn convince Sister Adams that his relationship with a student was not inappropriate? What factors might people with an F preference prioritize over hard truths?

      c. How do Father Flynn and Sister Adams express concern for each other? How do people with an F preference typically express concern for each other?

The Queen (2006; Helen Mirren, Michael Sheen): Following the death of Princess Diana in a car accident in August of 1997, Queen Elizabeth II faces a personal crisis as she is caught between reserved tradition and the needs of her grieving people.

1 (Ch 4, 0:22:09–0:26:34) In this scene, Queen Elizabeth II and Prime Minister Tony Blair express differing views about the appropriate response of the monarchy to the people of England.
   a. How does Queen Elizabeth II express her Thinking preference?
   b. How does Tony Blair express his Feeling preference?
   c. Can you identify other recent leaders with Thinking preferences? With Feeling preferences?

Sensing/Intuition

Intuitive/Sensors – Intuitives input information by relying on their sixth sense and seeing the larger picture. Sensors tend to be more down to earth and rely on their five senses to input information.

Unstrung Heroes (1995; John Turtorro, Andie McDowell, Michael Richards): This Diane Keaton directed movie tells the story of three brothers, inventor Sid (Turturro), pack rat Arthur (Maury Chaykin) and delusional Danny (Richards) whose lives are impacted by Sid's son Stephen (Nathan Watt) who lives with his two uncles when his mother (McDowell) develops cancer.

1 (Ch 1, 0:00:00–0:03:55) In this opening scene, we are introduced to Sid (Turturro), an inventor with a profound belief in the power of science ("science is the only heroic path"), while the opening credits unfold.
   a. What are the elements of the Sensing (S) preference illustrated by Sid?
   b. What would be the best way to convince Sid of something?
   c. How do Ss best learn? What are their strengths in intimate relationships? Their shortcomings?

Secretariat (2010; Diane Lane, John Malkovich, James Cromwell, Fred Thompson): This is the true story of Penny Chenery Tweedy's tenacity as she "risks it all" on her stallion Secretariat who, in 1973, wins the coveted Triple Crown of horse racing.

1 (Ch 4, 0:18:14–0:22:36) In this first scene, Peggy Chenery Tweedy (Lane) acts on behalf of her father, a horse breeder, who has bred two of his mares, Hasty Matilda and Somethingroyal, with the stallion Bold Ruler, owned by Ogden Phipps (Cromwell), one of the richest men in the world. When the mares deliver, one foal will belong to the Chenerys and the other will go to Ogden Phipps in lieu of a stud fee. Prior to the mare giving birth, the ownership of offspring is determined by a coin toss, the winner of which will have the first choice between the two foals. In a phone call to her husband, Peggy indicates her gut feeling about the horse she will choose, one who will eventually bear the name Secretariat.

2   In the second scene, Peggy disagrees with her brother about which foal to
    choose on the coin toss.
    a. How does Peggy Chenery exhibit the characteristics of an N?
    b. In their confrontation prior to the actual coin toss, Peggy's brother Hollis
        (Dylan Baker) challenges Peggy by saying "Ogden Phipps has the best
        horse people in the world. Do you think you know more than they do?
        How does an N explain her intuitive approach to an S who relies on facts?
    c. What problems might Ns encounter in working "from the gut"? How might
        they find balance through the development of their less well-developed
        S side?

Judging/Perceiving

Perceivers/Judgers – Perceivers tend to be spontaneous and open ended. Judgers
tend to be very goal directed and time conscious.

The Story of Us (1999; Bruce Willis, Michelle Pfeiffer): Two personality
    opposites, Ben (Willis) and Katie Jordan (Pfeiffer) marry and have children
together, with predictable clashes.
1   (Ch 3, 0:07:32–0:08:28) In this scene, Ben and Katie are driving their
    children to meet the bus that will take them to summer camp. A huge
    double-wide trailer pulls out in front of them and Ben and Katie respond very
    differently.
    a. What are the aspects of Ben's character that are typical of the Perceiving
        preference? What are the aspects of Katie's character that are typical of
        the Judging preference?
    b. What are some of the interpersonal challenges in the Perceiving (P) pref-
        erence? What are some of the interpersonal challenges in the Judging (J)
        preference?
    c. What feelings are triggered by Ben in Katie? What feelings are triggered by
        Katie in Ben? How are such feelings typical of mates with these particular
        differing preferences? How would you counsel couples who present with
        these particular types of problems?

The Notebook (2004; James Garner, Ryan Gosling, Rachel McAdams):
    During frequent visits to a female nursing home resident, an elderly man
reads a story about the blossoming love affair between Allie, a young woman of
privilege, and Noah, her relentless suitor.
1   (Ch 4, 0:12:26–0:17:58) Walking home from a movie, Allie and Noah discuss
    her busy schedule and plans for the future. Noah proposes some spontaneous
    fun and Allie deliberates if she will take the risk.
    a. How does Allie represent the J preference? How does Noah represent
        the P preference?

    b. There is a dictum in couple therapy that opposites attract, polarize, and repel. Given this dictum, what conflicts do you predict that this couple will have in ten years?

    c. Why are Allie and Noah attracted to each other?

Stranger Than Fiction (2006; Will Ferrell, Maggie Gyllenhaal, Emma Thompson, Dustin Hoffman): Living through a series of routines, IRS Auditor Harold Crick (Ferrell) wakes up one morning to the omniscient voice of a woman who is narrating his life. The woman, tragedy author Karen Eiffel (Thompson), interrupts Crick's structured life with the declaration that he will die very soon. Crick subsequently pursues his attraction to the tax-offender Ana Pascal (Gyllenhaal) and he tracks down the nameless author of his fate.

1 (Ch 3, 0:09:22–0:11:57) In this scene, Crick (Ferrell) meets the woman he is auditing: bakery-owner Ana Pascal (Gyllenhaal). In a passionate tirade, Pascal tells a reserved Crick why she decided not to pay all of her taxes.

    a. How do Pascal's actions in the scene demonstrate the personality traits of a P preference? How are Crick's priorities typical of the J preference?

    b. Are there moments in this scene that demonstrate the interpersonal flaws of the P preference? What are some of the interpersonal flaws of the J preference?

    c. Paying attention to Pascal's cookie-dough and her baking preparations, how does Pascal illustrate the "in the moment" P preference? If Crick were a baker instead of an IRS agent, how might someone with his J preference approach cookie-dough and baking?

2 (Ch 10, 0:35:09–0:37:02) Here we see writer Karen Eiffel (Thompson) sitting on a bench trying to think of ways to kill the subject of her book, Harold Crick. She chats in the rain with her perplexed assistant, Penny Escher (Queen Latifah).

    a. How does Eiffel hope to generate ideas for her book, and how does this method illustrate her P personality preference?

    b. How are Escher's writing suggestions more indicative of a J preference than a P preference?

    c. How might people with P preferences approach a creative task? How would people with J preferences approach a creative task? What are the pros and cons of both methods?

Temperaments

In their book *Please Understand Me*, Kiersey and Bates describe four temperaments that arise from combinations of personality preferences. These are the Sensing-Perceiving (SP), Sensing-Judging (SJ), Intuitive-Thinking (NT) and Intuitive-Feeling (NF) temperaments.

SP

SP individuals live for the moment. They value spontaneity and do not want to be tied down. They tend to be exciting and irresponsible, but can have great bursts of focused energy.

The Apostle (1997; Robert Duvall, Farrah Fawcett): Sonny (Duvall) is a charismatic Texan preacher with a dark side of rage and lust. After he commits a crime of passion, he creates a new identity for himself in hope of redemption.
1   (Ch 16, 0:46:35–0:49:24) After impulsively injuring his wife's lover, Sonny escapes town to build a new life for himself. With no plan, he heads out, hoping that instincts and The Spirit will lead him to the right place.
   a. How does Sonny manifest the common characteristics of the SP such as impulsivity and restlessness in this scene?
   b. What are the strengths of the SP temperament in terms of interpersonal relationships?
   c. To what kind of careers are SPs most suited?

The Fighter (2010; Mark Wahlberg, Christian Bale, Amy Adams): This is based on the true life story of two brothers who are both professional boxers. Micky Ward (Wahlberg) is the younger brother who has historically been upstaged by his older brother, Dicky (Bale), a local legend. Dicky, a crack addict now past his prime, offers to train Micky for a title bout, a partnership that elicits tension in their extended family.
1   (Ch 2, 0:07:13–0:10:20) In this sequence of scenes, we first see Dicky (Bale) acting out his videotaped fight with Sugar Ray Leonard from years ago while smoking crack with friends. He realizes that he is late for a training session with his brother, runs to the gym to meet Micky (Wahlberg) and immediately engages the entourage assembled there in light banter.
   a. How does this scene reflect key elements of the SP temperament (i.e. living for the moment; charisma; physicality)?
   b. Are SPs more prone to drug addiction that other temperaments? If so, why?
   c. Are SPs less time conscious than other temperaments? If so, why?

SJ

The SJ temperament is characterized by duty, tradition, and hard work. SJs are often drawn to fields of service where effort is expected, not rewarded. SJs are often characterized by loyalty and dependability.

The Remains of the Day (1993; Anthony Hopkins, Emma Thompson, Christopher Reeve): Stevens, played by Anthony Hopkins, is a fastidious butler who serves a diplomat's mansion in Great Britain after World War II. In his later years, he begins to question the sacrifices he made for his life of servitude.

1 (Ch 9; 52:55–56:50) Even as his own father is dying, Stevens (Hopkins) attends to his household duties during an important international summit.
   a. What characteristics of the SJ temperament are portrayed by Stevens?
   b. How do you imagine that Stevens's loyalties in carrying out his responsibilities, regardless of the tragic personal circumstances, are perceived by others?
   c. With regard to mental health hygiene and well-being, what are some of the drawbacks of the SJ temperament?

Gone With the Wind (1939; Vivien Leigh, Clark Gable, Olivia de Havilland, Leslie Howard): This American classic chronicles the turbulent life of a southern belle, Scarlett O'Hara (Leigh), through the Civil War and Reconstruction.
1 (Ch 21, 1:20:30–1:25:25) Scarlett (Leigh) and Ashley (Howard) are caught in an embrace. Scarlett fears how Melanie (de Havilland) and others will react later that evening at Ashley's birthday party.
   a. How does Melanie portray the SJ temperament?
   b. In addition to temperament, what are other psychological explanations why an individual such as Melanie would prefer to work behind the scenes, thereby avoiding acknowledgment and praise?
   c. What other personality types do SJs naturally connect with and/or complement and why?

The Queen (see earlier description)

1 (Ch 4, 0:22:09–0:26:34) In this scene, Queen Elizabeth II and Prime Minister Tony Blair express differing views about the appropriate response of the monarch to the people of England.
   a. How does Queen Elizabeth II embody the SJ temperament?

NT

NTs tend to be eccentric, somewhat interpersonally remote and original in their thinking. They are often drawn to fields involving research. The Intuitive Thinker (NT) is often characterized as competent, cerebral, and elitist. They are likely perfectionists and attempt to achieve power through knowledge and self-improvement.

Kinsey (2004; Liam Neeson, Laura Linney): A film biography of Alfred Kinsey (Neeson), a pioneer in the field of human sexuality. The film tells the story of Kinsey's ground-breaking efforts to study human sexuality as well as his marriage to Mac (Linney), a former student.
1 (Ch 3, 0:11:30–0:13:20) Here we see Kinsey giving a biology lecture at Indiana University on gall wasps. His future wife, Mac, sits enthralled.
   a. What elements of the NT temperament are portrayed by Kinsey?

   b. What are the strengths of the NT temperament? What are the limitations of the NT temperament? How might others perceive NTs?
   c. Why are NTs so uniquely gifted in research?

The Devil Wears Prada (2006; Meryl Streep, Anne Hathaway): A recent college graduate Andy (Hathaway) moves to New York and "settles" for a job at a high fashion magazine (that a million girls would kill for) when unable to find work in her chosen field of journalism. In her new position, she contends with her impossibly demanding boss, the magazine's legendary editor in chief, Miranda Priestly (Streep).
1   (Ch 9, 0:21:46–0:24:25) Andy is summoned to assist in her first fashion run-through. Priestly displays her savvy intuition regarding fashion trends (and their systemic implications) while simultaneously shaming Annie's ignorance and seeming naiveté.
   a. While Miranda Priestly is an admittedly harsh portrayal of this temperament, what characteristics of NTs contribute to their success?
   b. What are the various reactions to Priestley's brilliance and perfectionism?
   c. What attributes could NTs refine or cultivate to improve their leadership skills?

The Social Network (2010; Jesse Eisenberg, Andrew Garfield, Justin Timberlake): A dramatic movie based on real-life events, Mark Zuckerberg (Eisenberg) is a sophomore at Harvard when he creates the social networking site, Facebook. His incredible success is tainted by relational and legal complications.
1   (Ch 2, 0:8:41–0:13:05) After his girlfriend breaks up with him because of his condescending remarks, Mark Zuckerberg needs a project to distract him. In this scene, he hacks into Harvard's network and creates a new website, which gets 22,000 hits within its first 2 hours.
   a. List three attributes of an NT that Zuckerberg displays in this scene.
   b. What characteristics of NTs make them good at creating and executing ideas?
   c. In what vocations would NTs likely succeed?
   d. What are the strengths and weaknesses that NTs bring to their interpersonal relationships?

NF

NFs tend to be charismatic, interpersonally adept, and restless. They are often drawn to fields involving psychology, philosophy, or the arts and they make excellent leaders.

The Queen (see earlier description)

1   (Ch 4, 0:22:09–0:26:34) In this scene, Queen Elizabeth II and Prime Minister Tony Blair express differing views about the appropriate response of the monarchy to the people of England.

a. How does Tony Blair embody the NF temperament?

Iron Man (2008; Robert Downey, Jr., Gwyneth Paltrow, Terrence Howard): Following in his father's footsteps, Tony Stark (Downey) is a charming and brilliant inventor. After creating a suit of armor with prodigious capabilities, he attempts to fight against his former partner who has a secret nefarious plan.

1 (Ch 15, 1:53:22–1:57:10) After defeating his nemesis as Iron Man, Tony processes the events with his assistant, Pepper Potts (Paltrow) and a governmental/public relations official. He is encouraged to quell sensational rumors about these super-heroic events by "sticking to the official statement" during the press conference.
   a. What traits of an NF does Tony Stark exhibit?
   b. What specific characteristics do NFs possess that make them good leaders?
   c. In addition to those fields previously listed, to what other occupations would individuals with this temperament likely be attracted?

Invictus (2009; Morgan Freeman, Matt Damon): In the early days of his presidency, Nelson Mandela aspires to foster greater unity in postapartheid South Africa through the successes of the nation's 1995 World Cup rugby team led by Francois Pienaar (Matt Damon).

1 (Ch 7, 0:29:18–0:35:13) When Mandela received word that his new leadership team has just unanimously voted to disband the Springboks, the national rugby team composed largely of Afrikaners, he and his staff advisor rush across town to interrupt the national assembly where he makes an impassioned appeal to keep the team together as a sign of goodwill.
   a. What characteristics of the NF temperament does Nelson Mandela demonstrate in this scene?
   b. How does Mandela use empathy, approval, and identification to achieve his impact as an NF leader?
   c. Contrast the NF style of leadership, as portrayed by Mandela, with that of the NT, SJ, and SP temperaments.

Revolutionary Road (2008; Leonardo DiCaprio, Kate Winslet): A suburban couple of the 1950s looks for a way to escape their ordinary lives to pursue their dreams. Frank, trapped in his career, and April, longing for passion, explore the possibilities of running away from it all.

1 (Ch 6, 0:26:44–0:30:30) In this scene April engages Frank in a heartfelt discussion and pitches the idea of selling their home and moving to Paris so as to break free from the mundane rhythm of life they have created.
   a. How does April epitomize the NF perspective on life and love? How does April's idealism make Frank feel?
   b. How does Frank epitomize the SJ perspective on life and love? How does Frank's practicality make April feel?

    c. What are the strengths and challenges that exist in a committed relationship between an NF and an SJ?

    d. If this couple were in therapy with you, how would you help them best work together?

    e. How do NFs and SJs best work together in a professional environment? Do companies need employees with differing temperaments in order to best succeed?

References

1 CPP Products. Available at: www.cpp.com/products/index.aspx (accessed 4/14/12)

2 Kiersey D, Bates M. *Please Understand Me*. Del Mar, CA: Prometheus Nemesis Books; 1978.

3 Thompson B, Borello G. Educational and Psychological Measurement, Construct Validity of the Myers-Briggs Type Indicator. SAGE Publications; 1986.

4 Capraro R, Capraro M. *Educational and Psychological Measurement, Myers Briggs Type Indicator Score Reliability Across Studies: a meta-analytic reliability generalization study*. Thousand Oaks, CA: Sage Publications; 2002.

5 Schaubhut N, Herk N, Thompson R. *MBTI Form M Manual Supplement*. Available at: www.cpp.com/pdfs/MBTI_FormM_Supp.pdf (accessed 4/20/12)

20

More Personality Typing: The Enneagram

F. Scott Valeri & Anne Geary

THE ENNEAGRAM IS A POWERFUL TOOL TO UNDERSTAND PERSONALITY, providing numerous, practical, and often immediate applications. There are nine distinct personality types, which reveal the spectrum of perspectives that inform our approach to engaging in relationships. The Enneagram describes the strengths and potentials of each personality type as well as the unconscious patterns of perception and attention inherent to each type.

Working with the Enneagram can improve personal and professional relationships. Understanding the nine types opens the door to a deeper and fuller insight into oneself, while at the same time enabling a less judgmental and more appreciative approach to the diverse perspectives of others.

When we gain an understanding of our own habitual patterns of thinking and behaving, we can better our relationships with friends, colleagues, and patients. Insights from Enneagram typology can help providers develop quick rapport and insight into the worldview of clients/patients leading to improved empathy, increased compliance with diagnostic and therapeutic recommendations and, ultimately, improved outcomes.

The Enneagram personality system encompasses all levels of psychological development. Our intent is to represent typical or archetypal characteristics to portray each of the nine personality types. Several of the selected movie clips represent exaggerated character traits of the personality type being discussed.

Type One: The Perfectionist

Conscientious and ethical, Ones want to uphold the highest standards, be an exemplar to others and avoid feeling wrong. Ones tend to focus on being correct. When threatened Ones will justify their way as the right way. At their best, Ones can be discerning and morally heroic. The challenge for Ones is to learn to accept their imperfections and tolerate other people's points of view. We can support Ones by encouraging them to experience more pleasure, accept errors and differences, and detach their self-esteem from internal standards. We can also be an example to a One by owning our own mistakes.

- Strengths: Honest, responsible, improvement-oriented
- Challenges: Resentful, nonadaptable, overly critical
- Speaking style: Precise and detail oriented, with a tendency to sermonize or preach
- Famous One's: Hillary Clinton, Jerry Seinfeld, Elliot Spitzer, Martha Stewart, Mahatma Gandhi, Sandra Day O'Connor, Bill Moyers, Ralph Nader, Katherine Hepburn, Harrison Ford, Vanessa Redgrave, George Harrison, George Bernard Shaw, Margaret Thatcher, William Buckley, The "Church Lady" (*Saturday Night Live*), "Mr. Spock" (*Star Trek*)

Doubt (2008; Meryl Streep, Phillip Seymour Hoffman, Amy Adams): Sister Aloysius Beauvier (Streep) is highly suspicious of Father Flynn (Seymour Hoffman) who she perceives is paying too much attention to a young boy. She begins to build a case against him to support what she believes to be "the truth" without valid evidence, except her moral certainty.

1 (1:33.45–1:43:00) Sister Aloysius states her position with firm conviction then admits she distorted the truth while justifying her lie as acceptable because she was upholding the highest standards. Admitting being wrong or doubting a position held with certainty is a significant growth point for a One.

   a. As difficult as it might be, are you able to see the good in Sister Aloysius's intentions? Can you see how challenging it is to be compassionate to a One when they are in a judgmental mindset, but how important it is to "sit with them" in a nonjudgmental mindset while they process their logic and access their own self-compassion?

   b. In a therapeutic session, how might you shift a person's perspective into balance when they insist their black and white judgment is right and refuse to admit there is a middle ground?

The Social Network (2010; Jesse Eisenberg, Andrew Garfield, Justin Timberlake, Joseph Mazzello): The film is the story of the founders of Facebook. Mark Zuckerberg (Elsenberg), a computer genius, Edwardo Saverine (Garfield) his founding business partner and Sean Parker (Timberlake), a fellow entrepreneur, become entangled into what becomes a compelling story of betrayal and how the global social network came to be.

1 (09:088–10.41:00) Twin brothers, Cameron and Tyler Winklevoss, go to the Dean, insisting that Mark Zuckerberg stole their intellectual property and violated Harvard's code of ethics. Cameron does most of the talking, making his case from what he thinks are the highest ideals, but is discounted and belittled by the dean. He politely does the right thing by holding in his anger and maintaining his cool.

a. Can you recall a situation where another person believed they were doing the right thing, but their demeanor turned you off to the point where the conversation ended before a word was exchanged? How might you let them know while keeping in mind their good intentions?

b. How might you compromise a relationship while holding a rigid point of view and choosing to be "right" rather than be open to another's point of view? Are you aware of a circumstance where you held low-grade anger below the surface rather than completing a conversation to reach a middle ground, even if it is to agree to disagree?

Type Two: The Giver

Supportive and warm hearted, Twos wants to be appreciated and express their feelings for others and avoid feeling needy themselves. Twos tend to focus on relationships and are generous and self-sacrificing and put other's needs before their own. When unappreciated, Twos can over react emotionally. At their best, Twos are altruistic, unselfish and offer unconditional love for others. The challenge for Twos is learning to set boundaries and coming to terms that loving oneself is an inside job. We can support Two's by encouraging them to explore what it means to put themselves first, and overcome meeting the needs of important others as a way to be taken care of and loved.

- Strengths: Caring, popular, communicator
- Problems: Privileged, naïve, dependent
- Speaking style: Being nice and sympathetic, giving advice, flattering
- Famous Two's: Mother Teresa, Barbara Bush, Eleanor Roosevelt, Leo Buscalia, Bill Cosby, Kenny G, Luciano Pavarotti, Lillian Carter, Sammy Davis, Jr., Martin Sheen, Robert Fulghum, Bishop Desmond Tutu, and "Dr. McCoy" (*Star Trek*)

The Hours (2002; Meryl Streep, Nicole Kidman, Julianne Moore, Ed Harris): Clarissa Vaughn (Streep) is throwing a party for her friend Richard (Harris), a famous author dying of AIDS, and she is challenged to face her motivations.

1 (1:12:16–1:17:07) Richard asks Clarissa, "who is the party for? It's for you to cover the silence." He says he is staying alive to satisfy her and when he dies she will have to live her own life and think for herself. Richard triggered the Two's core issue which is being tuned into others' emotions and needs while being out of touch with their own.

a. How might you make Richard's point in a more balanced and compassionate manner without losing the impact? How would you "hold the space" if your insight to a client was met with a long silence? How would you feel if the client left upset?

2 (1:12:24–1:17:07) While sorting through her feelings about Richard's

comments, Clarissa says, "When I'm with him, I feel I am living and when I'm not with him everything does seem silly."

   a. Twos tend to believe putting themselves first is selfish. However, taking care of our own needs is the cornerstone of a healthy relationship. If you were with Clarissa at that moment, what might you have said to help her move deeper into her moment of truth? What practical suggestions would you make to open the door for her to explore what it meant to put herself first? What does putting yourself first mean to you?

   b. The fundamental challenge for the Two is interpersonal boundaries; giving and receiving in equal measures, nothing more and nothing less than is needed in any given situation. How do you feel when you are the recipient of an over giver? How do you communicate to a person who has crossed your boundary while being sensitive to their good intention and keeping the relationship on an even keel?

Type Three: The Achiever

Driven, image-conscious, and adaptable, Threes want to be recognized as successful and avoid feeling like a failure. Threes tend to focus on accomplishing tasks and looking good. When threatened, Threes have a low tolerance for incompetence and are prone to workalcholism while compromising their relationships and health. At their best, Threes are role models who inspire others towards success. The challenge for Threes is to step out of their roles and slow down to "smell the roses." We can support Threes by letting them know we appreciate them for who they are, not for what they do. Communicating what is really important to us is helpful as well.

- Strengths: Successful, energetic, high achiever
- Problems: Overworked, impatient, competitive
- Speaking style: Enthusiastic, motivating themselves and others for success
- Famous Three's: Oprah Winfrey, Jane Pauley, Tony Robbins, Tom Cruise, Barbara Streisand, Sharon Stone, Madonna, Sting, Paul McCartney, Dick Clark, Whitney Houston, Michel Jordan, Shania Twain, Sylvester Stallone, Arnold Schwarzenegger, Truman Capote, O. J. Simpson

American Beauty (1999; Kevin Spacey, Annette Bening, Thora Birch, Wess Bentley, Mena Suvari): Lester (Spacey) and Carolyn Burnham's (Bening) marriage is falling like a house of cards. Carolyn stays focused on keeping up appearances while Lester's infatuation with his daughter's friend, Angela (Suvari), is rocking his world. Daughter, Jane (Birch), is having an intense relationship with the shy boy-next-door named Ricky (Wes Bentley), who lives with a homophobic father (Peter Gallager).

1 (0:00:00–0:06:30) We see Carolyn as charming and delightful one moment and insensitive and impatient the next. While Lester's voice is in the

background saying, "Man, I get exhausted just watching her. She hasn't always been this way. She used to be happy. We used to be happy."

a. Given that appearances are important to support the perception of success, can you see how Carolyn's focus creates a barrier to her own emotional honesty and compromises her primary relationships?

b. How do you balance the stress of work and the time and attention you give to your most significant relationships?

c. If Carolyn and Lester came to you for couple therapy, how would you begin to unravel the patterns and habits they have developed over the years? Can you name three behavioral changes you might suggest to Carolyn to support her development?

Wall Street (1987; Charlie Sheen, Michael Douglas, Michael Sheen): Bud Fox (Charlie Sheen) finds himself swept into a world of shady business deals, the "good life," fast money, and fast women. This is at odds with his family including his estranged father (Martin Sheen) and the blue-collar values with which Fox was brought up.

1 (0:11:00–0:21:10) When Bud tells his father he is going to make it big and make him proud, his father replies, "you gotta make yourself proud kid." This is the "catch-22" for some Threes; while striving for what they believe success to be, they risk compromising their own values in their pursuit.

a. What does being successful mean to you? What is the price you are willing to pay for it? How do you support somebody close to you who has crossed the line and is driven to the point of loosing their connection to their own emotion life?

b. At times we all compromise our values. How do you resolve your internal conflict and regain your own sense of integrity? How easy or difficult is it for you to move on?

Type Four: The Individualist

Empathetic and intense, Fours want to distinguish themselves from others and be seen as unique and avoid feeling ordinary. Fours attention tends to go to what others have and they don't. When threatened, Fours tend to idealize other people and feel deficient. At their best, Fours inspire and transform others with their creativity and capacity to empathize with the suffering of others. The challenge for the Four is to balance sadness with the capacity for happiness and dissatisfaction, even if the relationship or the experience seems flawed or incomplete. We can support Fours by standing steady for them when their feelings are intense, show empathy, share our own feelings, and let them know they are loveable separate from their identification with being special.

● Strengths: Compassionate, idealistic, capable of emotional depth
● Problems: Moody, withdrawn, uncooperative

- Speaking style: Sometimes warm and full of feeling, sometimes flat and dry, they tend to be subjective and try to be aesthetically correct; often a tone of sadness or dissatisfaction
- Famous Fours: Ingmar Bergman, Paul Simon, Jeremy Irons, Patrick Stewart, Bob Dylan, Miles Davis, Jonny Depp, J. D. Salinger, Anais Nin, Marcel Proust, Tennessee Williams, Edgar Allan Poe, Annie Lennox, Prince, Michael Jackson, Virginia Woolf, Judy Garland, Thomas Merton

American Beauty (see earlier description)

1 (0:1:17–1:23:30) Jane (Thora Birch) whines about all that is missing from her life. Her parents are "weirdos," she feels abandoned by a father who pays more attention to her hot girlfriend, Angela, whose beauty she envies. Later in the scene, she then shows great pleasure in the emotional intensity of her relationship with her boyfriend, Rickey, who lets her know she's the most special person in his world. Just what a Four wants: to feel special in the eyes of another.
   a. Some of our deepest relationships are formed around shared losses and the vulnerability of expressing our feelings to another person. Can you relate a similar experience?
   b. Fours' ability to access their deeper feelings give them the capacity to empathize with others especially when others are vulnerable or in intense situations. Have you known somebody with this gift?

The Hours (see earlier description)

1 (0:17:35–0:27:45) Richard claims he is being honored for his work as an author because others feel sorry for him. He says he is a failure because he wasn't able to immortally express the specialness of the ordinary moments of life. This is a core insight for a Four: that uniqueness is present in the ordinary if we are open to appreciating it. In general, one of the Four's fears is of being seen as ordinary.
   a. Can you appreciate Richard's sense of longing and loss and why someone who feels so deeply is drawn towards artistic expression?
   b. The intense emotional life of Fours contributes to complex relationships and an understandable tendency towards depression. Have you experienced a relationship like this? How did you deal with it?
   c. How could you stand in and support the Four to balance his/her subjective emotionality to a more objective balanced perspective? How broad is your spectrum of emotions?

Type Five: The Observer

Perceptive and distant, Fives want to possess knowledge and avoid being perceived as uninformed. Fives' attention tends to go to protecting their boundaries. They can appear ill at ease in social situations and value their privacy and are sensitive to the intrusion of others. At their best Fives are visionaries, and able to see the world in an entirely different way. The challenge for Fives is to balance their tendency to withdraw or withhold from people by reaching out to others, even if that means discomfort of conflict. We can support the Fives in our lives by encouraging them to welcome their feelings in the here and now rather than intellectualize them, and respect their need for privacy while understanding it is not rejection.

- Strengths: Scholarly, perceptive, self-reliant
- Problems: Isolate, overly intellectual, stingy
- Speaking style: Rational and content oriented, most comfortable in their area of expertise; not big on "small talk," Fives want to know they can sustain self-sufficiency
- Famous Fives: Albert Einstein, Bill Gates, Georgia O'Keefe, John Lennon, James Joyce, Björk, Susan Sontag, Emily Dickinson, Jane Goodall, Bobby Fischer, Stephen King, Vincent Van Gogh, Kurt Cobain, Jodie Foster

The Social Network (see earlier description)

1 (0:0:00–0:5:24) This scene illustrates the challenges we can encounter when dealing with Fives. Fives can struggle with feelings of social isolation and often compensate with over intellectualization. Fives often process their feelings after the fact. This poses a challenge when trying to develop intimate relationships with others.
   a. How do you allow someone the space and time to explore their feelings? What if your preference is to be emotionally spontaneous? How might this difference create interpersonal challenges?

American Beauty (see earlier description)

1 (0:47:00–0:50:02) This scene illustrates the Five's proclivity for knowledge in a specialized area. In this case, Ricky is a connoisseur of grass and has a vast collection of music and video equipment.
   a. Establishing an intellectual connection before an emotional connection is the preferred style of the Five. Have you known somebody like this who might be misunderstood by others?
2 (Same scene) Ricky demonstrates his specialized knowledge of every type of grass and is also sensitive to being intruded upon by his father.
   a. Fives develop expertise in specific subjects and connect to others with their knowledge. Establishing an intellectual connection before an

emotional connection is the preferred style of the Five. Have you known somebody like this who might be misunderstood by others?

Type Six: The Loyal Skeptic

Loyal and trustworthy, Sixes want to feel safe and secure and avoid feeling anxious. Their attention tends to go to safety and security. When threatened, they hesitate. Other Sixes prefer to stay in the "strength mode" – they rush into action and seek to brace themselves physically or ideologically as a way of overcoming their fear. At their best, Sixes are internally stable and self-reliant, courageously championing themselves and others. The challenge for the Six is to learn to trust themselves as well as other people as they become more flexible and develop the courage to act, even in the presence of doubt or ambivalence. We can support the Sixes in our lives by encouraging them to notice the positives, develop trust, appreciate their own strengths and take positive action. Being consistent, trustworthy, and able to disclose personal feelings and thoughts can be a model for them to develop.

- Strengths: Loyal, courageous, attentive to people and problems, often strategic thinkers
- Challenges: Suspicious, pessimistic, doubtful
- Speaking style: Setting limits on themselves and others, having serious questions, and playing devil's advocate; by contrast, sometimes they are ideologically zealous
- Famous Sixes: Robert F. Kennedy, Malcom X, Princess Diana, George H.W. Bush, Tom Hanks, Bruce Springsteen, Candice Bergen, Gilda Radner, Meg Ryan, Helen Hunt, Mel Gibson, Julia Roberts, Phil Donahue, Jay Leno, Woody Allen, J. Edgar Hoover, Richard Nixon, "George Costanza" (*Seinfeld*)

The Social Network (see earlier description)

1 (1:05:32–c1:11:19) Sixes tend to give their power to others, rather than standing on their own two feet. Sixes can be suspicious and test their credibility as a means of feeling safe. During the meeting in the bar, Edwardo shows disdain for Sean's self-confidence. He has done his research to find that, on paper, Sean isn't as successful as he is making himself out to be.
   a. Can you see how Edwardo's gift might also be his curse? Can you see how taking a balanced stand with Sean and Mark with a sense of self-confidence rather than disdain would make Edwardo a more supportive and effective partner to Mark?
   b. Can you think of any situations in your life where you take on the position of a victim of authority rather than a stand for who you are and what you believe in?
2 (Same scene) Sixes focus on safety and security enables them to be excellent

strategists. However, when doubting themselves, they tend to imagine worst-case scenarios and might be perceived as pessimistic.

   a. How do you deal with a person who tends to be a pessimist? How do you help them to see positive scenarios so they don't feel judged or patronized by you? What are your coping strategies when you are in the grips of projecting a fear of what might happen?

The King's Speech (2010; Colin Firth, Geoffrey Rush, Helena Bonham Carter): This film tells the story of the man who became King George VI (Firth), the father of Queen Elizabeth II. After his brother abdicates, George ("Bertie") reluctantly assumes the throne. Plagued by a dreaded stammer and considered unfit to be king, Bertie engages the help of an unorthodox speech therapist named Lionel Logue (Rush). Through a set of unexpected techniques, and as a result of an unlikely friendship, Bertie is able to find his voice and boldly lead the country through war.

1 (1:38:31–1:49:23) In this scene Bertie demonstrates just about all the exceptional qualities of the Six: overcoming his fear and self-doubt and courageously speaking to his country out of a firm sense of duty and loyalty.

   a. It is said that true courage only arises through seeing and honestly dealing with one's own fears and being able to rise above them. Can you recall a situation in your life where confronting a deep fear resulted in tapping into your inner resources while accomplishing something you didn't think you could do?

Type Seven: The Epicure

Enthusiastic and optimistic, Sevens want to keep their options open and avoid feeling tied down. Sevens tend to focus on the bright side of any given situation. When Sevens feel limited, they generally find a way to get out of the situation. At their best Sevens are forward thinkers, imaginative, and innovative. The challenge for Sevens is to focus in depth and to stay the course in work and relationships. Slowing down, being in the moment, and learning to tolerate their own and other people's suffering can bring needed balance. We can support the Sevens in our life by providing a supportive framework to move into deep commitments and painful situations. One can also take a firm stand when communicating important feelings, wants, and needs.

- Strengths: Adventurous, fun loving, quick thinking
- Challenges: Self-absorbed, dispersed, uncommitted
- Speaking style: Personal storytelling, which can be either highly entertaining or simply self-absorbed; they also focus on the positive, and tend to ignore or quickly "reframe" the negative
- Famous Sevens: John F. Kennedy, Benjamin Franklin, Leonard Bernstein, Leonardo DiCaprio, Elizabeth Taylor, Wolfgang Amadeus Mozart, Steven

Spielberg, Timothy Leary, Robin Williams, Jim Carey, Cameron Diaz, Elton John, Sarah Ferguson, Larry King, Howard Stern, John Belushi, "Auntie Mame" (*Mame*)

The Social Network (see earlier description)

1 (1:05:32–1:11:19) Sean Parker reveals the multifaceted characteristics of the Seven: a visionary and a great storyteller while, at the same time, arrogant and self-absorbed. He reframes his defeats and rationalizes the ramifications of his reckless behaviors.
   a. How do you facilitate a capacity for resilience, while at the same time staying grounded and honest?
   b. Some say it is difficult to pin a Seven down as they tend to get distracted by their many and varied interests. How might this be an excellent capacity to have when creating a visionary enterprise?
   c. On the other hand, why might this be frustrating on an interpersonal level?

The King's Speech (see earlier description)

1 (0:34:24–0:38:40) This scene demonstrates Lionel's capacity to be innovative. For Sevens, difficult challenges can be turned into play and obstacles surmounted with fun and innovation.
   a. Unconventional thinkers at times can challenge our patience. How can you support a Seven to develop the grounding, organization and self-discipline they require to work well with others and to see an idea to completion?

Type 8: The Protector

Energetic and intense, the Eight wants to control others and avoid feeling defenseless. Their focus tends to go to fairness and justice, when they are wronged or the weak are taken advantage of, they will fight back. At their best, Eights are magnanimous and use their strength to improve the lives of others. The challenge for Eights is to combine assertion and control with interdependency and cooperation, as well as learn how to manage their excessive energy. We can support the Eights in our lives by encouraging them to accept their own vulnerability, distinguish it from weakness, and reduce excessive impulsive behavior. Be forthright, firm, and yet flexible.
- Strengths: Enthusiastic, generous, powerful
- Problems: Excessive, angry, dominating
- Speaking style: Eights usually speak assertively and exert strong leadership; they tend to be bossy and often get angry when something goes wrong
- Famous Eights: Martin Luther King, Jr., Franklin Roosevelt, Lyndon Johnson,

Mikhail Gorbachev, Pablo Picasso, Richard Wagner, Sean Connery, Susan Saradon, Glen Close, John Wayne, Charlton Heston, Norman Mailer, Mike Wallace, Donald Trump, Frank Sinatra, Bette Davis, James Brown, Courtney Love, Leona Helmsley, Sigourney Weaver, Fidel Castro, Saddam Hussein, John McCain

The Blind Side (2009; Sandra Bullock, Quinton Aaron, Tim McGraw, Cathy Bates): Oversized African-American Michael Oher, the teen from across the tracks and a broken home, has nowhere to sleep at age 16 and is taken in by an affluent Memphis couple, Leigh Anne and Sean Touey.

1   (0:46:50–0:48.39) In this scene Bullock marches onto the football field and grabs the young player by the face mask and bluntly tells him to protect his teammates the same way he protects the family he loves. In getting her point across, she gains the respect of the coach while also intimidating him.

   a. What strategies can one use to communicate with a well meaning and strong willed person who takes a position of leadership in an intimidating manner?

   b. How would you approach a person who is not in touch with his or her own vulnerability but masks it with an intimidating posture?

   c. How can you manage your own reactivity to a strong personality and understand his or her perspective?

Wall Street (see earlier description)

1   (1:14:45–1:18:56) Gekko (Michael Douglas) redefines fairness and justice according to his self-serving values and uses his power to turn the table on the board. This is the power of the Eight in action.

   a. How do you deal with an individual who welcomes and relishes a good fight?

   b. Can you see how matching the Eights' energy can gain their respect and put you both on equal footing?

Type 9: The Mediator

Easygoing and self-effacing, the Nine's attention tends to go toward understanding other points of view and wanting to avoid feeling conflicted. When threatened they withdraw and procrastinate while allowing enough time to let problems resolve themselves. At their best, Nines are great listeners, able to see others' points of view and are natural mediators. The challenge for the Nine is to know what they want, set clear goals and markers along the way to stay the course. We can support the Nines in our lives by encouraging them to speak up for themselves and voice their needs and wants. A solid system of accountability can support the Nine to maintain their momentum.

- Strengths: Inclusive, considerate, good listener
- Challenges: Stubborn, ambivalent, self-forgetful
- Speaking style: Inclusive and welcoming at their best; Nines may have trouble getting to the point; they can be linear and controlled, or quite scattered
- Famous Nines: Abraham Lincoln, Carl Jung, Ronald Reagan, Gerald Ford, Queen Elizabeth II, Princess Grace, George Lucas, Walt Disney, Sophia Loren, Gena Davis, Kevin Costner, Keanu Reeves, Ron Howard, Ringo Starr, Janet Jackson, Marc Chagall, Norman Rockwell

The Blind Side (see earlier description)

1 (1:54:00–1:55:19) LeAnne asks Michael how he made it out of the projects. He replies that he learned to close his eyes when something bad was about to happen and then after it was over, "the world is a good place." This is a core coping strategy for the Nine.
   a. In Michael's case, his ability to avoid was an effective survival skill and served him well. However, as an adult, it could limit his ability to fully participate in life. If you were guiding Michael to stay present with his conflicted feelings, what are three practical suggestions you would recommend to him?
   b. How do you stay present in a difficult conversation when you feel conflicting emotions? Are there any situations where you might be repressing your own anger and avoiding having a difficult conversation?

American Beauty (see earlier description)

1 (0:01:12–0:06:13) Lester tells us he is just going through the motions in his life and he knows that his wife, Carolyn, and daughter, Jane, consider him a loser. We also see that he is more aware of and expressive of his anger as when he lets his manager know how angry he is followed by an angry outburst with his wife while driving home.
   a. Like Lester, many people have not really explored their own needs or taken risks to find out what makes them feel alive. How would you point this out to another person while supporting their need to feel safe?
   b. Are there areas in your life where you don't really know what you want, and rather than making the effort to explore or take your own risks to find out, you just don't deal with it? What steps could you take to open that door?

Further Reading

- Daniels D, Price V. *The Essential Enneagram*. New York, NY: Harper Collins; 2009.
- Lapid-Bodga G. *What Type of Leader are You? Using the Enneagram system to identify and*

grow your leadership strengths and achieve maximum success. New York, NY: McGraw-Hill; 2007.

- O'Hanrahan P. *Enneagram Studies in the Narrative Tradition*. Enneagram Professional Training Program Brochure; 2007.
- Palmer H. *The Enneagram: understanding yourself and the others in your life*. San Francisco, CA: Harper; 1991.
- Riso DN, Hudson R. *The Wisdom of The Enneagram*. New York, NY: Bantam; 1999.
- Wagner J. *Nine Lenses on the World*. Evanston, IL: Nine Lens Press; 2010.
- www.enneagramworldwide.com [online test]
- www.enneagramwork.com [online test]
- www.enneagraminstitute.com [online test]
- www.theenneagraminbusiness.com/index.html [online test]
- www.vivianatrucco.com.ar/research [online test]

PART V

Movie Portrayals of Health-Care Professionals

21

This Won't Hurt a Bit: Novocaine and Other Sorrows

Edward Thibodeau, Lauren M. Consonni, Matthew Alexander, Amanda Kotis & Karen Likar Manookin

OVER THE PAST 100 YEARS OF CINEMATIC HISTORY, SOME OF HOLLYWOOD'S most famous actors have played the role of a dentist in movies that cross multiple genres, including action, comedy, drama, horror, western, and adult fantasy. In the past, the overwhelming majority of films depicted dentists in comedic or horror roles and many have featured them as incompetent, menacing, sadistic, unethical, or morally corrupt. The consequences of such portrayals have had a significant impact on public opinion and have led to society's commonly held stereotypes of the dentist and the profession.

Modern advances in cinematography have allowed filmmakers to enhance the visceral and somatic experiences of the movie-going audience. In addition, there has been some evolution in the way dentists are portrayed. More recent films have allowed for in-depth character development, often presenting dentists in a more dramatic and realistic light. Furthermore, the subject matter of many films has shifted from slapstick comedy and gore to complex interpersonal relationships, cultural issues, and societal commentaries. Hopefully, over the next 100 years, the cinematic image of dentistry will come to better reflect the true qualities of the profession and the important role it plays in the lives of patients.

Societal Stereotypes of Dentists

Living the Good Life

Snow Dogs (2002; Cuba Gooding, Jr., Sisqo, James Coburn): In this Disney comedy, Cuba Gooding, Jr. plays Dr. Theodore "Ted" Brooks, a successful, self-promoting Miami dentist. He seems to have it all until he finds out he is adopted and inherits a pack of Alaskan sled dogs, which sends him on a journey of personal growth and self-discovery.

1 (Ch 1, 0:00:00–0:03:47) In the film's first scene, a young Ted Brooks is in his father's dental office for career day. Fast-forward 25 years. Throughout the opening credits the audience gets a glimpse into the life of Dr. Ted Brooks as he goes about his privileged daily routine.

   a. What are the major influences or reasons for selecting a particular career? Are there gender differences in motivations behind career choices? Are there racial or ethnic differences in motivations behind career choices?

   b. Who played a role in your decision to enter a health profession? How important are parental influences in this process and can parental pressures have a negative role?

   c. In the case of this dentist, how is success portrayed? Does society's measure of success differ for different health professionals? How do you as health-care professional measure success? How important is job satisfaction to a successful career?

   d. How important is the "personal touch" philosophy of internal marketing versus external marketing and advertising for the growth of a practice?

Laughter is the Best Medicine

Little Shop of Horrors (1986; Steve Martin, Rick Moranis): This campy B-rated cult musical features Seymour Krelborn (Rick Moranis) and his coworker Audrey (Ellen Greene) as employees at a struggling flower shop. While shopping at a wholesale flower market, Seymour purchases an exotic plant that quickly captures national attention. Unfortunately, the plant relies on human blood to survive and thrive. In several cameos throughout the movie, Steve Martin plays the role of a sadistic dentist, Dr. Orin Scrivello, as Audrey's abusive boyfriend.

1 (Ch 11, 0:33:10–0:35:43) In this scene Dr. Scrivello (Martin) arrives at his office on his motorcycle, dressed as a 1950s James Dean wannabe. The audience gains insight into Scrivello's childhood and his motivations for becoming a dentist.

   a. Is personal appearance important in the doctor-patient relationship? Given this portrayal, how do you think Dr. Scrivello's community and peers would view him?

   b. What are some of the psychological characteristics of Dr. Scrivello and how do these contribute to society's fear of dentists?

   c. Discuss the use of dental instruments as props in this clip. Does their use reinforce common misconceptions about the delivery of dental care?

   d. Does Dr. Scrivello's shrine to his mother suggest deep-seated psychological issues that could impact his interpersonal relationships? Does this influence the quality of care he provides?

   e. Why does this film clip elicit a comedic response? Does this exaggerated portrayal of the dentist have any basis in truth?

Stress and Dentistry

The Secret Lives of Dentists (2002; Scott Campbell, Hope Davis): This independent film tells the story of two married dentists, Drs. David and Dana Hurst. The couple works in the same dental office and co-parent three daughters. During the course of the film, David comes to fear that his wife, an aspiring opera singer as well as fellow dentist, is unfaithful.

1   (Ch 1, 0:00:00–0:05:15) Dr. David Hurst (Campbell) shares his philosophy about teeth in the opening scene. The scene continues on to portray Dr. Hurst and his hygienist working with a difficult patient, Slater (Denis Leary), as well as Dr. Hurst engaging his wife (Davis) with some banter.

   a. Do you believe dentists have a special relationship with teeth? Is Dr. David Hurst's monologue consistent with stereotypes about dentists?

   b. What common stressors of dentistry are revealed in this clip?

   c. What common signs of dental anxiety are shown in this clip?

   d. How well do the dentist and hygienist handle the difficult patient? Is the relationship between dentist and hygienist also a stereotype?

   e. Would you have done anything differently with this difficult patient? What are some other types of difficult patients dentists are likely to encounter in their work?

   f. Contrast the different interpersonal styles of the married dentists. How would you describe these styles? What is your interpersonal style?

   g. What are the pros and cons of working with your mate, either as dentists or physicians?

   h. What are the benefits of health-care professionals having a hobby about which they are passionate?

2   (Ch 12, 0:36:12–0:40:07) At this point in the film, Dr. Hurst, the primary parental caretaker, is dealing with suspicions of his wife's infidelity. Furthermore, his youngest daughter is becoming unbearably attached to him and acting out towards her mother. This scene shows the difficult patient, Slater, returning to have a filling redone after having publicly humiliated Dr. Hurst over a lost filling at his wife's opera performance. As the dentist leaves his office, he fantasizes that Slater is sitting next to him in his car and engaged in dialogue with him.

   a. Have you ever had a patient "come home" with you in your mind's eye after a day at the office? What types of patients are most likely to remain in a health provider's consciousness after work?

   b. While working on Slater's mouth, Dr. Hurst fantasizes about punishing his wife for her assumed infidelity. How can health-care professionals, under personal stress, best balance work and home stress? What strategies can be most effective in this regard?

   c. What is the best way to handle patient dissatisfaction?

   d. Discuss the dialogue between Dr. Hurst and Slater that occurs in Dr

Hurst's car? What common stressors of and stressors and stereotypes about dentistry are verbalized by Slater?

    e. How is Dr. Hurst's anger at Slater revealed in this dialogue? How do dentists best handle the frustration associated with patients not caring for their own teeth?

Primal Fears, Phobias, and Terror

Marathon Man (1976; Laurence Olivier, Dustin Hoffman): In this dramatic thriller, Dustin Hoffman portrays Babe, a graduate student who inadvertently becomes involved in an international diamond conspiracy involving his brother "Doc," a US government secret agent, and a fugitive Nazi dentist, Dr. Szell (Laurence Olivier). Dr. Szell murders Doc and abducts and tortures Babe, mistakenly assuming that his brother gave him information on the diamond smuggling operation.

1 (Ch 33, 1:11:47–1:16:00) The scene opens up after the death of Babe's brother. Dr. Szell enters and begins his interrogation while laying out his dental instruments. He repeatedly asks Babe, "Is it safe?" referring to his ability to leave the country with the diamonds. Babe, unfortunately, does not know the meaning or answer to Dr. Szell's question.

2 (Ch 35, 1:20:25–1:23:30) In this scene, Babe is being interrogated a second time following a staged rescue attempt. Babe is still unable to answer Szell's questions, resulting in further torture.

    a. Discuss the significance of Dr. Szell's character in this film. How does this portrayal reinforce the stereotype of a dentist as a purveyor of pain and fear?

    b. What is unique about dental (tooth) pain compared with other types of physical discomfort?

    c. What is unique about the dental handpiece (drill) as used in the film that evokes an emotional or visceral response from the audience?

    d. How does Dr. Szell's "bedside manner" contrast with his actions?

    e. Many patients have moderate to severe "dentist" anxiety? What is the best way to handle patients' anxiety about coming to the dentist?

The Compassionate Healer

Thumbsucker (2005; Lou Taylor Pucci, Keanu Reeves): This quirky, coming-of-age film centers on Justin Cobb (Pucci), a 17-year-old with anxiety issues and a thumb-sucking habit. His "transcendental" orthodontist, Dr. Lyman (Reeves), attempts to help him deal with the problem. However, when Justin stops thumb sucking he copes with his anxieties through experimentation with sex and drugs.

1   (Ch 8, 0:20:04–0:23:53) Dr. Lyman confronts Justin about his thumb-sucking behavior. He is not only concerned about the dental consequences of Justin's habit, but also with the emotional and psychological basis for the dependency. Dr. Lyman tries to cure him through the use of hypnosis.
   a. How important is it for a health-care provider to be attuned to a patient's psychological or mental state? What obligations does a health-care provider have when concerned about a patient's emotional well-being?
   b. What important qualities should a compassionate health-care provider demonstrate?
   c. Is Dr. Lyman's unconventional approach to Justin's problem an acceptable modality of treatment? Does it matter that Justin is a minor?
   d. Discuss the role of alternative medicines or therapies and their place in the modern health-care system.

The Daily Grind

Novocaine (2001; Steve Martin, Helena Bonham Carter, Laura Dern): Steve Martin plays a successful dentist (Dr. Frank Sangster) whose upper-middle-class existence becomes a tangled web of sex, drugs, and murder from the moment the alluring, narcotic-seeking Susan Ivey (Bonham Carter) walks into his office.

1   (Ch 1, 0:01:38–0:04:17) In the film's opening scene, Dr. Sangster is treating his own lawyer, who is desperately trying to carry on a conversation with him about his business affairs. However, Dr. Sangster appears to be hurried and disinterested in the discussion. The scene also includes a romantic encounter between the dentist and his hygienist as played by Laura Dern.
   a. Is Dr. Sangster's approach to his patient an accurate depiction or a stereotype of the dental profession? Do these types of abrupt interactions occur in other health-care settings?
   b. How important are good communication skills in health-care provider-patient interactions?
   c. How is technology and equipment utilized for the patient's benefit and comfort? How does the use of dental technology and equipment in this film clip differ from the more common portrayal of dental instruments as inducing pain, torture, and fear?
   d. Discuss the appropriateness of personal relationships in the workplace. Under what circumstances are provider-staff romantic relationships acceptable? Under what circumstances are provider-patient romantic relationships acceptable?
   e. Is Dr. Sangster's treating his own lawyer a violation?

Drug-Seeking Behavior
· ·

1   (Ch 2, 0:5:15–0:9:15) This selection includes two scenes. The first scene depicts the patient, Susan, asking Dr. Sangster for a prescription of a strong narcotic to help manage her tooth pain. Dr. Sangster writes her a prescription for five tablets of Demerol. In the next scene, Dr. Sangster is consequently contacted by a pharmacy to verify the highly unusual prescription for 50 tablets of the potent drug.

   a. What tactics does Susan use to manipulate Dr. Sangster to get her prescription?
   b. What are signs that Susan is drug-seeking?
   c. Dr. Sangster attempts to stand his ground, but finally gives into Susan's demands. How often do you encounter drug-seeking patients and how do you handle them?
   d. Do you think that dentists are "easy marks" for drug-addicted patients? If so, why?
   e. What are some of the potential legal consequences of inappropriately prescribing controlled substances? How can one guard against a patient tampering with a prescription?

Further Reading
· ·

● Berry JH. Dentistry's public image: does it need a boost? *J Am Dent Assoc*. 1989; **118**(6): 686–92.
● Mandel ID. The image of dentistry in contemporary culture. *J Am Dent Assoc*. 1998; **129**(5): 607–13.
● Thibodeau EA, Mentasti LE. Who stole Nemo? *J Am Dent Assoc*. 2007; **138**(5): 656–60.

22

Beyond Nurse Ratched: Nursing

David Stanley

THIS CHAPTER GREW FROM A RESEARCH STUDY INVESTIGATING HOW nurses (male and female) were portrayed in feature films made between 1900 and 2007 with the nurse as the film's main or principle character and a story line specifically related to nursing.[1] The first part of this chapter will focus specifically on how male nurses are portrayed in feature films and the second part will address the portrayal of female nurses in film. The original research identified 280 feature films, and of these films, seven featured male nurses in significant roles. However, further investigation, a more focused review of films related to male nurses, and the consideration of films made since 2007 has resulted in a wider representation of male-nurse related feature films.

The film media has a significant and profound influence on how the public view male nurses and the nursing profession in general,[2–4] supporting, and in some cases promoting, stereotypical perceptions.[3] Indeed, stereotypical views such as nursing being a female-oriented profession, nurses being sex objects, the powerlessness of nurses, and the subservience of nurses to the medical profession are reinforced in many feature films. Male nurses, as well as being underexposed, are also viewed through a stereotypical lens.[2] Patients may not always accept male nurses, with some fearful or homophobic male patients, or shy female patients refusing or having difficulty with intimate care provided by male nurses.[6,9–12]

Nurses are required to be empathetic, compassionate, and supportive and as such, male nurses are commonly stereotyped as either "gay" or effeminate.[5] While some male nurses are homosexual, this labeling may be an effort to exert social control over male nurses because the nursing profession continues to be defined as a woman's profession[7] or it could be the result of sexism by peers, colleagues, or patients. Male nurses are also considered either to be aggressive and ambitious, or lazy, underachievers who were not up to admission to medical school.[8] (*See* dialog regarding the film *Meet the Parents* [2000] in this chapter for an example of this.)

The film media and most of the films reviewed for this chapter support all these stereotypical views. However, all the films identified offer a range of learning opportunities and insights that widen our understanding of male nurses.

Male Nurse–Patient Interactions

Magnolia (1999; Julianne Moore, William H. Macy, John C. Reilly, Tom Cruise, Philip Seymour Hoffman, Philip Baker Hall, Jason Robards): Set in the San Fernando Valley, the film is a mosaic of interrelated stories, where the key characters are each searching for love or forgiveness, reconciliation or happiness, or meaning. A central character is Earl Partridge (Robards) who is in the terminal stages of brain and lung cancer. He is dying at home with the support and care of a male nurse, Phil Parma (Hoffman). His wife Linda (Moore) struggles to deal with Earl's imminent death and it is left to Phil to initiate the reconciliation with Earl's estranged son Frank (Cruise). The interrelated nature of the stories in this film and the style of editing make it difficult to single out discrete scenes. The language and themes of the film are confronting throughout.

1 (2:03:36–2:13:10) In these scenes Earl talks to Phil about his first love, his son, and his regrets. "Life is long," he laments before asking Phil to help him. Phil becomes upset and cries as he prepares to give the morphine drops he knows will speed on Earl's death.
   a. The request to help someone to die would not be unfamiliar to many health professionals. If you have been in this situation or one similar to it, how did you act or respond?
   b. In your view how should health professionals act when placed in this position?
   c. Did Phil do the right thing?
2 (2:18:00–2:41:00). These scenes are intermixed with many other stories as the film draws to a close. They show Earl's son, Frank come to be at his side while Phil acts as a facilitator and concerned supporter, although at a distance.
   a. Phil has acted as a facilitator and mediator throughout this film. How do you rate his clinical performance in these competencies?
   b. Could Phil have done more to support Frank, Earl's son?
   c. Phil is a committed carer and gets caught up in the emotion of his work. How can health professionals retain their commitment to care without becoming emotionally involved?
   d. Does it matter if health professionals are affected emotionally when confronted by family tragedy or death? Why?

Talk to Her (*Hable con Ella*) (2002; Javier Camara, Dario Grandinetti, Leonor Watling, Rosario Flores): This Spanish film is about three relationships: that between Marco (Dario Grandinetti) and his girlfriend Lydia (Rosario

Flores), a bullfighter, who is injured during a fight; another between Benigno (Javier Camara) a male nurse and a dancer and Alicia (Leonor Watling), who is now his patient, in a deep long-term coma; and the friendship that forms between the two men as they care for the woman they love.

1 (0:03:37–0:07:36). These scenes show Benigno and another nurse caring for Alicia with skill and compassion. Benigno talks with Alicia, although she is unconscious. They also provide hair care, passive movement, skin care, nail care, and wash and dress Alicia. Benigno is also shown making clinical decisions and taking part in intimate personal care in a friendly, professional manner.

   a. These are fundamental clinical nursing skills and this film attempts to depict a male (and female) nurse engaged in these skills. Are they appropriate skills for a male nurse to be engaged in? Are these skills compatible with your understanding of a male nurse's duties and responsibilities?

   b. A number of publications[6,9,10,12] suggest that male nurses and female patients are confronted by the need to provide or receive intimate care. Why might this be the case?

2 (0:18:27–0:19:30). These scenes also show Benigno and another nurse caring for Alicia with skill and compassion. Benigno is cutting Alicia's hair while he again talks to her.

   a. Hair cutting has not traditionally been seen as a fundamental clinical nursing skill. Is this an appropriate skill for a male nurse (or any nurse) to be engaged in?

   b. Is this a skill you would see as compatible with your understanding of a male nurse's duties and responsibilities?

3 (0:37:29–0:38:50) These scenes again show Benigno providing essential clinical care, but they also offer an interesting dialog between Marco and Lydia's doctor about the chances of recovery from a persistent vegetative state. The other issue these scenes relate to are patient dignity, skin care, and eye care for comatose patients.

   a. When discussing the balance between scientific knowledge and the possibility of "miracles" do you feel the doctor gets the balance of the discussion right?

   b. How might you engage Marco in this discussion or answer his questions?

   c. These and previous scenes show Benigno providing essential care to a comatose patient. On a purely clinical level, how would you rate the quality of his care? What other care might he need to consider when caring for a long term comatose patient?

Meet the Parents (2000; Robert De Niro, Ben Stiller, Blythe Danner, Teri Polo): Greg (Ben Stiller), a male nurse, and Pam (Teri Polo) set off to meet Pam's parents, Jack (De Niro), an ex-CIA agent, and Dina (Danner), so that Greg can ask for Pam's father's permission to marry his daughter and to prepare for her sister's sudden wedding. A key theme of this film is that nursing is an inappropriate career for a male and it opens with a song that includes the line, "show me a man who is gentle and kind and I'll show you a loser."

1   (0:02:08–0:03:04). In the opening scenes Greg is practicing a marriage proposal with a male patient while he is inserting a urinary catheter.

   a. There are times when it may be appropriate to engage patients in conversations of a personal nature; however, does Greg cross the boundary of appropriateness with this conversation?

   b. Greg is dressed in scrubs and the patient mistakes him for a doctor claiming he has a gentle touch for a doctor. Uniforms seem now to be more generic with little to differentiate various professional groups. Does this matter and if so, what impact has this loss of uniform specificity had on the way patients and professionals interact?

Angels in America (2003; Patrick Wilson, Al Pacino, Meryl Streep, Emma Thompson, Mary-Louise Parker, Justin Kirk, Jeffrey Wright, Ben Shenkman): Described as a TV miniseries, this epic movie revolves around a group of individuals as they deal with the HIV/AIDS crisis in the mid to late 1980s in New York.

1   (Disk 2, 0:07:50–0:18:00) A doctor approaches the nursing station to inform an African-American, openly homosexual male nurse (Belize, played by Jeffery Wright) that a new patient is to be admitted. This patient's chart states that he has "liver cancer" but in fact he has AIDS. The scene shows the dialog between the doctor and nurse and then the nurse and patient (Roy Cohen, played by Al Pacino). Roy is hostile, prejudiced, and belligerent but Belize, with some restraint and frankness, talks honestly and explains the risks of taking part in a research trial.

   a. Belize is quite frank and confrontational at times both with the doctor and patient. Is this type of communication approach appropriate in these circumstances or could he have dealt with both the doctor and patient differently?

   b. Have you ever encountered a patient who was this hostile and offensive? How have you dealt with them?

   c. Should this behavior be tolerated and if so, under what circumstances?

   d. To what extent does Belize's sexuality influence how he deals with Roy?

2   (Disk 2, 0:46:30–0:53:10) In these scenes Belize, a male nurse, brings in medications to the new patient, Roy Cohen. Roy is hostile and abusive and reveals that he has a personal supply of azidothymidine. The drug is new, expensive, and rare. Belize asks for some of the drugs for his friend who has none and then, after a verbal dispute with Roy, Belize takes a number of bottles of the drug from Roy's large supply.

   a. Is Belize justified in taking some of Roy's azidothymidine?

   b. What might be an effective way to deal with Roy? Is there a way to support and care for this type of patient without engaging in conflict?

   c. Should health care be only for those who can pay or pull the right strings? How are health-care resources dealt with in other countries?

d. Review the 2007 film *Sicko* by Michael Moore for an interesting insight and comparison of health-care provision in a range of countries.

Male Nurse Clinical Skills

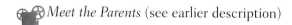

Meet the Parents (see earlier description)

1. (0:02:40–0:03:04) The male nurse, Greg (Ben Stiller), is attempting to insert a male urinary catheter.
   a. This clinical skill is commonly seen as a task appropriate for male nurses. Why should this be more so that some other clinical skills?
   b. Are there skills that should be gender specific or is care not an issue of gender?

Talk to Her (*Hable con Ella*) (see earlier description)

1. (0:03:37–0:07:36; 0:18:27–0:19:30) These scenes show Benigno and another nurse caring for Alicia with skill and compassion. The nurses provide hair care, passive movement, skin care, nail care, and wash and dress Alicia. Benigno is also shown making clinical decisions and taking part in intimate personal care in a friendly, professional manner.
   a. Is there anything in these scenes that makes you feel uncomfortable or question the masculinity of the male nurse involved?
   b. Is this even a reasonable question given that it would be very unusual to question the femininity of a female nurse?

Angels in America (see earlier description)

1. (Disk 2, 0:10:00–0:11:10) A male nurse (Belize, played by Jeffery Wright) undertakes a cannulation on an abusive and offensive patient (Roy Cohen played by Al Pacino). In the process he implies he can do it well or make it more painful for the patient.
   a. Roy is clearly abusive and offensive, but does this justify Belize's threat?
   b. Do health professionals have to tolerate this type of behavior and what other options are there?

Magnolia (see earlier description)

1. (1:20:00–1:21:08) Phil is on the phone trying to contact Earl's estranged son and he cannot hang up. As he waits Earl calls out in pain and Phil struggles to give him his medication, spilling the drugs all over the floor. One of the dogs (there are four in the room with Earl) eats some of the drugs while Phil goes on to administer the medication.

    a. Phil was placed in a dilemma, not wanting to hang up and having to administer the medication in a hurry. How might you have dealt with this situation?

    b. Could a more appropriate form of pain management have been used? If so what might you recommend or suggest?

    c. Is Phil responsible for the overdose and eventual death of the dog? What might be the consequences of this error?

Gender, Sexuality, and Care: Do they Matter?

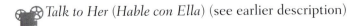 *Talk to Her* (*Hable con Ella*) (see earlier description)

1 (0:38:60–0:12:24) In these scenes Benigno is massaging Alicia's thigh. When her father (a psychiatrist) comes into the room, the father is clearly uncomfortable with a man providing such intimate personal care. He asks Benigno about his sexual orientation; Benigno lies and claims to prefer the company of men.

    a. Does the care provider's gender really matter for the provision of safe, effective, competent, and clinically relevant care?

    b. How would Alicia's father have reacted had Benigno been honest and claimed to have a heterosexual orientation?

    c. Why do you think Benigno felt the need to lie?

    d. Do you think patients are ever concerned about a health professional's sexual orientation?

    e. Have you had any experience where your sexuality was an issue in care provision or a concern for a patient?

    f. What factors do you think may have contributed to the stereotypical idea that male nurses are effeminate?

2 (0:58:20–0:59:22) Later in the film three of Benigno's female nurse colleagues are discussing his sexual orientation in the tea room. One leaves the room in protest at the character assault.

    a. Does a professional colleague's sexual orientation matter to the provision of safe, effective, competent, and relevant clinical care?

    b. Is there an appropriate way to discuss concerns colleagues might have about another colleague's clinical practice?

    c. Thinking back to the examples of clinical care offered in the earlier scenes, was the level of care Benigno provided too intimate or was he simply a competent and thorough nurse?

Meet the Parents (see earlier description)

1 (0:14:34–0:15:04) While Greg is meeting Pam's parents, Pam asks Greg what work he does and Greg explains that he has been transferred to triage.

Dina asks, "Oh, is that better than a nurse?" Pam explains that it is an area of emergency medicine where the top nurses work and Greg then has to agree that there are not "traditionally" many men in the nursing profession.

   a. Why do you think Pam's mother would hope that Greg was doing something "better" than nursing?

   b. From a historical perspective, have men been involved in providing care as male nurses?

   c. What percentage of the nursing profession is male? Try and consider a range of different countries and cultural groups as you think about this question.

2 (0:43:12–0:44:06) In this short scene Greg is introduced to Pam's relatives and friends. When Greg says he is a nurse the doctors in the group laugh because they think it is a joke. When it is clearly not so, there is stunned and embarrassed silence. Greg then goes on to explain that medicine wasn't for him and that he became a male nurse because he liked the freedom to work in a range of medical areas, to focus on patient care and avoid bureaucracy.

   a. What are the advantages of a career as a male nurse?

   b. What are the disadvantages of a career as a male nurse?

   c. Does doing nursing mean avoiding bureaucracy or is it just in a different form?

3 (1:34:00–1:34:10) This short scene towards the end of the film sees Greg and Jack confronting each other. Greg asks Jack to stop making fun of him for being a male nurse and Jack suggests that he could at least try another profession. Greg says "no."

   a. These scenes and the song at the start of the film ("show me a man who is gentle and kind and I'll show you a loser") support the idea that being a male nurse is not a masculine or desirable job and that it may only be fit for losers. What are the implications of these views for the nursing profession in general and male nurse recruitment in particular?

Angels in America (see earlier description)

1 (Disk 1, 1:19:01–1:23:10) An off-duty registered nurse (Belize, played by Jeffery Wright), who is a friend of the patient Prior Walter (Justin Kirk), visits him in hospital and provides advice, comfort, and a nontraditional "magic goop" cream that he applies while they talk.

   a. What are the implications of patient's using nonprescription medications while under medical care?

   b. Should Belize have known better or at least have notified the nursing team about his nontraditional medication? Why?

The Male Midwife
······················

Knocked Up (2007; Seth Rogen, Katherine Heigl, Paul Rudd, Leslie Mann): This comedy is about the relationship between two people, Alison (Heigl) and Ben (Rogen) who meet, have unprotected sex, and conceive a child. The film captures aspects of their adjustment to the pregnancy and the setbacks and hurdles they face in coming to know each other more fully. The film culminates in the child's birth.

1 (1:50:07–2:00:10) Ben and Alison arrive at the maternity hospital. They are greeted and introduced to their (male) nurse, Samuel. Ben says, "you're a nurse?" The male nurse proceeds to admit Alison and then takes a limited role in the labor and delivery while a doctor takes control of the birth process. The male nurse has difficulty with cannulation and apart from offering the doctor information (which is challenged) the male nurse plays only a limited part in the birth.

   a. Why would a competent and specifically trained midwife be unable to perform what appeared to be a normal delivery? Are there clinical concerns, professional issues or insurance considerations? These questions drive to the heart of health-care provision, professional roles and responsibilities, and a woman's right to choose the level of intervention in her birth.

   b. The doctor was very quick to assert his dominance over the birth process, even going as far as threats and fear mongering. For the mother to be in this vulnerable and painful state appeared inappropriate and it negated the opportunity for midwifery practice centered on the woman. Should the woman's rights to choose, or medical risk issues be more prominent in a normal birth situation?

   c. In these scenes it is left to the father to advocate for his partner. What is the male nurse's role (or, indeed, any nurse's role) in advocating for the laboring woman?

   d. The doctor in these scenes declared to the male nurse that they "were a team." What examples of teamwork did you see? What could have been done to enhance teamwork and include all parties in the decision-making process?

   e. Are there any advantages or specific disadvantages to having male midwives?

Meet the Fockers (2004; Robert De Niro, Ben Stiller, Dustin Hoffman, Barbra Streisand, Blythe Danner, Teri Polo): A follow-on from *Meet the Parents*, this film sees Greg (Stiller) and Pam (Polo) set off with her parents and her toddler nephew (Little Jack) to meet Greg's ex-hippie parents at the Focker home in Florida to discuss Greg and Pam's impending marriage. The film opens with Greg at work, delivering a baby. The main theme of the film is that Pam is pregnant – a fact they try to keep from everyone, especially Pam's ex-CIA father, Jack (De Niro).

1 (0:00:55–0:20:02) The film begins with Greg attempting to deliver a baby. There are no medical staff on hand to assist him so he delivers the child alone. Greg explains to the European parents that he is not a doctor, to which they reply, "you are a man and you are nurse? What kind of man is a nurse?" Greg then successfully delivers the baby.

   a. What kind of man is a nurse? Is there a "type"? Is there a stereotypical male nurse?

   b. What "type" of men enter the nursing profession?

   c. "What kind of man is a nurse?" Does this imply that being male and a nurse are incongruent? Are men and care incompatible or does this character reflect a wider view in society that men have no place in the "caring profession"?

   d. The film's writers (and those who wrote *Knocked Up*) clearly thought that having a male nurse deliver a baby was of comedic value, yet having male doctors deliver a baby is not seen as intrinsically funny. Why do you think there is this apparent disparity of gender-related professional roles in relation to the birth process?

Male Nurses and Terminal Care

Magnolia (see earlier description): Much of this drama deals with the final day of Earl Partridge's life, but the stories in the film are all very intertwined making it difficult to single out specific scenes. In my view it is the most positive film with a male nurse character.

1 (0:18:34–0:23:34) These scenes take place early on in the film. Earl is resting in bed, with Phil sitting in a chair beside him. Earl discusses his impending death, his current wife, the value of a good woman, and how he wishes he could meet his estranged son Frank (Tom Cruise). Phil listens quietly, offers encouraging comments and is left with the dilemma of whether or not to seek out Earl's son.

   a. Phil's dilemma is clear. What would you have done?

   b. Is it the health professional's responsibility to intervene on the patient's behalf and follow up on this request? If not what else could Phil have done?

   c. There is a lot of profanity used in this film. Is this acceptable because Earl is dying in his own home, or should nurses uncomfortable with the level of profane language used by the patient be able to object?

   d. Communication plays a vital role in health care. Can you identify aspects of "active listening" employed by Phil.

   e. What role does a nurse have in dealing with personal/potentially confronting information offered by a patient, particularly at this time in their care?

els in America (see earlier description)

;k 2, 1:41:30–1:47:10) In this scene the patient, Roy Cohen (Al Pacino), nes from his room with a drip, in a state of confusion induced by the morphine infusion. The male nurse, Belize (Jeffrey Wright), mischievously plays along with Roy's delusion before a female nurse leads him back to bed.

    a. What does the research say about supporting a patient who is delusional?

    b. Was Belize correct to play along with Roy's delusion in such a mischievous and potentially distressing way?

2   (Disk 2, 2:05:12–2:16:30) The patient, Roy Cohen (Al Pacino), is dying and he is found to be talking with the ghost of Ethel Rosenberg (Meryl Streep). Roy dies and the male nurse, Belize (Jeffery Wright) turns off the machines, steals a key from around the dead patient's neck and proceeds to take azidothymidine from Roy's large supply.

    a. Roy has many friends who are unable to access azidothymidine (which would have been a new drug and very expensive at the time the film was set). Was he right to steal it and therefore potentially help others suffering with AIDS?

    b. Roy's death was troubled and difficult. What else could Belize (or any nurse) have done to better support Roy's passing?

A Flawed Perception: The Feature Film Medium and Male Nurses

Most films that feature male nurses do little to counter the negative stereotypes common in the literature and public's perception. This category offers examples of films that do the least to negate the proliferation of the negative stereotypes.

Talk to Her (*Hable con Ella*) (see earlier description)

1   (0:45:26–0:58:20) Although this film begins with scenes that show excellent examples of male nurse care, these scenes outline the initial infatuation of Benigno with Alicia before her accident and his descent into obsession.

    a. Benigno has clearly crossed the appropriate boundary between a client and a professional's relationships. Where should the line be?

    b. What type or level of personal contact is appropriate between a client and a nursing professional?

2   (1:00:20–1:09:08) Here Benigno describes a strange black-and-white film and his infatuation is seen to grow into an obsession. This takes place at night and it is implied that he rapes Alicia, although it is not shown.

    a. What are the professional obligations of health professionals should they become aware of similar transgressions between a colleague and a client?

3 (1:20:00–1:22:14) In these later scenes a clinic meeting is shown where the nursing and medical team are discussing Alicia's pregnancy. It is clear that Benigno is the main suspect, as he has falsified the clinical notes and his obsession has become obvious.

    a. Is this team-based investigation an appropriate way to have investigated the issue?

    b. Should the police have been called or should the matter have been dealt with internally by the organization?

    c. How would you react if a colleague began describing their infatuation with a patient?

4 (1:23:30–1:43:15) The film draws to a close as it is revealed that Marco finds out that Benigno has been sent to jail. Marco also learns that Alicia has given birth to a stillborn child and awakes from her coma, but Benigno is unaware of this and commits suicide in jail, hoping to be reunited with Alicia who he thinks is still in a coma.

    a. Should the authorities have informed Benigno about the birth of Alicia's baby and her subsequent recovery?

    b. Did Benigno have a right to know about these events, given that it may have prevented his suicide?

    c. If Alicia came to you as her health professional and asked to know about the events of the previous four years while she was in a coma, and what happened to her to become pregnant and then recover, what would you tell her? What are the ethical implications of this situation and further implications for her future recovery?

    d. After starting the film as a sterling example of a caring and compassionate nurse, Benigno is found to be obsessed and morally corrupt. Garp's mother, in the 1982 film *The World According to Garp*, also rapes a patient in a persistent vegetative state, so she can conceive a child. Yet our sympathies for her may be quite different. What is it that sets the events in these two films apart? Is it just the fact that Benigno is a male?

Kill Bill: Vol 1 (2003; Uma Thrman, Lucy Liu, Vivica A. Fox, Daryl Hannah, David Carradine): In this action film a woman known only as "The Bride" (Thurman) wakes after a long coma and begins a killing spree in retribution for her attempted murder.

1 (0:26:40–0:30:60) A male care provider (it is not clear if "Buck" is a qualified nurse) has been facilitating, and taking part in the sexual abuse of The Bride while she has been in a coma. When she wakes she proceeds to murder an abuser and then Buck.

    a. While this sort of abuse seems far-fetched, what would be a health professional's responsibility if this or anything like it were to be suspected in their area of practice?

    b. All patients and especially those who are particularly vulnerable require diligent attention to ethical care and respect for any power imbalance that may be evident between the carer and the client/patient. How can health professionals engage the "voice" of the less powerful in our care?

c. As I watched this part of the film I wondered how this person even secured a job with these responsibilities. How can employers ensure that only people who are serious and actively committed to high-quality patient care inhabit our health-care facilities?

Killer Nurse (2008; Steve Robert Olson, Jaquelyn Aurora): Described as a "true story," this horror film is about an American male nurse (Charles Cullen) who killed between 35 and 40 dependant and vulnerable patients in his care.

1 Almost every scene in this film features the male nurse (Cullen), showing his involvement in the deaths of five women. The style of this movie is very repetitive and involves nudity, simulated rape, and patient's being tormented before their murder. The film is offered here as an example of this categorization, but it is a most unpleasant film to watch.

a. There are numerous cases of health professionals murdering some of the people in their care. Health professionals such as Harold Shipman, Dr. Patel and Beverly Alatt offer some disturbing examples, but what is it that motivates these murders and why don't colleagues recognize their crime or, if they do, why do they not act to stop them sooner?

b. One of Cullen's stated motives was that he was ending his patients' "suffering," but what measures are in place or should be in place to support the physiological well-being of health-care staff that may be unable to deal with their patients' suffering?

c. Cullen was able to move from facility to facility with his crimes virtually undetected. It is speculated that a lack of reporting mechanisms and inadequate legal protection for employers facilitated this. What is needed in the health service to ensure reporting mechanisms are in place and to better support employers with similar suspicions?

d. As a result of Cullen's crimes stronger laws are now in place, but how would you react if you suspected a colleague of similar criminal behavior?

Female Nurses in Feature Films

Films that feature female nurses or nursing in general are evident in significant numbers. They offer a unique insight into and reflection on the image of nurses. They portray nurses in romantic and military roles often represented with a self-sacrificial or heroic sub-plot. However, more recent films show nurses as strong practitioners who have grown both professionally and on the screen. There are a significant number of films that feature nurses in key roles with story lines that relate to nursing. These films are predominantly produced in the United States and focus on the dramatic, romantic and comedic genre. The story lines feature nurses at war, in love, or dedicated selflessly to their duty.

It is clear that the early films featuring nurses focused heavily on the self-sacrificial, heroic work of nurses, although more recent films are appearing from a wider range of countries and featuring nurses (both male and female) who are portrayed as strong, self-confident, and professionally aware. This portrayal is effected without losing elements of the theme that has dominated nurse-related films throughout the years: selflessness and self-sacrifice. Nurses are no longer appearing as one-dimensional "angels in white," selfless and meek, but they are increasingly emerging multi-dimensional professionals, caring and confident.[1] The following themes are offered as examples of the types of films that portray nurses on the "big" screen.

The Self-Sacrificial Angel

There are a large number of feature films made explicitly to celebrate the self-sacrificial aspects of nursing. For example, *Nurse Marjorie* (1920), *The White Angel* (1936), *Nurse Edith Cavell* (1939), *Cry Havoc* (1943), *So Proudly We Hail* (1943), *They were Expendable* (1945), *Sister Kenny* (1946), *The Lady with the Lamp* (1951), and *Florence Nightingale* (1985). While any of these films could offer a bountiful assortment of clips and scenes showing nurses in self-sacrificial roles, only a few films have been detailed here.

The English Patient (1996; Ralph Fiennes, Kristin Scott Thomas, Willem Defoe, Colin Firth, Juliette Binoche, Naveen Andrews): This film is about a nurse caring for a critically burned man (Ralph Fiennes) known only as "the English patient." Hana (Binoche) cares for him in a ruined Italian monastery. The patient is in fact a Hungarian geographer who has been injured in a plane crash during World War II. The film offers insights into the patient's past and the events that led to the plane crash in a series of "flashbacks." The film also deals with Hana's romance with Kip, an Indian sapper in the British Army.

1 (0:12:00–0:18:00) After her friend is killed by a mine, Hana leaves the security of the military convoy to care for the "English patient" alone in a ruined Italian monastery. Although the war is coming to a close there are very real dangers for her, and yet she decides to stay behind.
   a. Why might she choose to do this? Why would she put herself at risk (or why do health professionals put themselves are risk) to care for patients?
   b. Why might a health professional single out one patient's needs over another?
   c. What are the implications for health professionals when care is directed to one client over others?
   d. It could be argued that nothing is achieved without some degree of risk. But is taking a risk acceptable when deciding how far to take our care of others over self?
2 (0:42:50–0:46:20) Hana meets Kip while playing Bach on a booby-trapped

piano and she invites the sappers to stay with them in the grounds of the monastery. Hana is glad of the extra company and security the sappers add as she continues to care for the "English patient" in the villa.

a. Hana becomes close to the "English patient" as she cares for him, but does this type of special attention put her at risk of developing too close a relationship with this patient?

b. Is there such a thing as being "too close" to a patient?

c. Have you ever been in a position where you were tempted or close to crossing your professional boundaries? Doses this matter in terms of the outcome at the end of the film?

Paradise Road (1997; Glenn Close, Frances McDormand, Pauline Collins, Cate Blanchett): This film tells the story of a group of women who are imprisoned by the Japanese during World War II. While it highlights the atrocities of war and suffering as a result of man's inhumanity to man, it also celebrates the capacity of people to rise above their adversity and find moral strength and support in one another. These women do so both by individual acts of courage in the face of danger and by starting a voice orchestra that focuses them and lifts their spirits. A doctor (McDormand) and a small group of Australian nurses (one of whom is played by Blanchett) support the group physically.

1 (0:33:00–0:38:50) In these scenes, the nurses are caring for frail prisoners in a makeshift hospital, with a German doctor overseeing their efforts. An Asian woman sneaks medications into the camp so that some of the patients can be treated.

a. These scenes highlight self-sacrifice on a number of levels. But the doctor is thought to be doing her duty to avoid work on other more unpleasant tasks. Can altruism ever be a selfish act?

b. All of the women are starving and struggling for rations. Given the dreadful circumstances that they find themselves in are these precious resources wasted on the ill and infirm? What parallels are there with resources allocation in the current health system or global health profile?

2 (1:21:00–1:25:50) After being accused of speaking during an assembly, nurse Susan McCarthy is tortured and tested, but remains defiant and proud.

a. Courage is a key factor in the act of self-sacrifice. The example in the film is extreme, but what acts of courage do you recognize in the health service or by your colleagues today?

The Lamp Still Burns (1947; Rosamund John, Stewart Granger, Godfrey Teale, Sophie Stewart, Cathleen Nesbitt): This is a remarkable film about a successful architect (John) who decides to become a nurse. The film details her experiences as she learns how hard the profession can be. As well, she falls in love with one of her patients (Granger) and must choose between her career and potential marriage. She chooses her career. While an old film, it has some stark lessons and parallels for today's professional nursing issues.

1 (0:17:40–0:35:00) The whole film is a celebration of self-sacrifice and from the moment nurse Hilary Clarke enters nurse training she is called upon to give of herself to her "calling."

   a. How is this different from how nurses are trained/educated today?

   b. Is nursing still seen as a "calling" or has the road to professionalism driven the vocational roots of nursing away?

   c. The film romanticises the nursing road that nurse Hilary has taken. Has this been lost and what might be the costs and advantages of the changes to nurse education in recent years?

2 (0:44:30–0:47:30) During an air raid nurses are asked to volunteer to remain on the ward with the sickest patients while others are escorted to the air raid shelter. One nurse (Hilary) is assigned to look after a patient recovering from surgery.

   a. It is the nurses who are asked to stay behind and care for the patients who cannot be moved. How would you feel if you were asked to place yourself in harm's way for your patient's care? Do you already do this? If so, in what way are nurses currently placed at risk?

3 (1:10:50–1:25:00) Nurse Hilary Clarke and Nurse Christine discuss Christine's impending marriage and the impact it will have on her career. Christine is offered the post of "sister," but when Hilary congratulates her, the Matron is upset at their joyful celebration. Hilary has an outburst about the hospital rules and is sacked. Later she confronts the Board of Governors and argues for her post by outlining her dedication to her profession, as she was prepared to give up "everything she valued most."

   a. Nurses today are not called upon to "give up everything" they value most in order to become a nurse. But what do nurses have to sacrifice in order to follow their career paths, study and work in today's health service?

   b. After watching these scenes, if you had the authority, would you have given Hilary her job back? If you were Hilary, would you have even wanted it back, given the attitude of the Matron and the hospital board?

   c. Could the issues Hilary raised before the Board be an issue in today's health service, or are these issues also a thing of the past? If so, what are the current issues facing nursing?

The Caring Professional

There are a number of films that show nurses as the caring professional, some controversially so, such as *The World according to Garp* (1982), *Talk to Her* (2002), and *14 Hours* (2005). However, this type of film is appearing more frequently, as Stanley's[1] study showed, with the emergence of films showing nurses as the "strong woman" and in roles that celebrated the nurses' more autonomous and professional role in health care. These include films such as *Whose Life Is It Anyway?* (1981), *Intimate Strangers* (1986), and *Angels in America* (2004).

The following films offer a glimpse into this aspect of the nurse's role in feature films.

Wit (2001; Emma Thompson, Christopher Lloyd, Eileen Atkins, Audra McDonald, Jonathan M. Woodward): This film offers an insight into the patient's perspective of dealing with being diagnosed and treated for ovarian cancer. The patient (Vivian) (played brilliantly by Thompson) deals, often alone, with the assault of the illness, finding support only in the professional and compassionate attention of her nurse Susan (McDonald). This is a realistic film, but rich with amusing soliloquies and glimpses into the patient's perspective of being dealt with by the health system and health professionals.

1 (1:00:30–1:09:00) Vivian occludes her intravenous line so that the alarm sounds and the nurse will come. She does this because she is feeling scared. While the nurse is there, they share a popsicle and the nurse (Susan) comforts Vivian as they talk about what will happen toward "the end."

   a. Have you ever been the health professional a patient has turned to for comfort and advice? What do you think they want from you really? How did you feel about being placed in this position?

   b. Have you ever had to have a similar conversation with a patient? To what extent has your training prepared you for this type of conversation? Where do you gain the insight and experiences to know how to deal with this type of situation?

2 (1:29:30–1:34:00). Vivian dies and the doctor calls a code blue, even though she is "no code." The nurse (Susan) comes in ahead of the crash team and tries to cancel the code, but they arrive and continue to try to resuscitate Vivian. The result is basically an assault on the patient with only the nurse trying to care for the patient and keep to her wishes.

   a. All of the health professionals are trying to do their "job" but, without recourse to the patient's wishes, how professional do they appear?

   b. How could this situation have been avoided?

   c. Which is more important, trying to save a patient's life or caring for the patient the way they want to be cared for?

The English Patient (see earlier description)

1 (2:21:00–2:25:00) The "English patient" is nearing death, Kip leaves and as Hana prepares some analgesia, the patient pushes all the vials to her and pleads to be euthanized. Hana sobs, but agrees, injects him, and then reads to him as he drifts off to "sleep."

   a. After caring for this patient alone in the monastery is Hana's act of euthanasia another selfless act?

   b. This clip raises the issue of role boundary violations again. Given their relationship, her sacrifice, and the circumstances, was Hana right to agree to the patient's wishes? Issues of legality aside, is this ever right?

c. Hana found time to care for herself while also caring for the "English patient." How difficult or easy is this in the modern health service and how important is self-care for health professionals to foster.

The Sex Object: Sexuality and Care

There are a plethora of feature films that portray nurses as sex objects or in sexually explicit ways, with Kalishch *et al.*[5] suggesting that as many as 73% of nurse roles in feature films up to 1980 could be characterised as sexually provocative or flirtatious. In Stanley's[1] research, 26.4% of the films reviewed feature nurses in overtly sexual roles. These types of films include *Night Nurse* (1931), *Operation Petticoat* (1959), *The Student Nurses* (1970), *The Hot Box* (1971), *Rosie Dixon: Night Nurse* (1978), *Young Nurses in Love* (1986), and *Yes Nurse! No Nurse!* (2002). Only a few examples have been outlined here.

Carry on Nurse (1959; Kenneth Connor, Shirley Eaton, Hattie Jacques, Terence Longdon, Bill Owen, Leslie Phillips, Joan Sims): Set in Haven Hospital, a ward of male patients causes all sorts of headaches for the medical and nursing staff. Love blossoms between one of the patients (Longdon) and nurse Denton (Eaton); chaos reigns as a result of a bumbling student nurse and when the patients take their treatment into their own hands. Sexual innuendo permeates the film and even a female doctor is seen in a sexually provocatively way.

1 (0:08:05–0:01:04) A staff nurse prepares a patient for surgery, and the patient later grabs a nurse and kisses her. She is "rescued" by a colleague who gives the patient sleeping medication.
   a. Is it ever appropriate for a nurse to kiss a patient?
   b. Does the film's depiction of nurses as sexually available and the reality of practice ever cross? Have you ever had any experience of a patient making sexually overt suggestions or gestures?
   c. If so how do you deal with them? Is sexual harassment an issue because of the way male patients view nurses, and does the media image of nurses have any impact on this?

2 (0:33:54–0:35:15) A new patient is admitted and the nurse looks longingly at the doctor as he discusses his plan of care. Another patient looks on jealously as the nurse reveres the doctor. The nurse follows the doctor who looks on another nurse flirtatiously. Then a patient gets sexually excited during a back rub.
   a. These scenes suggest that there is an almost natural romantic connection between medical staff and nurses. Do you agree?
   b. As professional colleagues is it reasonable or appropriate that doctors and nurses should become romantically involved. What might be the advantages and disadvantages of these liaisons?

    c. Can work and social activities be divided? Can our professional roles be left behind at work to allow post work social/sexual liaisons to flourish?

M*A*S*H (Donald Sutherland, Elliot Gould, Tom Skerritt, Sally Kellerman, Robert Duvall): M.A.S.H stands for Mobile Army Surgical Hospital. This comedy recounts the experiences of two young army surgeons (Skerritt and Sutherland) sent to a M.A.S.H unit during the Korean War. Their arrival coincides with the arrival of a new head nurse (Kellerman) and the film details a series of antics and events that explore how they deal with the horrors of working so close to the front.

1 (0:07:15–0:09:50) Forest and Hawkeye arrive at their M.A.S.H unit and immediately flirt and regard the nurses as sexual objects, setting the tone and an example for their behavior toward the female nurses for the rest of the film.

    a. *M*A*S*H* was made in the 1970s and reflects the moral standards of the day, but are these attitudes still evident in the current health service?

    b. Is there anything that excuses their behavior toward the female nurses? Because they are at war, because they are away from home, because they are nurses? Do these things matter?

2 (0:37:44–0:44:15) The staff celebrate while the commanding officer is away. Trapper demands sex from Margaret, but Burns and Margaret have sex and the camp listen in on their passionate encounter over the camp radio.

    a. Margaret, even with her senior rank and vast experience is predominantly viewed as a potential sexual conquest. She is batted, embarrassed, and undermined. What do these scenes say about nursing as a profession and how the medical and army professions view nursing?

    b. Are these views the same today? If they have moved on, why is this?

3 (1:09:00–1:14:20) The surgeons are talking about the hair color preferences they have in females and they bet to find out the color of Margaret's hair. The surgeons set up the shower tent and gather about like it's a theatrical event, to so that Margaret is revealed naked. Margaret then protests to their commander and hysterically threatens to resign her commission.

    a. Margaret is shown to respond hysterically to the embarrassment of her torment but her concerns and issues are ignored. Does this mean women remain powerless and are viewed as hysterical in response to a crisis?

    b. What can women do when faced with intransient, male dominated responses to their appeals to be heard and respected?

    c. Do women, and nurses in particular, face the same issues today or do the military and health service have processes in place to deal with people equally? Has the power shifted?

Carry on Matron (Sid James, Kenneth Williams, Charles Hawtrey, Joan Sims, Hattie Jacques, Bernard Bresslaw, Kenneth Connor, Barbara Windsor): In this 1972 comedy a gang of thieves plots to steal a consignment of contraceptive pills from a maternity hospital. To do so one of them dresses as a nurse, but the Matron (Hattie Jacques), who is being "wooed" by the obstetric consultant (Kenneth Williams), and a flirty nurse (Barbara Windsor) foil the gang's attempt to pull off the perfect crime.

1   (0:20:50–0:23:50) A criminal dressed as nurse tries to infiltrate the hospital and is pestered by randy doctor Prod.

  a. Is the idea that nurses are sexually pursued by doctors or vice versa still an issue in the modern health-care work place? If so, how is it manifest?

2   (0:40:30–0:43:30) The criminal dressed as a nurse goes to Dr. Prod's office to get the plans of the hospital. Here, Dr. Prod has a collection of photos of his "conquests" on his wall and he attempts to seduce the criminal dressed as a nurse.

  a. Throughout the film nurses are presented as sexually available. Here Dr. Prod has the evidence on his wall. There is something of the "doctor/nurse game" played by both parties as they grapple for power. Is flirting and sexual banter still used as currency in the battle for power between nurses and doctors in hospitals?

  b. Should this be the case? Or is this type of "game" become so entrenched in the health service culture that "sexy" nurse and "cheeky" doctor remains the way nurses and doctors relate.

The Dark Nurse

Sadly there are also a significant number of feature films that show the darker side of nurses' behavior or place nurses in roles that provoke fear or distress. These films, such as *Catch-22* (1970), *Talk to Her* (2002), and *Killer Nurse* (2008) show nurses in a less than caring role.

One Flew Over the Cuckoo's Nest (1975; Jack Nicholson, Louise Fletcher, William Redfield, Michael Berryman, Peter Brocco: The film depicts the story of McMurphy (Nicholson) who, in order to avoid time in jail, has convinced a psychiatrist that he is mentally unstable and is transferred to a secure psychiatric unit. There he plays cards, basketball, and generally fires up his fellow "patients." However, the aloof and apparently uncompassionate nurse Ratched (Fletcher) maintains a firm and authoritarian domain over the unit and the men's lives with disturbing consequences for them all.

1   (0:37:50–0:46:45) Nurse Ratched runs a number of therapy sessions throughout the film. In this one she presses one of the patients about his problems and is challenged on a previous issue to allow the men to watch a baseball game. The men vote to watch the game on TV and although they eventually get the required votes she is too inflexible to allow them to watch the game. McMurphy defies her by calling an imagined game and getting his fellow patients excited, much to nurse Ratched's annoyance.

    a. Mental health nursing has struggled for years to be seen as acceptable and compassionate in its dealing with mentally ill patients. There are some remarkable mental health nurses, but the legacy of the Victorian asylum hangs over the specialty. Treatment methods have improved and attitudes toward people with mental health problems have moved forward. What impact do films about people with mental health issues have on our perception of mental illness and care processes for those who suffer?

    b. How can health professionals overcome any lingering negative perceptions of mental health care?

    c. Locate another film about nursing and mental health care (there are a few others available). How do these portray mental health issues and care services?

2 (1:07:50–1:16:20). In another therapy session nurse Ratched loses control over the patients and they demand their rights, such as access to cigarettes. Nurse Ratched struggles to keep the group focused but the group ends up in chaos and a fight ensues. Nurse Ratched remains stony faced and unsympathetic throughout.

    a. The film can be seen as a battle between McMurphy and Nurse Ratched for the loyalty and attention of the patients and in many ways McMurphy can be seen to do more to empower and liberate them from their illness and circumstances. Were Nurse Ratched's dealings with the patients in any way beneficial? What else could she have done to care for or treat these patients?

Misery (1990; Kathy Bates, James Caan, Richard Farnsworth, Frances Sternhagen, Lauren Bacall): When novelist Paul Sheldon (Caan) crashes his car on a snowy road he is discovered by his number-one fan Annie Wilkes (Bates), an ex-nurse. Badly injured, Annie imprisons him, instead of helping him to medical aid, and while at first she is caring, she soon realizes that her favorite character from his books (Misery Chastaine) is to be killed off. Annie then drugs Paul and after finding he has tried to escape ties him up and breaks his ankles. She plans to kill Paul after he writes another "Misery" novel but Paul fights back.

1 (1:12:25–1:19:50) Paul is out of his room looking for ways to escape and he finds Annie's scrap book. In it he sees clippings of Annie's nursing career highlights and hints about her previously unstable and murderous past behavior. He steels a knife and hopes to ambush Annie. Instead she drugs him and ties him to the bed, trapping him. She goes on to break his ankles with a sledgehammer.

    a. Nurses are often placed in positions of responsibility. Does behavior from a few nurses that challenges a commonly held perception that nurses can be trusted, damage nursing and the image of nursing.

    b. Are nurses ever cruel? Have you ever witnessed nurse colleagues being physically, emotionally, or mentally cruel? If so, what have you done about it? What can you do about it?

🎥*Where the Money Is* (2000; Paul Newman, Linda Fiorentino, Dermot Mulroney, Susan Barnes): Henry Manning (Paul Newman), a safecracker, fakes a stroke in order to be transferred from prison to an elderly care home. Once in the home, Carol (Linda Fiorentino), a nurse, cares for Henry but she is immediately suspicious of him. She attempts to arouse him from his stupor and, once she does so, she recruits him for a series of robberies.

1 (0:08:00–0:18:56) A nurse has sex with her husband while at work in front of a patient she thinks has had a stroke. She begins to suspect the patient is pretending to be ill and sets about testing his symptoms by dropping instruments, lap dancing for him, and ultimately she throws him in a canal. Another nurse takes advantage of him by stealing his possessions.

   a. This "dark nurse" torments and assaults her patient. While far-fetched (although not in the context of this film), elder abuse and cruelty by nurses is (sadly) not uncommon. Are there ever circumstances when tormenting, teasing or abusing patients is acceptable?

   b. In these scenes a nurse steals from a patient. Is this common? Is this ever acceptable? Have you ever encountered nurses stealing and what have you done about it?

References

1 Stanley DJ. Celluloid angels: a research study of nurses in feature films 1900–2007. *J Adv Nurs*. 2008; **64**(1): 84–95.

2 Meadus RJ, Twomey JC. Men in nursing: making the right choice. *Can Nurse*. 2007; **103**(2): 13–26.

3 Hereford M. *Exploring the Reel Image of Nursing: how movies, television and stereotypes portray the nursing profession* [dissertation]. Moscow; University of Idaho; 2005.

4 Ward C, Styles I, Bosco A. Perceived status of nurses compared to other health care professionals. *Contemp Nurse*. 2003; **15**(1–2): 20–8.

5 Kalisch BJ, Kalisch PA, McHugh ML. The nurse as a sex object in motion pictures, 1930–1980. *Res Nurs Health*. 1982; **5**(3): 147–54.

6 Chur-Hansen A. Preferences for female and male nurses: the role of age, gender and previous experience: year 2000 compared with 1984. *J Adv Nurs*. 2002; **37**(2): 192–8.

7 Evans J. Men in nursing: issues of gender segregation and hidden advantage. *J Adv Nurs*. 1997; **26**(2): 226–31.

8 Fisher MJ. 'Being a chameleon': labour processes of male nurses performing bodywork. *J Adv Nurs*. 2009; **65**(12): 2668–77.

9 Genua J. The vision of male nurses: role, barriers and stereotypes. *InterAction*. 2005; **23**(4): 4–7.

10 Gilloran A. Gender differences in care delivery and supervisory relationship: the case of psychogeriatric nursing. *J Adv Nurs*. 1995; **21**(4): 652–8.

11 Harding T. The construction of men who are nurses as gay. *J Adv Nurs*. 2007; **60**(6): 636–44.

12 Inoue M, Chapman R, Wynaden D. Male nurses' experiences of providing intimate care for women. *J Adv Nurs*. 2006; **55**(5): 559–67.

Additional Reading
· ·

- Keogh B, Gleeson M. Caring for female patients: the experiences of male nurses. *Br J Nurs.* 2006; **15**(21): 1172–5.

23

Let's Analyze Everything: Individual, Couple, and Group Therapy

Matthew Alexander

PSYCHOTHERAPISTS UTILIZE A VARIETY OF APPROACHES IN WORKING with individuals encountering mental, emotional, spiritual, and relational problems. While methodological problems often make it difficult to "prove" the benefits of psychotherapy, two types of individual therapy, cognitive-behavioral and interpersonal, consistently show good outcomes.[1,2]

Couple therapy is considered by many to be one of the most challenging forms of psychotherapy. Success rates vary widely, from about 20% to 75% stable improvement after two to five years.[3–5] Emotionally focused couple therapy appears to be linked with the best outcomes.[6] Movies very frequently deal with relationships and so are optimal vehicles for teaching couple therapists.[7] (*See* Chapter 4, Two to Tango: Couples in the Cinema, for additional movie clips to use in the education of couple therapists.)

Child and adolescent therapy, group therapy, and ethical dilemmas are other topics covered in this chapter. Ethical issues such as boundary crossing[8] and inappropriate self-disclosure[9] are paramount to address with psychotherapists and other health-care professionals in training. Movies provide fertile ground for such discussions, in part because boundary violations make for good drama, if not good therapy.[10]

Several of the movies used in this chapter are older. These have been included because they illustrate classic examples of good (and not so good) psychotherapy.

Individual Therapy

Historical Perspectives

It has been estimated that there have been over 500 movies made that portray some aspect of psychotherapy since the first "psychiatric" film, *Dr. Dippy's Sanitarium* (1906). Sadly, most movies portray psychotherapists and psychiatrists in a negative light, so much so that an American Psychological Association committee was formed in 1998, Media Watch, to establish an ongoing rating system to rank the different ways mental health professionals are portrayed in film.[11]

Gabbard and Gabbard[12] identified three common stereotypes in pre-1950 films; namely, the "Alienist" (*His Girl Friday*, 1940), a forensic psychiatrist who is an expert on the criminal mind; the "Quack" (Fred Astaire as the dancing psychiatrist in *Carefree* [1938]); and the "Oracle," an intelligent, mystical psychotherapist (*Blind Alley*, 1939).

Psychiatrist Irving Schneider[13] has identified three additional categories of therapist stereotypes portrayed on screen, namely:

- "Dr. Dippy," who is as psychologically unstable as his or her patients (i.e. Mel Brooks in *High Anxiety* [1977]).
- "Dr. Evil,'" who is controlled by destructive or even homicidal tendencies (Anthony Hopkins's portrayal of Hannibal Lecter in *The Silence of the Lambs* [1991]).
- "Dr. Wonderful," who is ever present, ever knowing, and often able to cure patients with relative ease (the Judd Hirsch character in *Ordinary People* [1980]).

Psychologist Harriet T. Schultz[14] has suggested even more categories; namely:

- "Dr Rigid," who stifles joy, nonconformity, and free expression (the psychologist in *Miracle on 34th Street* (1994) who attempts to commit Santa Claus to an insane asylum).
- "Dr. Line Crosser," who crosses ethical boundaries and becomes sexually involved with a patient (Barbara Streisand as Dr. Lowenstein in *Prince of Tides*; Dr. Elizabeth "Libbie" Bowen, as played by Lena Olin, who treats Mr. Jones [Richard Gere] in *Mr. Jones* [1993]) or who becomes physically abusive with a patient and/or reveals excessive personal information to them (Robin Williams as Dr. Sean Maguire in *Good Will Hunting* [1997]).

Of all these categories, it is probably the last one, "Dr. Line Crosser," that is the most dangerous in promoting negative stereotypes in the public eye and the most vexing to mental health professionals.

Despite their penchant for misleading stereotypes, all such films can potentially be useful in cinemeducation when used with care and consideration. For example, clips that show therapists too readily accessible to patients can be used to discuss self-care, and clips that show easy solutions to complex client problems can be used to discuss the realistic pace of change in psychotherapy.

Historically speaking, the vast majority of films show Caucasian psycho-therapists with the exception of (at least) two portrayals of African-American psychologists (Danny Glover in *Dead Man Out* [1989]; Morgan Freeman in *Kiss the Girls* [1997]), at least five portrayals of African-American psychiatrists (i.e. *Benny and Joon* [1993], *Death Becomes Her* [1992], *Mad Love* [1995], *Antwone Fisher* [2002], and *She's So Lovely* [1997]) and at least one Latina psychiatrist (*Mr. Jones*). For a historical (and deservedly critical) review of the portrayal of female psychotherapists in film, the reader can reference an excellent article by Dr. Laurel Samuels.[15]

I have chosen two films to include in this first subsection on historical per-spectives. Both provide wonderful snapshots of psychotherapy as practiced in America in the 1970s and 1980s. More importantly, however, they illustrate some timeless issues that pertain to the practice of psychotherapy.

An Unmarried Woman (1978; Jill Clayburgh, Alan Bates): This movie tells the story of Erica (Clayburgh) a woman in the midst of adjusting to single life during a painful separation.

1 (Ch 14; 49:01–52:47) Erica has her initial visit with a therapist. The therapist is masterful at listening, reflecting, and comforting her client.
   a. How does this therapist establish rapport with the patient?
   b. How does the therapist show the patient that she is truly being listened to?
   c. How does the therapist balance listening with thoughtful advice?
   d. How does the therapist express hope and confidence? Is this realistic?
   e. What thoughts do you have about the physical setup in this office? Does this accurately reflect current standards? It appears that the office is in the therapist's home. What are the advantages and disadvantages of seeing clients in one's home?

Ordinary People (1980; Donald Sutherland, Mary Tyler Moore): This award-winning movie tells the story of Beth (Mary Tyler Moore), her husband Calvin (Donald Sutherland), and their son Conrad (Timothy Hutton) coping with the loss of Conrad's brother in a boating accident. While this movie has been covered extensively in the literature as a tool to teach family dynamics and psychotherapy, I decided to include it in this chapter nonetheless, both for its historical perspective and the fact that it offers one of the best, if not exaggerated, cinematic examples of the healing power of the psychotherapeutic alliance ever portrayed. As previously elucidated in this chapter, even movies that distort the basic realities of psychotherapy can be enormously useful in teaching student therapists.

1 (Ch 3, 0:15:12–0:20:23) In this scene, Calvin (Hutton) has his first meeting with a therapist Dr. Berger (Judd Hirsch) after being released from the hos-pital following a suicide attempt. As with the clip from *An Unmarried Woman*, this scene provides a "time capsule" about psychotherapy as practiced in an earlier time as well as providing insights into the therapeutic process.

  a. What aspects of this clip reveal "physical" characteristics (i.e. office set-up) of psychotherapy that are currently "outdated" (i.e. smoking, an old reel-to-reel tape player, sitting with a desk between you and the client)? What aspects of the clip are still relevant in this regard?

  b. How accurately does this scene illustrate the ambivalence and anxiety some clients feel upon first entering therapy? How well (or poorly) does Dr. Berger (Hirsch) address these and make his client feel comfortable?

  c. Are there significant differences in how therapists conduct therapy with adolescents versus adults? If so, what are these?

  d. Are therapists more likely to have looser boundaries (i.e. conducting therapy on a basketball court) with teens than with adults?

2 (Ch 8, 1:38:50–1:45:40) In this pivotal scene, Calvin calls Dr. Berger who meets him late at night for an emergency session in which Calvin experiences a dramatic emotional breakthrough.

  a. Is Dr. Berger an example of a "Dr. Wonderful" stereotype?

  b. Would most therapists meet with a client in distress in the middle of the night?

  c. How common is the type of therapeutic breakthrough we see depicted in this scene? Does this scene set up false expectations for therapists and their clients?

  d. Is it appropriate for a therapist to be a "friend"?

  e. When is it appropriate to hug a client?

  f. How does Dr. Berger show empathy? How is his advice to Conrad useful in a broader way to clients suffering from immense guilt over a personal tragedy?

Child Psychotherapy

The Sixth Sense (1999; Bruce Willis, Haley Joel Osment): This haunting movie tells the story of a troubled 8-year-old boy, Cole Sean (Osment) who is isolated and depressed because of his ability to talk to the dead. An equally troubled psychologist, Dr. Malcolm Crowe (Willis), is treating the boy.

1 (Ch 3, 0:12:24–0:15:09) In this scene, Dr. Crowe (Willis) follows the boy into a church and they have a brief interaction/session.

  a. This session takes place in a church. Is it common for child and adolescent psychotherapy to be more flexible than adult psychotherapy in terms of setting? If so, how might this flexibility with younger clients be helpful in establishing trust and therapeutic rapport?

  b. Dr. Crowe uses the boy's toy soldiers to establish communication? In what ways is indirect interviewing (i.e. having a child communicate his or her feelings indirectly through puppets, drawings, or toy soldiers) often a better way to promote disclosure in children than more standard interviewing techniques?

2   Ch 7, 0:32:20–0:32:54) In this brief scene, Dr. Crowe engages the boy in discussing his therapeutic goals.

   a. Cole (Osment) appears to be playing hide and seek with Crowe. How is play therapy useful in child psychotherapy?

   b. Discuss the important role of therapeutic goal setting with children or adults.

Boundaries

Antwone Fisher (2002; Denzel Washington, Derek Luke): This movie is based on the true story of Antwone Fisher, who also wrote the screenplay for the movie. Fisher is an African-American sailor in the Navy required to see a Navy psychiatrist, Dr. Jerome Davenport (Washington), after an angry altercation with another sailor. The movie is rife with boundary crossings, arguably a therapeutic choice by the treating psychiatrist who hopes to "re-parent" his client.

1   (Ch 3, 0:05:34–0:08:14) In this scene, Fisher has his first session with Davenport. It is clear that Fisher is an unwilling client.

   a. Fisher notices a photo of Davenport's wife that is present in the office. What are the risks of having personal photographs in one's professional office?

   b. Fisher has been forced to see Davenport. What are the challenges in developing rapport with clients mandated to see a therapist? What models and approaches are most useful in working with clients who have been mandated to seek counseling (i.e. motivational interviewing)?

   c. At what "stage of change" is Fisher? What is the role of the therapist in working with clients at this particular stage of change?

   d. Does Davenport succeed in developing rapport with his reluctant client? What would you have done in his situation?

   e. Clients often assume that psychiatrists do "talking therapy" when, in reality, this is often not the case. Do you know any psychiatrists who practice psychotherapy in your community? Why is it important to help clients distinguish between the role of a medication prescribing psychiatrist and that of a therapy providing psychologist?

2   (Ch 12, 0:36:27–0:39:33) In this scene, Fisher discusses his anxiety about an upcoming romantic date. Davenport role-plays the situation with him, provides reassurance and then gives him his personal phone number, encouraging Fisher to call "anytime, day or night" in the event of any problems.

   a. Are there instances where it is appropriate to give out your home or cell phone number to a client? Is this always a boundary violation? What types of wrong messages might be invoked by providing your home or cell phone number?

   b. How useful is Davenport's use of role-play with Fisher? Have you tried role-playing with your clients? When is role-playing indicated?

    c. Do you believe that Davenport is guilty of false reassurance when he tells Fisher, in effect, that everything is sure to go well on his date? Have you ever provided false reassurance to a client? If so, why have you done so?

3 (Ch 14, 0:44:34–0:47:30). In this scene, Fisher shows up unexpectedly at Davenport's home.
    a. How well do you believe Davenport handles Fisher's surprise visit? How would you have handled such an occurrence?

4 (Ch 17, 1:00:56–1:04:44) Davenport sees Fisher for a therapy session in his home. The scene ends with Davenport informing Fisher that his wife has invited him to Thanksgiving dinner.
    a. What are the pros and cons of seeing clients for psychotherapy in one's home?
    b. What violations of confidentiality and the therapeutic bond occur in this scene in which Davenport's wife can overhear the session?
    c. How did this scene make you feel? What are the drawbacks in having a desk between you and a client?
    d. Are there ever cases where inviting a client into one's home for a holiday dinner would be considered part of the therapy? What are the dangers involved in such a boundary crossing?

It's Complicated (2009; Meryl Streep, Alec Baldwin): This romantic comedy tells the story of Jane (Streep) and her ex-husband Jake (Baldwin) who have an "affair" despite the fact that Jake has remarried a younger wife, Agness (Lake Bell).

1 (Ch 10, 0:54:39–0:57:35) In this scene, Jane shows up unexpectedly at her therapist's office. He has only 20 minutes before his first session but agrees to fit her in. She is desperate for him to tell her what to do about her affair with her ex-husband and he, somewhat reluctantly, offers her advice.
    a. What are the pros and cons of meeting a client's urgent request for an unexpected consultation, either by phone or in person?
    b. How would you have handled this situation?
    c. What is it like for you, as a therapist, when clients ask you to tell them what to do in terms of a major life choice?
    d. What do you make of the therapist's advice? Would you have given similar advice or held your counsel?
    e. What are the ramifications of giving advice under "duress"?
    f. What are some effective ways that the therapist might have set better boundaries with this patient?

The Prince of Tides (1991; Barbara Streisand, Nick Nolte): This movie, based on the Pat Conroy novel of the same name, tells the story of Tom Wingo (Nick Nolte), his dysfunctional family and his romantic relationship with his sister's psychiatrist, Dr. Susan Lowenstein. Prior to this scene, Wingo has met with Lowenstein in her office to discuss his sister.

1 (Ch 11, 0:40:44–0:43:33; 0:43:33–0:46:19) In the first of these two scenes, Wingo (Nolte) and Dr. Lowenstein (Streisand) see each other at a party. In the second scene, Wingo accompanies Lowenstein home from the party and they begin to develop a romantic attachment.
    a. What is the appropriate protocol if health-care providers bump into clients in public?
    b. What are the ethical implications of Dr. Lowenstein developing a romantic relationship with Tom? In terms of ethical standards, does it matter that Lowenstein is the psychiatrist of Wingo's sister and not his own psychiatrist? How do you think that Wingo's sister, Savannah, would react if she knew that her psychiatrist was involved with her brother?
    c. What are the current guidelines for social contact with current or ex-clients?
    d. How did you feel as you watched the second scene? Do you believe that romantic involvement between clients and their health-care provider (as depicted in this movie) is a Hollywood exaggeration or a true problem? What percentage of psychiatrists and psychologists become romantically involved with their clients? What types of clients are most likely to evoke such inappropriate liaisons?

Women in Trouble (2009; Caitlin Keats, Sarah Clarke): This movie tells the story of six women whose lives become intertwined over the course of a day.
1 (Ch 3, 0:11:33–0:15:42) In this scene, psychiatrist Maxine (Clarke) is having a session with Charlotte (Isabella Gutierrez), the daughter of one of her adult clients, Addy (Keats). Charlotte informs Maxine that her mother is having an adulterous relationship with Maxine's husband, Travis (Simon Baker).
    a. Charlotte refers to her psychiatrist by her first name. Is this appropriate?
    b. How effectively does Maxine respond to Charlotte's beliefs about ghosts and hypnosis? What are optimal ways to respond to clients' beliefs about paranormal experiences?
    c. Maxine begins a therapeutic relationship with Charlotte after already having an established psychotherapeutic relationship with her mother. What are the potential problems in "adding" members of a family to one's client roster if a therapeutic relationship has already been established with another individual in that family?
    d. Although Charlotte has found out about Addy's therapy sessions by reading her mother's diary, Maxine still expresses alarm that Addy might have shared details of their sessions with Charlotte. How can a therapist best encourage clients to set boundaries with intimate partners about sharing the details of their psychotherapy sessions?

Transference
• • • • • • • • • • • • • • • • •

Bloom (2005; Mara Monserrat, Jessi Perez): This film weaves together the interlocking stories of Letty (Perez), the youngest daughter of an upwardly mobile Latino family in Chicago who has two children (one with cerebral palsy) and a drug dealing boyfriend, and Dr. Sharon Greene (Monserrat), her court appointed therapist, who is dealing with problems of her own (i.e. infertility and a terminally ill mother).

1   (Ch 12, 1:27:00–1:31:12) Dr. Greene has returned from a leave of absence necessitated by the death of her mother and a recent miscarriage. Despite the fact that Letty had been informed of this leave of absence, she still expresses anger at Dr. Greene for not being there when she needed her.
   a. How realistic is this scene in terms of transference issues related to perceived abandonment?
   b. Have you ever had a client be angry at you for taking a medical leave or vacation? What is the best way to handle such feelings?
   c. Discuss the countertransference issues revealed here. Is it appropriate for Dr. Greene to "scold" her client for not listening to her mother more often?
   d. Given that Dr. Greene recently had a miscarriage, might some of her negative countertransference be related to the perception that Letty is an uncaring mother? When do therapists need their own therapy to help them separate their personal issues from their professional work?
2   (Ch 13, 1:34:45–1:35:06) A year after treatment, Dr. Greene enters her pediatrician's office with her newborn baby only to encounter Letty, employed there as part of the front office staff. Both seemed pleased to see each other.
   a. What is it like for clients to bump into their therapists, by chance, in public? What is it like for therapists to run into clients in public?
   b. What is the proper protocol for running into clients outside the office? What HIPPA issues are involved in such situations?

Countertransference
• •

Analyze This (1999; Robert De Niro, Richard Dreyfuss): This "older" but timeless film tells the story of Paul Vitti (De Niro), a crime racketeer with panic disorder, and his unwilling therapist, Ben Sobel (Crystal).

1   (Ch 3, 0:05:31–0:07:32) In this scene, Dr. Sobel (Crystal) is listening to a client "whine" about her primary love relationship. Sobel fantasizes about getting angry at her for being so neurotic and appears to act out his feelings.
   a. Have you ever felt this type of irritation toward a client? Would you classify Sobel's internal dialogue (and acting out fantasy) as an example of sadomasochistic countertransference? If so, how can an awareness of countertransferences such as this be useful in the therapeutic process?

   b. What are some other types of negative countertransference (i.e. erotic, bored)?

   c. How does Sobel manage to reorient himself to the room after his internal dialogue and adopt a therapeutic tone?

   d. What are productive ways of coping with negative countertransference?

   e. What are some risk factors for burnout in therapists?

Ira and Abby (2006): Ira (Messina) and Abby (Westfeldt) marry a week after meeting. The film tells the story of their relationship as they navigate a tortuous journey that involves too many therapists, neurotic parents, and multiple, complicating factors.

1 (Ch 12, 1:11:32–1:12:26) In this scene, we see two analysts, married to one another, both becoming very distracted while listening to their patients. In fact, the husband and wife are both tense because of the wife's infidelity, a situation that impairs their ability to focus on their clients who are facing similar situations.

   a. How can therapists most effectively deal with countertransference issues triggered by client stories that mirror their own life situations?

   b. When, if ever, is it appropriate to share one's own story with clients who are in similar life situations?

   c. What is the ethical standard for therapists if a personal crisis interferes with their capacity to be effective caregivers?

Medication Versus Therapy

Garden State (2004): This film tells the story of Andrew Largeman (Zach Braff) who returns to his New Jersey home from Los Angeles after the death of his mother. Largeman has struggled with depression for most of his life.

1 (Ch 8, 0:31:06–0:34:20) Andrew sees a neurologist, Dr. Cohen (Ron Liebman), for his headaches. Dr. Cohen uncovers the fact that Andrew's psychiatrist father has been prescribing him psychotropic medicines for years. Largeman has been on a host of mood disorder medications since he was a child (Lithium, Paxil, Zoloft, Celexa, and Depakote). Because of the sudden nature of his trip home, Largeman has left his medications behind in Los Angeles.

   a. Are Largeman's symptoms (i.e. a surge of electricity and lightning in his head) attributable to his abrupt cessation of his psychotropic medications? What is the best way to educate patients about the dangers of "discontinuation syndrome"? What is the best way to wean clients off of medications, when necessary, such as antidepressants?

   b. When are psychotropic medications warranted? When do they help the psychotherapeutic process and when do they hinder it? What do you make of Cohen's assertion that sooner or later Largeman will need therapy?

    c. What impact does Dr. Cohen's self-disclosure about his wife's infidelity have on the doctor-patient relationship? Is such self-disclosure warranted or does it, instead, serve as a distraction?

    d. Is it ever ethical for a psychiatrist to treat members of his or her own family?

    e. Discuss Dr. Cohen's use of humor? Does it help build or hinder rapport?

    f. Is it helpful for clients on psychotropic medications to have a drug holiday? Why or why not?

Termination

Ira and Abby (see earlier description)

1 (Ch 1, 0:00:20–0:03:10) In this opening clip, Ira's psychoanalyst, Dr. Friedman, "fires" him (Messina) after 12 years of analysis.

    a. What is the ethical approach to take with clients who are no longer benefiting from therapy/analysis?

    b. When and how should one bring up termination with patients?

    c. What do you make of Dr. Friedman's obvious discomfort with his client?

    d. Is there research support for psychoanalysis as a change agent?

Antwone Fisher (see earlier description, section on boundaries for movie description)

1 (Ch 21, 1:14:52–1:17:59) In this scene, the treating psychiatrist Davenport (Washington) terminates his sessions with Fisher (Luke) in a very unusual setting, a men's lavatory. Davenport believes that his work with Fisher to date has been successful but that further treatment is useless unless Fisher takes the next step of contacting his family in Ohio to resolve family of origin issues.

    a. What are the clear boundary violations in addressing such a serious issue as termination in a public facility?

    b. In this scene, Davenport's termination of Fisher triggers serious abandonment issues. How should termination be handled to minimize such powerful emotional reactions in clients?

Couple Therapy

Therapeutic Process in Couple Work

Couples Retreat (2009; Vince Vaughn, Kristin Davis): Four couples, who are friends with one another, attend a couple retreat on an island resort. Only one of the couples, however, is there to work on their marriage; the other three don't realize until it is too late that couple therapy was "part of the package."

1 (Ch 8, 0:38:36–0:45:10) Here, we are exposed to four different couple

therapists conducting intakes with the four different couples. Each couple is dressed in a different color suit provided them by the retreat center. Only the couple in the green suits, however, is prepared to work on their marriage. The four couple therapists take different approaches in their intake procedure. In discussing these clips, it might be helpful for students to break down into groups of four, with each group focusing on the therapeutic style of a different couple therapist.

    a. Contrast the four intake styles. Can you attach each therapist to any particular type of couple therapy approach?

    b. Is note taking a distraction in therapy? Please discuss.

    c. When should a therapist introduce the topic of sex during a couple therapy intake? How is this best done?

    d. Can couple therapy sometimes make a couple feel worse about their relationship? Is this outcome a reflection of the therapy or the couple? Is there a useful distinction between clients "feeling better" and "getting better"?

2   (Ch 12; 0:59:50–0:1:02:20) In these clips, we see the same couple therapists who were shown in the previous clips conducting couple therapy during follow-up sessions.

    a. How long should a couple therapist allow a couple to fight in session before intervening? If you were the therapist working with the "orange" couple, how would you have intervened in their fight? What toll does such intense in-session fighting take on couple therapists?

    b. Do female partners have an advantage in couple therapy given that the focus of couple therapy is often on verbal communication, an arena in which women are traditionally stronger? How can a couple therapist "level the playing field" between the genders when it comes to communication (i.e. by validating unappreciated aspects of male communication and intimacy that don't involve language)?

Ira and Abby (see earlier description)

1   (Ch 8, 0:44:24–0:46:30; ch 9, 0:48:33–0:49:14) Ira and Abby consult with Dr. Morris Sapenstein (Jason Alexander) because Ira wants Abby to show more ambition in her life. Dr. Sapenstein appears to take sides with Abby. After the session, the couple argues about who "won" the therapy.

    a. While this scene is more parody than reality, how does the scene speak to the critical importance of neutrality when it comes to couple therapy?

    b. What suggestions can the couple therapist make to help prevent couples from fighting about the session once it is over?

    c. What are some communication techniques that would help this couple talk productively about their personal differences?

Attachment Theory and Couple Therapy
· ·

Sue Johnson, a thought leader in couple therapy and frequent public speaker, showed the following clip at a national conference on psychotherapy. Johnson is the developer of emotionally focused couple therapy[16] a couple therapy approach based on the understanding that attachment issues are at the heart of most, if not all, couple fights.

The Hours (2002; Julianne Moore, Meryl Streep, Nicole Kidman): A movie about three women whose lives are connected in some way with the novel *Mrs. Dalloway* by Virginia Woolf.

1   (Ch 15, 0:01:26–0:01:28) Laura (Moore) is a depressed housewife who plans to kill herself. She leaves her son with a caretaker in order to commit suicide but then changes her mind and returns, hours later, to pick up her son. He is waiting at the window and has an emotional meltdown when he sees her arrive in her car (Sue Johnson would say that he is engaging in "attachment protest"). However, once in the car Laura is able to soothe her son by reassuring him that he is, quite simply, "her guy."

   a. In what ways are adult attachment bonds between committed couples similar to the attachment bonds in childhood between parents and offspring? How would you communicate this understanding to a couple in couple therapy? How might such a perspective help a distressed couple?

   b. Discuss the concept of "attachment protest" and how it relates to this scene.

   c. How does this scene speak to the important issue of emotional regulation, both as it impacts parenting and coupling?

   d. How do underlying attachment issues sabotage a couple's attempt to resolve content issues? How does one help couples identify their attachment issues in couple counseling?

   e. Why is Laura able to soothe her son with the reassurance she offers? How can therapists apply the mother-son dynamic shown here to couples who are attempting to heal after suffering attachment wounds as caused by such issues as infidelity and neglect?

Group Therapy
· · · · · · · · · · · · · · · · · · · ·

Manic (2001; Joseph Gordon-Levitt, Don Cheadle): A movie about Lyle Jensen (Gordon-Levitt) who is admitted to a juvenile psychiatric hospital ward after using a baseball bat to beat another teen. Jensen's mother has committed him against his will. Dr. David Monroe (Cheadle) attempts to get him to open up in group therapy.

1   (Ch 2, 0:6:22–0:9:56) This scene shows Jensen's first day in group therapy. Dr. Monroe (Cheadle) is leading the group therapy.

   a. How accurate a depiction of group therapy is provided in this scene?
   b. How effectively does Monroe deal with "cross talk"?
   c. Discuss the group process as it unfolds in this scene?
   d. When is group therapy warranted? When is it contra-indicated?

Fight Club (1999; Edward Norton; Brad Pitt): Edward Norton plays a nameless narrator alienated from his white-collar job as a traveling salesman. Norton suffers from insomnia and seeks medication for this problem from his doctor. However, the physician refuses to prescribe him medicine and instead encourages him to attend support groups so that he can see others who are in worse shape than he.

1   (Ch 5; 0:06:20–0:11:05) Norton pretends to have testicular cancer so that he can attend a support group for those who actually suffer from the disease. He is encouraged by the group to "let go." We then see him attend other support groups, also under false pretense.

   a. How do support groups differ from more traditional psychotherapy groups?
   b. What is the best way to deal with emotion in a group context? Is in-session physical touch between group members to be encouraged or discouraged?
   c. Can one become "addicted" to support groups?
   d. For what psychological conditions might group therapy be superior in efficacy to individual therapy (and vice versa)?
   e. How would you best encourage an individual client to attend group therapy and/or a support group? What are some common resistances to group work?
   f. In your community, what is the best way to find out about support groups and/or group therapy (i.e. where they meet, how often they meet, whether or not they are still meeting, cost, and so forth)?
   g. Do individuals sometimes attend support groups under false pretenses (i.e. to meet members to date)? How might this be a problem?

References

1 Butler AC, Chapman JE, Forman EM, *et al*. The empirical status of cognitive-behavioral therapy: a review of meta-analyses. *Clin Psychol Rev*. 2006; **26**(1): 17–31.

2 DeMello MF, deJesus MF, Bacaltchuk J, *et al*. A systemic review of research findings on the efficacy of interpersonal therapy for depressive disorders. *Eur Arch Psychiatry Clin Neurosci*. 2005; **255**(2): 75–82.

3 Gurman A, editor. *Clinical Handbook of Couple Therapy*. 4th ed. New York, NY: Guilford Press; 2008.

4 Christensen A, Atkins DC, Baucum B, *et al*. Marital status and satisfaction five years following a randomized clinical trial comparing traditional versus integrative behavioral couple therapy. *J Consult Clin Psychol*. 2010; **78**(2): 225–35.

5 Gottman JM. *Marital Therapy: a research-based approach*. Seattle, WA: Gottman Institute, 2000.

6 Johnson SM, Hunsley J, Greenberg L, *et al*. Emotionally focused couples therapy: status and challenges. *J Clin Psychol*. 1999; **6**: 67–79.

7 Alexander M. The couple's odyssey: Hollywood's take on love relationships *Int Rev Psychiatry*. 2009; **21**(3): 183–8.

8 Zur O. To cross or not to cross: do boundaries in therapy protect or harm? *Psychother Bull*. 2004; **39**(3): 27–32.

9 McDaniel SH, Beckman HB, Morse DS, *et al*. Physician self-disclosure in primary care visits. *Arch Intern Med*. 2007; **167**(12): 1321–6.

10 Gutrell T, Gabbard B. The concept of boundaries in clinical practice. *Am J Psychiatry*. 1993; **155**: 409–14.

11 Sleek S. How are psychologists portrayed on the screen? *APA Monitor*; **29**(11): 1998.

12 Gabbard GO, Gabbard K. *Psychiatry and the Cinema*. 2nd ed. Arlington, VA: American Psychiatric Press; 1999.

13 Schneider I. The theory and practice of movie psychiatry. *Am J Psychiatry*. 1987; **144**(8): 996–1002.

14 Schultz HT. Hollywood's portrayal of psychologist and psychiatrists: gender and professional training differences. In: Cole E, Daniel JH, editors. *Featuring Females: feminist analyses of media*. Washington, DC: American Psychological Association; 2005. pp. 101–12.

15 Samuels L. Female psychotherapists as portrayed in film, fiction and nonfiction. *J Am Acad Psychoanal*. 1985; **13**(3): 367–78.

16 Johnson S. Emotionally focused couple therapy. In: Gurman A, editor. *Clinical Handbook of Couple Therapy*. 4th ed. New York, NY: Guilford Press; 2008. pp. 107–37.

24

Call Me in Some Hydrocodone, Please: Pharmacy

Shay Phillips

PHARMACISTS PLAY A VITAL ROLE IN HEALTH CARE. ALTHOUGH PHAR-macists are most visible preparing prescriptions in community pharmacies, numerous other job opportunities exist. For example, pharmacists work in hospitals, doctors' offices, clinics, colleges/universities, pharmaceutical companies, home infusion centers, and managed care facilities, to name but a few. Regardless of the physical location of a pharmacist, the fundamental responsibility remains to provide a patient the right medicine for the correct disease at the accurate strength and dosing schedule to maximize effectiveness and safety according to the most recent evidence-based literature and/or to manage this intricate process. Despite the importance of pharmacists to real-life multidisciplinary health-care teams, their depiction in cinema is often omitted, abbreviated, or lessened. While an enormous complement of cinema depicting health-care professionals is available, rarely are pharmacists shown in a leading or supporting role. Even more unusual is cinema footage conceptualizing the specialized training of pharmacists or the expertise required to be a competent pharmacist. The comprehensive view of pharmacists in cinema needs to expand to match the multifaceted nature of the profession.

Despite these challenges, many films are useful in teaching topics relevant to pharmacy education. Whether the films perpetuate stereotypes of the pharmacy profession or exploit illogical practices, a lesson can often times be learned. Because of the paucity of pharmacist depictions in movies, the author has elected to include scenes from two popular television series.

Substance-Related Disorders
• •

It's a Wonderful Life (1946; James Stewart, H. B. Warner): A celestial angel is sent to show a kindhearted, yet discouraged businessman, George Bailey (Stewart), how life would have been had he never existed.

1 (Chs 3–4, 0:5:24–0:11:37). In the opening scenes of the movie, a young George Bailey assists an intoxicated pharmacist, Mr. Gower. Because of his overwhelming grief over a telegraph announcing his son's death, Mr. Gower makes an egregious mistake of compounding tablets with poison. George Bailey, recognizing that anguish and intoxication are impairing Mr. Gower's level of functioning, is tasked with how to respectfully bring the medication error to Mr. Gower's attention.

   a. According to DSM-IV-TR criteria, how would you diagnose Mr. Gower?
   b. What characteristics of alcohol dependence does Mr. Gower demonstrate? What behavioral complications of alcohol abuse does Mr. Gower exhibit?
   c. What are the rates of drug abuse and addiction among pharmacists? Are these more or less than those seen in other health-care professions? In what ways are pharmacists particularly vulnerable to becoming addicted or dependent on medications?
   d. What is the pharmacologic treatment of alcohol and drug abuse dependence?
   e. What is your responsibility as a health-care professional if you know that a colleague is having drug or alcohol problems that are interfering with his or her ability to work without endangering patients? What programs are available to treat pharmacists and other health-care professionals with substance abuse issues?
   f. How do you think loved ones of substance abusers feel? Why do you think George Bailey left the pharmacy with the poison-filled tablets instead of informing Mr. Gower immediately of his mistake? What would have been a different way of bringing this error to Mr. Gower's attention?
   g. As a profession, how well do pharmacists deal with the issue of prescription error? What factors may contribute to prescription errors? Have you known any colleagues who are paralyzed by the fears of making a prescription error? How would you counsel them?

Don't Shoot the Pharmacist (2008; Ben Bailey, Edwin Matos, Jr.): A comedy depicting work challenges of one community pharmacist during his shift at Goodyear Drugstore.

1 (Ch 5, 00:18:22–00:21:12) In this scene, pharmacist Zack Wright (Bailey) is faced with the dilemma of whether or not to supply insulin syringes to a non-diabetic patient who is a known substance abuser currently under the influence of an illicit substance.

   a. If you were the pharmacist in this scene, would you have responded differently to the patient's request for needles?

   b. How did you feel when the patient approached the counter? As health-care professionals, do we sometimes harbor discriminatory feelings or stereotypical judgments of substance abusers? If so, does this interfere with our ability to care for such patients? From where do such judgmental beliefs originate (i.e. our own family backgrounds; societal messages; etc)?

   c. Have you ever worked with patients who are substance abusers? What is the best way to treat patients in your practice who are known substance abusers?

   d. Health-care professionals are often interfacing with patients who claim to have chronic pain but are, in reality, drug seeking. How do health-care professionals, in general, best maintain the delicate balance between optimal pain management and risk of enabling medication addiction? What is the difference between drug tolerance, drug dependence and drug addiction?

Stereotypes

House M.D.: "Occam's Razor" (2004): *House M.D.* is a US television medical drama that follows the professional life of Dr. Gregory House (Hugh Laurie), a medical genius, as he and his diagnostic team hypothesize diagnoses and treatment of multiple disease states.

1   (Season 1, episode 3, title 3, ch 5; 0:07:56–0:09:11; Hugh Laurie, Joshua Wolfe Coleman): In this episode of *House*, a college student is rushed to the hospital suddenly suffering from seven symptoms unrelated to one single diagnosis. While several physicians rule out causes, one postulates that the student's original symptom was cough; and that a prescription for colchicine was accidentally given in place of the intended cough medicine at the pharmacy. The physician further explains that colchicine could cause the other six symptoms from which the patient is suffering. The plot continues as physicians try to uncover whether a pharmacist mistakenly gave colchicine in place of a cough medicine, and inadvertently caused the student's sudden onset of symptoms. In this following scene, physicians, a concerned mother, and girlfriend visit the community pharmacy where the alleged prescription error between cough medicine and colchicine could have taken place. The pharmacist defends his accuracy in filling prescriptions as the physician demands a visible comparison between the tablets found in the cough medicine bottle to the pharmacist's stock of colchicine.

   a. How did you feel when the pharmacist made the statement: "I'm just a pharmacist?"

   b. Name a few of the stereotypes surrounding the profession of pharmacy. From where do you think these stereotypes originate? What role, if any, did the pharmacist in the scene play in perpetuating stereotypes of pharmacists?

c. If you were the pharmacist in this scene, how would you have respectfully handled the situation? Discuss diplomatic ways to handle professional conflict.

d. Do you feel that other health-care professionals stereotype pharmacists according to their job location or the amount of postgraduate training/ education they received?

e. What is your opinion regarding standardizing pharmacy training to include postgraduate education? Would stereotypes of the pharmacy profession by the professional and lay public be curtailed if residency training with strict accreditation standards became a requirement after passing the NAPLEX (North American Pharmacist Licensure Examination) and before pharmacists could legally practice?

Seinfeld: "The Sponge" (1995; Jerry Seinfeld, Julia Louis-Dreyfus, Peter Mehlman): Seinfeld is a US sitcom that depicts the lives of Jerry Seinfeld and his close friends in various comedic situations.

1 (Season 7, disk 2, title 3, ch 2; 0:06:27–0:07:32) After learning that her prophylactic of choice, the Today's Sponge, is being removed from the market, Elaine (Louis-Dreyfus) goes on a hunt from pharmacy to pharmacy to secure as many of the sponges as she can possibly find. In this series of scenes, Elaine visits many pharmacies, interfacing with several pharmacists, to try to find the Today's Sponge. She is grateful to the pharmacist (played by Peter Mehlman) at Pasteur Pharmacy for selling her a large quantity of sponges.

a. What stereotypes of a pharmacist are depicted in these scenes? How is the reality of the profession different from what is portrayed on film? Do different stereotypes exist for male versus female pharmacists?

b. What are the job responsibilities of community pharmacists? How is the role of the community pharmacist depicted in the scenes? Compare and contrast the stereotypes of community pharmacists with real-life job responsibilities.

c. Discuss the issue of professional liability in pharmacy. Is it necessary for pharmacists to have professional liability/malpractice insurance? How does professional liability vary among different health-care specialties (nurses, physicians, respiratory specialists, etc)?

d. How would you recreate these short scenes to reflect a more realistic view of the pharmacy profession today? Using the same amount of time allotted for the scenes, how could you accurately portray the expertise and training required to be a pharmacist?

Ethics
....

Magnolia (1999; Julianne Moore, Tom Cruise): *Magnolia* colligates the life and experiences of several different characters in search of happiness and life's purpose. One of the characters, Linda Patridge (Moore), is under immense stress as she deals with her older husband's illness, imminent placement in hospice care, and pending death.

1   (Ch 5, 1:03:31–1:04:20; 1:11:40–1:13:47) Physicians have suggested placing Mrs. Partridge's elderly husband on liquid morphine as a palliative measure and have explained the irreversible impairment he will suffer as his chronic neoplastic pain is adequately managed. Overwhelmed by the ethical implications of this management strategy and the stress of his illness, Partridge experiences an increase in anxiety. In this scene, she visits her neighborhood pharmacy to get her and her husband's prescriptions prepared. She interfaces mostly with a young pharmacy technician and briefly with the pharmacist.

   a. Review the "Code of Ethics" and "Oath of a Pharmacist." (Both can be found on the American Pharmacists Association website, www.pharmacist. com). Discuss violations of both the "Code of Ethics" and the "Oath" in this scene.

   b. How might the pharmacy technician have handled the situation differently? Should the pharmacist have intervened earlier? Discuss the role of the pharmacist in maintaining a patient's dignity.

   c. As health-care professionals, how do we maintain the delicate balance between beneficence (i.e. "do good [acts] by the patient") and non-maleficence (i.e. "first, do no harm")? As an example, consider the use of liquid morphine to adequately manage pain and at the same time cause irreversible impairment in a patient. Discuss why this dilemma may have led to increased anxiety for Mrs. Partridge.

   d. Discuss the conflict between beneficence and non-maleficence specifically in this scene. Think on a broader scale and discuss specific conflicts encountered by health-care professionals.

   e. Discuss the pharmacist's ethical responsibility in providing care for the patient and, at the same time, protecting the integrity of his license. Who do you think the pharmacist called when he picked up the phone immediately after viewing the medication names written on the prescriptions?

   f. Explain the importance of confidentiality when cultivating the patient-pharmacist relationship. Discuss specific examples when confidentiality – and the desire to maintain it – pose ethical challenges for health-care professionals.

   g. Do you feel Mrs. Partridge was justified in the way she reacted to the pharmacy technician and the pharmacist? Have you ever encountered an emotional outburst by a patient? What are appropriate ways to handle emotional outbursts by patients and other health-care professionals?

Don't Shoot the Pharmacist (see earlier description)

1 (Ch 9, 0:47:00–0:48:55) In this scene, pharmacist Zack Wright (Bailey) is approached by a regular female patron of Goodyear Drugstore requesting the contraceptive morning-after pill. After informing the woman of the price, Zack discovers she does not have enough money to pay for the prescription. He then makes the ethical decision to pay for the woman's prescription.
   a. If you were the pharmacist in this scene, would you have paid for a prescription for your patient? What are the pros and cons of such an action?
   b. Discuss why some pharmacists may experience an internal conflict when their legal obligation to help patients clashes with their individual moral objection to a particular "mode of help" (i.e. contraception).
   c. Discuss easily accessible nonprescription medications that you feel pose ethical dilemmas in terms of safety, abuse potential, misbranding, and so forth.
   d. Have you ever experienced a situation where a pharmacist or other health-care professional withheld medication or failed to render care due to reasons of religion or conscience? How did this make you feel? Are such actions justifiable?

Drugstore Cowboy (1989; Matt Dillon, Kelly Lynch): A crime drama depicting the lives of drug addicts Bob Hughes (Dillon) and his friends as they rob several pharmacies in support of their prescription drug habit.
1 (Chs 2–3; 00:03:18–00:07:42; ch 18, 00:44:00–00:45:27) Bob and his friends contrive extravagant subterfuges to distract pharmacists on duty in order to steal controlled substances from the pharmacy. After one heist, they discuss the inventory of stolen medications.
   a. Discuss the definition of drug diversion. Which medications are more likely to be diverted and why?
   b. What pharmacokinetic/pharmacodynamic properties of opioids make it highly desirable by Bob and his friends?
   c. When diversion happens in the pharmacy, what are the appropriate steps to take and the appropriate agencies to notify? Discuss ways to prevent drug diversion.
   d. Discuss the different ways drug diversion can occur. Have you ever witnessed drug diversion? How should pharmacists handle patients suspected of diversion? How should pharmacists handle pharmacy technicians, pharmacists or other health-care professionals suspected of diversion?
   e. Discuss the ethical balance between (i) clinicians treating pain and law enforcement stopping diversion and (ii) clinicians avoiding contributing to diversion and law enforcement avoiding interfering in medicine and patient care.

Further Reading

- American Pharmacists Association, Academy of Student Pharmacists, Leadership and Professionalism/Professional Development. Code of Ethics for Pharmacists. Available at: www.pharmacist.com/Content/NavigationMenu2/LeadershipProfessionalism/ProfessionalDevelopment (last accessed, 4/18/12)
- American Psychiatric Association (APA). *Diagnostic and Statistical Manual of Mental Disorders: DSM-IV-TR*. 4th ed, text revision. Washington, DC: APA; 2000.
- Buerki R, Voterro L. *Ethical Responsibility in Pharmacy Practice*. 2nd ed. Madison, WI: American Institute of the History of Pharmacy; 2002.
- Controlled Substances Act. Title 21: Food and Drugs. Chapter 13 Drug Abuse Prevention and Control. www.fda.gov/RegulatoryInformation/Legislation/ucm148726.htm (last accessed 4/18/12)
- Farre M, Bosch F, Roset PN, *et al*. Putting clinical pharmacology in context: the use of popular movies. *J Clin Pharmacol*. 2004; **44**(1): 30–6.
- Ferri M, Amato L, Davoli M. Alcoholics Anonymous and other 12-step programmes for alcohol dependence. *Cochrane Database Syst Rev*. 2006; **3**: CD005032.
- Veatch R, Haddad V. *Case Studies in Pharmacy Ethics*. 2nd ed. New York, NY. Oxford University Press; 2008.
- Ventura S, Onsman A. The use of popular movies during lectures to aid the teaching and learning of undergraduate pharmacology. *Med Teach*. 2009; **31**(7): 662–4.
- www.deadiversion.usdoj.gov/index.html

25

Vets and Pets: Domesticated Animals and the Veterinarians Who Care for Them

LaTasha K. Crawford

VETERINARY MEDICINE IS A WIDE-RANGING FIELD THAT PLAYS A CRUCIAL role in food safety, animal welfare, and public health. In addition to general practitioners and board-certified specialists who practice medicine in animal hospitals, there are lab animal vets who support and conduct translational biomedical research, comparative pathologists who provide critical expertise to preclinical trials in pharmaceutical companies, farm animal vets and US Department of Agriculture representatives who are crucial for the prevention of food-borne illness, specialists in zoonotic disease who work for the Centers for Disease Control and Prevention (CDC), and wildlife vets who help monitor emerging diseases and treat life-threatening illness in wild animals after natural (or man-made) disasters. The challenges of providing a unified education for such a wide range of careers is further complicated by the need to incorporate elements of pharmacy, dentistry, surgery, and medicine that differ not only between species but also often between breeds of a single species.

It is common for the depiction of veterinarians to overlook many of the nuances of our field[1,2] but a closer look at our portrayal in the media can bring those inaccuracies to light and help us to shape our role in the public forum. Cinemeducation can also enable discussion of the facets of veterinary medicine that are not easily taught in textbooks, including legal and ethical issues as well as the intricacies of the human–animal bond.

Though a love for animals is a common driving force for any veterinarian, much of the satisfaction of being a vet is garnered not only from improving the health of our patients but also from relationships formed with the clients who have come to love and rely on our patients. Veterinarians uphold a unique relationship with our human clientele and the animals that play important roles in their owners' lives as assistance animals that help the physically disabled, protectors of the home, labor animals on a farm, mainstays of economic sustenance, or simply the pets that owners come to love as members of the family. Client communication is therefore an invaluable skill that helps with every component of the visit from taking a full history to ensuring compliance with discharge instructions.[3–5] It is especially important when dealing with the sensitive subjects of poor prognosis and euthanasia.

Several other chapters that highlight the challenges of human medicine can be translated to veterinary medicine to some degree. The clips selected for this section address some of the unique skills and resources beyond medical knowledge that form a crucial part of veterinary education.

The Role of the Veterinarian in Society

Free Willy 2: The Adventure Home (1995; Jason James Richter, Michael Madsen, Elizabeth Peña, Francis Capra): In this sequel, we pick up with Jesse, the young boy who helped Willy the orca jump to freedom in the original film. He reunites with Willy and Willy's two younger siblings Luna and Littlespot, who all come to visit a local cove. However, after an oil spill threatens the lives of the whales, Jesse must use the bond he has developed with Willy to save Willy and his family. Dr. Kate Haley, a wildlife veterinarian, is called to help treat the whales affected by the oil spill.

1 (0:50:08–0:53:04) Dr. Haley (Peña) arrives at the site of an oil spill that threatens the lives of Willy and two other orca whales in his family that were visiting a local cove. Willy's past experiences with abusive keepers have sparked a distrust of strangers and he instinctively tries to protect his sibling Luna when strangers approach them in a boat. This, unfortunately, prevents Dr. Haley and her crew from being able to treat Luna, the whale who has the most extensive illness as a result of the oil spill. Dr. Haley and the owner of the oil company appeal to Jesse (Richter) to help them as they try to approach the whales, since Jesse has developed a close bond with Willy.

2 (0:54:30–0:57:58) Jesse coaxes Willy by playing his harmonica and offering fish. This calms Willy and allows Dr. Haley and her team to approach Luna and administer the antibiotics she needs.

 a. Discuss the portrayal of Dr. Haley and her approach to treating Luna. Is it medically accurate?

 b. Discuss the role of the veterinarian in environmental catastrophes that threaten wildlife.

 c. What are the potential dangers of an oil spill to marine mammals? Birds? Sea turtles? Other wildlife?

Quarantine (2008; Jennifer Carpenter, Steve Harris, Columbus Short): A television reporter (Carpenter) and her cameraman find themselves among the tenants trapped inside an apartment building when an outbreak of a contagious virus causes the building to be quarantined by the government. In this unusual interpretation of a zombie thriller, filming firefighters in response to a routine 911 call provides inadvertent documentation of the spread of a viral disease that renders its victims neurologically inappropriate, blood-thirsty, and unusually violent. Viewers should be warned that some scenes contain violent, graphic content, and coarse language.

1 (0:19:46–0:20:30) In this scene a police officer has just been attacked by a violent, infected Mrs. Espinosa and is in need of medical attention. However, the exits have been locked from the outside and there are no paramedics present. The familiar call "is there a doctor in the house?" is answered by one of the tenants of the building, Lawrence (Greg Germann), a veterinarian who provides first aid to the injured officer.

2 (0:38:00–0:38:44) In this scene a reporter is interviewing Lawrence about the people who have been attacked by Mrs. Espinosa and who are now under his care. He states that, as a veterinarian, all he can do is to dress their wounds and try to comfort them.

   a. Discuss the portrayal of a veterinarian as demonstrated in these clips.

   b. Discuss the public opinion of veterinarians that you have experienced. How does it compare with the depiction of Lawrence in these scenes?

   c. Why is the public perception of veterinarians important? How might it affect your interaction with clients?

3 (0:40:15–0:42:15) In this scene, a fireman who was attacked earlier in the night now experiences the peak effect of the disease and charges violently into the lobby before being sedated by Lawrence. In the next room, Lawrence starts to piece together the patterns of signs shown by all the infected victims and notices a striking similarity to rabies, except this disease progresses in a matter of minutes.

4 (0:48:07–0:50:48) The CDC arrives in full containment suits. They gather everyone for a roll call of all the building tenants but avoid giving full disclosure of the suspected infectious agent and the test needed for definitive diagnosis.

5 (0:57:05–0:57:50) The lone surviving CDC representative finally reveals the reason for the quarantine – namely, an outbreak of a mutated rabies virus that causes rapid disease progression. A series of dog attacks at a local veterinarian's office was traced back to a sick dog owned by a tenant of the building.

   a. Discuss the role for veterinarians in educating the public about zoonotic disease.

   b. Discuss the potential role for vets in managing zoonotic disease outbreak.

   c. What are other zoonotic diseases that your clients may need to be informed about?

   d. Why is it particularly important to educate the public about rabies?

   e. What are the signs of a rabies infection? What would you do if you were suspicious that a patient has a rabies infection? What information do the owners need to know?

f. What would you do if a patient presented with bite wounds from a stray dog whose rabies status was unknown?

Legal and Ethical Issues for the Practicing Veterinarian

Treating Human Patients

1 (0:19:46–0:20:30) In this scene a police officer has just been attacked by a violent, infected woman and is in need of medical attention. However, the exits have been locked from the outside, and there are no paramedics present. The familiar call "is there a doctor in the house" is answered only by one of the tenants of the building, Lawrence, a veterinarian who provides first aid to the injured officer.

  a. What are the laws regarding medical treatment of human patients? What if it is an emergency?

  b. What are the potential risks for Lawrence in terms of liability or licensure once he decides to provide first aid? analgesia? sedation?

Drug Storage and Regulations

Terminator 3: Rise of the Machines (2003; Arnold Schwarzenegger, Nick Stahl, Claire Danes): In the third movie of the Terminator series, John Connor (Stahl) is living "off the grid" with an impending sense that someone or something is trying to track him down to kill him. Arnold Schwarzenegger returns as a robot from the future, this time reprogrammed to protect John Connor and his new companion Kate Brewster (Danes) from the new and improved terminator robot that is hunting them down.

1 (0:12:42–0:13:35) In this scene, John Connor has just been injured in a motorcycle crash and needs to seek medical treatment. He hitchhikes into town and his attention is caught by a veterinary clinic that is closed for the night. He limps across the street toward the vet clinic. We then see him break into the drug cabinet, grab a bottle of medication, and swallow two pills.

2 (0:17:57–0:20:58) John Connor is seen laying on the floor of the vet clinic, surrounded by first aid materials and the bottle of drugs we saw him take in a previous scene. The scene cuts to Kate Brewster receiving a phone call from a client whose pet needs emergent care. Kate heads to the vet clinic to prepare for the arrival of the client and the ill patient. Upon her arrival to the clinic, Kate sees that the drug cabinet has been broken into, discovers John Connor, and assumes he is a drug addict who broke in to steal drugs. The client arrives with her ill pet and Kate places her in an exam room while she returns to deal with the intruder she has trapped in a crate in the back room.

  a. How should drugs be stored in a veterinary practice?

b. What are the regulations regarding storage and record keeping of controlled substances? How do these differ for other types of drugs found in a veterinary practice?

c. What steps should you take if you discover that a controlled substance is unaccounted for?

d. Why might veterinary clinics be more vulnerable to theft that human pharmacies?

Lien Laws

Dark Horse (1992; Ed Begley, Jr., Mimi Rogers, Ari Meyers): Allison is the new girl in town who is having a tough time fitting in to her new high school and starts to hang out with the wrong crowd. After she gets into trouble and gets arrested, she is sentenced to community service at a horse ranch owned by Dr. Susan Hadley, an equine veterinarian. While there, Allison (Meyers) finds a connection with Jet, a troublesome horse who, like herself has been misunderstood. Through her budding relationship with Jet and the handicapped children that visit the ranch, we see a vivid portrayal of the mutual benefit of the human–animal bond. We also see some of the challenges Dr. Hadley faces as the owner of an equine veterinary practice.

1 (0:21:10–0:22:52) Dr. Hadley (Rogers) arrives at her ranch to find that Jet, a patient who is still healing from injury, is being ridden without her approval. While galloping, Jet falls down as he has worsened his leg injury. Dr. Hadley becomes angry that the client has not heeded her instructions to limit Jet's activity and the client storms off. He removes Jet from Dr. Hadley's care without paying for services rendered with the intention of taking Jet to another veterinarian.

2 (0:33:51 to 0:37:44) In this scene, Jet and his owner return to Dr. Hadley's ranch to seek treatment once again. Dr. Hadley agrees to admit Jet, but only on three conditions: (i) that the client pay off some of his bill, (ii) that the client yield to her treatment and training plan, and (iii) that the client reveal the names of the other equine vets that have seen Jet since he left her care. The client begrudgingly agrees and writes a check for part of his outstanding bill. Jet proves to be unruly when he is unloaded from the trailer and the client deals with him harshly. Dr. Hadley has a calmer approach as she leads Jet inside and begins to treat his leg injury.

a. What are some strategies you can use to address a client who continues to seek your services but refuses to pay the bill?

b. What are lien laws and how might they apply to veterinary medicine? Are there lien laws in your state?

c. What would be the potential repercussions if Dr. Hadley decided to hold Jet against the wishes of his owner?

Neglect, Animal Abuse, and Animal Cruelty

Turner and Hooch (1989; Tom Hanks, Mare Winningham, Craig T. Nelson):
Scott Turner is an uptight small-town cop who is working his last case before taking a new job in the city. Things change when Scott responds to the call of an old man who complains of suspicious noises heard from across the pier in the middle of the night. The following night the old man is murdered, and his slobbery, hard-to-handle dog, Hooch, is the only witness. Turner unwillingly adopts Hooch with hopes of using him to find the old man's murderer. The bond between Turner and Hooch grows stronger as the police get closer to finding the murderer and his coconspirators.

1 (0:25:44–0:29:07) After taking Hooch away from the scene of his owner's murder, Turner (Tom Hanks) decides to take him to the local vet, Dr. Emily Carson (Mare Winningham), with hopes that they will help find him a new home. Hooch drags Turner in through the doggie door where they are discovered by Dr. Carson. Dr. Carson expresses her concern about the poor condition that Hooch is in and accuses Turner of neglect.
   a. What is the difference between neglect, animal abuse, and animal cruelty?
   b. What elements of a patient's history would make you suspicious of passive neglect? of active maltreatment or abuse?
   c. What clinical signs would make you suspicious of neglect? animal abuse?
   d. How would you approach a client who you felt was guilty of neglect?
   e. What are your legal obligations if you suspect your patient is the victim of neglect?
   f. What are some of the reasons a veterinarian might feel reluctant to report animal abuse?

Amores Perros (2000; Emilio Echevarría, Gael García Bernal, Goya Toledo):
Three stories of the complexities of love and life are interconnected by way of a car accident. Octavio (Bernal) starts to use his pet Rottweiler in a dog-fighting ring to raise money to run away with his brother's wife. A couple's rocky relationship is tested after their pet dog gets trapped beneath the floorboards of their apartment. El Chivo (Echevarría) is a homeless man who befriends stray dogs and revisits his old former trade as a murderer for hire. Viewers should be warned that some scenes contain graphic content and coarse language.

1 (0:00:40–0:03:01) In this scene Octavio and his friend are fleeing the scene of a dog fight gone wrong. His dog, Cofi, was shot in the left flank during a dog fight and lies bleeding in the back seat of Octavio's car as they speed away from the men who shot Cofi. Octavio runs a red light and causes a car accident.

2 (1:43:16–1:45:11) In this scene El Chivo, the homeless man, has just witnessed the car crash and watches as the ambulance arrives to care for the people injured in the crash. He sees patrons carry Cofi away from the car

and then return to aid the people injured in the crash. He approaches Cofi, takes him in, and cares for his wounds.

3   (1:54:55–1:57:42) Cofi has recovered from his wounds and has become one of El Chivo's faithful canine companions. In this scene, Cofi's past as a vicious dog is brought to light when El Chivo arrives home to find that Cofi has attacked and killed the other dogs that cohabited El Chivo's make-shift home.

   a. If this were your patient, what types of clinical signs would make you particularly suspicious that this patient has been involved in dog fighting?
   b. What types of wounds may be more indicative of involvement with dog fighting rather than a single attack by another dog?
   c. What resources are available to you if you suspect that your patient is the victim of animal abuse or cruelty? What are your legal and ethical obligations as a veterinarian?
   d. What are the potential risks of adopting out dogs that were previously used in dog fighting? What can you do to manage those risks?

The Human–Animal Bond

The Long Shot (2004; Julie Benz, Marsha Mason, Paul Le Mat): Annie, her daughter, and her horse relocate with her husband who has to move in order to take a new job. Once he learns that his job is unavailable, he abandons his family. To provide for her family, Annie takes a job mucking out stalls and helping out at a local stable. As she works her way up to a position as a riding teacher, the bond with her daughter and with her horse, Tolo, grows stronger.

1   (0:53:10–0:54:16) In this scene Annie (Julie Benz) has just learned that her horse Tolo is blind. As she contemplates euthanasia, she sits with Tolo and talks to him, giving the audience a glimpse into the bond she has developed with Tolo through the years and especially through the recent difficult phase of her life.

   a. What is the human–animal bond?
   b. Why does the human–animal bond seem to get stronger when people go through a stressful phase of life or a traumatic event?
   c. How does the bond between the patient and the client and affect you as a veterinarian?

Dark Horse (see earlier description)

1   (0:42:35–0:43:08) In this scene, Jet refuses to eat from Allison's hand.
2   (0:47:41–0:48:45) Jet still has difficulty trusting people and refuses to eat from anyone's hand. Allison has visited Jet's stall several times to talk to him and offer food, which he usually rejects. In this scene, Jet finally trusts Allison enough to eat directly from her hand.

a. How can the human–animal bond help you as a veterinarian?
b. Discuss the use of food or treats during appointments or when providing performing treatments on in-patients.
c. How can the human–animal bond be used to benefit patient care?
d. How can the human–animal bond be used to benefit the relationship between the veterinarian and the client? How can it benefit the relationship between a veterinary practice and the community at large?

3 (1:21:32–1:25:06) After a car accident leaves Allison in a wheelchair and Jet with a fractured leg, Allison refuses to return to the ranch. She endures a period of self-pity and helplessness and, being unable to ride, begins to loath reminders of Jet. In this scene she finally returns to the ranch on the day that handicapped children come to visit as part of a therapy riding program. Though Allison is reluctant, her father (Ed Begley, Jr.) and Dr. Hadley force her to spend time with Jet; she finally reestablishes a bond.

4 (1:28:56–1:35:50) In this scene, an unattended tractor crashes into the stall where Jet was slung while recovering from his orthopedic injuries. The sling breaks, leaving Jet on the floor of the stall, seemingly unconscious. Roused by Allison, Jet stands up pulling Allison onto her feet. As she watches Jet run in the nearby field, Allison stands for the first time under her own strength.

The Horse Boy (2009): Rowan Isaacson is an autistic child who has very limited social interaction with others. Raising Rowan has been a challenge for his parents who are sometimes at a loss for ways to calm him down when something upsets him; that is, until they find that he has a unique connection with horses. His contact with horses provides a sense of calm and increased responsiveness. The documentary follows Rowan and his parents as they embark on a journey to Mongolia to obtain a spiritual understanding of his condition and his unique connection to horses.

1 (0:06:17–0:09:50) In this scene, we see examples of Rowan's tantrums. As his father narrates, we see the unique, calming effect that contact with horses has on Rowan. In addition, Rowan's presence seems to have a calming effect on the horses with whom he interacts.
a. Why do you think interacting with animals can be beneficial for physically or mentally handicapped people?
b. What effects can community outreach have on a veterinary practice? How could it benefit you and your staff?

Wild Horse Redemption (2007): In this documentary, incarcerated criminals at a correction facility in Colorado work closely to tame wild mustangs that are to be adopted out to the public. Despite limited experience with horses, many who volunteer for the program learn the techniques of horse whisperers. As they face creatures wilder, stronger, and more dangerous than they are, the inmates learn patience and focused determination as training horses proves to help in their own rehabilitation.

1 (Ch 2, 0:00:42–0:02:39) In this scene two inmates speak about the connection they feel to the wild mustangs and why the program appealed to them. They see striking parallels between their own incarceration and rehabilitation and the wild horses who become approachable, trusting, faithful companions over the course of the 90-day program.

   a. What benefit might the human–animal bond have for at-risk youth or the incarcerated?

Client Communication

Marley and Me (2008; Owen Wilson, Jennifer Aniston): In this heartfelt film based on the autobiographical novel by John Grogan, a young couple finds love and inspiration after adopting a troublesome Labrador retriever, Marley. The ups and downs of building a relationship and a career evoke both laughter and tears as Marley becomes an integral part of the Grogan family.

1 (1:27:15–1:32:56) In these scenes, Marley shows signs of illness at home, including decreased activity, lethargy, and flatulence. John (Wilson) takes her to the vet who diagnoses Marley with gastric dilatation and volvulus (GDV). Because Marley is not a surgical candidate, the vet explains that they can only provide supportive care and hope that Marley lasts through the night.

   a. Critique the vet's approach to client communication.

   b. What are the benefits of using layman's terms in lieu of medical terminology?

   c. How would you communicate the contributing factors and potential outcomes of GDV to a client?

   d. What discharge instructions would you provide to a client whose pet just recovered from an illness as serious as GDV?

Dark Horse (see earlier description)

1 (0:21:10–0:22:52) Dr. Hadley arrives at her ranch to find that Jet, a patient who is still healing from injury, is being ridden without her approval. Jet falls down while galloping, as he has worsened his leg injury. Dr. Hadley becomes angry that the client has not heeded her instructions to limit Jet's activity and the client storms off. He removes Jet from Dr. Hadley's care without paying for services rendered with the intention of taking Jet to another veterinarian.

2 (0:33:51–0:37:44) In this scene, Jet and his owner return to Dr. Hadley's ranch to seek treatment once again. Dr. Hadley agrees to admit Jet, but only on three conditions: (i) that the client pay off some of his bill, (ii) that the client yield to her treatment and training plan, and (iii) that the client reveal the other equine vets that have seen Jet since he left her care. The client begrudgingly agrees and writes a check for part of his outstanding bill. Jet proves to be unruly when he is unloaded from the trailer and the client deals

with him harshly. Dr. Hadley has a more calm approach as she leads Jet inside and begins to treat his leg injury.

a. What would you say to an owner who you feel is handling your patient inappropriately?

b. Critique the methods that are used to manage the unruly client. What are some strategies you can use to address a client who continues to seek your services but refuses to pay the bill?

c. What are some strategies you can use when the client does not agree with your diagnosis or your treatment plan?

d. Why did Dr. Hadley want to know where else the horse has been?

e. Discuss the positive and negative repercussions of Dr. Hadley's willingness to treat Jet despite the difficulty she has had getting the owner to pay his bill?

Euthanasia

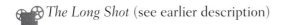

The Long Shot (see earlier description)

1 (0:50:25–0:53:10) In this scene Annie discovers that her horse Tolo's reluctance to move lies in his sudden inability to see. The vet is called out and determines that Tolo's retinas have detached and his blindness is irreversible. He mentions the option of euthanasia but Annie elects to think about it before making any decisions.

a. Critique the veterinarian's discussion of euthanasia.

b. What are potential risks associated with bilateral blindness in a horse?

c. What would you do if you felt euthanasia was in the patient's best interest but the client refused?

Turner and Hooch (see earlier description)

1 (1:30:01–1:33:03) Hooch is shot in the neck during an altercation with the criminals that Turner has been investigating for the murder of Hooch's owner. Turner takes Hooch to the local vet, Dr. Carson, whom he is now dating. Though Dr. Carson tries to provide emergency care, she is unable to save Hooch's life and he dies on the table.

a. How would you prepare a client who may witness these final, and perhaps agonizing, moments of their pet's life?

b. If you were Dr. Carson, would you advise the owner to euthanize Hooch, rather than let him die on the table?

c. How would you respond to an owner in your exam room who is wailing after observing the death of their pet? What are some ways to help a grieving owner?

Marley and Me (see earlier description)

1   (1:40:31–1:48:24) Marley has a second episode of GDV and is taken to the vet. Because of the degree of illness and poor prognosis, the decision is made to euthanize Marley. John spends a few last moments with Marley and stands by his side as the vet euthanizes him in the exam room.

a. What are some ways to broach the topic of euthanasia with a client?
b. How would you respond to a client who would prefer to let the patient "die at home" in lieu of euthanasia?
c. Critique the veterinarian's approach to prepare John for observing Marley's euthanasia.
d. What are some of the things you should warn an owner about prior to observing their dog's euthanasia? How would this differ for a reptile? A horse?

References

1   Campbell H. The portrayal of veterinary medicine in films. *Vet Herit*. 1999; **22**(2): 35–7.
2   Pulfer DM. President's message: veterinary medicine – our public image. *Can Vet J*. 1993; **34**: 391–2.
3   Cornell KK, Brandt JC, Bonvicini KA, editors. Effective communication in veterinary practice. *Vet Clin of North Am Small Anim Pract*. 2007; **37**(1): 1–202.
4   Lue TW, Pantenburg DP, Crawford PM. Impact of the owner-pet and client-veterinarian bond on the care that pets receive. *J Am Vet Med Assoc*. 2008; **232**(4): 531–40.
5   Shaw JR, Adams CL, Bonnett BN. What can veterinarians learn from studies of physician-patient communication about veterinarian-client-patient communication? *J Am Vet Med Assoc*. 2004; **224**(5): 676–84.

Further Reading

● Babcock SL, Neihsl A. Requirements for mandatory reporting of animal cruelty. *J Am Vet Med Assoc*. 2006; **228**(5): 685–9.
● Benetato MA, Reisman R, McCobb E. The veterinarian's role in animal cruelty cases. *J Am Vet Med Assoc*. 2011; **238**(1): 31–4.
● Hannah HW. Liens for veterinary service: how effective are they? *J Am Vet Med Assoc*. 2001; **218**(12): 24–5.
● Hannah HW. Dead animals, abandoned animals, and animals held for payment of fee: a veterinarian's options. *J Am Vet Med Assoc*. 2002; **221**(5): 641.
● http://vet.tufts.edu/ccm/
● Kaiser L, Smith KA, Heleski CR, *et al*. Effects of a therapeutic riding program on at-risk and special education children. *J Am Vet Med Assoc*. 2006; **228**(1): 46–52.
● Manette CS. A reflection on the ways veterinarians cope with the death, euthanasia, and slaughter of animals. *J Am Vet Med Assoc*. 2004; **225**(1): 34–8.

- Morris A. Reporting animal abuse: a vet's responsibility to society? *Vet Rec.* 2010; **167**(17): 638–9.
- Yoffe-Sharp BL, Loar LM. The veterinarian's responsibility to recognize and report animal abuse. *J Am Vet Med Assoc.* 2009; **234**(6): 732–7.
- www.tufts.edu/vet/cfa/hoarding/
- www.americanhumane.org/
- www.vetmed.ucdavis.edu/whatsnew/article.cfm?id=2201 Web delivers lessons in international animal health: USCA grant supports interactive case studies on food animals (last accessed 12/1/11)
- www.vetmed.ucdavis.edu/whc

PART VI

Specialties

26

Blood, Sweat, Tears and Fears: Sports Medicine and Sports Psychology

Laura J. Schrader & David E. Price

PEOPLE OF ALL AGES ENJOY THE PLEASURE AND BENEFITS OF PARTICI-
pating in sporting events and different forms of exercise. Health-care providers
are continually extolling the many benefits of physical activity. Exercising regularly decreases the risk of cardiovascular disease, diabetes, strokes, and it helps
maintain a healthy weight. Along with the many benefits of exercise, there are
unique health issues and injuries that can occur in athletes. Therefore, sports
medicine is an important area for physicians receive training in. Athletes can
suffer from acute injuries and also overuse injuries. Physicians must be aware of
specific issues that may arise with female athletes, children and adolescent athletes, and athletes from different cultures. The history and physical exam are both
important in proper diagnosis and management of athletes. Attention should be
paid to training regimens, diet, supplement usage, and past injuries. Participating
in sports can have many psychological benefits, but physicians should also be
alert to the psychological stresses that may be unique to this population.

Sports-Related Injuries

Friday Night Lights (2004; Billy Bob Thornton, Jay Hernandez, Derek Luke):
In Odessa, Texas, everyone lives for Friday night high school football. The
members of the Permian Panthers are under a lot of pressure to be perfect. Led
by coach Gary Gaines (Thornton), the team struggles to make a comeback after
star Boobie Miles (Luke) suffers an injury.

1 (0:47:00–0:50:03) In this scene, Boobie Miles (Derek Luke), the star quarterback, has suffered a knee injury and is going to the hospital for an MRI.
After the doctor examines his knee, he tells Boobie there is a significant injury

to his anterior cruciate ligament (ACL). The doctor says that, based on the MRI and exam, he does not feel that Boobie should play football anymore. He says, "[when healthy] you can run and cut and hammer people and you don't hesitate because you have a solid knee, but when you don't have this ligament you can't do that, so it's really out of the question." When told the news, Boobie reacts with anger, denial, and disbelief.

   a. What is the anterior cruciate ligament and what is its function?
   b. Describe the classical mechanism of injury for a torn ACL. What are risk factors for this type of injury?
   c. Discuss the physical exam findings of a torn ACL.
   d. Boobie has a very emotional reaction to the news that he can no longer play football. Discuss the psychological effects that injury can have on athletes.
   e. Significant life events can sometimes precipitate episodes of depression. For serious athletes, an injury can be a significant life event. Discuss how you might screen injured athletes for depression.

Any Given Sunday (1999; Al Pacino, Dennis Quaid, Cameron Diaz, Jamie Fox): The Miami Sharks are a professional football team led by coach Tony D'Amato (Al Pacino) and owner Christina Pagniacci (Diaz). After quarterback Cap Rooney (Quaid) is injured, little-known quarterback Willie Beaman (Fox) takes over. This is an inside look at the world of professional football and the lives of the players.

1   (0:00:50–0:03:50) Quarterback Cap Rooney is seen taking a hard hit. The doctors rush onto the field to assess him. We find out later he suffered an L5 herniated disk. The pressure to keep up appearances is seen when the doctor asks him, "Are you too old to walk off?"
2   (0:10:30–0:11:20) This second scene takes place in the locker room. We see the internist speaking to the orthopedist. The internist is worried because Cap is losing strength in his ankle and the orthopedist brushes him off. We then see the orthopedist look at an X-ray and he tells Cap he is fine, "It's just a bruise." Cap tells him that something is definitely not right and the orthopedist finally says they will order an MRI of his back.

   a. Back pain is one of the most common presenting complaints in a primary care office. Discuss the appropriate history and physical examination.
   b. Often back pain can be treated conservatively with anti-inflammatories and physical therapy; further workup is unnecessary. What are some "red flags" that would prompt you as a doctor to evaluate the patient further?
   c. In the second scene, the internist is concerned about loss of ankle strength. Why would this worry him?
   d. Professional athletes have extraordinary pressures placed on them from coaches, teammates, trainers, and the public. Many times these pressures can put the athletes' health at risk. Discuss whether Cap should have been pressured to walk off the field without further assessment of his back.

e. Discuss all the ways this orthopedist did not act like an ideal sports medicine physician.

Concussion

Varsity Blues (1999; James Van Der Beek, Jon Voight, Paul Walker, Ron Lester): John Moxon (Van Der Beek) is a second-string high school football quarterback who suddenly becomes the leader of his team after the star quarterback Lance Harbor (Walker) suffers an injury. The movie follows these young athletes as they deal with intense pressure to win from their coach Bud Kilmer (Voight) and the entire community.

1 (0:11:45–0:13:00) Billy Bob is a high school football player who we see in this clip taking a hard hit. He loses consciousness for a short time and is awakened by smelling salts. We see the trainers ask Billy Bob how many fingers he is holding up and he appears to be having some visual disturbance and confusion.
   a. Discuss the signs and symptoms that are consistent with concussion.
   b. Ideally what should happen medically for Billy Bob at this point?
   c. Discuss whether this situation is common enough to be seen in a primary care office and how you would treat this patient if he came to you.

2 (0:27:00–0:31:00) In this scene we see Billy Bob feeling poorly in class and passing out. The nurse says Billy Bob should not play football because of his recent concussion. The coach pressures Billy Bob into playing even though we clearly see he is not feeling well. The result is that Billy Bob has blurred vision and dizziness, and he passes out on the field. Subsequently, another player is injured.
   a. Why does the nurse feel Billy Bob should not participate? What are the risks to Billy Bob?
   b. Discuss the motivation of the coach and whether Billy Bob should have been allowed to play.
   c. Discuss ways in which health-care providers can be advocates for protecting athletes.

Any Given Sunday (see earlier description)

1 (1:09:55–1:11:10) Team orthopedist Dr. Ollie Powers (Matthew Modine) is seen speaking with team owner Christina Pagniacci (Cameron Diaz) about football player Shark Lavay (Lawrence Taylor). The doctor says that Shark is having migraines and postconcussive syndrome. He has suffered three concussions in the last 5 months and no one can predict what another hit will do to this player. The team owner puts pressure on the physician to let Shark play for her own financial gain.
   a. What are the signs and symptoms of postconcussive syndrome?

b. What are the risks involved in multiple concussions?

c. Discuss the medical ethical issues brought up by this clip.

Training

Rudy (1993; Sean Astin): Rudy's ultimate dream is to play football for the University of Notre Dame. Although he has poor grades, minimal athletic ability, and is half the size of the other players, Rudy works his way onto the team. Because of his determination, he becomes a beloved member of the team, showing that drive and spirit can bring success.

1 (1:14:00–1:19:25) In this scene Rudy (jersey number 45) is at football practice. He is seen taking very hard hits. The training is grueling. Rudy can be seen with a bloody nose, wrapped wrist, and shoulder and ankle injuries. Later there is a scene with the trainer dealing with Rudy's training injuries.

a. Training is necessary for athletes, but there is a point when an athlete can overtrain. Injuries are a sign of overtraining and can be detrimental to an athlete. Discuss other signs and symptoms of overtraining syndrome.

b. Football is notorious for traumatic impact injuries. Sports medicine physicians and trainers see these frequently. Discuss prevention and treatment strategies for these injuries.

Performance Enhancing Drugs

The Wrestler (2008; Mickey Rourke): Randy Robinson (Rourke) is a professional wrestler forced to retire after an illness. The movie follows his return to wrestling to try to defeat his longtime rival. During this time he also starts a new relationship and tries to reconnect with his daughter.

1 (0:23:28–0:25:15) Randy is in the locker room at the gym meeting with a dealer to purchase illegal steroids and other performance enhancing drugs. He says that he just needs to get big and strong. He is then seen injecting the steroids and lifting weights.

a. Besides anabolic steroids, what are some other performance enhancing drugs that are used by athletes?

b. What motivation do athletes have to use steroids?

2 (0:33:30–0:37:03) Randy is in the locker room after a professional wrestling match and appears ill. He vomits then grabs his chest and collapses. In the next scene he is in the hospital and a doctor reveals he has had a cardiac bypass surgery. The doctor says, "the stuff you are putting in your body, you need to cut it out."

a. What are the possible risks and side effects of anabolic steroids and other performance enhancing drugs?

b. If an athlete comes into the office asking for something safe and effective to help enhance his training, how would you respond? What advice would you give the athlete?

Cultural Issues for the Athlete

Bend It Like Beckham (2002; Parminder Nagra, Keira Knightley, Jonathan Rhys Meyers): Indian teenager Jess (Nagra) aspires to be a professional soccer player, but her family does not approve of females playing the sport. Jess goes behind her parents' back to join a team.

1 (0:20:47–0:23:30) In this scene, Jess's mother catches her playing soccer with some boys in the park. Her mother is upset because, as an Indian female, she does not believe it is appropriate for Jess to be playing soccer. She voices several cultural concerns including that girls should not show their legs, girls should not stay out in the sun because their skin will darken, and girls should not play sports with boys. She says soccer is OK for little girls, but now Jess should be concerned with learning to cook and finding a husband. She says Jess is bringing shame on the family by participating in sports.

   a. As physicians it is always important to be culturally sensitive. If this family came into the office and these issues came up, how would you respond?
   b. Discuss the benefits of exercise and the benefits of team participation.

The Female Athlete

Center Stage (2000; Amanda Schull, Zoe Saldana, Susan May Pratt): This movie follows three young ballet dancers as they study at the American Ballet Academy. Jodie (Schull) struggles with her technique, Eva (Saldana) works on her bad attitude, and Maureen (Pratt) has issues with her body.

1 (1:15:00–1:17:00) Maureen is one of the ballet dancers who we have seen earlier in the movie becoming quite preoccupied with body image and food restriction. In this scene Maureen's boyfriend catches her making herself throw up. He confronts her about her anorexia and Maureen reacts with anger and denial.

   a. Certain sports encourage female athletes to have a thin physique. Discuss which sports these might be and why.
   b. What additional history questions and physical exam components might a physician include when seeing a female athlete?
   c. What is the female athlete triad?
   d. Discuss whether you would be concerned about this condition in Maureen. How might you approach her if you saw her in your office?

Psychological Stresses in the Athlete

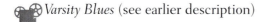 *Varsity Blues* (see earlier description)

1 (0:18:48–0:24:07) The scene starts out with the football team practicing. The fathers of players John Moxon and Lance Harbor are watching. We see John get yelled at by the coach, who screams in his face and says "You're gonna be second string your whole life." We then see the boys and their fathers at a barbecue. The two fathers seem to be very competitive with each other and are bringing the two boys into it. The fathers make the boys try to hit a can off the top of their heads and John throws the ball in his father's face in frustration.
    a. During the interaction with his coach, what do you think John is feeling? If he is treated like this day after day do you think this would bring significant stress into his life?
    b. We see John's frustration with his father later in the scene. If pressure is also being put on John at home, this would very likely add to his stress level. Discuss how stress can affect health.
    c. Huge amounts of pressure are put on athletes whether from coaches or parents and this can lead to depression and anxiety. As physicians, it is important to speak with the athletes alone to ensure these issues can be brought up. Discuss some signs and symptoms of depression and anxiety.

Black Swan (2010; Natalie Portman, Mila Kunis, Vincent Cassel): Ballet dancer Nina (Portman) wins the lead role in the production of *Swan Lake*. As opening night approaches Nina tries to capture the essence of both the White Swan and the Black Swan. The pressure builds and Nina slowly loses her mind.
1 (0:18:20–0:23:35) Nina meets with her ballet instructor to ask for the part of the Swan Queen. He tells her that he sees her obsessing about each move. She says that she just wants to be perfect. To this he says that perfection is not always about control, but about letting go. He then kisses her and she bites him. The next scene shows Nina getting the part, but her fellow dancers being angry with her. She is so happy she cries … then she sees someone has written WHORE on the bathroom mirror.
2 (0:48:45–0:54:35) This scene begins with Nina upset after a difficult practice session. She is tearful and talks to a fellow dancer. She then goes home to take a bath and we see some of the first signs of the stress effecting Nina's psychological well-being. She begins hallucinating and self-mutilating. We then see a scene with Nina's instructor being hard on her again and Nina becoming upset.
    a. These scenes are good examples of instructors/coaches pushing athletes too hard. Discuss the effect this instructor is having on Nina and her health.
    b. These are also good examples of the personal pressure athletes put on

themselves to be perfect. Discuss the effect that perfectionism can have on a person's health and well-being.

c. Discuss what you would do as Nina's physician if she told you about the abnormal hallucinations she is seeing.

d. What is self-mutilation? Why do patients do it and what can be done to help them?

e. What could you do to help support Nina if you were her physician? If you know an athlete has an important event coming up, what preventative measures could you take to help them cope with the stress?

f. In the athlete who already has a known anxiety disorder, obsessive-compulsive tendencies, or perfectionist qualities, how would this change your management?

Further Reading

- Cimino F, Bradford SV, Setter D. Anterior cruciate ligament injury: diagnosis, management, and prevention. *Am Fam Physician*. 2010; **82**(8): 917–22.
- Harmon KG. Assessment and management of concussion in sports. *Am Fam Physician*. 1999; **60**(3): 887–94.
- Jenkinson DM, Harbert AJ. Supplements and sports. *Am Fam Physician*. 2008; **78**(9): 1039–46.
- Joy EA, Van Hala S, Cooper L. Health-related concerns of the female athlete: a lifespan approach. *Am Fam Physician*. 2009; **79**(6): 489–95.
- Kopes-Kerr C. Preventive health: time for change. *Am Fam Physician*. 2010; **82**(6): 610–14.
- McKinley J. New challenges in assessing and managing concussion in sports. *Am Fam Physician*. 2007; **76**(7): 948–9.
- Patel AT, Ogle AA. Diagnosis and management of acute low back pain. *Am Fam Physician*. 2000; **61**(6):1779–86, 1789–90.
- Stephens M. Supplements and sports: honest advice. *Am Fam Physician*. 2008; **78**(9): 1025.

27

Better Safe Than Sorry: Medical Malpractice

Darin Kennedy

Introduction

IN WRITING THIS CHAPTER IN A BOOK WHERE READERS GLEAN THEIR education from mass media, I thought it appropriate to pull the definition of medical malpractice from the most trusted source for information on the Internet: Wikipedia. The article on the subject there begins with the following statement: "Medical malpractice is professional negligence by act or omission by a health care provider in which care provided deviates from accepted standards of practice in the medical community and causes injury or death to the patient."

This chapter is not meant to be an exhaustive read on what does or does not constitute malpractice nor is it meant to discuss the ethics behind litigation either for or against physicians. My goal in this chapter is to provide some good examples of malpractice from the cinema and use these scenes to help learners discuss and learn about this important area. As evidenced by the examples given here, it is far easier to find cinematic examples representing acts of commission rather than the equally dangerous acts of omission. Most of these movies are from the early 1990s, as I was unsuccessful in finding examples from more recent films. Still, the lessons from these scenes are still applicable today. Special thanks to physician assistant Lindsay Kuhn for remembering the medical malpractice facet of *The Fugitive* (1993) and helping me incorporate that classic movie into this chapter.

The God Complex

Malice (1993; Alec Baldwin, Nicole Kidman, Bill Pullman): In this tale of deception and betrayal, Dr. Jed Hill (Baldwin) and Tracy Safian (Kidman) perpetrate an elaborate and cruel fraud in an effort to bilk $20 million from Dr. Hill's malpractice insurance, and in the process, devastate Tracy's loving husband, Andy. There are multiple examples of malpractice in this movie, as will be evidenced in several sections of this chapter.

1   (Ch 16, 0:49:30–0:55:01) In what is probably the most famous scene from this movie, Dr. Hill faces the lawyers in the lawsuit, and when accused of having a "God Complex," he responds in a memorable way.

   a. The arrogance shown by Dr. Hill is over the top, clearly meant to make him appear as the villain in his and Tracy's scheme, but to a degree this attitude/behavior can occur in medical professionals as well as in other professions (professional athletes, entertainers, and so forth). What are the dangers of a person truly believing they are incapable of being wrong?

   b. How would one go about identifying someone with such narcissistic tendencies? What kind of training or therapy might they participate in to help them obtain a more realistic view of their role in society?

2   (Ch 2, 0:06:17–0:07:08) Dr. Hill and his associate Dr. Robertson have a pointed conversation regarding comments Dr. Robertson made in the operating room.

   a. Is there a role for the "God Complex" to some degree? Can such utter confidence actually prove useful? Could his refusal to admit an outcome other than success potentially be a boon to his patients?

Flatliners (1990; Kiefer Sutherland, Julia Roberts, William Baldwin, Oliver Platt, Kevin Bacon): A group of five medical students decide to explore what lies beyond death by conducting a dangerous experiment where each of them, one by one, allows the others to stop their heart for a short time while in a "controlled" environment. As you might expect, their little experiment goes awry and they get answers to questions they wish they had never asked.

1   (Ch 3, 0:07:00–0:11:50; ch 4, 0:14:01–0:24:04) Alec Baldwin's arrogance in *Malice* is in some ways trumped by Kiefer Sutherland's performance of Nelson Wright in *Flatliners*. In this movie, the "God Complex" becomes quite literal as he and the other medical students play with life and death. In the first scene, Nelson manipulates the others to aid in the experiment by appealing to their various personality quirks. In the second scene, his four classmates perform the insane experiment by cooling his body down, then stopping his heart with defibrillator paddles, all in the name of "science."

   a. While some of the aspects of this procedure are not medically accurate, it does raise some interesting philosophical points. Are there lines in medicine that should not be crossed? Is it acceptable for science to pursue answers, regardless of the cost? Apply this thought to issues like stem cell research, end of life, and so forth. Does "can" equal "should"?

   b. *Primum non nocere* First do no harm. Most research trials have the potential to do harm. How do medical professionals who do not know the outcome of their studies ahead of time rationalize the fact that the very treatments/procedures they are testing could in fact be harming the research participants?

Performing Medical Duties While Under the Influence of Alcohol or other Substances

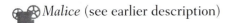*Malice* (see earlier description)

1   (Ch 12, 0:35:43–037:34; ch 13, 0:37:35) Dr. Hill drinks several shots of bourbon while on call, then proceeds to the operating room while under the influence of alcohol to operate on Tracy.
   a. Though this was clearly part of the plan to ensure he would be viewed as guilty, it is unfortunately not unheard of for physicians and other health-care providers to show up for work under the influence of a substance. What are the repercussions on patients and their families of this kind of behavior? On the provider? On the institution?
   b. What programs are available for health-care providers with substance abuse problems?

Molestation

The Hand that Rocks the Cradle (1992; Annabella Sciorra, Rebecca De Mornay, Matt McCoy, Ernie Hudson, Julianne Moore, Madeline Zima, John de Lancie): Although the main story from this film is Rebecca De Mornay's spot-on portrayal of a vengeful manipulating nanny who threatens to tear a family apart, the inciting event of the story is perpetrated by the husband of de Mornay's character.

1   (Ch 3, 0:02:05–0:08:04) In this scene, Dr. Victor Mott, played by the talented John de Lancie, is a gynecologist who molests Claire Bartel (Sciorra) during a routine gynecological exam. Claire tells her husband about the incident and they report Dr. Mott to the authorities. As the story breaks, four other women come forward reporting similar events and Mott commits suicide rather than face public disgrace.
   a. This example goes beyond simple malpractice and enters the realm of assault. What specific actions of Dr. Mott constitute medical malpractice?
   b. This scene is striking in that not only does the doctor send the nurse away but also that she agrees to leave the room knowing he is about to do a pelvic exam. Why is it important to have a chaperone present during examinations of sensitive areas? How does this protect the patient? How does this protect the physician?
   c. Had he not committed suicide, what actions would most likely have been taken against Dr. Mott by the medical board? The police?

 d. How might a malpractice lawyer prosecute such a case?

 e. Similarly, how might Mott's defense attorney have presented this case to shed a different light on his client?

Intentional Maiming

Malice (see earlier description): In the three scenes below, Dr. Hill's less than noble actions and how they fit into the overall plan are revealed.

1 (Ch 13, 037:35–043:46) Dr. Hill performs lifesaving surgery on Tracy by removing the hemorrhaging ovary, only to discover the second ovary has torsed (twisted on its own blood supply) and now appears necrotic (dead). Refusing to wait until he can get pathologic confirmation of the viability of the ovary, he proceeds with removing the ovary.

2 (Ch 14, 0:44:21–046:50) Here, we learn that the ovary was in fact viable and that Tracy plans to sue. Dr. Hill seems appropriately concerned about this, but as evidenced previously in the scene from the lawyer's office, not exceptionally worried.

3 (Ch 25, 1:34:40–1:34:50) Here, we learn that Dr. Hill himself torsed the ovary intentionally to further his and Tracy's plan.

 a. Questions regarding this sequence of scenes seem almost rhetorical, as intentional maiming of patients is clearly unethical, but what about medical treatments that are warranted? Chemotherapy harms the patient even as it treats cancer. Amputation of a gangrenous limb can save a life, though the procedure is forever life changing. Discuss the ethics of such drastic procedures and where the line should be drawn.

 b. When Dr. Hill realizes that Tracy is pregnant, he clearly has a crisis of conscience. Later in the movie, she accuses him of considering letting her bleed out, though his reticence to continue could be also be interpreted as unwillingness to continue with the plan. Consider his motivations and discuss the probable inner debate Dr. Hill dealt with.

Inappropriate Relationships with Patients

1 (Ch 22, 1:20:34–1:21:35) In this scene, Andy learns that Dr. Hill and Tracy are in fact lovers, and he continues to unravel the web of deception at the root of their plan.

 a. What are the ethics, rules, and laws that prohibit sexual relationships between health-care providers and their patients? How are these implemented and policed?

 b. What potential harm can come from such relationships?

Falsifying Data
. . . .

The Fugitive (1993; Harrison Ford, Tommy Lee Jones, Sela Ward, Andreas Katsulas, Jeroen Krabbé): Dr. Richard Kimble (Harrison Ford) is falsely accused of murdering his wife and flees Deputy Samuel Gerard of the US Marshals (Tommy Lee Jones) as he seeks the mysterious "one-armed man" who is the actual murderer.

1 (Ch 18, 1:50:04–1:54:36) In the ultimate confrontation of the movie, Dr. Kimble confronts his friend, Dr. Charles Nichols (Krabbé), as he gives a speech about the new medicine Provasic. In the process of finding the one-armed man, Kimble discovers that he was the target of the murder, not his wife. He also discovers that Nichols planned the murder as part of a plan to cover up the dangerous side effects of Provasic. Nichols, the primary investigator on the drug, is set to receive a financial windfall from Provasic's success. Kimble had investigated the drug and the corresponding pathology slides and had discovered the medicine caused liver damage.

a. What does this confrontation say about the state of the pharmaceutical industry?

b. Should investigators of a drug be in a position to benefit financially when a drug succeeds, or should the research be conducted by independent researchers?

28

Make Me Like New:
Rehabilitation Medicine

Kimberly Romig

SIMPLY STATED, REHABILITATION MEDICINE IS THE ART OF USING multiple therapies in order to restore or maximize a patient's functional ability. The goal is to assist patients in community and vocational reintegration. When such is not possible, the focus becomes to try to lessen a patient's impairment, and to continue to foster skills of autonomy and independence.

Upon closer examination of this process, however, one may find patients dealing with issues of loss of dignity and hope and re-defining their sense of purpose.[1] This search for meaning is often intertwined with one's individual definition of quality of life, a construct that is difficult to measure and to agree upon.[2] The multidisciplinary health-care team is central to the resolution of this struggle. These members are in a position to be active participants in the empowerment, education, and facilitation of patients' self-reliance. Through a bond of trust and mutually agreed upon goals, patients have the opportunity to regain a sense of self-worth and overall well-being.

Yet, this work is not without challenges for the professionals. Health-care providers often struggle with how to communicate that delicate balance between hope and reality and must be mindful of keeping their own emotions in check. Nowhere is this more beautifully depicted than in some of the selected scenes from *The Diving Bell and the Butterfly* (2007).[3] In addition, working with patients whose injuries have caused impairment in insight and preparing families for a change in family relationships are also aspects of the challenge.[4-5]

This chapter has attempted to include films that illustrate different aspects of the rehabilitation process. Viewers are encouraged to explore the various elements of communication and existentialism on the part of both patient and clinician.

The Diving Bell and the Butterfly (2007): Mathieu Amalric (as Jean-Dominique Bauby), Marie-Josée Croze (as Henriette Roi), and Anne Consigny (as Claude) star in this docudrama that exquisitely portrays the life of Jean-Dominique Bauby, editor of Elle fashion magazine, following his massive stroke and diagnosis of locked-in syndrome. Jean-Do, as he is referred to, is paralyzed and unable to communicate in any manner other than to blink one eye. With the support of an extraordinary speech therapist, Henriette, and scribe, Claude, Jean-Do painstakingly dictates the story of his experience through an interactive eye-blink-alphabet system. Please note that the film is in French with subtitles. Jean-Do's inner dialogue is in italics.

Communication and Empathy

1 (0:02:37–0:06:27) Jean-Do wakes from a coma and is initially addressed by physician Dr. Cocheton.
2 (0:08:08–0:11:23) The neurologist, Dr. Lepage, informs Jean-Do that he has locked-in syndrome.
   a. Compare and contrast the communication styles of the physicians.
   b. What are your thoughts on promising recovery to a patient?
   c. What do you think is happening for the neurologist when he asks Jean-Do to "think of him as a friend"?
   d. Comment on Jean-Do's response, "just be a doctor."
   e. Comment on the two physicians' attempts to identify with Jean-Do's experience by making statements such as "you'll be fine," "I know how hard this is for you," and "there's hope." How might patients perceive these statements?
   f. What are the various definitions of hope?

Human Responses in the Health-Care Provider

1 (0:32:39–0:35:11) Jean-Do communicates to the speech therapist, Henriette, that he wants to die. Henriette responds with anger, leaves the room but returns to apologize.
2 (0:39:01–0:40:06) The professional relationship continues …
   a. As a health-care professional, how do you separate your personal and professional values from those of your patients?
   b. What is it like for you as a health-care professional to listen and respond to a patient's emotional pain?
   c. Discuss Henriette's ability to take responsibility for her behavior.
   d. How would you suggest moving forward in a patient-professional relationship following a mistake in professional judgment?
   e. Who is available to you for support following a difficult interaction with a patient?

Loss of Control

1 (0:24:51–0:26:25; 1:04:34–1:04:57; 1:07:49–1:08:29) These scenes illustrate just some of many experiences Jean-Do has with feeling a loss of control.
    a. As a health-care provider, how can you remain cognizant of a patient's need for control?
    b. In what ways can you communicate to a patient that you are aware of their sense of helplessness?
    c. What steps can you take to ensure that a rehabilitation team also remains vigilant to the issue of loss of control?
    d. For those who regularly work with patients in this capacity, comment on how you keep yourselves from becoming immune to patients' concerns.

Finding Meaning

1 (00:37:20–00:43:13) Jean-Do begins to reframe his thoughts and attitudes in an attempt to find meaning in his life.
    a. What are some of the elements of an existential crisis?
    b. What are some of the spiritual concerns that patients with locked-in syndrome or other medical situations might be experiencing?
    c. How do you encourage a patient's search for meaning in the midst of a despairing situation?
    d. Which disciplines might you engage to assist a patient with these concerns?
    e. It is sometimes inferred in the medical community that the development of pneumonia in an incapacitated patient may be a welcomed event as it usually leads to the patient's demise. Discuss this concept in the context of Jean-Do's accomplishments. Is Jean-Do's experience the norm? What other forms of "meaning" exist for patients and who should determine what is a meaningful existence?
    f. Discuss your own experiences with patients and their search for meaning.

Beyond Medical Rehabilitation: Living With a Disability

Rory O'Shea Was Here (*Inside I'm Dancing*) (2004): James McAvoy (as Rory O'Shea), Steven Robertson (as Michael Connolly), and Romola Garai (as Siobhan) star in this film about Rory O'Shea, a rebellious wheelchair-bound young man with multiple sclerosis. He moves into an institutional congregate living home where he befriends Michael, who is also wheelchair bound. Michael has cerebral palsy and his speech and motor skills are severely impaired. Only Rory seems to be able to understand what Michael tries to communicate. Together, Rory and Michael strive for independence and some sense of normalcy in a world where they are defined by their disabilities and limitations.

1 (000:12:30–0:13:56) Rory wants to "be like everyone else" despite his limitations.
2 (0:28:55–0:32:27) Rory applies for independent living benefits and must defend his position in front of a panel of evaluators.
3 (0:33:11–0:33:46) Michael applies for independent living status as well.
4 (0:34:11–0:36:36) Because of Michael's communication limitations, Rory interprets for Michael as he goes before the evaluation panel.
5 (1:32:37–1:36:12) Michael advocates for Rory's right for independent living despite the fact that Rory is actively dying.
   a. How would you expand your definition of rehabilitation to include living with a disability?
   b. At what point during the acute rehabilitation phase is a determination of long-term disability made?
   c. Following the acute rehabilitation phase, what types of social or medical rehabilitation programs are available in your community for patients with disabilities?
   d. What are the eligibility requirements for Medicaid and Supplemental Security Income? How does a disabled person under the age of 65 qualify for Medicare?
   e. How do you help a patient and family make the physical, social, and emotional transition from having rehabilitation potential to being disabled?
   f. Discuss a disabled person's desire to "fit in" with the nondisabled population.
   g. How would you motivate a disabled patient to move toward or sustain his or her autonomy and productivity?
   h. Discuss the Americans with Disabilities Act of 1990.

Regarding Henry (1991): Harrison Ford (as Henry Turner) Annette Bening (as Sarah Turner), Mikki Allen (as Rachel Turner), and Bill Nunn (as Bradley) star in this movie depicting the life of an ambitious, driven lawyer (Henry Turner) whose self-absorption has cost him his relationship with his wife (Sarah Turner) and daughter (Rachel Turner). Henry leaves home one night to buy a pack of cigarettes, interrupts a robbery in progress, and suffers a gunshot wound to the head. He experiences an anoxic brain injury and amnesia. He must then put the pieces back together of a life he does not remember and no longer functions well in. With the assistance of his physical therapist and the patience of his family, he must reconcile with the person that he was prior to the injury and find new meaning in his life. Although the relationship with his physical therapist is key, one is reminded that the most difficult part of rehabilitation takes place outside of the medical setting during the arduous process of reintegration into professional, family, and social life.

Scenes have been grouped so as to offer more logical and thorough discussions.

Communicating Prognosis

1 (0:17:19–0:19:17) The physician explains Henry's condition and prognosis for recovery to Sarah.
2 (0:19:17–0:19:56) Sarah explains Henry's condition and prognosis to their daughter.
   a. Assess the physician's communication skills in relaying this information.
   b. Discuss the balance between hope and reality when having to communicate prognosis.
   c. Contrast the physician's delivery of information to Sarah with Sarah's delivery of the information to her daughter.
   d. How, as health-care professionals, can we assist families in communicating difficult news to their children or other family members?

The Role of the Physical Therapist

1 (0:23:08–0:25:43) Henry begins therapy and meets his physical therapist, Bradley.
2 (0:27:56–0:30:40) Breakfast with Bradley.
3 (0:32:00–0:34:00) Henry begins working with the walker.
4 (0:34:00–0:35:14) Henry practices on his own.
5 (0:35:14–0:35:53) Bradley makes personal disclosures to Henry.
   a. Comment on the style/approach of the physical therapist, Bradley.
   b. What is the impact of unconventional methods on the relationship between patient and health-care worker? Does this impact the ability to motivate patients in general?
   c. As a health-care provider, what techniques can you use to motivate behavior change in a patient?
   d. What are the parameters for sharing personal information with patients? Is it ever permissible, and, if so, what kind of information and under what circumstances?

Facing Uncertainties

1 (0:35:54–0:38:10) Henry is being discharged from the rehabilitation unit and tells Bradley he does not want to go.
2 (0:38:10–0:39:43) Family arrives to take Henry home, but he is resistant.
3 (0:39:43–0:40:40) Physician expresses reservations about Henry's readiness to return home, and Bradley attempts to talk with Rachel.
   a. What do you think Henry fears most about returning home?
   b. Would you expect the family's concerns to be the same or different?

    c. What do these scenes say about the value of multidisciplinary family meetings?

    d. If this were your patient, how would you facilitate a family meeting? How would you address Henry's feelings of dependence on the physical therapist?

    e. On what opportunities did Bradley miss out when talking with Rachel?

Changes in Roles

1 (0:40:40–0:41:54) Rachel teaches her father how to tie his shoes.

2 (0:45:48–0:46:29) Recognizing that family dynamics will be different.

3 (0:53:57–0:55:44) Rachel teaches her father about library etiquette.

    a. What other roles would you expect to change in a family when a member is impaired?

    b. What emotions would you anticipate arising for both patients and families?

    c. Are there any other interventions that the physical therapist could have utilized to assist the patient and family in preparing for future role changes?

Depression and Social Judgments

1 (1:23:40–1:29:00) Henry sinks into depression following a party where he overhears "friends" being insensitive about his impairments. Sarah asks Bradley to intervene.

    a. As a health-care provider, how do you facilitate patients' coping with new limitations?

    b. Bradley comments on his feelings of professional and personal satisfaction for his part in Henry's recovery. Recount one patient encounter that has made you feel glad you chose to be a health-care provider.

Cultural Considerations

1 How might things have been different if Henry and his family were of another ethnicity and culture (e.g., consider the patient population in your area of practice) in terms of:

    a. the delivery of health care?

    b. a philosophy of and expectations for recovery?

    c. comfort level of expressing fears and concerns?

2 As a health-care provider, what can you ask that would open the door for cultural dialogue with any given patient and his or her family members?

The Ballerina and the Physical Therapist
. . . .

Black Swan (2010): Starring Natalie Portman (as Nina Sayers), Vincent Cassel (as Thomas Leroy), Mila Kunis (as Lily), and Barbara Hershey (as Erica Sayers), *Black Swan* is a psychological thriller set in the world of professional ballet. Emotionally fragile Nina, who lives under the rigid control of her former-ballet-dancer mother, is chosen to play the principal role of Swan Queen in Tchaikovsky's *Swan Lake*. Nina becomes obsessed and consumed by the dual role, loses her grip on reality, and pays both the physical and emotional price for elusive perfection.

1 (0:45:54–0:46:34) During film production, Natalie Portman sustained a dislocated rib and was treated by real physical therapist Michelle Rodriguez. The session was filmed and included in the final production. Compared with the other movies in this chapter, this scene has a markedly different feel as one observes the genuine intimate nature of work between a professional ballerina and her physical therapist.

   a. Discuss the level of trust that must exist between a professional dancer and a physical therapist.

   b. Discuss the goal of returning an injured dancer back to performance level.

   c. What must the physical therapist or other health-care provider understand about the mind-set, characteristics, and expectations of both a professional dancer and the ballet world itself?

   d. As a health-care provider, to what additional resources besides physical therapy might you refer for an injured professional dancer?

   e. What advice or education would you give to the parents of a young ballet dancer on injury prevention and early treatment?

The Unique Nature of a Sports Injury
. . . .

Just Wright (2010): Starring Queen Latifah (as Leslie Wright), Paula Patton (as Morgan Alexander), Common (as Scott McNight), and Phylicia Rashad (as Scott's mother), *Just Wright* is a romantic comedy about a physical therapist (Leslie Wright) who falls for a professional basketball player (Scott McNight) while helping him recover from an injury that is predicted to end his career. Included are action scenes from some professional games.

1 (0:32:56–0:34:24) Scott gets injured during a game.

2 (0:34:27–0:35:35) The diagnosis, treatment plan, and reactions of family and coaches.

   a. What are the various issues that arise in treating a professional sports player?

   b. Are the goals of therapy the same for a professional sports player as they are for a layperson?

   c. How do you imagine that team physicians, sports trainers, and allied

health-care professionals maintain their composure and objectivity immediately following a player's injury?
   d. How does a health-care professional protect an injured player's well-being
   when those around him/her might have a different agenda?
   e. What psychosocial concerns are present for an injured minor/professional
   sports player?

The Hard Work

1 (0:37:34–0:39:19) Leslie begins as Scott's physical therapist and impresses
   his mother with her knowledge of basketball.
2 (0:39:19–0:40:25) Physical therapy in progress.
3 (0:40:32–0:40:54) Leslie has professional doubts.
4 (1:29:16–1:30:50) Scott credits Leslie on national television for his recovery.
   a. What characteristics make up the unique relationship between a patient
   and a physical therapist?
   b. How does personality (both the therapist's and the patient's) impact the
   therapy?
   c. As a health-care professional, how do you cope with the enormous sense
   of responsibility for your patients' outcomes?

Coping with Difficult News

1 (0:41:56–0:43:09) A teammate tells Scott there is a rumor that he will not
   be re-signed.
2 (0:43:15–0:44:17) Scott hears the rumor in a public forum.
3 (0:46:57–0:47:44) Leslie's attempt to provide emotional support is met with
   Scott's anger.
   a. Within your particular scope of practice, how do you support someone
   who is grappling with difficult news?
   b. What are some ways to deal with anger specifically? How do you protect
   yourself emotionally?
   c. In this film, Scott's fiancé copes through avoidance, shopping, and ultimately breaks off the relationship. What other coping mechanisms might
   present in family members or close friends?

Moving Through and Out of Depression

1 (0:47:49–0:50:00) Leslie remains consistent in her attempts to work with
   Scott.
2 (0:51:51–0:54:36) Scott finds his motivation.

a. What is the prevalence of depression in the occupational and physical therapy patient population?
b. Within your own health-care discipline, how would you intervene with a depressed patient?
c. Do drastic measures (such as Leslie throwing a bucket of ice on Scott) have any merit?
d. What are some techniques that can be used to encourage frustrated patients?
e. How do agreed-upon goals between the patient and the health-care professional influence behavior?

References

1 Chisholm N, Gillett G. The patient's journey: living with locked-in syndrome. *BMJ*. 2005; **331**(7508): 94–7.
2 Tulsky DS, Rosenthal M. Measurement of quality of life in rehabilitation medicine: emerging issues. *Arch Phys Med Rehabil*. 2003; **84**(4 Suppl. 2): S1–2.
3 Alexander M. Movies in medical education. *Fam Med*. 2009; **41**(3): 215.
4 Conan N. Setting goals, rehabilitation after brain injury [interview transcription]. *Talk of the Nation*. National Public Radio. 2011 May 16. Available at: www.npr.org/templates/story/story.php?storyId=136363460 (last accessed 12/01/11).
5 Schmidt S, Bullinger M. Current issues in cross-cultural quality of life instrument development. *Arch Phys Med Rehabil*. 2003; **84**(4 Suppl 2): S29–34.

Additional Films for Consideration

- *My Left Foot* (1989)
- *The Horse Whisperer* (1998)
- *The Waterdance* (1992)
- *Soul Surfer* (2011)

29

Bringing the War Home:
Military Medicine/Psychology

Douglas McGeachy & Michael Metal

STUDIES SUGGEST THAT 5%–15% OF SERVICE MEMBERS MAY RETURN from combat with posttraumatic stress disorder (PTSD) and between 2% and 14% will suffer from major depression.[1] Whether brought on by vicarious trauma or direct injuries, it is estimated that there are more than 300 000 service members suffering from PTSD or severe depression.[1] The consequences of mental health conditions may grow more severe, especially if left untreated.[1]

Although physical injuries can be devastating, improved medical treatments and technology have helped many of these patients make significant recoveries. Not surprisingly, however, the enormous impact that "invisible injuries" such as PTSD, depression, and traumatic brain injuries have on our service personnel is well documented.[1] Linkages also have been found between chronic pain and PTSD, which may result in increased levels of anger, irritability, negativity, and anxiety. Individuals with physical injuries may be at a higher risk of developing PTSD if their pain is not controlled effectively. Therefore, a comprehensive treatment plan including pain management is needed.[2]

A disproportionate number of army soldiers and marines are at increased risk for PTSD or depression since these branches of the military are exposed most often to combat areas. In addition, individuals serving in reserve units, people who are no longer on active duty, enlisted personnel, women, and Hispanics also have higher rates of PTSD or major depression.[1] While there is a correlation between PTSD and/or major depression and those military personnel who either have served extended combat tours ranging from 12 to 15 months in duration or have had more-extensive exposure to combat traumas,[1] there is additional evidence that dose exposure impacts the successful treatment of PTSD. Service members who have sustained high doses of traumatic exposure have a reduced chance of PTSD remission and are more likely to develop lifetime PTSD symptoms.[3]

If not treated in an efficient and effective manner, these conditions can be complicated by the patient's inability to reintegrate into relationships or society as a whole. Left untreated, these factors will ultimately produce unintended consequences such as strained relationships, self-destructive behavior (self-medicating, overeating, high-risk sexual behavior, and so forth) and increased risk for suicide. Anger and aggression are commonly manifested in those service personnel who have experienced military-related trauma or who have been diagnosed with PTSD. These behaviors not only restrict social interaction but also serve to alienate the family members who are most likely to provide help. Sometimes the families themselves become the target of the veteran's aggressive behavior.[4] Veterans with heightened hyperarousal levels and a history of alcohol problems have demonstrated a higher frequency of aggression.[4]

There are significant factors affecting the effective treatment of PTSD. First, veterans who are experiencing distress that threatens their masculinity may be more likely to avoid behaviors consistent with trauma recovery. This may contribute to the high treatment dropout rates of Operation Iraqi Freedom and Operation Enduring Freedom veterans.[5] Second, studies have shown that family functioning levels impact the veteran's progress during treatment. Current research suggests that veterans and their partners benefit from couple or family therapy where the involved partners gain a greater understanding of PTSD to increase internal family support mechanisms.[6] In particular, studies show that as relationship adjustment improves and intimacy increases, not only were significant others more likely to participate in treatment options but also veterans themselves were more likely to utilize treatment services.[7] This is particularly important since support from family, significant others, and military peers tends to have the greatest positive influence on the veteran over other support systems.[8]

There are several areas where the available health-care system could improve to achieve greater success in the treatment of our veterans. First, the continuity of care must be improved. Due to the frequency of comorbidity among service members, the various treatments must be coordinated in a way that ensures doctors and clinicians work together toward a common goal while reducing the impact on the patient. Second, family members must be included in the treatment process. Third, the ability to discretely access mental health services needs to be improved. When surveyed, service members indicated overwhelmingly that some of the reasons they do not seek out mental health services include the notion that they would be perceived as weak, leadership might treat them differently, and peers would have less confidence in them. Fewer respondents, although still in significant numbers, indicated they believed mental health treatments could harm their careers (e.g. prevent them from obtaining a security clearance), it was too difficult to make an appointment, they were too embarrassed, or there was a lack of trust in mental health professionals.[1]

Treating our military veterans is a difficult but extremely important task. They have been asked to serve in some of the most difficult conditions and have witnessed unthinkable tragedies. Often these sacrifices have occurred at young ages where the service member had minimal life experience, making events even more difficult to comprehend, particularly when the negative experiences involve the significant injury or death of their friends. Taking steps to close some of these gaps will help to increase the treatment rates of our military veterans. These young men and women have contributed significantly to the safety and security of our country so the least we can do is provide them with the best possible care upon their return so they may assimilate back into society and lead successful lives.

Years of training, deployments, and combat tours only add to the plethora of experiences that have required military personnel to work long hours, spend months away from their families, and endure hardships that most cannot even imagine. Understanding these warriors is critical and some of the movie clips in this chapter provide the viewer with a glimpse into that world where the true warriors of our time live.

Public Views and Understanding of Posttraumatic Stress Disorder: From World War II to the Korean Conflict

Chattahoochee (1989; Gary Oldman, Dennis Hopper, Frances McDormand): Emmet Foley (Oldman) is a combat decorated Korean War veteran who returns home suffering the effects of PTSD. His difficulties readjusting to society culminate in his attempted "suicide by cop" which results in his imprisonment in an asylum for the criminally insane.

1 (0:01:30–0:01:50) The movie begins with a monologue talking about expectations of a person returning home with combat decorations.
   a. What do you feel are common expectations of how a person decorated for valor in combat should behave? What are the societal expectations?
   b. What impact do these expectations potentially have on someone struggling with the trauma that resulted in their decorations?
   c. What do you think the differences are between survivor guilt and PTSD? What treatments would be most effective?

2 (0:03:10–0:03:50) A monologue from Emmet's wife (McDormand) questions how things occurred. She asks if and how she could have seen it coming.
   a. What are the potential warning signs of the onset of PTSD?
   b. How can those close to a military combatant become more aware of the signs?
   c. If signs are seen by those in contact with someone suffering from PTSD, what can they do to help that person?

3 (0:33:35–0:36:15) A preacher is praying for the evil to be banished from Emmet.
   a. How was PTSD viewed during the Korean War era?
   b. How has/hasn't the perception of mental health treatment changed since this time period?

4 (0:42:00–0:44:11) Emmet fights to defend a weaker inmate from abuse at the hands of the prison guards.

a. How does helping others appear to help Emmet appease his own stress disorder?

b. Is the defense of a weaker person in keeping with what you know of combat PTSD? Why?

5 (1:19:00–1:22:53) Emmet is subjected to shock therapy.

a. What were the common therapies utilized in this era?

b. How has the role of social workers changed?

c. What stigmas existed surrounding those who sought or received therapy?

d. What role does electroconvulsive therapy have currently?

Windtalkers (2002; Nicholas Cage, Adam Beach, Peter Stormare, Jason Isaacs). Nicholas Cage plays Sgt Enders, a troubled marine fighting in the Pacific during World War II. After being the lone survivor of a bloody campaign, he is given a grim assignment that will test his abilities.

1 (0:15:20–0:16:25) The Major (Isaccs) tells Sgt Enders that he has done better as a marine than he did as a civilian.

a. How is the idea that the military "straightened out" Sgt Enders consistent with popular concepts of the effect of the military on misguided youth?

b. What factors do you think play into this transformation?

c. How can these factors be applied in a traditional household?

d. What negative effects can this transformation have on a person?

2 (0:26:38–0:30:25): The Gunnery Sgt (Stormare) gives a speech to motivate the troops while Sgt Enders has a flashback.

a. Why does the Gunnery Sgt need to give a motivational speech before going to war?

b. What factors contribute to the onset of the flashbacks for Sgt Enders?

c. Private Yahzee (Beach) is turned away from Sgt Enders when attempting to help him. How is this behavior consistent with PTSD and how can it be circumvented?

3 (0:48:00–0:52:17) The marines sit around after combat action reminiscing about places and women back home.

a. What protective factors are displayed in this scene?

b. What does storytelling do for people?

4 (0:59:00–0:60:10) In this scene the marines are reading mail and writing letters.

a. What is the impact of correspondence from home on a service member? Does it have a beneficial or harmful effect on a service member's mental state?

b. What is the potential positive and negative impact of the increase in technology on the service members?

c. What is the potential impact of technology on the families of the service members?

Indoctrination into the United States Marine Corps (or Military Service in General)

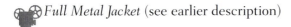 *Full Metal Jacket* (1987; Matthew Modine, Adam Baldwin, Vincent D'Onofrio, Arliss Howard, Lee Ermey): This is a provocative movie describing the experiences of young men as they enter the United States Marine Corps during the Vietnam War era. Beginning with the rigorous boot camp indoctrination at the hands of Gunnery Sergeant Hartman (Ermey), the recruits with colorful nicknames like Joker (Modine), Animal Mother (Baldwin), Gomer Pyle (D'Onofrio), and Cowboy (Howard) try to survive as the hardened drill instructor prepares them for the realities of war. Following a tragic end to boot camp when Pyle suffers an emotional breakdown and kills Gunnery Sergeant Hartman, the remaining recruits are deployed into the combat theater where they experience harsh conditions while fighting a formidable enemy combatant.

1 (0:00:00–0:07:31) In this segment, the initial experiences of boot camp unfold. While the "reality check" that new recruits experience is accurately portrayed, the viewer must be cautioned that the actions of the drill instructor are exaggerated in this "made for Hollywood" version of Marine Corps boot camp. Nevertheless, boot camp is certainly one of the toughest and most life-changing experiences a person can endure.

   a. How do the expectations of the new recruits correlate to their prior civilian lives?
   b. What preparation did the recruits have for this experience?
   c. How will boot camp serve to change these individuals in the short and long term?
   d. How can someone that has never undergone such an experience relate to a person that has completed boot camp?

The Trials of Combat

Full Metal Jacket (see earlier description)

1 (1:19:44–1:22:53) In this series of interviews with the characters, they express their feelings and opinions about serving in the Marine Corps during a combat tour in Vietnam.

   a. How do the marines feel about their service?
   b. Do they feel as though their sacrifices are appreciated?
   c. What are some of the difficulties they express? Do those same difficulties still exist now?

A Look Back

• • • • • • • • • • • • • • • •

Full Metal Jacket (see earlier description)

1 (1:51:50–1:52:30) Joker reflects back on his boot camp experience in light of what he has learned during combat.
  a. How does Joker view his boot camp experiences in hindsight?
  b. Is it common for people to look back at past experiences and have a greater appreciation for the lessons they learned than they had at the time?

The Destiny of War

• •

Forrest Gump (1994; Tom Hanks, Robin Wright, Gary Sinise, Mykelti Williamson, Sally Field): The movie chronicles the life of Forrest Gump (Hanks), who may not have the highest IQ but certainly has determination and a moral compass like no other. Beginning as a disabled boy, Forrest is cared for by his loving mother (Field) as he grows to be a great runner and football star, all the while in love with his childhood sweetheart Jenny Curran (Wright). Forrest then joins the Army to serve his country during Vietnam and meets his best friend Benjamin Buford "Bubba" Blue (Williamson) and their platoon leader, Lieutenant Dan Taylor, aka "Lt. Dan" (Sinise). Forrest utilizes his talents as he rescues several members of his platoon after coming under heavy fire that kills Bubba. Forrest returns from war a hero but continues to deal with adversity in his relationships with his mother, Jenny, Lt. Dan, and Bubba's family. Forrest Gump is an instant classic that gives hope that everyday people can achieve greatness.

1 (0:44:14–1:01:58) Forrest arrives in Vietnam with Bubba where they meet Lt. Dan. During a patrol, the platoon comes under heavy fire injuring several in their unit. Destined to be an unintentional hero, a wounded Forrest carries several soldiers to safety including Lt. Dan. After being evacuated, Forrest and Lt. Dan share a hospital room, where they discuss the consequences of his actions.
  a. How did Forrest and Lt. Dan fulfill their destinies?
  b. How did this affect each of them?
  c. How might these competing views be applied to current service members serving in times of combat?

The Tale of Two Warriors

• •

Taking Chance (2009): Starring Kevin Bacon, this is a powerful and heart-wrenching tale of Lieutenant Colonel Michael Strobl (Bacon) who is serving in a stateside administrative assignment while in the United States Marine Corps. Lt. Col. Strobl finds himself on an emotional rollercoaster as he fights his own personal battle against feelings of inadequacy because he has not been deployed to the combat theater, along with a sense of guilt that he chose to remain with his wife and children rather than to be with his fellow Marines. Lt. Col. Strobl volunteers to escort the body of fallen Lance Corporal Chance Phelps to his home town in Wyoming. During the journey, Lt. Col. Strobl experiences the sorrows of the entire nation that will forever change his life.

1   (0:00:00–0:20:05) During this opening segment of the movie, the viewers are introduced to the two main characters of the movie. The first is Lt. Col. Strobl and the other is L/Cpl. Chance Phelps. The movie switches back and forth between these two very different characters. Strobl is a senior marine officer serving in the United States. He works in an office and goes home every night. Phelps, on the other hand, is making the journey home after being killed in action during Operation Iraqi Freedom.

    a. How does Strobl view his role as a marine serving in an administrative assignment during a time of war? How do others view him in the Marine Corps?

    b. How does Strobl view the competing interests of his sense of duty to the Marine Corps and his commitment to his family?

    c. How did Phelps' introduction into the movie impact those assigned to bring him home to his family with dignity and honor?

The Consequences of War on the Civilian Population

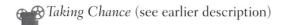 *Taking Chance* (see earlier description)

1   (0:20:05–0:29:50; 0:34:48–0:39:21) While service members may believe there is a disconnect between themselves and the general public, the reality is that a lot of civilians truly appreciate their service and the sacrifices they make on behalf of our country. These scenes demonstrate the many ways in which Strobl encounters civilians that fit this bill.

    a. How do the consequences of war affect the general public?

    b. How can the actions of civilians help or hinder those serving in the Armed Forces?

    c. Was Strobl prepared for the treatment he received? How did it make him feel?

    d. Does the response of the public in *Taking Chance* differ from that of past wars? How can we use this positive response to help our returning veterans?

The Importance of Being Part of the Team

Success in the military is often gauged by a person's leadership and teamwork. Being able to support the mission of the team in a positive way is essential. Conversely, failure can often lead to alienation and personal feelings of failure and/or inadequacy. This is particularly true during times of adversity or combat when members of a military unit depend on one another.

Difficulty Fitting In

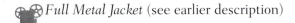*Full Metal Jacket* (see earlier description)

1   (0:08:39–0:09:57) Private Pyle (D'Onofrio) experiences difficulties performing rifle drills with his platoon, subjecting him to severe criticism and abuse from Gunnery Sergeant Hartman (Ermey).
    a. How important is it for Pyle to fit in?
    b. How does Pyle respond to the feedback provided by Gunnery Sergeant Hartman?
    c. Have the expectations of Pyle been made clear to him?
    d. What effects does this treatment have on Pyle?
    e. While the overarching goal of Gunnery Sergeant Hartman is to make Private Pyle a team player, is his "one-size-fits-all" approach effective?

Building Teamwork?

1   (0:13:20–0:17:32) In this scene, we see how difficult it is for Private Pyle to adapt to the Marine Corps' standards. While the viewer doesn't know if Pyle is working as hard as he possibly can to achieve success, we can tell that he falls short more often than not. This not only becomes frustrating to the drill instructor but also to Pyle's peers in his platoon.
    a. How do Private Pyle's failures affect others in the platoon?
    b. Does the boot camp experience, as portrayed in *Full Metal Jacket*, encourage teamwork?

Enough is Enough

1   (0:28:11–0:30:11) After numerous failures by Private Pyle, the platoon members have reached their wits end and finally decide to take matters into their own hands.
    a. How does the platoon express their displeasure with Pyle?
    b. How effective is their message?

   c. Do their actions serve to make Private Pyle a member of the group?

Casualties of War May Have a Far-Reaching Impact

Taking Chance (see earlier description)

1 (0:29:50–0:32:36) During a flight layover, Strobl (Bacon) encounters an army sergeant (Noah Fleiss) who is also escorting a deceased serviceman home. At the onset he thinks they have something in common, but he quickly learns that is not the case.
   a. Strobl initially felt he had something in common with the army sergeant. How did that change during their conversation?
   b. How does this scene take vicarious trauma to a new level?
   c. How well do we understand the selflessness of families throughout our nation that have multiple children serving their country during a time of war?

Meeting the Family

1 (1:00:46–1:04:32) Strobl meets Phelps's family and returns Phelps's property to them. During the meeting, Strobl has an opportunity to tell the family how proud they should be of Phelps and also communicate his experiences while escorting Phelps home.
   a. How does this experience impact Strobl? Will this encounter end up being a positive or negative event in Strobl's life?
   b. What affect does the meeting have on the family?
   c. Does Strobl try to make the family part of the Marine Corps team?

The Impact of Losing a Parent to Military Service and Role Reversal

Grace is Gone (2007; John Cusack, Shélan O'Keefe, Gracie Bednarczyk, Doug James): The movie tells the story of a military family whose parent is killed in combat. This film is different because it focuses on the issues faced by the surviving spouse, a father (Cusack), who now must tell his two young daughters that their mother is never coming home.
1 (0:01:50–0:4:00) Stan (John Cusack) is sitting in a military spouse support group. It becomes clear that he is both the only and the first man to be in this group.
   a. What are the common ideas of a military spouse and how does this scene run contrary to them?
   b. The wives in the group engage in conversations that make Stan feel

uncomfortable. How is this scene different from commonplace society? How are Stan's feelings different from or similar to those that a woman may feel?

2   (0:06:55–0:10:05) The army chaplain (James) comes to the house to notify Stan of Grace's death. He tells Stan that he has 45 days to remain in base housing and offers assistance.

   a. What is the impact of placing timelines on a person who is dealing with trauma?

   b. In what ways could things have been done differently and how would these changes likely have changed the outcome?

   c. What role does emotional support play in helping a family through trauma?

   d. What impact does losing a parent at war have on a child?

   e. What do Stan's actions indicate may be happening and what impact could this have on the family?

3   (0:45:23–0:48:30) Stan and Heidi talk about Grace being deployed but her death is still unknown.

   a. How does open communication aid family resiliency?

   b. What role does gender play in talking about feelings?

   c. How does this conversation appear to help both Stan and Heidi?

The Effects of Compounding Trauma

Compounding trauma refers to traumatic experiences, caused by wartime experiences such as seeing a dead body, handling remains, or knowing someone who has been killed. As demonstrated in the literature review, compounding trauma can be a significant trigger for PTSD symptoms. The clips below depict some examples of compounding trauma and the effects they have on the subjects of those experiences.

The Mental Breakdown

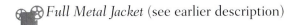 *Full Metal Jacket* (see earlier description)

1   (0:30:11–0:35:50) Private Pyle clearly begins to disconnect from the rest of his platoon. His actions cause Joker to become concerned for Pyle's mental health but has this realization come too late?

   a. How clear is Pyle's disconnect to the rest of his platoon?

   b. How do the members of Pyle's platoon try to help him? Did they do enough?

   c. Are there any key indicators that should have raised a red flag for the drill instructor or the others in Pyle's platoon?

The End of Boot Camp

1   (0:40:00–0:45:22) Despite successfully completing boot camp, the damage to Private Pyle has been done. While standing fire watch, Joker encounters Pyle and finds himself in a position for which he is unprepared.
   a. How clear is it to Joker that Pyle is in distress?
   b. How effective is Gunnery Sergeant Hartman's approach to this problem?
   c. What will be the potential impacts, both immediate as well as long-term, on Joker and the rest of his platoon?

The Lack of Control

1   (1:25:30–1:51:00) The platoon comes under sniper fire and must figure out a way to eliminate the threat, among fears that additional forces are in their midst. As a result, platoon members are killed before they are able to capture the sniper. Because of the trauma they were exposed to, the members of the platoon then find themselves facing an ethical dilemma once the sniper is captured.
   a. What impact may we expect of service members who are subjected to seeing their peers killed in action?
   b. How does this situation prompt some individuals to act while others cannot? What lasting effects can either of these courses of action have on those involved?
   c. How does the team approach the ethical dilemma of dealing with a wounded sniper? As she begs them to shoot her, the marines wrestle with the idea but if they choose to, will their actions be merciful or murderous? How will their actions impact them in the long term?

The Path of Self-Destruction

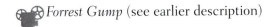 *Forrest Gump* (see earlier description)

1   (1:15:21–1:23:44) Lt. Dan seeks out Forrest and renews their already strained relationship. During their time together, Forrest watches as Lt. Dan battles his demons and as he tries to cope with life and being a double amputee.
   a. How does Lt. Dan deal with the physical and emotional scars of combat?
   b. How likely is it that this path will lead him to successfully overcome his disability?
   c. What can be done to prevent this self-destructive behavior?

Looking in the Rearview Mirror

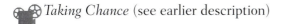*Taking Chance* (see earlier description)

1   (0:50:50–0:58:58) Strobl attends an event at the local VFW where he meets many of Phelps's friends as well as a few marines including Phelps's recruiter and a sergeant that was with Phelps when he died. They all share stories with Strobl about how Phelps lived before and during his time in the Marine Corps. Strobl also learns how the events unfolded leading up to Phelps's death.
    a. How does this event personalize the mission for Strobl?
    b. How did Phelps's death impact those in his unit?
    c. Why does Strobl question his worth as a warrior? Why does he feel guilty that he has been able to remain at home with his family while others are fighting a war?
    d. How do the competing interests of duty and family affect our service members?

The Emotional Toll of Combat

Restrepo (2010): This is a documentary about a US Army platoon from Battle Company, 2nd of the 503rd Infantry Regiment, 173rd Airborne Combat Team assigned to the Korengal Valley in Afghanistan during a planned 15-month deployment. The movie, named for the platoon's medic who was killed in action, chronicles the experiences of the soldiers serving in one of the US military's most dangerous duty assignments. This film is unique because it provides an actual glimpse at the harsh realities experienced by service members assigned to a combat tour. This is the closest viewers can get to combat without enlisting themselves. This movie not only presents live footage of combat action but also powerful interviews with soldiers in the midst of combat operations. *Restrepo* is a must-see for any health-care provider who truly wants to understand military or combat experience.

1   (Ch 4, 0:12:40–0:14:05; ch 10, 1:00:38–1:08:52; ch 11, 1:12:15–1:13:20) In these three scenes, interviews with various members of the platoon describe the extreme difficulties associated with losing peers during combat operations.
    a. Do the soldiers interviewed in these scenes have a higher propensity to suffer from PTSD or major depression when compared to other service members assigned to areas that were not subjected to the same level of combat in the Korengal Valley?
    b. Do any of these soldiers demonstrate masculine traits that may inhibit their ability to deal with these experiences or seek treatment?
    c. What type of treatment plan would be most effective for the various soldiers interviewed in this scene?

Dealing with Trauma at an Organizational Level

Significant traumatic events and the resulting effects, whether physical or emotional, not only impact the person but also the organization as a whole. In order to carry out the mission, the organization must also address these issues on a global scale to ensure service members are capable of carrying out the tasks at hand. In the following movie segments, assess the level of success in which the organization attends to traumatic events and how well they balance the competing interests between mission success and sustained healing.

Dealing with Repeated Failure

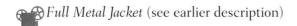 *Full Metal Jacket* (see earlier description)

1   (0:23:47–0:27:40) Private Pyle continues to fail in his quest to fit in with the standards and requirements of the United States Marine Corps. As a result, the platoon is punished for Pyle's transgressions because they have not helped him achieve success. Pyle clearly understands the difficulties he experiences and asks for help.
    a. How do Pyle's failures affect the rest of his platoon?
    b. As a representative of the organization, does Gunnery Sergeant Hartman effectively deal with these issues in a way that will encourage unit harmony?
    c. Does Pyle effectively ask for help? How likely is it that his audience will understand the call for help he is trying to make?

A Sense of Duty

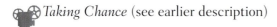 *Taking Chance* (see earlier description)

1   (Ch 6, 0:32:37–0:34:36) During an overnight layover, Strobl decides to spend the night in the warehouse with Phelps instead of going to his hotel.
    a. How does this sense of duty and service differ from that of the average organization or worker?

Vicarious Trauma

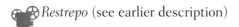 *Restrepo* (see earlier description)

1   (Ch 12, 1:19:40–1:22:51) News arrives that nine soldiers from a sister Company were killed and 25 others were wounded during combat operations.

This information clearly spurs an emotional response from the troops. In an effort to deal with this issue, Captain Kearney addresses the platoon to provide them with information, discuss the incident, and bring perspective to their mission.

  a. Understanding that resources were probably not available in this remote area, was the manner in which Captain Kearney handled this briefing appropriate for the situation?
  b. If available, what resources may have been helpful to address such a tragedy?
  c. Recognizing the leadership necessity to deal with this incident, how important is it to provide military leaders with basic psychological training?

Sustained War Effort, Loss, and Effects of Stress on Soldiers
• • • • • • • • • • • •

The Hurt Locker (2008; Jeremy Renner, Evangeline Lilly, Brian Geraghty, David Morse): This movie tells the story of a team of army explosive ordinance disposal soldiers in Iraq, the stressors that they face, and the effects on them mentally.

1 (0:11:00–0:12:32) Sgt James (Renner) deploys a smoke grenade, obscuring the view of his team.
  a. How do standardized procedures assist those in stressful situations to both perform and cope with stress?
  b. In what ways does violating these procedures exacerbate the stress felt and limit the coping abilities of those enduring it?
  c. How would you assess the behavior of Sgt James in this situation?
2 (0:27:32–0:28:30) Specialist Eldridge (Geraghty) talks with an army social worker about his thoughts.
  a. What mental health disorders should be considered in this situation?
  b. How can social workers effectively treat those who remain in high-risk fields?
  c. What intervention would you effect in this situation and why?
3 (Ch 12, 1:22:36–1:26:11) Sgt James finds his friend, murdered, with a bomb inside of him.
  a. What impact would losing someone close to you have on a soldier already exhibiting PTSD symptoms?
  b. How does James's relationship to the boy appear to affect his handling of the explosive?

Returning to a "Normal" Life

Studies and experience have taught us that many people involved in traumatic experiences have difficulty assimilating back into their "normal" lives. The members of our Armed Services are clearly affected by these challenges given the horrific challenges of war, whether experienced personally or vicariously. Understanding these challenges and providing help so they can assimilate is a huge step toward success.

A Renewed Sense of Control and the Beginning of the Healing Process

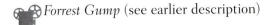 *Forrest Gump* (see earlier description)

1   (Chs 12–13, 1:31:3–1:38:16) Lt. Dan works with Forrest while on his shrimping boat. Forrest helps Lt. Dan transform himself from the angry person to a person that finds peace and builds hope for a recovery from his physical and emotional scars.
    a. Why is the peace found by Lt. Dan so critical to his recovery?
    b. How can helping someone find a purpose for their lives help them rebuild after a traumatic event?

Finally ... Something to Live For

1   (Chs 18, 2:04:40–2:06:33) Lt. Dan attends Forrest's wedding with new legs and a fiancée.
    a. How have these turn of events in Lt. Dan's life impacted him?
    b. What has he overcome to get to this point in his life?
    c. Does this scene help us to understand the literature's contention that positive family functioning can have a significant influence on treatment and recovery?

Strobl Returns Home

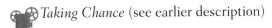 *Taking Chance* (see earlier description)

1   (Ch 11, 1:10:53–1:12:40) Strobl returns to his family without witnessing the attention he received during the trip to Wyoming. As he arrives home, we immediately see how he must return to his normal life in spite of the events he has recently endured.

a. How easy will it be for Strobl to assimilate with his military unit or family after his experience?
b. Can we really expect those that have been subjected to life changing experiences to quickly return to their normal routines?

The Hurt Locker (see earlier description)

1 (2:01:00–2:02:18) Sgt James (Renner) is in the grocery store with his wife (Lilly) and young son. He seems to be having difficulty managing the everyday task of shopping. His wife's cart is full while his is empty. She asks him to pick out some cereal.
   a. What is the significance of the bright colors and Sgt James's inability to focus?
   b. To what other symptoms of stress disorders might he be susceptible?
   c. What interventions would be most useful in treating these disorders? What are the strengths and weaknesses of each one?
2 (Ch 17, 2:02:54–2:04:10) Sgt James talks to his son about the "facts of life."
   a. How are the effects of combat displayed in this interaction?
   b. How can repeated exposure to trauma change a person's ability to relate to others?

How Soldiers Deal with Adversity

Restrepo (see earlier description)

1 (Ch 3, 0:07:40–0:08:02) In an interview with Staff Sergeant Joshua McDonough, he cites the lack of experience and information available to treat him and his fellow soldiers for PTSD. McDonough uses dissociative language such as "they haven't had to deal with people like us since World War II and Vietnam."
   a. The language used by McDonough is very powerful. What is he trying to communicate? Does he see himself as being different than everyone else?
   b. Is McDonough simply frustrated with an inadequate mental health-care system or are his statements indicative of difficulties reintegrating with society following his combat tour?
   c. What treatment options might help McDonough deal with his sense of alienation?

Coming Home for the Holidays
· ·

Nothing Like the Holidays (2008; Alfred Molina, Elizabeth Pena, John Leguizamo, Freddy Rodriguez, Vanessa Ferlito): This film focuses on the Rodriquez family living in Chicago. Family secrets and dysfunctions are revealed as they make their preparations to celebrate Christmas and the arrival of all their children returning for Christmas, including their son who is home from Iraq.

1 (Ch 6, 0:30:50–0:32:20) Eddy (Molina) moves into the bedroom with his son, Jesse, who has returned from combat. He sits on the bed and tells Jesse that he and his mother are worried about him. Eddy says: "We rented *Coming Home*." Jesse retorts that he's surprised they didn't rent *Black Hawk Down*. Eddy says they did.

   a. How can family members be assisted in understanding the re-entry process for their loved ones?

   b. What expectations of combat did Eddy and his wife have based on watching war movies?

2 Eddy tells Jesse that it isn't good to keep things bottled up. "You saw some really bad things. We know you've been through a lot." Jesse tells his Dad that it should have been me, not Lenny. Eddy tries to reassure him, telling him that he knows he did his best. Jesse replies that he can't imagine that Lenny's folks are having too many laughs now. When his father suggests that Jesse gives them a call, Jesse turns out the light.

   a. What is the impact of survivor guilt?

   b. How do holidays and special festivities affect these feelings?

3 (Ch 7, 0:45:15–0:47:28) Jesse is walking with his old girlfriend, Roxanna (Ferlita). They sit on a bench and he tells her that a guy he knew died because of him. He described Lenny as a funny kid from Wisconsin who always wore his baseball shirt under his fatigues. Jesse says that he was on lookout at the window and Lenny wanted to switch places with him. Jesse said that an RPG was launched through the window and Lenny's body was blown back into the table. Jesse asks Roxanna: "Do you know how I felt? Happy … happy to be alive." Roxanna asks Jesse if he has spoken to Lenny's family. Jesse tells her that it wouldn't make a difference because Lenny was an only child.

   a. What feelings is Jesse trying to convey?

   b. How can family and friends assist a returning soldier cope with their trauma exposures?

   c. How would you interpret Jesse's statement that he is happy to be alive and his admission to his Dad that it should have been me?

References

1 Tanielian T, Jaycox L. *Invisible Wounds of War: psychological and cognitive injuries, their consequences, and services to assist recovery.* Santa Monica, CA: RAND Corporation Center for Military Health Policy Research; 2008.

2 Otis J, Gregor K, Hardway C, *et al.* An examination of the co-morbidity between chronic pain and posttraumatic stress disorder on U.S. Veterans. *Psych Serv.* 2010; **7**(3): 126–35.

3 Kolassa I, Ertl V, Eckart C, *et al.* Spontaneous remission from PTSD depends on the number of traumatic event types experienced. *Psychol Trauma.* 2010; **2**(3): 169–74.

4 Taft C, Kaloupek D, Schumm J, *et al.* Posttraumatic stress disorder symptoms, physiological reactivity, alcohol problems, and aggression among military veterans. *J Abnorm Psychol.* 2007; **116**(3): 498–507.

5 Garcia HA, Finley EP, Lorber W, *et al.* A preliminary study of the association between traditional masculine behavioral norms and PTSD symptoms in Iraq and Afghanistan veterans. *Psychol Men Masculinity.* 2011; **12**(1): 55–63.

6 Evans L, Cowlishaw S, Forbes D, *et al.* Longitudinal analyses of family functioning in veterans and their partners across treatment. *J Consult Clin Psychol.* 2010; **78**(5): 611–22.

7 Meis L, Barry R, Kehle S, *et al.* Relationship adjustment, PTSD symptoms, and treatment utilization among coupled National Guard soldiers deployed to Iraq. *J Fam Psychol.* 2010; **24**(5): 560–7.

8 Wilcox S. Social relationships and PTSD symptomatology in combat veterans. *Psychol Trauma.* 2010; **2**(3): 175–82.

Further reading

● Possemato K, Wade M, Andersen J, *et al.* The impact of PTSD, depression, and substance use disorders on disease burden and health care utilization among OEF/OIF veterans. *Psychol Trauma.* 2010; **2**(3): 218–23.

● Taft C, Street A, Marshall A, *et al.* Posttraumatic stress disorder, anger, and partner abuse among Vietnam combat veterans. *J Fam Psychol.* 2007; **21**(2): 270–7.

30

Going Under the Knife: Surgical Interventions

Meghann Kaiser

THE VERY IDEA OF SURGERY, OR INFLICTING SO-CALLED "CONTROLLED trauma" to bring about later healing, is inherently unnatural and confusing – so much so, in fact, that the classic Hippocratic oath expressly forbade it among physicians.[1] Performing (and to a greater extent, undergoing) invasive operations demands a tenacious faith to prioritize an abstract science over flesh-and-blood instinct.[2] This is all the more magnified when complications occur, and surgeons are given the option to re-examine, reconstruct, blindly follow or utterly deny that faith.[3,4]

In order to play the necessary roles of surgeon and surgical patient, society has adopted both conscious and subconscious methods to justify their philosophies and behaviors. Such methods classically entail some effort to distance surgeon and patient, whether by tacitly subverting the "humanness" of patients or, conversely, deifying an infallible surgeon-self.[5–7] Both tactics minimize the perceived consequences of the trauma caused by surgeons, but exact a toll on the physician-patient relationship, and, over time, can undermine the integrity, ethics, and very person of the surgeon herself. Many are familiar with Alec Baldwin's infamous monologue in the fictional film *Malice* (1993): "if you're looking for God, he was in operating room number two on November 17, and he doesn't like to be second-guessed. You ask me if I have a God complex. Let me tell you something: I am God."[8]

The Surgical Patient as Human

Never Let Me Go (2010; Carey Mulligan, Keira Knightley, Andrew Garfield): This science-fiction drama tells the story of a subclass of human clones, raised within society for the sole purpose of donating their organs in stages over time, ultimately culminating in their planned death to prolong the lives of non-clones.

1   (Ch 18, 59:54–1:03:29) In this scene Kathy (Carey Mulligan) and Ruth
    (Keira Knightley), two clones raised together as children, are reunited in a
    hospital as Ruth is recovering from a recent donation. Kathy is a "carer," or
    clone who has not yet begun the donation process herself, whose job it is to
    guide and counsel other clones throughout the surgery experience. The set-
    ting and dialogue both explore the dehumanization of the surgical patient,
    Ruth, as she progresses from her pre-operative self to her anticipated death.

 a. What is Kathy preparing herself for as she enters Ruth's room? What is
    the significance of the toys at Ruth's bedside?

 b. Surgical patients often remember the moment when they were wheeled
    from their rooms toward the operating room. In this scene, how does the
    setting and mood of the hall differ from the patient room? Why did the
    director set the bulk of the dialogue in the hall? What are they walking
    toward?

 c. Ruth talks about illness and dying in inanimate, passive terms. What is
    the effect of referring to oneself as "broken" versus "sick"? Why does Ruth
    refer to being dead as "technically completed" and "switched off"? What
    euphemisms for death, both technical and otherwise, do surgeons use
    with their patients, their colleagues, and themselves, and how does that
    affect each party's perception of the process?

 d. Ruth and Kathy both downplay the drama of the scene: Ruth saying she
    doesn't "fancy" her fate; Kathy chuckling and mocking the finality of
    Ruth's statement "one last time." Both the health-care provider, Kathy,
    and the patient, Ruth, insist on minimizing the weight of the moment for
    the benefit of the other. Do health-care providers sometimes expect their
    patients or their patients' families to reciprocally comfort them when they
    have poor outcomes?

 e. Like Kathy, health-care providers will eventually confront the same mor-
    tality as the patients they care for. How would this realization affect a
    surgeon's willingness to empathize? How might this affect their patients'
    willingness to confide in them or unburden themselves?

 f. Ruth's monologue hypothesizes the experience of the surgical patient as
    she is stripped of her human comforts and dignity ("no more recovery
    centers, no more carers"), when the world around her believes she no
    longer has awareness or self-worth. Many health-care professionals who
    deride unconscious (or apparently unconscious!) surgical patients in their
    presence unwittingly capitalize on such vulnerability.[6]

 g. Anecdotally, when health-care providers care for a colleague or friend, they
    do not generally exhibit these sorts of behaviors, even with patients under
    general anesthesia. Why is this? If, despite Ruth's fears, the patient is *not*
    conscious, is there "no harm, no foul" associated with demeaning treat-
    ment, or is there a minimum expectation of human dignity, which should
    not be conditional on any other factor? How can such a policy positively
    or negatively impact both surgeon and patient?

2 (Ch 24, 1:20:05–1:21:03) In this scene, Ruth makes her final donation and dies on the operating room table. Once again, the contrast between "person" and "thing" is explored.

   a. How does the changing camera angle – from Ruth's face, to the back of her head, to across the room – give us insight into Ruth's experience as the scene unfolds?

   b. The scene preserves some elements of the traditional operating room setting – masks, lighting, audible monitors, sterility – but others are noticeably absent. Ruth's eyes are open, her hair uncovered, her breathing tube does not obscure her mouth and her face is well lit and undraped, clearly visible to the surgeons. If real-life surgeons operated in similar settings, how might it improve or impair their skills and decision-making processes?

   c. Multiple health-care professionals attend to Ruth, but, as the scene closes, the surgeon concludes harvesting and abandons her. While this is obviously an extreme case, patients often feel their surgeons have somewhat differing endpoints for their therapy. Surgeons may consider a successful operation a job well done, but patients still hope to "get better" during an often prolonged recovery process. Thus patients often feel betrayed and deserted by their surgeons halfway through healing, even when their immediate needs are adequately addressed. How can surgeons more effectively prevent and confront both perceived and real discrepancies?

   d. Brain-dead organ donors are typically sutured closed at the conclusion of the operation, but Ruth's surgeon simply leaves the room. Does our commitment to our patients also end when they die? In what ways can we continue to care for our patients in the port-mortem period? How do these efforts affect our future physician-patient relationships?

   e. Ruth dies the moment her organ is removed. This implies a comforting physicality and logical equation to life and death, which is not always so apparent in the actual practice of surgery. The definition of "brain death," for example, is different in the United States and the United Kingdom.[9] Likewise, cardiac electrical activity may continue for several minutes after time of death is officially declared. What is the effect of these uncertainties on surgeons and family members? Should we feel compelled to discuss with families the vagaries in our man-made definitions? Why or why not?

The Surgeon as Human

*M*A*S*H* (1970; Elliot Gould, Robert Duvall, Donald Sutherland, Tom Skerritt): This Korean War comedy/drama focuses on a group of reluctant military surgeons attempting to retain normalcy in their lives while providing optimal care for their patients under very adverse circumstances. The often unrealistic expectations of surgeons that society, and the expectations surgeons have for themselves, are a recurring theme throughout this film.

1 (Ch 10, 0:27:47–0:28:58) In this scene, cardiothoracic surgeon Major Frank Burns (Duvall) tends to a postoperative patient, and enlists the help of an unprepared orderly, Boone. Another surgeon, Captain John McIntyre (Gould), observes their interaction.

   a. As the scene opens, Burns is pounding on the patient's chest and calling for help. The other health-care professionals present hear him but return to their activities. Why do they not offer immediate help? How does Major Burns feel at this moment? How is this similar to a surgeon's mind-set and mood in the operating room?

   b. At what point does Burns realize the patient has died? Why does he ceremoniously wait to cover the patient's face until there is another person present?

   c. Boone makes it clear that he is not a nurse, and retrieving the medications and supplies is neither his responsibility nor within his field of expertise. Does Burns realize this? Does it matter to him? Was it unfair to ask for Boone's help when no other suitable health-care professional was available? If you were in either Burns's or Boone's shoes, how might you have handled the situation differently?

   d. Rather than using passive language, e.g. "the patient has died," Burns tells Boone, "You killed him." Why does he feel it necessary to assign blame and a clear cause-and-effect relationship to this tragedy? Does blaming Boone exonerate Burns? Conversely, does excusing Boone imply that Burns himself is at fault?

   e. Traditional surgical morbidity and mortality conferences hypothetically assume human error whether or not it is likely, because human behavior, not the natural course of the disease itself, is a variable we can theoretically improve upon. In your opinion, is this practice helpful or harmful for the surgical community? How can the surgeon prevent this artificial "blame" construct from evolving into perceived fact?

   f. Boone is at first incredulous but then apparently accepts responsibility for the poor outcome. He knows Burns's demands of him were unfair, so why does he still feel guilty?

   g. Boone does not attempt to defend himself in the face of Burns's accusations. Burns apparently does not expect him to and walks away immediately. Should Boone have argued his innocence? What could he say to persuade Burns? How would Burns have reacted? How might the scene have played out differently had Boone returned with the correct supplies?

   h. McIntyre clearly disapproves of Burns's behavior. Rather than reprimand Burns immediately or comfort Boone, he instead pauses to review the patient's chart. What do you think he's looking for specifically? Does McIntyre empathize and/or identify with Burns, Boone, or both? What, if anything, would you have said or done if, like McIntyre, you had witnessed a similar scene?

2 (Ch 39, 1:52:23–1:53:22) Captain Hawkeye Pierce (Sutherland) interrupts

Captain Duke Forest (Skerritt) in the middle of brain surgery with the exciting news that they will be going home.

a. The dialogue takes place during brain surgery, presumably a very intense time. Why does Pierce ask Forest if he's busy, when he clearly is, and why does Forest ask if he can leave "right now," when he clearly can't? Do Forest and Pierce consciously prioritize their own needs above the patient's? Do their offhand comments make them more or less likable as human beings? As surgeons?

b. Upon learning he will soon be going home, Forest pauses briefly in the midst of the operation to fantasize about his homecoming. Are we meant to feel critical of him for this momentary lapse in attention? Would you feel differently if he were operating on your loved one?

c. Forest calls his senior surgeon a "perfectionist," a term with both positive and negative connotations in this situation. How do you think Forest intends it?

d. Athletes often "borrow the will" of their coaches to keep striving even when they are sore or exhausted. Congregations "borrow the will" of religious teachers when they are tempted to stray from their beliefs. Surgeons sometimes "borrow the will" of other surgeons, when making the right clinical decision means working harder or longer, especially when it conflicts with their personal lives. In this scene from *M*A*S*H*, Forest subtly asks permission to leave during the operation and is denied by a more objective surgeon. Was this the answer he was expecting? Do you think he would have left if he had been allowed? When surgeons "borrow the will" of others, is it because they are weak or incapable of the necessary commitment? Do you/their colleagues think less of them as a result?

From One Human to Another

City of Angels (1998; Meg Ryan, Nicholas Cage, Dennis Franz): Maggie (Ryan), a young cardiothoracic surgeon at the top of her game, must make peace with the concept of mortality as she struggles with forces outside her control and discovers both the extent and limitations of her abilities. Throughout the film, Maggie and her various patients interact in scenes that illustrate the shared humanity between a surgeon and her patients and their families.

1 (0:08:07–0:14:37) In this extremely realistic portrayal of cardiac bypass surgery, Maggie performs what begins as a (relatively) uneventful operation but concludes with her patient dying on the table despite vigorous attempts to resuscitate him. She is now faced with telling his family the unfortunate news.

a. Maggie is surprised that her patient wants to meet her prior to the operation. Why does he want to meet her? Why does this request catch her off guard? Shouldn't she want to meet him too? Why or why not?

b. Maggie says nothing at all to her patient while he is still conscious, but after he codes she addresses him directly, by his first name, "Tom." In her mind, has their relationship changed? How so?

c. The writer and director go to great lengths to portray the normal, human characteristics of the surgical team in a very "un-normal" environment. They listen to Jimi Hendrix, they read *People* magazine, they discuss doubts regarding their own parental fitness. What other clues to their "human side," both positive and negative, are layered throughout the operating room scene? Would you have developed a different opinion of the characters without these subtle details? How so?

d. Tom's spirit appears in the background as the action slows, reminding us that he is as much a character in this scene as the surgeon and her team. How does his presence – and visible face – affect us as viewers? Is it easy to forget that he has been there the entire time, and should be, in fact, the center of attention? Do you think his surgeons have forgotten? There is a suggestion that Maggie can perceive certain aspects of the afterlife. If she could sense his spirit, how would this affect her?

e. Prior to entering the waiting room, Maggie briefly observes Tom's family through the glass. Why does she pause? What is she looking for? Is she preparing herself, or allowing his family an opportunity to prepare?

f. Typifying a very common scenario in everyday clinical practice, Tom's widow is somewhat surprised to learn her husband's surgeon is a woman. How does this brief interchange affect an already difficult conversation? Should Maggie be offended? Would you be? Unfortunately, sexism in our society continues to be a very real issue, and Maggie has clearly encountered similar prejudice before. What steps can she take to alleviate potential awkwardness, address preconceived notions, and feel validated as a female surgeon, without alienating patients and their family members?

g. As the scene opens, Maggie is discussing the patient's history with her colleague. The patient collapsed and suffered a massive heart attack while jogging, his EKG and echocardiogram reveal advanced disease, and his blood pressure is dangerously low, prompting emergent surgical intervention. Despite all this, as Maggie enters the waiting room, his wife and children are smiling and chatting, apparently utterly unprepared for the news of his death. It is unclear whether they fully understood how grave his condition was prior to the operation. Should they have been told? How would this have affected their perception of the surgeon and situation, if at all? In times of crisis, which *should* and which *does* typically play a greater role in decision making, facts or hope? Is it the surgeon's responsibility to both *inform* and *convince* patients and families of poor prognoses?

h. Giving bad news is a skill that must be observed, practiced, and perfected, no different in some ways than taking a history or suturing. We can safely assume in her line of work that Maggie has had this responsibility more than once. She chooses to announce Tom's death to his family bluntly, at the outset, without benefit of euphemisms: quite simply, "He didn't survive." Thereafter, she briefly recounts the events leading up to his death, although she apparently doesn't expect them to absorb all this. When Tom's widow protests that she doesn't understand, Maggie only responds "I'm sorry," and allows the family time and space to grieve. Does Maggie take this approach for her own benefit, for the family's, or both? Is this the "right" way to tell someone his or her loved one has died? What might she have done differently? Is there anything she could have done to ease their pain or change their reaction?

2 (0:22:10–0:23:17) In this scene, Maggie greets Mr. Messenger (Dennis Franz) after his surgery has been rescheduled because of her illness. Her interaction with him and his wife is a classic example of the skepticism that the medical community and laypeople often harbor for one another.

 a. Both parties spend the conversation alternately correcting and ignoring one another. Mrs. Messenger indignantly informs Maggie that she has mispronounced the family name. Maggie indifferently repeats the mistake. She upbraids Mr. Messenger for noncompliance and he shrugs unapologetically. Why the mutual reluctance to give ground? In what ways are Maggie and Mr. Messenger on the same team? In what ways are they opponents? What are their respective goals?

 b. Maggie does not give Mr. Messenger a specific reason for rescheduling, saying only that "circumstances were not optimal for the procedure." Should she feel obligated to tell him details of her personal life since it did impact his care? Why doesn't she? Would telling him she was sick affect his perception of her, either negatively or positively?

 c. Mr. Messenger seems very invested in ensuring his surgeon sees him as a human being: "I ain't 'the procedure,' my name is Nathan Messenger, and I'm sitting right here." Why is this so important to him? How could Maggie assure him she recognizes and respects his humanity and person?

 d. Maggie informs Mr. Messenger that his surgery is "a big deal," but rather than quantifying this in terms of risk, pain, or effort, she instead assigns it a dollar amount: "If you're going to continue to eat in this manner, you might as well skip it. Save yourself the thirty grand." How might this comment affect his perception of her? Why does she choose these particular units of measurement?

 e. Maggie goes to the closet to hand Mr. Messenger a new gown after he spills ice cream on himself. Recalling other media portrayals of health-care professionals and/or your own personal experience, is this the sort of behavior physicians and surgeons are known for? What does this gesture say about Maggie? Why did Mr. Messenger not acknowledge her help more favorably? Did you yourself even notice this small act of kindness when you watched the scene? Why or why not?

 f. Health-care professionals, and, in particular, surgeons, often bemoan the fact that patients and families are no longer grateful for their services, as presumably they once were. Mr. and Mrs. Messenger certainly seem to be examples of this, and it clearly annoys Maggie. Should paying customers – as Maggie acknowledges they are – be grateful? Why or why not? Why do surgeons treasure this quality in their patients? Does a grateful attitude on the part of patients alleviate or exacerbate the classical discrepancy in standing commonly felt between surgeon and patient? Should surgeons, in turn, also be grateful to their patients? Why or why not? How can this be expressed in a professional manner?

References

1 Miles, Steven H. *The Hippocratic Oath and the Ethics of Medicine*. Oxford: Oxford University Press; 2004.
2 Hall JC, Ellis C, Hamdorf J. Surgeons and cognitive processes. *Br J Surg*. 2003; **90**(1): 10–16.
3 Gerber LA. Transformation in self-understanding in surgeons whose treatment efforts were not successful. *Am J Psychother*. 1990; **44**(1): 75–84.
4 Ballentine CJ, Ayanbule F, Haidet P, *et al*. The patient-physician relationship in surgical students. *Am J Surg*. 2010; **200**(5): 624–7.
5 Newton BW, Barber L, Clardy J, *et al*. Is there hardening of the heart during medical school? *Acad Med*. 2008; **83**(3): 244–9.
6 Baillie L, Ilott L. Promoting the dignity of patients in perioperative practice. *J Perioper Pract*. 2010; **20**(8): 278–82.
7 Rady MY, Verheijde JL. General anesthesia for surgical procurement in non-heart-beating organ donation: why we should care. *Anesth Analg*. 2010; **111**(6): 1562–3.
8 Beckett H (director). *Malice* [motion picture]. United States: Columbia Pictures; 1993.
9 Zamperetti N, Bellomo R, Defanti CA, *et al*. Irreversible apnoeic coma 35 years later: towards a more rigorous definition of brain death? *Intensive Care Med*. 2004; **30**(9): 1715–22.

31

Trauma and Toil: Emergency Room Medicine

Hans House, Amy E. Cassidy, Anna Pavlov & Patricia Lenahan

THE TELEVISION SERIES *ER* HAS GIVEN THE GENERAL POPULATION A glimpse of what life may be like for the health-care professionals who work in that environment as well as offering viewers a look at the personal lives of those who choose to work there. Newer television shows also have shown examples of emergency medicine. One of the newest series to look at trauma care is *Combat Hospital*. Movies also have provided powerful examples of emergency care.

The practice of emergency medicine encompasses a vast field of knowledge, in specialties as diverse as neonatology to geriatrics, from psychiatry and substance use to surgical skills. The pace of the work can be grueling, as can be the hours of practice. The physicians, nurses, social workers, chaplains, and ancillary staff must work in concert in order to provide the best possible care to individuals while offering information, guidance and crisis-related support to their families.

Generally, health-care providers in the emergency department do not establish and foster long-term relationships with the patients or their families. The goals are to diagnose emergent conditions, stabilize the patient and determine the appropriate level and source of care. The scenes described below can be used to provide various aspects of emergency medicine and the populations seen.

Daily Life in the Emergency Department

Just Like Heaven (2005; Reese Witherspoon, Mark Ruffalo): Reese Witherspoon is an ambitious emergency medicine resident who is hoping her diligence and skills will earn her an attending physician position after residency. She has an accident while driving home after more than 26 hours on duty and becomes a patient, albeit a comatose patient, in the hospital where she works. 1 (Ch 1, 0:1:15–0:4:20) Dr. Elizabeth Masterson (Witherspoon) triages and examines various patients (a young male who has been using illicit drugs, an older gentleman who asks her repeatedly to marry him, a patient with a urinary tract infection, and so forth). She gets a quick cup of coffee in between suturing wounds and managing the patients. At one point she is in the bathroom when a male nurse calls for her to see an X-ray. In the bathroom, one of the other residents says that she is lucky because "all you have to worry about is work,"a reference to the fact that Elizabeth isn't married or dating.

    a. What aspects of emergency medicine does this scene illustrate?

    b. How can emergency medicine residents learn to multitask effectively?

    c. What is the impact of working long shifts? Does this impact clinical judgment?

    d. How does medical school and residency affect a trainee's personal life?

2 (Ch 1, 0:05:35–0:06:40) A nurse calls Dr. Walsh, the attending physician, and announces that a patient with a gunshot wound has arrived. He looks at Elizabeth and another resident, Dr. Rushton, asking both of them how long they have been on duty. Dr. Rushton says he's been working for 12 hrs. Elizabeth replies "a little more than that." Dr. Walsh tells Elizabeth that she has been working for 26 hours and to go home. He asks Dr. Rushton to see the patient. Elizabeth looks disappointed. Dr. Walsh calls to her and tells her that he was going to make the announcement the next day, but shares with her that he has selected her as an attending physician. He adds: "You do what is best for the patient rather than kiss my behind like some of the others." Elizabeth beams, thanks him, and prepares to go home.

    a. How would you interpret Dr. Walsh's comments?

    b. How does an individual's ambition affect professionalism? Patient care? Can this be both positive and negative?

Duty Hours

1 (Ch 2, 0:06:50–0:07:05) Elizabeth leaves the hospital when one of the nurses stops her as the elevator doors are closing. He says "there is a bowel obstruction in Room 6. Can you take a peek?" Elizabeth agrees to see the patient.

    a. The nurse refers to a patient as "the bowel obstruction in Room 6." Does this de-personalization of an individual affect providers in an emergency department? Does this occur in other areas of clinical care? What purposes may it serve? How does this affect the patient?

    b. Why would the nurse prefer to stop Elizabeth than ask for help from another provider?

    c. How might Elizabeth establish boundaries and foster self-care/wellness? How would a refusal to stay and see the patient affect the professional relationship between Elizabeth and this nurse?

2 (Ch 8, 0:48:30–0:49:00) This scene shows a resident asleep in the break

room, a salad in her lap. The scene shifts quickly to a couple of staff in the supply room, engaging in heavy kissing.
   a. Does this scene portray a realistic view of emergency medicine?
   b. How might this scene affect a patient's sense of confidence in being treated in an emergency room?

Trauma
. . . .

Three Kings (1999; Mark Wahlberg, George Clooney, Ice Cube): At the close of the first Gulf War, three soldiers follow a map to one of Saddam Hussein's hidden bunkers to steal a treasure in gold.
1   (Ch 6, 0:19:00–0:20:38) Archie Gates (Clooney) explains to his team the nature of gunshot injuries and why many bullet wounds result in sepsis. Then, when practicing their assault on the bunker, a cow activates a leftover cluster bomb and the team experiences a concussive blast injury.
   a. The bullet is seen tracking through some abdominal organs. What organs do you think are injured? What would be the clinical result from the injury depicted?
   b. Which abdominal wounds require operative exploration? Blunt force? Penetrating? What is an example of a high-velocity wound? A low-velocity wound?
   c. How does the force from an explosion cause injury? What injuries can you expect from the pressure wave?
2   (Ch 26, 0:1:32:00–0:1:34:00) Troy Barlow (Mark Wahlberg) is hit in the chest with a bullet and develops a tension pneumothorax. He is saved by the quick actions of Gates as Chief Elgin (Ice Cube) assists.
   a. Does a tension pneumothorax result in pulseless electrical activity? Describe the pathophysiology. What are other causes of pulseless electrical activity?
   b. Describe the technique for a needle thoracostomy, including landmarks. Describe the technique for a tube thoracostomy.
   c. Inserting a chest tube is very painful. Describe how you could provide anesthesia for the procedure.

Return to Me (2000; Minnie Driver, David Duchovny, Carrol O'Connor, Robert Loggia, Joely Richardson): A building contractor donates his wife's heart after she is tragically killed in an accident. A year later, he falls in love with a waitress, only to discover that she received a heart transplant at the same time and place.
1   (T5C7; 0:14:06–0:15:02) Paramedics burst in the emergency room with a 34-year-old female with head trauma secondary to a motor vehicle accident. Bob (David Duchovny), the patient's spouse, is alongside the moving stretcher. He appears to be in shock as he tries to answer the doctor's basic

questions. Bob is told he has to wait outside. The scene ends with Bob looking through the glass with a blood stained shirt. A song about love is playing in the background.

a. Bob is alone and in a blood stained shirt. What care could be/should be provided to him?

b. How can Emergency Department personnel attend to the needs of family members as well as to the identified patient?

The Medicine Show (2001) Taylor Darcy (Jonathan Silverman), a cynical young man is diagnosed with colon cancer which his father also had. During his stay in the hospital, he meets a rambunctious young leukemia patient (Natasha Gregson Wagner) who more than matches his distaste for intravenous drips and forced sentiment. Kari Wuhrer and Annabelle Gurwitch costar.

1 (T2 C1, 0:01:33–0:03:00) Taylor, with fear in his eyes, is lying flat on a gurney as a nurse asks him in rapid fire succession if he, "takes any of the following: ASA, anticoagulants, blood thinners, anti-depressants, MAO inhibitors, anti-hypertensives …" The nurse then asks in a similar pace, "Do you or does anyone in your family have a history of pulmonary disease, diabetes, hypertension, heart disease, blood disease …?" At the same time, another nurse is putting in an intravenous line in an insensitive manner. The first nurse continues the history questions and includes, "unexplained vaginal discharge?"

a. What is your reaction to this scene?

b. Patients and accompanying family members often feel overwhelmed in the Emergency Room. While obtaining a history is paramount, how can we minimize the negative effect demonstrated in the scene?

c. How can teaching and the need for repetitive questioning by multiple doctors contribute to a negative experience in the ER and over the course of a hospitalization?

d. What pressures do health-care providers experience to obtain all that is required and work at a brisk pace?

Toxicology

Pulp Fiction (1994; John Travolta, Uma Thurman, Eric Stoltz): Quentin Tarantino's asynchronous tale of gangsters and violence consists of three linked stories. One story follows Mia Wallace (Thurman) going on a date with Vincent Vega (Travolta).

1 (Ch 11, 0:53:00–0:54:45) Mia, wearing Vincent's jacket, discovers a pouch of white powder in one of the pockets. Thinking it is cocaine, she snorts a line. It is actually pure heroin and she immediately overdoses.

2 (Ch 12, 0:58:50–1:01:00) Vincent, panicking over Mia's impending demise, takes her to the home of his drug dealer, Lance (Stoltz). Lance has a vial of epinephrine that he uses to resuscitate Mia.

   a. What clinical signs do you observe in Mia's overdose? What are the expected symptoms and signs of a heroin overdose?

   b. Describe an opioid toxidrome. What are the features of some other toxidromes?

   c. In the actual practice of medicine, intra-cardiac injections are not used. What is the dose and the route for epinephrine when treating cardiac arrest? What is the dose and route when treating anaphylaxis? Why are these different?

   d. Epinephrine would stimulate a patient with a severe opiate overdose, but there is a more effective antidote. What is it? What is the dose? Name some other toxins and their antidotes.

   e. Vincent does not take Mia to a hospital out of fear of prosecution and vengeance from Mia's husband. How would you handle the situation if Vincent brought Mia into your emergency department? How would you balance the physician's responsibility for confidentiality versus society's requirement for justice?

The Rock (1996; Sean Connery, Nicolas Cage): This is a wild action-thriller about renegade marines capturing Alcatraz prison (aka The Rock) and threatening to release chemical weapons on the population of nearby San Francisco.

1 (Ch 13, 1:26:00–1:28:00) Dr Goodspeed (Nicolas Cage) explains to John Mason (Sean Connery) the nature of VX nerve gas while he defuses one of the rockets.

2 (Ch 20; 2:03:00–2:04:30) Dr Goodspeed shoves a container of VX into the mouth of a villain, killing his foe but exposing himself to the deadly gas. He treats himself with a syringe of antidote. Note his pupil size at the end of the clip.

   a. What class of agent is VX? What other chemicals and medications also act this way?

   b. Describe the mechanism of action of cholinesterase inhibitors.

   c. Which patients are likely to present with an accidental overdose of cholinesterase inhibitors?

   d. How are these agents used in agriculture?

   e. What are the symptoms and signs of a cholinergic toxidrome? And the anti-cholinergic toxidrome?

   f. What is the antidote for cholinesterase inhibitor overdose? What is the role of 2-PAM? After Nicolas Cage gives himself the antidote, why do his pupils appear the way they are? How do you titrate the antidote for cholinesterase inhibitors?

Emergency Nursing

Little Fockers (2010; Ben Stiller, Robert De Niro): Family patriarch Jack Burns (De Niro) wants to appoint a successor. He continues to put his son-in-law, male nurse Greg Focker (Stiller), to the test. Through miscommunication, assumptions, and sarcasm, the plot ultimately leads to bringing the family closer together.

1   (Chs 18–19, 1:26:01–1:37:50) In this clip, Greg, the male nurse of the family, performs the Heimlich maneuver on the family cat to expel a lizard from his mouth. His father-in-law (De Niro) then proceeds to collapse with chest pain. Greg instructs his wife to call 911, and has a neighbor retrieve some aspirin.
   a. What are the "basic" steps to perform when a patient presents with chest pain?
   b. Review the acronym MONA (morphine, oxygen, nitroglycerin, aspirin).
   c. What other patient interventions are important before the patient with chest pain presents to the emergency department?

Emergency Nursing in War and Combat

Pearl Harbor (2001; Ben Affleck, Kate Beckinsale, Josh Hartnett, Alec Baldwin): The movie starts in 1923 when best friends, Rafe and Danny (Affleck and Hartnett), play as children. They act as though they are already pilots in a war against the Germans. The story of the Japanese attack on Pearl Harbor is then told through the eyes of these two boyhood friends. They grow up to become Army Air Corps pilots. It is during the routine physical exams for the soldiers that Rafe falls head over heels for Nurse Lt. Evelyn (Beckinsale). The two become lovers for a short time before Rafe leaves the country when he volunteers to join the RAF Eagle Squadron. Evelyn and Danny find themselves reassigned to Pearl Harbor in mid-1941. When Rafe is reported killed in action, Evelyn and Danny form a close romantic relationship, only to learn months later that Rafe is alive and well. In the midst of this love triangle comes the Japanese attack on Pearl Harbor when Rafe and Danny are eventually assigned to Col. Jimmy Doolittle's raid on Tokyo.

1   (Ch 24, 1:37:12–1:38:09) In this scene, the victims of the attack on Pearl Harbor are flooding into the hospital. Soldiers, now turned patients, are seeking all levels of care from localized burns, to traumatic limb amputations.
   a. Besides the obvious, what are some signs and symptoms that are important to recognize when triaging patients?
   b. What signs need the most emergent treatment?
   c. The nurse practices patient safety when she moves the patients away from the windows as there is an external disaster outside. What are some basic emergency preparedness guidelines for external disasters within your local hospitals?

2 (Ch 25, 1:44:29–1:46:26) As there are hundreds of level 1 trauma victims entering the grounds of the hospital, there is an apparent loss of sense of control in this situation. The lead nurse, Evelyn, continues to triage patients.
   a. Discuss some ways to refocus yourself, or others around you, when you are presented with an overwhelming situation.
   b. One patient has an apparent carotid artery bleed. Discuss if you would do anything different than the nurse did in the scene. Did her treatment seem to be effective?
3 (Ch 30, 1:59:27–2:01:55) At this point in the severity of the attacks, there is an insurmountable number of victims that need emergent care. This is when triage plays the most important role. The physician tells the head nurse that only the patients that can be saved should be brought into the hospital.
   a. Discuss the effectiveness of the new triage system developed by the head nurse?
   b. What does M, C, and F stand for? Are there any other categories you would have added besides these three?
   c. The majority of the injuries appear to be burns. What medical treatments do you see being used that are still applicable today?
4 (Ch 31, 2:04:45–2:05:36) In the beginning of this scene, you see the chaplain with a dying patient. As the scene progresses, you can hear the words the chaplain is saying over the patient as he dies.
   a. Discuss your personal views of the role of the chaplain in the emergency department.
   b. What are some examples of patient situations in the emergency department where having a chaplain is beneficial?
   c. When would the chaplain be a resource for the nursing staff?

Marginalized Populations and Childhood Emergencies

John Q (2010; Denzel Washington, James Woods, Ray Liotta, Robert Duvall, Kimberly Elise, Daniel E. Smith, Anne Heche): Underemployed and financially strapped, John Quincy Archibald (Denzel Washington) finds that his meager insurance won't cover the heart transplant his son, Mike (Daniel E. Smith) needs to survive. When his distraught wife (Kimberly Elise) demands that he do something, John, in desperation after fundraising as much as possible, holds a hospital emergency room hostage until doctors agree to perform the surgery. Meanwhile, police chief Gus Monroe (Ray Liotta) and hostage negotiator Frank Grimes (Robert Duvall), try to diffuse the situation amid a media frenzy.

1 (T1C4, 0:12:20–0:15:53) Mike (Daniel E. Smith) is playing Little League while his parents watch from the stands. Mike goes up to bat and, after one strike, he hits the ball hard. While running the bases, Mike grabs his chest and suddenly falls to the ground. His parents rush to him, grab him, and drive

him to the hospital. They burst into the emergency room announcing that Mike is not breathing. The ER technician asks for a doctor immediately. We see Mike's shirt being cut open and the physician asking about allergies to medications. The doctor states that Mike's liver is enlarged. His father asks: "He's going to be all right, isn't he?" The mother becomes hysterical and asks. "What's wrong with him?" The physician says they are going to admit their son. The parents are taken outside to do the paperwork at which point John is asked for his insurance card.

a. Describe the response of the emergency room staff.
b. We see terror in both parents' reactions. What do you do to comfort parents in emergency situations? Is there anything that can be done to assist them?
c. Is there a difference in the emergency room ambiance with a child patient versus an adult or a geriatric age patient? What do you notice?

Violence in the ER

1   (T1C8, 0:33:10–0:38:26) When the hospital plans to release Mike, John's wife demands that he do something. John enters the hospital. We hear the cardiologist making fun and engaging in small talk with an older transplant patient and his wife. This patient is clearly receiving different treatment. John walks in on this. He tells the cardiologist that he paid the hospital $6000 yesterday and wants to talk. John swears that he will pay the money back. The cardiologist asks John: "Can you take your hands off me, please?" John pushes him and points a gun to his throat. They then walk into the emergency room. Dr. Turner (James Woods) tells John that the patients are not part of this.
a. Have you ever encountered a violent patient/client? How did you handle the situation? Can violence be predicted?
b. What safeguards are usually in place in emergency rooms to protect the public and the staff? Do you think they are foolproof?
c. What is the prevalence of situations of workplace violence?
d. What security procedures operate within the facility where you work?

2   (T1C9–10, 0:44:05–0:48:50) Helicopters and sirens are heard. John sees that police have swarmed the outside. The police chief (Robert Duvall) is briefed and makes contact with John. He asks if anybody is hurt. John replies that it's an emergency room … everybody is hurt. When the chief asks John what he wants, John responds that he wants his son on the donor list.
a. What are recommended precautions when confronted with a dangerous situation such as this? Are emergency rooms at a higher risk for violence? What are the sources of this risk?
b. Have you ever been in a patient/client care situation in which you felt unsafe? If yes, how did you handle the situation? Would you have done anything differently?

    c. What should you do if a patient/client is extremely angry or agitated and is threatening bodily harm?

    d. Have you ever had a patient engage in threatening behavior when opioid medication was not refilled or provided?

Further Reading

- Jones M. ER: *The Unofficial Guide*. New York, NY: Contender Entertainment Group; 2003.
- Newton MF, Keirns CC, Cunningham R, *et al*. Uninsured adults presenting to U.S. emergency departments: assumptions vs data. *JAMA*. 2008; **300**(16): 1914–24.
- Ross AD, Gibbs H. *The Medicine of ER; or, How We Almost Die*. New York, NY: Basic Books; 1996.

32

What Do Nerves Have to Do With It? Traumatic Brain Injury

Allison K. Bickett

ACCORDING TO THE CENTERS FOR DISEASE CONTROL AND PREVENTION (CDC), a traumatic brain injury (TBI) is "caused by a bump, blow or jolt to the head or a penetrating head injury that disrupts the normal function of the brain."[1] Individuals who sustain a TBI often experience myriad physical, cognitive, behavioral, and emotional changes often resulting in altered functionality, lifestyle, and relationships.

Personality changes and behavioral problems are often the most difficult challenges for TBI patients to handle. Behavioral sequelae of TBI include depression, apathy, anxiety, irritability, anger, paranoia, confusion, frustration, agitation, and mood swings. Those who have sustained a TBI may become aggressive, display impulsivity or disinhibition, and sometimes demonstrate socially inappropriate behavior. Cognitive changes after a brain injury may include impairments in attention, memory, reasoning, judgment, and communication, as well as alterations in sensory perception.

Medical practitioners are currently witnessing a spike in the incidence of TBI, in part, because soldiers with serious battle-related trauma are experiencing vastly improved emergency intervention and rapid evacuation to medical centers, which allows them to survive rather than succumb to their injuries. The Iraq war alone could produce a generation of veterans with life changing brain injury, affecting thousands of service men and women across the country. Reports from Walter Reed Army Medical Center indicate that nearly 30% of all patients with combat-related injuries from 2003 to 2005 sustained a traumatic brain injury.[1] The reports also revealed that blast injuries are a significant cause of brain injury in combat.

Diagnosis can be difficult even when TBI is apparent or the patient is able to describe a concussive head injury to their doctors.[2] As with more severe traumatic brain injury, a mild brain injury often has profound consequences, sometimes leading to depression, impaired cognitive functioning, sleep disturbance, erratic behavior, and mood swings, though these effects usually last no longer than 3 months. Such impairments are exacerbated by misdiagnosis, lack of treatment, and public misperception about brain injury and mental illness.[3] For veterans with brain injuries, the lack of physical signs and the vagueness of their complaints often trigger skepticism in medical professionals who may wrongly conclude that their symptoms are evidence of psychological problems or a desire to malinger.

Despite the multitude of symptoms that brain injury can cause, the cinematic portrayal of traumatic brain injury is limited to a general focus on memory loss or amnesia. Indeed, posttraumatic amnesia is common after a head injury, and deficits in the learning and retention of new information are often seen in the early stages of recovery. Hopefully, future films will explore other aspects of TBI.[3]

Memory Loss

The Lookout (2007; Joseph Gordon-Levitt, Jeff Daniels, Matthew Goode, Isla Fisher): Chris Pratt (Gordon-Levitt) was a promising high school athlete whose life was turned upside down following a tragic accident, in which two friends were killed and he was left with a debilitating traumatic brain injury. As he tries to maintain a normal life, he takes a job as a janitor at a bank, where he is manipulated into helping with a planned heist.

1   (0:03:05–0:05:09) In this clip, we hear daily life described from the perspective of one who has sustained a brain injury. Pratt (Gordon-Levitt) has lived with the consequences of his injury long enough to develop an awareness of his current level of impairment and has come to rely on cognitive strategies to help him remember routines, important information, and his life's purpose.
   a. What cognitive strategies does Pratt use to help him remember routines and important information? How helpful do the strategies appear to be?
   b. What sort of emotions would accompany the type of lifestyle described by Pratt? If Pratt were your client, how would you work with his emotions in therapy? How would you support and expand his use of coping strategies to help him function adequately?
2   (0:14:50–0:17:00) This scene depicts Pratt attempting to assert himself in his workplace, insisting that he is ready for new challenges and responsibilities.
   a. As a supervisor or colleague, would you trust someone like Chris Pratt with increased responsibility in the workplace? What emotional and practical factors would impact your decision? How might management best approach similar types of impairment in the workplace?
   b. How is Chris impacted by the reaction of his boss? How could this encounter be improved on both of their parts? What did Chris do right in the encounter with his boss?

Memento (2000; Guy Pearce, Jo Pantoliano, Carrie-Anne Moss): The audience is led to believe that Leonard Shelby (Pearce) suffered a traumatic brain injury during an attack on him and his wife by an unknown assailant, which left his wife dead and Shelby with amnesia. Following this devastating loss, Shelby's new mission in life is to get revenge against the person who killed his wife and ruined his life. This task is made exceedingly difficulty by his inability to form new memories. He relies on photographs, information from others, and his own tattoos to help him find the killer.

1 (0:08:15–0:10:30) Leonard describes his "condition" to a motel worker, who has heard Shelby's story before.
   a. What are the primary causes of traumatic brain injury?
   b. Describe the road blocks in communication presented in this clip.
   c. Describe additional memory and communication strategies that could improve Leonard's interactions with others.
   d. How would you react to Leonard's description of his "condition"? how would his self-report impact your interaction with him?
   e. What percentage of individuals with TBI have amnesia?
2 (0:36:39–0:38:50) Leonard Shelby is confronted with the reality of his memory loss, thereby eliciting a quagmire of emotions.
   a. What emotions do you see represented in this clip?
   b. If Leonard were addressing these questions to you, how might you answer, either as a therapist or friend?
   c. What are the most common treatments for memory loss as a function of TBI?
3 (0:40:35–0:44:00) The scene begins with Leonard waking up, and not knowing how he arrived in the situation in which he finds himself.
   a. Describe the emotions and thoughts that would go through your head if you awoke to a similar situation, without any recollection of the preceding events?
   b. What cognitive strategies and coping skills might someone employ upon finding themselves in an amnesic state?
   c. What percentage of individuals post-TBI experience amnesia? How treatable is this condition with medications? Psychotherapy?

Personality Change

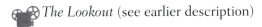 *The Lookout* (see earlier description)

1 (0:05:56–0:08:29) In this clip, Chris interacts with his female case worker, and displays emotional impulsivity, social inappropriateness, and sexually explicit comments that are common consequences of TBI.
   a. What comments from Chris serve as evidence that he is unable to filter his thoughts?
   b. How does the case manager's reaction help Chris? How could both Chris and the case manager improve their encounter?

    c. What emotions might be triggered in Chris by his interaction with the case manager?

    d. What percentage of individuals experience personality changes after their TBI?

Memento (see earlier description)

1 (0:28:50–0:31:51) Leonard interacts with Natalie, a woman he does not remember but with whom he has had an obvious previous connection.

    a. How might Natalie feel as a result of her encounter with Leonard? What assumptions might she make about herself and about Leonard?

    b. Leonard sometimes appears "matter-of-fact" and detached from the consequences of his injury. What emotions might he be hiding, ignoring or repressing? Why might he avoid expressing his true emotions?

    c. What is it like for clinicians to work with TBI patients who have had similar personality changes? What are the challenges and rewards of such work?

    d. If you were a relationship therapist working with a couple in which one member struggled with amnesia, how would you proceed?

Combat and TBI

The Hurt Locker (2008; Jeremy Renner, Anthony Mackie, Brian Geraghty): This film presents the conflict in the Middle East from the perspective of soldiers witnessing the fighting firsthand. An elite army explosive ordnance disposal team attempts to render present-day Iraq a safer place for American soldiers and Iraqis by disarming deadly improvised explosive devices. Each second spent dismantling a bomb puts the three American soldiers on the team at risk for severe injury and possible death. This responsibility weighs heavily on them and they struggle with dark emotions and constant tension.

1 (0:70:21–0:75:00) Sanborn (Mackie) and James (Renner) respond to a bomb report wherein an Iraqi civilian has a bomb attached to his person with padlocks. The man pleads for his life, saying he has a family. The locks are too complex, and James must leave the man behind. Seconds later, the bomb goes off, killing the man and throwing James in his bomb suit out of the blast area. James is merely stunned and quickly recovers consciousness, but he is shaken from the event.

    a. What physical and psychological consequences could James have suffered from the blast?

    b. What measures could the military implement to identify and treat such blast injuries?

    c. Why is it important to screen soldiers for brain injury upon their return from combat situations?

2 (1:25:00–1:31:00) James's tour in Iraq ends, and he returns to his home and family. He is unable to adjust to home life and his relationship with his wife and daughter becomes increasingly strained.

    a. What is the prevalence of combat-related TBI? Of combat-related PTSD?

    b. Aside from physical aspects of injury, what other problems could be caused by a combat-related TBI?

    c. What are the direct and indirect costs of combat-related TBI to our country?

    d. How would you counsel James's wife and daughter? What type of medical and psychological conditions are often experienced by family members of traumatized veterans?

References

1 Centers for Disease Control and Prevention (CDC). *Traumatic brain injury*. Atlanta, Georgia: U.S. Department of Health and Human Services, CDC (2012).

2 Okie S. Traumatic brain injury in the war zone. *N Engl J Med*. 2005; **352**(20): 2043–7.

3 Trudeau DL, Anderson J, Hansen LM, *et al*. Findings of mild traumatic brain injury in combat veterans with PTSD and a history of blast concussion. *J Neuropsychiatry Clin Neurosci*. 1998; **10**(3): 308–13.

33

More than Sex Education: Sexuality and Health

Gurvinder Kalra, Crystal Wilson & Dinesh Bhugra

Introduction

HUMAN SEXUALITY IS A FUNDAMENTAL DRIVING FORCE OF LIFE, AND is still, to a great extent, misunderstood. Sexuality, as originally conceived by Freud, begins in infancy and may continue until death. While a Freudian may view sex as a means to gain pleasure, a Darwinian may view sex as an evolutionary imperative meant to ensure the reproduction of one's species. Both male and female sexuality have been the focus of worldwide interest, scrutiny, and debate, both by "lay" people and experts, perhaps more than any other aspect of human behavior and experience.

The broader term sexuality includes an individual's sexual experiences and expressions, sexual desire, fantasy, orientation, behavior, and various other aspects of their lives as a sexual being. An individual's sexuality may be affected by many socio-cultural and religious factors, as well as by individual variations.

Any program on sex education may begin with an introduction to the anatomical and physiological make-up of the sexual organs and then move on to the more detailed description of other aspects of sexuality, such as masturbation, sexual intercourse and related dysfunctions, sexual variations, and various paraphilias. This chapter includes a collection of movie clips portraying all the aforementioned topics pertaining to human sexuality and can be included in various sex education programs.

Masturbation
• • • • • • • • • • • • • • • • • •

American Pie (1999; Jason Biggs, Chris Klein, Thomas Ian Nicholas, Seann
William Scott, Eddie Kay Thomas, Tara Reid): In this comedy classic, four
teenage boys enter a pact to lose their virginity by prom night.

1 (Ch 1, 0:00:21–0:01:39) In this scene, Jim (Jason Biggs) is trying to masturbate to blocked television pornography when he is caught by his parents.
   a. How common is masturbation? Is it normal?
   b. How young is too young to start masturbating? Discuss sexual explora-
       tion in children. What types of sexual behaviors/interests in a young child
       might suggest possible sexual abuse?
   c. How would you counsel a teenager who asks about masturbation?
   d. What are the benefits of masturbation? Are the benefits different in men
       versus women?
   e. Is too much masturbation possible? How often is too often?
2 (Ch 10, 0:36:46–0:38:02) After catching Jim masturbating in a pie, Jim's dad
   talks to him about masturbation. He discusses how he used to masturbate as
   a teenager in order to normalize the behavior. Jim's dad ends his speech by
   saying, "It can be fun, but it's not a game."
   a. How have views of masturbation changed over time?
   b. How would you help parents talk to their pre-teen or teen children about
       sex and masturbation?
   c. What is the best (and worst) way for parents to respond if they uninten-
       tionally catch their child masturbating?

Black Swan (2010; Natalie Portman, Mila Kunis, Vincent Cassel, Barbara
Hershey): In this psychological thriller, Nina (Natalie Portman) is an emotionally dysfunctional and somewhat frigid ballerina who desperately wants to
play the lead role in *Swan Lake*. The role requires the lead dancer to portray the
White Swan and the Black Swan. While she masters the role of the sweet, innocent White Swan with ease, she has difficulty portraying the darkly sensual Black
Swan. Her struggle to become the perfect White/Black Swan leads her down a
path of psychological destruction.

1 (Ch 10, 0:36:00–0:37:32) In this scene, Nina decides to masturbate after the
   ballet director encourages her to "touch herself" in order to loosen up.
   a. Are there any psychological benefits to masturbation?
   b. What fears may individuals have regarding masturbation?
   c. How would you deal with an individual who has guilt over masturbation?
   d. How would you counsel someone who is interested in exploring
       masturbation?
   e. How do you think Nina's mother would have reacted if she would have
       seen her "in the act"?
   f. How would you counsel a parent concerned with his/her child
       masturbating?

The 40-Year-Old Virgin (2005; Steve Carell, Seth Rogen, Catherine Keener, Paul Rudd): Andy (Carell), a 40-year-old man, feels increasing pressure from his coworkers to lose his virginity.

1   (Ch 8, 0:49:51–0:54:41) In this scene, Andy's friend brings over a box of pornography to help him masturbate. Andy does not want it because he says he does not masturbate often. Andy then has difficulty masturbating while watching the pornography.

   a. Describe scenarios when masturbation may be harmful or distressing.

   b. How can masturbation be used as a tool to enhance sexual activity with a partner?

   c. How old is "too old" to masturbate?

American Beauty (1999; Kevin Spacey, Annette Benning, Mena Suvari): Lester Burnham (Spacey) is a depressed, middle-aged father who starts developing an infatuation with his daughter's friend.

1   (Ch 11, 0:42:27–0:46:07) Lester masturbates to a fantasy he has of Angela (Suvari), his daughter's friend. His wife inadvertently catches him masturbating.

   a. Comment on the wife's reaction to Lester's masturbation. Comment on his response. What issues can masturbation bring up in their marriage?

   b. How common are disparities in sex frequency preference in married couples? How may this create a problem?

   c. How might masturbation benefit Lester and Angela's marriage? What harm could it cause?

   d. Is masturbation common in marriage? What is mutual masturbation?

   e. What is your emotional reaction to the content of Lester's masturbatory fantasy?

There's Something About Mary (1998; Ben Stiller, Cameron Diaz, Matt Dillon, Chris Elliot): In this romantic comedy, Ted (Stiller), a down-to-earth guy tries to reunite with Mary (Diaz), his high school dream girl, years after a disastrous and embarrassing first date. Little does he know that Mary has quite a few admirers pining for her affection!

1   (Ch 19, 1:19:04–1:20:47) Dom (Elliot) talks to Ted about "cleaning the pipes" prior to his date with Mary.

   a. Does masturbation prior to partner sex prevent premature ejaculation? Does it lead to delayed ejaculation or, in some instances, erectile dysfunction?

   b. Discuss myths surrounding masturbation.

Sexual Intercourse
Stages of Intercourse

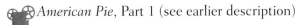 *Unfaithful* (2002; Diane Lane, Richard Gere, Olivier Martinez): Constance (Lane) is in a loving marriage with Edward (Gere). After an accidental run-in with a handsome, young book dealer named Paul (Martinez), Constance finds herself in a passionate affair with Paul that threatens to change Constance and Edward's lives as they know it.

1   (Ch 8, 0:30:47–0:36:30) Constance comes over to Paul's apartment where she begins a sexual affair.
   a. Masters and Johnson[1] proposed four stages of the human sexual response cycle. This includes excitement, or initial arousal stage, the plateau phase (when an individual is at full arousal, but not yet at orgasm), orgasm, and resolution. What are the phases of sexual intercourse noted in this clip?
   b. What other nonphysical factors can influence the sexual experience?

The First Time

American Pie, Part 1 (see earlier description)

1   (Ch 2, 0:03:10–0:06:17) Victoria (Tara Reid) discusses sex with her friend. Jim (Jason Biggs) and his friends discuss the possibility of losing their virginity at their friend Stiffler's (Seann William Scott) party.
2   (Ch 6, 0:15:45–0:20:28) Jim, Chris, Kevin, and Finch make a pact to lose their virginity by prom night after one of their classmates, Sherman, gets lucky.
   a. How would you counsel a teenager seeking advice about losing his/her virginity?
   b. What are your views on sexual intercourse in teenagers? How might your views/perceptions on sex influence your discussion?
   c. Would you encourage parents to speak to their teenagers about sex? When? How? How would you approach this topic with parents?

Sex and Marriage

Why Did I get Married? (2007; Tyler Perry, Janet Jackson, Malik Yoba, Jill Scott, Michael Jai White): In this comedy/drama, four married couples who have been friends since college explore marital troubles that are exposed during a group vacation to the mountains.

1   (Ch 6, 0:21:00–0:23:45) Marcus (Jai White) and Terry (Perry) discuss their marriages. Terry confides in Marcus that he and his wife have not had sex in months; Marcus tells Terry he has cheated on his wife and contracted a sexually transmitted disease.
   a. How important is sexual intercourse in marriage? What are common rates of sexual intercourse for committed couples?
   b. How common are disparities in the preference of sex frequency amongst

committed couples? What problem may arise amongst sex-frequency-discordant couples? How would you manage such problems in couple therapy?

c. Does sex frequency change during the course of marriage? Does sex satisfaction change during the course of marriage?

d. How would you counsel a patient who is presenting with concerns for a sexually transmitted disease from an adulterous relationship?

2 (Ch 8, 0:29:45–0:33:40) The men discuss infidelity in marriage. Mike (Jones) says, "If your wife ain't giving it to you, you have the legal right to get some."

a. Comment on this statement made by Mike.

Unfaithful (see earlier description)

1 (Ch 5, 0:17:15–0:19:20) Constance and Edward start to become intimate but are interrupted.

2 (Ch 10, 0:43:45–0:46:38) Constance takes a bath after having midday intercourse with Paul. Edward joins her in the bath and attempts to initiate intimacy with Constance but she refuses.

a. What external factors can influence the frequency of sex in marriage?

b. What suggestions would you give a couple trying to incorporate more sexual intercourse into their relationship?

Sex During Pregnancy

Knocked Up (2007; Seth Rogen, Katherine Heigl, Paul Rudd, Leslie Mann): When a drunken one-night stand between Allison (Heigl) and Ben (Rogen) ends in a pregnancy, the couple tries to deepen their connection and make the relationship last.

1 (Ch 10, 1:08:19–1:10:50) In this scene, Ben and Allison have sex when she is 5 months pregnant.

a. Is sexual intercourse safe during pregnancy? Do you know of special sexual positions that can be taken by couples in pregnancy?

b. Discuss Allison's frustration with Ben and Ben's hesitancy to have sex. How would you counsel a couple regarding having sex during pregnancy?

c. What are the myths associated with sex during pregnancy?

d. Does sexual desire change during pregnancy? If so, in what ways?

Sex and Aging

Something's Gotta Give (2003; Jack Nicholson, Diane Keaton, Keanu Reeves, Amanda Peet): Middle-aged playboy Harry (Nicholson), who has a taste for young women, falls in love with Erica (Keaton), who is closer to his age.

1 (Ch 5, 0:17:00–0:19:55) Harry has chest pain while getting ready to have sex with Marin (Peet). In the hospital, we learn that he has taken Viagra.

2 (Ch 12, 0:33:08–0:35:40) Harry meets with his doctor for a follow-up and discusses how soon he can have sex.

    a. What changes in sexual response patterns occur as an individual ages?
    b. What medications/aids/supplements are available to facilitate sexual activity, particularly in the older population?
    c. Discuss the various factors that can impede sexual activity in the elderly.
3   (Ch 17, 0:57:55–1:05:012) Erica and Harry consummate their relationship.
    a. What are the benefits of sex in older age?

Use of Sex Toys

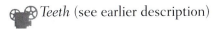 *Teeth* (2007; Jess Weixler, John Hensley, Hale Appleman, Ashley Springer): This movie is roughly based on the mythological concept of *vagina dentata*, wherein Dawn (Weixler) has teeth in her vagina, an adaptation that she believes is a curse, but later in the film is able to turn into an asset.
1   (Ch 14, 1:04:30–1:05:24) This clip shows Ryan (Ashley Springer) stimulating Dawn with a sex toy.

The Oh in Ohio (2006; Parker Posey, Paul Rudd, Keith David): This movie is about Priscilla Chase (Posey) who has been married for 10 years to Jack (Rudd) but has never attained orgasm. She later turns to vibrators and even becomes promiscuous with other men and one woman after dealing with her sexual dysfunction.
1   (Ch 5, 0:25:18–0:27:13) This clip shows Jack having a talk about sex toys with his friend Coach Popovitch (David), wherein Coach advises him to use sex toys as important tools in sexual intercourse.
3   (Ch 5, 0:21:32–0:23:23) In this clip, Priscilla goes to shop for vibrators at a sex shop, asking for a sex toy that would give her a 100% guarantee for orgasm.
    a. What is the role of sex toys in a sexual relationships? How would you handle questions by a couple regarding sex toys?

Sexual Dysfunction

Male

Teeth (see earlier description)

1   (Ch 8, 0:33:36–0:37:00) This clip shows Tobey (Hale Appleman) trying to force himself upon Dawn but in the process getting his penis cut off by the teeth in her vagina.
    a. What are the psychodynamics involved in sexual aversion disorder in the male?
    b. What psychodynamics are involved in male erectile disorder?
    c. What are common treatments for sexual aversion disorder? How effective are these?

Female

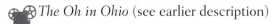 *The Oh in Ohio* (see earlier description)

1 (Ch 1, 0:2:25–0:3:03) This clip shows Priscilla's friend reading out an article from a magazine which points out that 30 million American women suffer from sexual dysfunction.

2 (Ch 2, 0:8:22–0:10:35) In this clip, Jack talks to Priscilla and tells her what her sexual dysfunction has done to him as a sexual being.

3 (Ch 3, 0:13:12–0:15:40) In this clip, Jack and Priscilla consult a therapist for their sexual dysfunction during which they have a talk on every issue that concerns them from penis size to orgasms. The clip also shows how focused Jack is on his inability to bring his wife, Priscilla, to orgasm for almost 10 years. Priscilla does not find it important at all to reach orgasm.

   a. What are the different sexual response cycles experienced by women? What are the different factors that affect sexual desire and activity in women?

   b. How would you go about dealing with such a couple where one partner is preoccupied by the other partner's sexual inability or dysfunction?

   c. What is meant by "invested partner"?

Sexual Variation: Male Homosexuality

History of Homosexuality

Un Amore A Taire (A Love to Hide) (2005; Jérémie Renier, Louise Monot, Bruno Todeschini): Set against a 1940s background during World War II, this powerful and yet disturbing movie is about the travails of Jean Lavandier (Jérémie Renier) and how his life changes when his own brother gets him arrested by the police to teach him a lesson. Things, however, don't go the brother's planned way and Jean lands up in the concentration camps for being gay.

1 (Ch 7, 0:28:00–0:30:54) Jean lies in the lap of Sara (Louise Monot), his childhood friend who loves him but has recently realized that Jean is in love with his friend Phillipe (Bruno Todeschini). Sara tries to kiss Jean, but then he pulls back and tries to explain exactly what he feels about her, himself, and Phillipe. What follows is an intense and a powerful dialogue between the two.

   a. Is it alright for Sara to allow Jean to lie down in her lap even though she knows her emotions for him and what he feels about her and Phillipe?

   b. Analyze the talk that Sara and Jean are having and present both their sides of the story.

   c. How would you counsel a woman like Sara who comes to you with the issue of falling in love with a gay man who is already in love with another man and quite clear about what he wants in life?

2 (Ch 9, 0:40:10–0:45:35): Jean's brother Jacques (Nicholas Gob) finds out

that he is gay when he sees Jean kissing Phillipe. He then confronts Jean and finds it difficult to accept "not that he is gay, but that he is a liar and a coward who passes himself off."

a. Express your emotions and feelings on seeing the kissing scene between Jean and Phillipe.

b. If you get a client like Jacques who is finding it difficult to accept his brother's homosexuality, how would you go about talking to him and help him in the process of accepting his brother for who he is? Are there organizations that help family members cope with their feelings regarding another family member's sexual orientation?

3   (Ch 18, 1:16:45–1:18:31): This scene shows the burning alive of a gay inmate in the concentration camp by the Nazi officers, while Jean tries to protect him.

4   (Ch 22, 1:34:19–1:42:17): Jean returns from the concentration camps but has been operated upon by the psychiatrists at Dachau. The surgery has rendered him almost akinetic and on the verge of dying.

a. What emotions do these two scenes evoke in you, keeping in mind that this was the way that the Nazi psychiatrists dealt with homosexuality in the past?

b. How would you deal with a gay client who has come to you with coming out issues in a country that has legal restrictions against homosexuality?

c. How has psychiatry's attitude and knowledge about homosexuality changed over the years?

d. Do you know the legal status of homosexuality in different countries around the world?

Religion and Homosexuality

Priest (1994; Linus Roache, Tom Wilkinson, Robert Carlyle): This movie is a story about Father Greg Pilkington (Roache), a priest who comes in conflict with his faith, sexual orientation, and love for another man, Graham (Carlyle), and has to choose between them.

1   (Ch 4, 0:23:34–0:28:20) Greg goes to a gay bar and then picks up Graham to have sex at Graham's place. After they have had sex, Greg is taken aback when Graham unexpectedly asks him if he is a Catholic. He does not answer the question.

2   (Ch 11, 0:46:25–0:55:05) Greg talks about God and his faith to Graham. This scene is followed by an intense kissing scene between them and then a silent confrontation between the two in the church. Graham unexpectedly ejaculates, and Greg is not able to give him communion. Later Greg discusses his conflict with one of his mentors who encourages him to "come out."

a. What role does religion play in one's sexuality?

b. In what ways can an individual's faith affect his or her sexual orientation?

c. What is the position taken by different religions on homosexuality?

3   (Ch 16, 1:02:43–1:05:24) Greg goes to meet Graham at his place but finds

him with another man. Later they settle things and express their love for each other in a parked car. But here police catch them in the act. On being asked about his occupation, Greg has to face taunting remarks from the policeman, "you little devil."

    a. How will you deal with a client like Greg who comes to you for help at the point of being caught between religion, law and sexual identity?

    b. Some people may interpret this clip as suggesting that homosexual men are often promiscuous and unfaithful to their partners. Discuss this stereotype.

4 (Ch 24, 1:27:46–1:35:10) Father Matthew (Tom Wilkinson) brings Greg back to the church after he is proven "guilty" of kissing Graham in a car on the roadside, but faces the opposition of the conservative church members who walk out and refuse to accept communion from Father Greg.

    a. What emotions can you expect in a patient like Greg who is in conflict between his homosexuality and faith?

    b. How would you deal with a conservative religious member who comes to you with the issue of not being able to accept the homosexuality of his or her family member?

Sexual Variation: Female Homosexuality

Bound (1996; Jennifer Tilly, Gina Gershon): This movie is a story of a torrid love affair between two women, Corky (Gina Gershon) and Violet (Jennifer Tilly), who risk their safety to steal $2 million from the Mafia.

1 (Ch 8, 0:18:14–0:21:00) This clip shows an intimate physical contact between Corky and Violet, wherein Violet brings Corky to orgasm by masturbating her.

    a. What are the various techniques used by lesbians during sexual intercourse?

    b. What is tribadism? Do you know of a somewhat similar technique that is used by gay men who do not wish to have penetrative sex?

    c. What is meant by dyke, butch, and femme?

    d. What is meant by sexual fluidity?

Transsexuality

Childhood with Gender Identity Disorder

Ma Vie En Rose (*My Life in Pink*) (1997; Georges Du Fresne, Michèle Laroque, Jean-Philippe Écoffey): This movie portrays the childhood of a boy, Ludovic (Du Fresne), son of Pierre Fabre (Écoffey) and Hanna Fabre (Laroque), who suffers from gender identity disorder (GID), as seen through the eyes of the child. The movie follows the child's daily life and brings out the hardships that the family as a whole faces because of their child's gender-variant behavior.

1 (Ch 3, 0:06:45–0:09:12) Pierre introduces his family to all the neighbors who have come in for a get together arranged by the Fabre family. Ludovic comes downstairs dressed as a girl in a pretty pink dress. This elicits various responses from different family members.
   a. What are the usual responses of other children and adults towards individuals with gender dysphoria? How is the childhood of a child with GID different from that of a child without GID?
   b. What emotional reactions might the family have as a result of being ridiculed because of their child's gender dysphoria? Do you think there would be a difference in the reactions of the male and female members of the family? What would be these differences?
   c. How can you help the family members deal with a child with GID?
   d. What is the role of a psychiatrist in a case of GID?
2 (Ch 9, 0:30:46–0:32:46; ch 17, 0:51:15–0:52:28; ch 23, 1:04:23–1:06:00) These clips show Pierre and Hanna taking Ludovic to a psychologist for therapy to "cure" him of his gender variant behavior that's becoming a problem for them. The clips show Ludovic's consultation in different stages, with the therapist warning the parents not to expect any miracles from the therapy, Ludovic calling himself a "girlboy," the parents having issues between themselves while coping with their child's therapy and, ultimately, the mother (Hanna) giving up on any expectations from the therapy.
   a. What is the etiology of Gender Identity Disorder?
   b. What is meant by the terms, sex, gender, gender identity, and gender role?
   c. What are the gender differences in GID?
   d. Do you know of any scales or inventories that can be used in cases of GID?
   e. How commonly have you dealt with a childhood case of GID?
   f. How would you deal with a child of Ludovic's age who is brought by the family for his or her gender dysphoria?
   g. What would you tell the parents of a child with GID if they ask about the disorder's prognosis and the future of their child and child's gender?
   h. How do you handle the blame-game between parents of a child with gender dysphoria, who put the responsibility of their child's gender-identity issues on each other?

Families of Transsexuals

Transamerica (2005; Felicity Huffman, Kevin Zegers): This movie follows a preoperative male-to-female transsexual Bree Osbourne (Felicity Huffman) who realizes that she has a teenage son, Toby Wilkins (Kevin Zegers), just a week before her surgery. Her son has lost his biological mother and has been estranged from his stepfather and supports himself by hustling on the New York streets.
1 (Ch 1, 0:2:00–0:4:12) This clip shows a psychiatrist interviewing Bree about her psychiatric history, surgical history, and other aspects of her life before she goes in for surgery. At one point he asks her if she considers herself a happy person to which Bree replies in the negative and then corrects herself

to an affirmative response but, she predicts, only after the surgery. Bree also makes a point on how plastic surgery can cure a mental disorder in her case.

   a. What do you think of the consultation between Bree and the psychiatrist?

   b. What is the protocol to be followed for transsexual individuals prior to undergoing sex reassignment surgery?

   c. What are the different types of surgeries that a transsexual individual undergoes as part of the whole sex reassignment procedure?

   d. As a mental health professional, what are the important points that you would like to focus on in terms of the history and mental status examination while interviewing a transsexual individual preparing for sex reassignment surgery?

2 (Ch 11, 1:06:54–1:12:03) In this clip, Bree (still preoperative) goes to meet her family for the first time. The clip shows the reactions of her parents to her as an individual and to her decision for sex reassignment; with the mother telling her that they love her but don't respect her and that things would have been different had Bree attended church when she was little.

   a. How do you think the parents of transsexual individuals cope up with the decision of their child to undergo sex reassignment surgery? What do you make of Bree's mother's perspective about the Church and sexual development?

3 (Ch 12, 1:22:34–1:24:36) Toby discusses the suicide attempt of Bree, in which she took half a bottle of Nembutal.

   a. How common are suicidal tendencies and attempts in transsexual individuals?

   b. How would you deal with a transsexual individual who comes to you with suicidal tendencies?

4 (Ch 14, 1:29:38–1:33:24) This clip shows Bree entering the hospital for surgery and then shifts to show her post surgery. Margaret (Elizabeth Peña), Bree's psychologist, pays her a visit in the hospital and senses that she is not as happy as she should be. The clip shows the emotional turmoil of Bree, not from her surgery but from what has happened in her life.

   a. What happens to the sexual functioning of a transsexual individual in the postoperative stage?[2,3]

   b. What is the overall satisfaction of transsexuals with their self-image, post surgery?

Normal (2003; Jessica Lange, Tom Wilkinson): This movie is about Roy Applewood (Tom Wilkinson), who announces that he is a woman trapped in a man's body and hence wants to undergo a sex change operation despite having been married to his wife Irma Applewood (Jessica Lange) for 25 years. The wife, although initially opposing her husband's decision, later supports him in his journey to becoming a woman.

1 (Ch 2, 0:4:45–0:10:30) In this clip, Roy reveals his secret to his wife and the Reverend of his congregation. The clip portrays the difficulty of the Reverend

to discuss this "strange declaration" of Roy and his religious exhortation to be "happy with the form that God chooses you to be in."

a. What are your impressions of the consultation of Roy with the Reverend?

b. What do you make of the Reverend expressing his inadequacy when it comes to dealing with such cases?

c. How comfortable are you discussing intimacy issues with couples who come in for consultation?

d. What do you think are the possible outcomes of such relationships where one partner decides they need sex reassignment?

2 (Ch 8, 0:51:31–0:54:26; ch 15, 1:35:23–1:40:37) These clips show the response of the daughter and the son when the father tells them his decision to cross his gender lines. The daughter raises specific questions about the physical changes that would be seen in the father post surgery, while the son has issues coming to terms with his father's decision.

a. What would be your strategy in dealing with children of a parent who has decided to undergo sex change surgery? How would this strategy change if the children are pre-adolescent, adolescent or young adult?

b. What psychopathology can be found in family members of transsexual individuals?

Paraphilias

A Dirty Shame (2004; Tracey Ullman, Johnny Knoxville, Selma Blair, Chris Isaak): This comedy movie is about Sylvia Stickles (Tracey Ullman), a conservative middle-aged lady who, together with her mother, leads a group of people who call themselves "neuter" that promote decency in their neighborhood. When Sylvia suffers from an accidental head injury, she turns into a sex addict and later comes to know of another such group that is full of sex addicts suffering from different kinds of paraphilias and about to take over their neighborhood.

1 (Ch 9, 0:31:02–0:36:30) This clip shows different individuals acting out their paraphilic acts. All these individuals have suffered head injury in the past, which is a part of the plot of the movie. Post concussion, these individuals become paraphilic sex-addicts.

a. What is meant by salirophilia and mysophilia?

b. What is infantilism and anaclitism? Are they similar or different?

c. What is meant by Wet and Messy fetishism (WAM)?

d. What is meant by sitophilia and botulinonia? How is food used by some people during sexual intercourse?

Sleeping Dogs Lie (2006; Melinda Page Hamilton, Bryce Johnson): The movie is about Amy (Hamilton) who has oral sex with her dog in her schooldays. When her boyfriend John (Johnson) later insists on being honest in their relationships with no secrets, Amy tells him of this secret and this leads to their breakup.

1 (Ch 6, 0:34:42–0:39:05) In this clip, Amy tells John of her dark secret when she had oral sex with her dog during her schooldays. This honesty on the part of Amy, however, does not go well with John.
   a. What is the difference between zoophilia and bestiality?
   b. What is the relationship between childhood and adolescent bestiality and adult interpersonal violence?[4]
   c. What do you know of the prevalence of bestiality in psychiatric in-patients?[5]
   d. Do you know of the use of animal tissue rather than animals for erotic purposes?[6]

References

1 Masters WH, Johnson VE. *Human Sexual Response*. Toronto, ON: Bantam Books; 1966.
2 Klein C, Gorzalka BB. Sexual functioning in transsexuals following hormone therapy and genital surgery: a review. *J Sex Med*. 2009; **6**(11): 2922–39.
3 Weyers S, Elaut E, De Sutter P, *et al*. Long-term assessment of the physical, mental and sexual health among transsexual women. *J Sex Med*. 2009; **6**(3): 752–60.
4 Hensley C, Tallichet SE, Dutkiewicz EL. Childhood bestiality: a potential precursor to adult interpersonal violence. *J Interpers Violence*. 2010; **25**(3): 557–67.
5 Alvarez WA, Freinhar JP. A prevalence study of bestiality (zoophilia) in psychiatric in-patients, medical in-patients, and psychiatric staff. *Int J Psychosom*. 1991; **38**(1–4): 45–7.
6 Randall MB, Vance RP, McCalmont TH. Xenolingual autoeroticism. *Am J Forensic Med Pathol*. 1990; **11**(1): 89–92.

34

Gender Agenda:
Women in Medicine

Susan Fleming McAllister

SUCCESSFUL WORKING WOMEN IN THE TWENTY-FIRST CENTURY HAVE often been depicted in movies as strong-willed and driven, even ruthless at times, reluctant to show their weaknesses and vulnerability. Such portrayals are typical especially of female physicians, from the surgeon who literally holds a patient's heart in her hands to the oncologist who announces to her patient that the cancer once thought to be in remission has recurred. Peter Dans, in his book *Doctors in the Movies: boil the water and just say aah*,[1] suggests that the image of the female physician has changed throughout the twentieth century from a meek character type at the beginning of the century to a more aggressive character type toward the end of the century.

In most movie portrayals of female physicians of the late twentieth and early twenty-first century, the characters are staunchly independent, financially secure, and overtly tenacious. Most of them do not have families, or, if they do, the family members have died or are distanced. The female physician is thus alone and, as a result, is sometimes vulnerable, but never weak. The films explored in this chapter, while not exhaustive on the subject, give a good sampling of images of female physicians as portrayed through the eyes of Hollywood and our culture at large.

Each of the films discussed in this chapter involves female physicians who, for the most part, are strong-willed and self-sufficient. Some general questions to consider regarding each film would be the following: do you think that women have had to take on some of the typically male gender roles in our society in order to succeed (i.e. goal oriented)? How would you define these gender roles? Now that more women are practicing medicine, have you noticed a shift in the image of female physicians in the media in general? Or do the character types in this chapter seem to be upheld?

The female physicians in these movies exhibit certain characteristics that make them distinct character types, usually stereotypes, of the successful working woman. The movie's plot then works to either question or support these images.

The purpose of this chapter is to examine several character portrayals of the female physician in order to discuss the implications of such portrayals on you and your colleagues as practicing and/or future physicians. These character portrayals include the superstar, the vulnerable, the lone ranger, and the hard-nosed and are as follows:

- The superstar is an overachiever, never wincing at the most difficult of encounters.
- The vulnerable often shrinks back as the result of the clash between her personal loss with the reality of her work demands
- The lone ranger remains self-absorbed and aloof, often ill-prepared to handle emotions and matters of the heart. Nevertheless, she remains able to swoop in and take over the situations that arise.
- The hard-nosed remains especially intense about work, domineering and even rude.

None of these categories is exclusive of the other; there may be obvious overlap. The following scenes and corresponding questions about the character types should be discussed within the context of workplace, personal life, and professional identity.

Hopefully this chapter will at least make you, the female reader, more aware both of the way Hollywood portrays female physicians and of the images your patients may have of you even before you walk in the room. As you plan and consider your career, how might you work to allay any of these images that you feel are unfair? How might you incorporate your femininity (for example, nurturing) into helping your patients cope with their illnesses? Or how might you use any of these images to your advantage?

Even though the discussion questions here are inherently framed toward a female audience and with the intent of female-only discussion groups, please feel free to modify them to include male perspectives and participants.

The Superstar

Just Like Heaven (2005; Reese Witherspoon, Mark Ruffalo): Dr. Elizabeth Masterson (Witherspoon), a successful emergency room resident physician, is in a coma after being in a head on collision with a truck. She is present only in spirit form to male lead character David (Ruffalo), whose wife has died. He rents her abandoned apartment after her head on collision. In her spirit form, she convinces him she loves him. He eventually saves her life.

1 (Ch 1, 0:01:15–0:07:50) Elizabeth, vying for a position as an attending physician, goes above and beyond her colleagues to achieve her goals. After working more than 24-hour shifts at a time, her diligence is finally recognized by the department head and she is offered the attending position. In these scenes the young doctor is shown being all things to all patients. She sutures,

she diagnoses, she comforts, she entertains, she speaks Spanish, and she even promises to marry a demented elderly patient. Yet the stress of her work shows on her face and she catches herself looking in the mirror wondering if her hard work is worth it.

a. Have the demands of medical school and residency caused you to try to be all things to all people? Describe some of the roles you play (if you are a woman) or that you see your other classmates and/or colleagues playing who are female physicians.

b. Do you think there are still inequities between male and female physicians? If so, what are some of them? Do women residents work harder than male residents? If so, why?

City of Angels (1998; Nicholas Cage and Meg Ryan): The movie is about a death angel, Seth (Cage) who falls in love with Dr. Maggie Rice (Ryan) after he sees her in the operating room. He eventually makes the choice to be with her over being an angel.

1 (Ch 3, 0:06:53–0:13:15) Dr. Rice (Ryan), a female hotshot cardiovascular surgeon who regularly performs open heart surgery, has an encounter with Seth (Cage). After riding her bike across town to work, she attempts a bypass surgery on a male patient. Her male colleague comments to the others in the operating room, "She's getting good." This perspective is reiterated by another employee in the operating room suite, "She's gettin' that attitude."

a. Can you think of a time that you did something well as a female physician? How did that make you feel? Were you ever afraid that you would end up somehow messing up the accomplishment? What did you do to try to ensure that you wouldn't mess it up?

2 Later in the scene, the patient suddenly begins to "crump" and Dr. Rice is called back into the operating room. She ends up losing the patient. No matter how hard she tries to massage the heart, the patient cannot be revived.

a. Have you ever been proud of an accomplishment in your work and then suddenly had something go wrong with your patient? How did that make you feel? How did you cope with it?

b. Have you ever failed at a procedure? How did you feel? How did your other colleagues respond?

The Vulnerable

Beyond Rangoon (1995; Patricia Arquette, Frances McDormand): Dr. Bowman (Arquette) and her sister Andy (McDormand) are female physicians on a trip to Burma. Their trip occurs during the time of the infancy of the political uprising of Aung San Suu Kyi, Nobel Peace Prize winner in 1991 for her political activity against the military regime of Burma. Andy offers moral support to Dr. Bowman (whose husband and son have just been murdered during a burglary in their home). She was at work when the incident occurred and found them on her arrival home. Devastated, she feels she can no longer work as a physician and decides to take the trip with her sister to help recover. She finds herself in situations that call her to exercise her ability and knowledge as a doctor, yet she cannot rise above her pain to react.

1   (Ch 1, 0:03:01–0:04:54) In this scene, a child of one of the tourists falls from the Buddha he is exploring.

   a. How does the jungle setting and the stone Buddha set the stage for the main character's response to the little boy's fall?

   b. Notice what Dr. Bowman says, "Nothing stirred in me. I was stone myself." Are there times when past personal experiences have caused you to freeze in your work when faced with difficulties? Or maybe contribute to your work becoming mechanical in carrying out tasks?

   c. How does Dr. Bowman's experience of tragedy in her own life serve to distance her from her sister in this scene? What is Andy's response to her? Does she seem sympathetic?

   d. Andy assumes the role of the physician immediately, after Dr. Bowman calls her. She runs to the patient to assess him. She reassures the worried parents: "I'm a doctor – it's OK." As a female physician, if you were faced with an emergency, how might establishing your position as a doctor help bystanders feel more comfortable? In what ways would making such a statement make you vulnerable? Can you think of a time where you had to assert your medical expertise over your role as a woman in a certain situation? If so, did you feel empowered or vulnerable or both?

2   (Ch 2; 0:06:01–0:08:32) Dr. Bowman (Arquette) has nightmares and tells her sister, "I never should have been working … I should have been spending that time with Nick and our boy."

   a. How might you handle dividing your time between family and work as a female physician? How might male physicians as your coworkers help you to achieve balance between work and family? Would you, as a female physician, feel guilt about the amount of time you have to spend away from family? What sort of strategies in the workplace might help to afford female physicians the opportunity to spend more time with their families? Do you feel that maternity leave is long enough? Why or why not?

   b. Andy reminds Dr. Bowman that her husband and son were proud of her: "They wanted so much for you to be a doctor." How does Dr. Bowman respond? Have any of you had to deal with the loss of a loved one while pursuing your career in medicine? How did the demands of your studies affect your grieving process? What is implied through Dr. Bowman's assertion that her role as a wife and mother should have superseded that of her role as a female physician? Can you identify with her sense of guilt over being absent from her family and home?

The Lone Ranger
······················

The female physician's work often calls her away from her family for long hours. Many women feel a conflict between their dedication to profession and family.

Beyond Rangoon (see earlier description)

1 (Ch 23, 1:34:00–1:35:30) Dr. Bowman (Arquette) finally makes it to the Thai border with the political refugees. In these last two scenes, Dr. Bowman watches as all the Burmese work to get their families across the river to Thailand. Some of them do not make it. She intensely feels her own solitude at this point in the film. Yet this is the turning point for her. She walks immediately into the Red Cross camp. Just as her sister Andy had spoken up and told the parents of the child she was trying to help that she was a doctor, Dr. Bowman (Arquette) finally speaks up: "I'm a doctor; can I help?" In the midst of her solitude, she has found her voice again as a female physician and takes charge triaging patients.
    a. Can you think of a time when you felt alone and sad but felt solace in your work as a physician?
    b. Have you ever lost a family member close to you? How might that experience help you relate to your patients?
    c. How would Dr. Bowman be especially suited to work with refugees? How might her gender help her in the refugee camp? How might it hinder her work?
    d. What are some of the dangers and/or challenges Dr. Bowman faces as a now single again woman working as a physician in this setting? Which ones might be specifically related to gender and how might she overcome them?

City of Angels (see earlier description): Dr. Rice (Ryan) finds herself alone after a very difficult surgery. She has spent many hours operating on her patient who then crashes and codes. She holds the patient's heart in her hands, but despite her heroic efforts, the patient dies anyway.

1 (Ch 3, 0:13:16–0:15:50) Faced with telling the family of the loss of their loved one, Dr. Rice resorts to medical jargon.
    a. How does Dr. Rice do in conveying the news? How might she have phrased her news differently?
    b. Dr. Rice runs to the stairway and bursts into tears, a distinctly feminine response to stress and difficulty. She is all alone, ruminating over the events: "What happened? It was textbook. It was textbook. I'm so sorry .... How did I get so small?" She admits, "I lost it." Have you ever "lost it" or watched a female colleague "lose it"?
    c. How might her response have differed from a male physician's response?
2 (Ch 10; 0:23:50–0:27:28) Dr. Rice (Ryan) and another female pediatrician

discuss that she is hiding from her patient's wife so she will not have to tell her about her husband's death. She confesses to her colleague, "None of this is in my hands."

    a. Can you think of a time in which you felt utterly alone as if none of your actions as a physician mattered? How did that make you feel?

    b. When Dr. Rice tells the family about the patient's death, what do you notice about her interaction with the family? Is it what you would expect from a female physician? Why or why not?

Just Like Heaven (see earlier description): The bathroom scene explores the difficulties female physicians have in maintaining relationships.

1 (Ch 1, 0:03:24–0:05:25) Elizabeth (Witherspoon) notes that she has not married or had a family because of work. Throughout the movie, we hear from observers that she was "always working." No one knows her in her apartment complex.

    a. Her friend tells her, "All you have to think about is work." Has choosing medicine as a career caused you to lose opportunities to develop relationships with others? How so?

    b. Her sister's homemaking atmosphere is juxtaposed with Elizabeth's busy life. How does your work schedule compare with those of your family members or friends?

2 (Ch 8, 0:42:06–0:52:18) Elizabeth laments in a later scene that she went through her whole life not knowing what she was missing until she had a wreck and ended up in a coma.

    a. How do you maintain professional distance from your patients and your coworkers? How might this help or hurt you psychosocially?

    b. Does Elizabeth's work seem worth the many hours of solitude she spent as a doctor?

    c. Do you have any regrets about becoming a physician? If so, what are they?

Stepmom (1998; Julia Roberts, Susan Sarandon): The main characters, Isabel Kelly (Roberts) and Jackie Harrison (Sarandon), fight to gain the affections of Jackie's son and daughter in the aftermath of divorce. Jackie discovers that her cancer has returned after being in remission. In the aftermath of her divorce, she must face losing her life and the prospect of having her children be raised by their new stepmother, Isabel.

1 (Ch 8, 0:40:14–0:42:05) Jackie gets bad news from her female oncologist, mainly that her cancer has recurred. The oncologist, Dr. Sweikert (Lynn Whitfield), maintains professional distance and matter-of-factly tells the mother, "Let's give it [chemotherapy] our best shot." She decides to take the chemotherapy, which later fails.

    a. What do you think is the best way to encourage a treatment plan you have to your patient and his/her family?

2 (Ch 23, 1:37:05–1:37:59) The oncologist desperately asserts optimistic

alternatives and suggests that Jackie can go to Paris or Switzerland for cutting-edge treatments. However, Jackie opts to not undergo any more treatments. Suddenly, Dr. Sweikert finds herself speechless and quietly accepts the patient's decision.

a. Describe a time when your patient or the patient's family member disputed a treatment you recommended. How did that make you feel? How did you react?

The Hard-Nosed

The Doctor (1991; William Hurt, Christine Lahti): Jack MacKee (Hurt) is a doctor with it all: he's successful, he's rich, and he has no problems – until he is diagnosed with throat cancer. After experiencing medicine, hospitals, and doctors from a patient's perspective, he realizes that there is more to being a doctor than surgery and prescription. Often, in the male's world of surgery, the female surgeon must be hard-nosed. In *The Doctor*, Leslie Abbot (Wendy Crewson) is the female ear, nose, and throat specialist who discovers the main character's laryngeal cancer.

1 (Ch 3, 0:20:14–0:23:39) She walks in saying, "Sorry to keep you waiting … busy day." These are the exact words the main character had used earlier to address his patients. After a few minutes, she announces, "Doctor, you have a growth." Dr. Mackee is left trying to process the information that he likely has cancer. She continues the exam without dropping her curt professional guard.

a. How might Dr. Abbot's (Crewson) training in surgery contributed to the way she acts toward Jack (Hurt) here?
b. Is Dr. Abbot the stereotypical female surgeon? In what ways?
c. How could she have broken the news in a softer way?

Blood Work (2002; Terry McCaleb, Jasper "Buddy" Noone): Terry (Eastwood) has just had a heart transplant. His doctor, Dr. Bonnie Fox (Anjelica Huston), wants to make sure he survives and has a strong opinion about his desire to chase and catch a serial killer.

1 (Ch 11, 0:32:55–0:35:50) Dr. Fox (Huston), Terry's cardiologist, maintains a hard-nosed attitude toward him. He wants to investigate a recent crime, but she reminds him, "You are 60 days post transplant. As your doctor, I'm ordering you not to do this." However, the main character decides to go ahead with his investigation.

a. Describe a time where you felt strongly about negative behaviors your patient was engaging in and what you did to stop it?
b. Dr. Fox dismisses Terry from her practice. How might her emotions have impacted her decision? Have you ever had to dismiss a patient from your practice? If so, how did the patient react? How did you react and feel?

2   (Ch 19; 1:04:38–1:09:30) The cardiologist later in the movie becomes even more concerned about the main character. After Dr. Fox has already told Terry she can no longer be his doctor, Terry goes back to see her anyway. He wants to talk with her, but she tells him, "You have 5 minutes." She tells him she will listen if he will allow her to do another biopsy of his transplant. He agrees.

   a. Describe a time when you felt you were short with a patient – what might have provoked you to that stage?

   b. How might the cardiologist have addressed the patient differently? Does he try to take advantage of her? In what ways might patients try to take advantage of their female physicians and approach them differently than they would their male colleagues?

Reference

1 Dans P. *Doctors in the Movies: boil the water and just say aah*. Bloomington, IL: Medi-Ed Press; 2000.

35

More Than a Prayer: Pastoral Care and Psychotherapy

James Pruett & David Carl

STATISTICS SHOW THAT FULLY HALF OF ALL AMERICANS PRAY OR meditate in private on a daily basis.[1] The efficacy of prayer in research studies is well summarized in the book *Be Careful What You Pray for … You Just Might Get It*, by Larry Dossey, MD.[2] This evidence provides the support for the widespread belief that the work of pastoral caregivers and psychotherapists primarily involves a "holy" person praying for those in need. It is the belief of the coauthors for this chapter that every thought is a prayer. Given this perspective, it is safe to say that, on average, humans "pray" 80 000 times per day. The questions that we would then pose are the following: what is one praying for one's self and what is one praying for others?

However, chaplains and pastoral psychotherapists incorporate far more into their work than invoking formal/informal and spoken/unspoken prayers. These health-care professionals work to remind patients of the interface between mind, body, and spirit. In addition, chaplaincy and pastoral psychotherapy come from a common heritage that is steeped in the following components:

- designation by one's faith group as specialized ministry
- professional training and supervision in the application of a select body of knowledge
- utilization of one's personhood as central to the fostering of health, healing, and wholeness of all four levels – physical, mental, emotional, and spiritual
- adherence to professional codes of ethics and standards of practice mandated by regulatory bodies and cognate groups.

Thus, the interventions of the pastoral care provider, chaplain, and pastoral psychotherapist establish them in a long tradition of specialized health-care providers who assess, develop care plans, implement congruent interventions, and evaluate outcomes.

The common denominator for all these health-care disciplines is the constructive use of the clinical alliance. Movies often mirror this dynamic but unfortunately most tend to portray mental health-care providers as simplistic, unprofessional, unethical, and incompetent. And almost none focus on the specialized fields of pastoral care/psychotherapy. A few, however, are well done and can be used to introduce clinical residents from various disciplines to some major principles and techniques of chaplaincy and pastoral psychotherapy.

Pastoral Care/Chaplaincy: "Interface of Mind, Body, and Spirit"

Up (2009): This is a Pixar Animation Studios film presented by Walt Disney Pictures. Carl Fredrickson is a retired balloon salesman who is inspired from childhood to seek and find Paradise Falls, which is described as "a land lost in time." Ellie is the childhood sweetheart who is both a dreamer and a doer and stimulates Carl to remain on track with his ongoing dreams.

1 (0:09:05–0:11:30) In this scene Carl and Ellie discover they cannot have children. Their ongoing dream to get to Paradise Falls continually gets dashed with financial crises. They grow old together with much love and affection present. Ellie then gets weaker, sick, and is in need of hospitalization. Ellie dies, leaving Carl alone.

   a. As energized as Carl and Ellie were as children and as in love as they were as adults, emotional, psychological, and spiritual questions must have arisen when they learned they could not have children. What would you imagine their questions might be?

   b. As Ellie becomes sick, what difference might it have made if the couple had been surrounded by family and an interactive neighborhood of friends?

   c. When Ellie dies, there seemingly is no one for Carl to turn to and so he becomes reclusive in his home. How vital is it that we have a support system to assist us at times of such loss and deep grief?

2 (0:11:35–0:19:40) In this scene we find Carl in his solitude and isolation. Metaphorically his neighborhood gives way to high rises. He refuses to sell his home and "let go" and so his house becomes the only one left on the block. A knock at the door reveals Russell, a helpful 8-year-old boy scout. Russell is over-eager to earn his Wilderness Explorer badge, which he would get if he were to help someone elderly. Carl dismisses him and sends him on a wild-goose chase. Later, Carl gets aggressive with a construction worker who accidently backs into his mailbox. Because of age and his eccentric behavior, Carl goes to court and is ordered to leave his house to receive specialized care in a retirement home.

   a. What unhealthy grief dynamics contributed to Carl's ill-advised behavior?

   b. How often do we see patients turning away others who are seeking to assist them in their healing process?

    c. How often do we see families and friends use unhelpful ways to attempt to help a patient recover from their illnesses or problems?

    d. How can we provide support for patients like Carl who must face the developmental crisis of growing older and becoming more dependent?

3 (0:19:45–0:27:31) Carl returns home after his court appearance. While there, Carl finds a scrapbook that Ellie had put together over the years. There is a picture of their house superimposed on Paradise Falls (their shared dream spot for retirement). Carl is inspired by these memories and Ellie's determination, as well as his own sense of integrity, to fulfill a promise he made to Ellie about getting to Paradise Falls. Consequently, he rigs balloons from the roof and windows of his house that lift the house up off the foundations and up and over the skyscrapers. Now aloft in a time of peaceful satisfaction, he sets course. Surprisingly, he hears a knock at the door: it is Russell the boy scout again. After Carl invites his unexpected company into the house, the house encounters a violent storm.

    a. In our work with patients, how can we best notice what gives them inspiration, hope, and determination? Is this part of our treatment assessment?

    b. Just when we think we know how things will go for those for whom we care, we are often surprised and delighted to see our patients pursue a whole new course? Have you ever had this experience with a patient?

    c. Which member of the health-care team has the task of exploring with patients in their last years of life the unexpected events that occur which lead them to more positive outcomes?

    d. As our own "temples" take a beating through storms that potentially throw us off course, how is it that we nonetheless survive and at times thrive in such difficult circumstances?

4 (0:31:38–0:49:20) These scenes show what happens when Carl's house actually lands in the area of Paradise Falls, an outcome due, in part, to Russell's navigation while Carl was unconscious as a consequence of the storm's turbulence. Carl realizes the placement of the house is not exactly where he and Ellie had pictured it would be, so he begins "walking" the house, still held aloft by balloons, toward that imagined spot. Carl estimates there are only 3 days' worth of air left in the balloons. Along the way, Carl and Russell meet Dug the dog – Dug can talk by way of a special collar. At a particular scene toward the end of this segment, the characters share a ritual "crossing of their hearts."

    a. How often do you observe that the worst of storms can still land you in places where dreams come true?

    b. How do we support patients who, like Carl, find that where they have landed is not perfectly where they want to be?

    c. Dug the dog represents a miracle of science, in as much as he has a collar around his neck invented by his owner that allows him to speak English. What miracles of medicine have you noticed in recent months and years?

    d. The "cross my heart" ritual is one that touches Carl's heart because he shared such an exchange with Ellie when he was a young boy. What rituals have you noticed patients and/or families utilizing to assist them in their healing?

  e. What resources do patients and families call upon to help them cope when all does not go perfectly or as planned?

5 (1:12:45–1:27:56) In this series of scenes, Carl has arrived at his special place but, in so doing, has lost his relationship with Russell, Dug, and their newfound friend, Kevin (a rare bird). After Carl completes his scrapbook with the picture of the house finally being where he and Ellie had imagined, he turns to a new page entitled "Stuff I am going to do." Carl is touched to read that after living together for those many years, Ellie wrote, "Thanks for the Adventure! Now go and have a new one." When he sees Russell and Dug running off to help their friend Kevin, Carl decides to help. In order to rescue them, he empties his house of all the precious belongings so that it becomes lighter, allowing it to float again. He completes a daring rescue but then sees his house floating away. However, when he sees it floating away he says: "It's just a house." The scene then switches to Carl and Russell having returned to the United States. Russell is at a scout ceremony receiving his final badge. When his father doesn't show up for the ceremony, Carl steps in to give him the "Ellie badge" (a grape soda on a pin). The movie closes with a final picture back at Paradise Falls where the house that had floated away from Carl has landed in the picture-perfect place right next to the falls, just as Carl and Ellie had always imagined it.

  a. When Carl reads over his scrapbook for the last time, he reframes his understanding of what the book has meant to him; not just something to complete, but rather as an encouragement to have a new adventure. Have you noticed patients reframing their crises and circumstances to allow them to get on with their lives?

  b. Carl had to "let go" of all of his precious belongings in order to be in the moment of his new adventure. Another phrase for letting go is to forgive. What do patients and families wrestle with in terms of letting go? What do such individuals need to be forgiven for and/or whom do they need to forgive and for what?

  c. The final frame of the movie shows the house perfectly placed on Paradise Falls, symbolizing endings not only beyond our control but also beyond our wildest dreams. As a caregiver, when was the last time you had to let go of control and rely on faith, only to see the outcome being far better than any you could imagine?

Attending to the Extra Ordinary

Dragonfly (2002; Kevin Costner, Suzanna Thompson): Dr. Joe Darrow (Costner), an emergency room physician, is in a deep grief process over the violent death of his wife Emily (Thompson) during a mission trip to South America. While pregnant, Emily, also a physician, had gone to fulfill her calling to care for children in a remote village far from the hospital where she and Joe worked.

1   (0:06:36:40–0:09:16:00) In this scene we see Joe trying to manage his grief by overworking in the ED. His stress is apparent as he dismisses a suicidal patient inappropriately, then goes back to round on the same patient when staff members tell him he was out of line. Despite their input, Joe still informs this patient that there is no life after this life, telling her, in essence, that she better live as best she can now. As he is making this statement a priest walks in. Joe quips: "Time for rebuttal?"

   a. How often do we find health-care workers denying their own emotions during times of crisis and grief by trying to literally lose themselves in their work?

   b. It is important that staff give each other feedback when inappropriate behavior arising out of unresolved issues begins influencing best practice. How well does such important feedback occur in our given units of care?

   c. Joe imposes his own belief onto the patient about the afterlife. How might a declaration like his serve to shut off a patient's sharing of his or her own beliefs?

   d. Joe's quip to the priest, "Time for rebuttal?" might symbolize the schism between science and religion. How well do science and religion integrate themselves into best practices in our various clinical settings?

2   (0:12:26–0:17:27) Joe begins experiencing things out of the ordinary. As his home lights flicker, a prism dragonfly mobile intended for his baby gets delivered to the house and Joe recalls Emily's birthmark on her right shoulder that resembled a dragonfly. This was her symbol for life. While Joe is reflecting on these memories, a heavy dragonfly paperweight falls off the table and rolls across the floor. As these scenes continue, Joe now starts seeing dragonflies everywhere.

   a. How open are we as clinicians to that which is extra ordinary and beyond reason?

   b. How well do we as clinicians notice the power of symbols in clients' lives and how well to we utilize these in their healing?

   c. Can we listen closely to the meaning and mystery of symbols in clients' lives when they try to talk to us about them? If so, how?

3   (0:19:30–0:36:00) To fulfill his promise to Emily, Joe starts rounding on children in her oncology unit. A dying boy catches his eye and waves as he goes past the room. One night Joe hears his name being called while sleeping at the hospital. He awakens in the hospital corridor to see this boy (Jeffrey) being rushed down the hallway as clinicians perform CPR on him. The boy dies on the table (or at least flatlines). As Joe approaches his still body, Jeffrey wakes up and the team rushes in to stabilize him. As the story unfolds, we learn that this child has had a history of heart stoppage and he has many stories to tell

about what he experienced during those times. Joe learns that Jeffrey was one of his wife's favorite patients (perhaps because of his openness to talk to her about his near-death experiences). So Joe goes to visit Jeffrey to let him know that he saw him during resuscitation. Jeffrey tells him that he had seen him too as when he looked down from the ceiling. Jeffrey adds that he saw Emily yesterday, as well, when he was under CPR. Jeffrey describes how he was about ready to make a transition to the other side when she met him and flew him back through the rainbow in order to tell Joe, "Joe, can't you hear me?" As is the case with many near death patients, no one believes Jeffrey's paranormal encounters, including his own parents. Finally, Joe experiences another child possessing a similar symbol to one that Jeffrey was drawing (a wavy cross).

    a. How open are we as clinicians to hear client stories about experiences beyond the ordinary such as near death experiences and other nonexplainable phenomena? According to the Gallup Poll, 35% of Americans experience phenomena they cannot explain. When and with whom can patients discuss such experiences?

    b. Why does science too often quickly dismiss such events as near death experiences, visions, out of body experiences, divine messages through dreams, and so forth?

4 (0:36:54–0:44:36) Joe meets another pediatric patient. The patient, Ben, tells Joe that Emily told him to tell Joe to go to the place of the "wavy cross." Ben states that he dreamed of Emily coming to him and even though he had not met her, he had been able to identify her as Dr. Darrow from a picture he had seen in the hall. Ben tells Joe, "She wants you to go there" and points to the rainbow (yet another symbol). Ben tells Joe that Emily showed him Joe's face (in his mind) and asked him to tell Joe to "go to the rainbow." Joe later goes home and begins to recount some of these experiences to his neighbor who is a lawyer. She reminds Joe that nothing is real without evidence. Some photos arrive in the mail from Emily from South America. In these photos, Emily is seen standing near a waterfall under a rainbow. As Joe looks at this photograph, a dragonfly comes to the window.

    a. Why do you think Joe's neighbor thinks Joe is out of his mind and tries to convince him that nothing is real without evidence?

    b. What do you say to someone who believes there is no such thing as coincidence in the light of occurrences such as Emily's photos coming in the mail and dragonflies tapping on windows?

5 (0:45:42–1:06:06) This series of scenes begins with the introduction into the movie of an embattled elderly parrot who had been a pet of Joe and Emily's for years. The parrot loved Emily and, apparently, merely tolerated Joe. The parrot had a ritual when Emily would walk in the door saying, "I am home." Joe is in the house and hears the parrot saying precisely that: "I am home." Joe runs down only to find the parrot in a frenzy slamming into the kitchen, hitting the ceiling light and knocking things off the counter. Joe sees Emily's apparition

in the window and then sees the same "wavy cross" in the soil spilled from the pot of flowers knocked down on the kitchen floor. In continued wonderment, he sees the same "wavy cross" symbol in all the windows. At this juncture Joe remembers that there was a chaplain named Sister Madeline who had been fired for helping the children talk about their extra-ordinary experiences. He meets with her and she tells him "Belief gets us there." Joe confesses that he thinks he is going crazy and asks Sister Madeline her opinion. She states, "As nuts as Christopher Columbus who thought there was another side of the world." As if this is not enough, Joe then goes back on duty in the emergency department and sits with a man who is a potential organ donor. While Joe is in the room alone with the body, the patient's heart rhythm comes back on the monitor. Joe hears his name called but it is Emily's voice. The dead man grabs him to confirm that Emily is speaking through him. Once again, Joe goes on to confidentially share this with his lawyer neighbor who advises him to grieve like she herself did.

a. Sister Madeline was fired from a hospital as a chaplain who encouraged patients to talk about extra-ordinary experiences. Would this type of pastoral care be allowed in your clinical setting?

b. Joe's neighbor advises him to grieve like she did. What happens to Joe when she advises him in this way? As health-care providers, we might better understand that everyone has their own unique grief process and that, even with best intentions, we need not require others to grieve like we do.

6 (1:07:32–1:38:00) In this segment Joe is now selling his house. While packing, the lights flicker as he is cleaning out Emily's closet. Joe then hears noises and, while he goes to investigate, the same dragonfly paperweight that he had packed away securely is now out again on the table and the clothes he had set aside are re-hung in Emily's closet. Joe's eyes divert to a rafting map given him by friends who wanted him to accompany them on a trip. As he studies the maps, he sees the symbol of the "wavy cross" and learns that it now symbolizes a waterfall. Joe then connects the picture Emily sent him in her last mailing to a waterfall. Joe flies to South America and finds his way to where the village graves are dug. He sees the waterfall in the picture and starts to run towards it. This takes him to a secluded village where the indigenous people lived. He dives into the river and the swift current carries him to the partially submerged bus in which his wife and others were riding before being washed into the river. While in the bus he gets trapped and begins drowning. Joe sees a light and sees Emily coming towards him. They touch hands. In this state he learns that she lived through the accident. The guide rescues Joe by jumping in and pulling him from the water. After Joe regains consciousness he goes to the village where he shows the villagers Emily's picture and learns from them that while they could not save her body they were able to save her "soul." They lead Joe to a hut where they enter and show Joe a Caucasian baby in a basket. The baby has a birthmark of a dragonfly on her ankle. The movie concludes with advice to trust, have faith, and a reminder that it is

belief that gets us there. The final scene closes with a rainbow over the waterfall.

   a. Joe's actions as a scientist fly in the face of orthodoxy when he has the courage to trust symbols and extra-ordinary signs that come his way. How often do health-care providers miss this dimension of who we are?

   b. Beliefs are powerful. Do we value the cross-cultural beliefs of our patients? How can Board Certified Chaplains identify and attend to such beliefs during spiritual assessments?

Integration of Projective Objects to Hold Reality

For those unfamiliar with ego psychology, we offer some definitions of terms used in this following section. Projective objects are aspects of one's inner world, often based on early childhood experiences with parents, that are recognized in others. While the other person(s) may carry similarities to these internal aspects, differences remain. The person who projects these inner aspects onto others usually sees these individuals in a way that is similar to how their own inner world functions. For example, a man who had a critical father when he was a child might adopt critical attitudes toward himself. When such a man encounters an authority figure, such as a physician, the man might assume, or project, that the physician is critical of him when this might not be the case. Such projections may be a step toward integration of the personality toward the end of wholeness if the individual who projects learns to "reclaim" his or her projections. Psychological wholeness occurs when individuals learn to be for themselves what they seek to gain from others (e.g. love or approval).

Split self-objects occur when the person projects their rewarding self-object unit, or internal aspect, (the "blessing") and their withdrawing self-object unit, or internal aspect, (the "curse") within themselves onto one or more persons in an attempt to blend the two in the service of balance and wholeness. The "other" may then be seen alternatively as a bad or good person at any given time until this split is resolved.

Agnes of God (1985; Jane Fonda, Anne Bancroft, Meg Tilly): When Agnes (Tilly), a naïve novice nun, is discovered with a dead newborn in her convent quarters, a court-appointed psychiatrist, Dr. Martha Livingston (Fonda), investigates her case, trying to help Agnes get a stronger grip on reality in order to find the truth. In the process, Dr. Livingston becomes involved in a conflictual relationship with Mother Superior Miriam Ruth who is also Agnes's maternal aunt (Bancroft) and wants Agnes to be left alone.

1   (0:12:23–0:14:07) This scene depicts the conflict between Dr. Livingston and Mother Superior Miriam Ruth regarding how Agnes will be treated. These early transference dynamics impact not only Agnes's overall care but also whether the world of science or religion will predominate.

    a. What is your view of projective objects and how might that be applicable to the diagnosis and treatment of Agnes?

2 (0:14:56–0:24:35) In this scene, Dr. Livingston initially meets Agnes who is standing, looking out the window in a room and singing a beautiful song as if in a trance. Dr. Livingston affirms her on many levels, all of which Agnes dismisses, saying it is not really her.

    a. What projective objects are introduced in this scene and how might their integration form the basis for treatment? What split self-object relations are evident? How might this split inform diagnosis and treatment?

    b. Dr. Livingston admits that her smoking is an obsession that needs to be replaced by a more desirable obsession. How does Dr. Livingston's identification with Agnes's obsession inform how she will treat Agnes?

    c. How do we measure such gifts of song as either belonging to the singer or as being generated by a Higher Power?

3 (0:28:30–0:30:01) In this scene Dr. Livingston visits her own mother who has dementia and is in a care facility. The mother confuses Dr. Livingston with her sister Marie who had previously died in a convent.

    a. How can the psychotherapist's integration of his/her own self-projective objects further the work with clients?

4 (0:34:09–0:35:00) This scene between Dr. Livingston and Mother Superior demonstrates not only power and control issues for treatment but also how splitting science and religion compromises the best care for a client.

    a. How might Dr. Livingston have helped hold or provide a clinical container for Agnes's projective world by utilizing a different response in order to integrate her position and that of Mother Superior

    b. To what degree have the split self-object relationships within the convent reinforced Agnes' internal splits?

    c. To what degree did Dr. Livingston's own split self-object relations interfere with that of the convent to impair the best care and treatment for Agnes?

5 (1:36:08–1:34:36) This closing scene depicts Agnes in her "secret place" within the convent. Dr. Livingston's interpretation of Agnes, her treatment, and the treatment outcome are heard as Agnes plays with and releases a white dove.

    a. What might the white dove symbolize?

    b. How does psychiatrist Dr. Livingston's experience of a personal miracle in working with Agnes inform her approach with Agnes?

References

1 Gallup Poll reported in *Life* magazine. March 1994.
2 Dossey L. *Be Careful What You Pray For … You Just Might Get It*. San Francisco, CA: Harper Collins; 1997.

36

Mind Your Peas: Food, Nutrition, and Weight

Kimberly Romig & Katrina Saunders

THE RELATIONSHIP BETWEEN NUTRITION AND CERTAIN DISEASE STATES has long been established.[1] Patients who are provided with nutritional education have an opportunity to make lifestyle changes in their diet. However, there is a general understanding that diet and nutrition are best explored from a multidimensional point of view. Indeed, the American Academy of Family Physicians encourages family medicine residency programs to include the identification of patient factors that influence nutrition such as culture, socioeconomic status, and mental health conditions in their nutrition curriculum.[2] Genetics, industrial practices, and the stigma associated with obesity are additional factors that deserve consideration when educating health-care professionals about nutritional guidance and discussing behavior change with patients. Given such factors, the authors have made attempts to select films and scenes that illustrate these important issues.

Cultural practices, in particular, are important to understand when assisting patients in making lifestyle changes. Education about historical perspectives of various food traditions can assist providers to better appreciate the meaning of food and what is being asked of patients to change. For example, with respect to African-American food traditions, Anne L. Bower's collection of essays entitled *African American Foodways: explorations of history and culture*[3] gives an account of the incredible complexities involved in understanding the relationship between what has been termed "soul food" and the expression and preservation of sociocultural identity. How easy is it to make adaptations to recipes and food selections that have historical significance and hold the collective memories of generations?

Taking a comprehensive nutrition history[4] and exploring the various factors impacting food choices may be one way to strengthen the patient-provider relationship and open the door to ongoing dialogue that encourages increased self-awareness and healthier living for patients and perhaps even the provider. Clips have been chosen to illustrate these teaching points, as well.

Impact of Fast Food
· ·

Fast Food Nation (2006): This movie stars Greg Kinnear, Wilmer Valderama (as Raul), and Catalina Sandino Moreno (as Sylvia). As head of marketing for Mickey's fast food chain, Don Anderson (Kinnear) is responsible for investigating when an independent research lab finds feces in the beef. In order to inspect the main supplier for Mickey's, Don heads to the fictitious town of Cody, Colorado. While there, Don discovers the ugly truth about the meat industry and its impact on everyone, from the cows, to the illegal factory workers, to the consumers eating Mickey's bestselling burger, "The Big One."

1 (0:01:00–0:01:45) Families enjoy the food in the crowded Mickey's dining area.
2 (1:10:07–1:10:46) People discuss changes in Cody, Colorado, over the past few years.
3 (1:44:24–1:45:37) Illegal migrants arrive in the United States and are greeted by an individual who has helped them be smuggled into the country, and are given child meals from the local Mickey's restaurant.
   a. What are some factors that have contributed to the high rates of fast food consumption in the United States?
   b. How do you address nutrition with a patient who consumes or allows his or her children to consume fast food regularly?
   c. As a health-care professional, how do you address a patient's argument that fast food is more affordable than more nutritious choices?
   d. How do you encourage patients to incorporate fresh fruits and vegetables into their diets when they live in the inner city and/or low socioeconomic status neighborhoods with limited access to such foods?
   e. How do you work with a patient to choose "healthier" fast food options when they are unwilling to eliminate fast food from their diet?
   f. What health risks are associated with high levels of fast food consumption? How do you communicate these concerns to patients who are at high risk and for those who are already experiencing some of the related health issues?

Cultural Norms, Healthy Weight, and the Meaning of Food
· · · · · · · · · · · · · ·

Real Women Have Curves (2002): This movie stars America Ferrera (as Ana Garcia), Lupe Ontiveros (as Carmen Garcia), and George Lopez (as Mr. Guzman). *Real Women Have Curves* depicts the coming-of-age story of Ana, a young Latina growing up in East LA. Newly graduated from high school, Ana struggles to resolve the conflict between her own ambitions to attend college and her traditional family's expectations that she help provide for the family by working in her sister's sewing shop. During her time spent at the shop, Ana learns to appreciate her family and herself, which translates to following her own dreams.

1 (1:08:35–1:12:20) While working in the sewing shop, Ana and her coworkers show off their cellulite and weight and embrace their beauty.

   a. As a health-care professional, how do you counsel a patient about nutrition when the patient is satisfied with their physical appearance despite not meeting standards for healthy weight?

   b. When working with patients of different cultural groups, how do you respect cultural standards of health and beauty while promoting proper nutrition and health?

   c. How, as a health-care professional, can you facilitate proper nutrition for your patients, while incorporating traditional cultural foods?

Soul Food (1997; Irma P. Hall, Vanessa Williams, Nia Long, Vivica Fox, Brandon Hammond): A family's strong matriarchal figure, Big Mama Joe (Hall), suffers from complications of diabetes and subsequently dies. The film is narrated from the perspective of her grandson, Ahmad (Hammond), who discusses the family dynamics from the perspective of food traditions. In the first two mouth-watering scenes, Ahmad attributes his family's closeness to their 40-year ritual of Sunday family dinners. The film clips speak to this African-American family's cultural traditions around food, to the etiology and meaning of those traditions, and hints at the African-American struggle to maintain their original culture through food.

1 (0:08:48–0:11:14) The opening scene features Sunday dinner with the extended family.

2 (1:34:45–1:38:37) This is one of the final dinner scenes following Big Mama's death.

3 (1:48:00 –1:50:35) In this final scene, Ahmad addresses his understanding of "soul food."

   a. What is the possible relationship between the historical information referenced in the introduction to this chapter and the importance of this family's traditional Sunday dinners?

   b. Is it possible for food to have the sole (no pun intended) purpose of being a source of nutrition? Why or why not?

   c. Explain the connection between food and cultural identity as well as food and relationships. To what other issues might food be connected?

   d. What happens when food becomes a source of comfort rather than nutrition?

   e. How can you intervene when patients explain that the most affordable food items are the least nutritious?

   f. What culinary traditions and the cultural significance of such in other cultures have you come in contact with as a health-care provider?

Impact of Weight on Child/Adolescent Peer Interactions
· · · · · · · · · · · · · · · ·

To Be Fat Like Me (2007): This movie stars Kaley Cuoco (as Alyson), Caroline Rhea (as Madelyn), and Melissa Halstrom (as Ramona). Alyson is a beautiful, popular, high school athlete who seems to have it all until an injury sidelines her for the rest of the softball season, preventing her from being scouted for a full scholarship to a state university. In an attempt to win tuition money, Alyson decides to enter a film contest, documenting her experiences as she goes undercover as an overweight high school student with the use of a fat suit. Although Alyson begins the documentary believing that overweight people are treated the same as everyone else, she quickly learns that this is not the case. By putting herself in someone else's body, Alyson not only learns what it's like to be overweight but also learns a lot about herself.

1 (00:5:45–00:6:51) Alyson's younger brother, who is overweight, is harassed by some of his peers.
2 (0:25:52–0:27:00) Alyson has her first experience in the school cafeteria as a "fat" high school student.
3 (0:27:57–0:31:39) While Alyson is playing basketball with her male friends, they discuss the "mom test," referring to the notion that if you want to know how your girlfriend will age, look at her mother.
4 (0:34:25–0:35:11) Alyson faces taunting from peers while at school.
5 (0:52:10–0:54:00) Alyson and her friends face taunting while bowling.
   a. What is the potential impact of teasing on overweight children and adolescents?
   b. What emotional/psychological issues should be taken into consideration when working with overweight youth?
   c. Given the rise in pediatric obesity rates, how can you educate parents about providing proper nutrition for their children? How might your education change if the parents of your client/patient are overweight/obese?
   d. If you witnessed the taunting shown, would you intervene? Under what circumstances might you intervene and in what way? How would you counsel a child or teen about how to respond to taunting/bullying.

Discrimination and Confronting Stigma
· ·

1 (0:39:10–0:41:06) Alyson wears a "fat suit" and has befriended Ramona, an obese high school student. Together, they experience rudeness and discrimination as they step into a trendy boutique.
2 (1:15:00–1:19:23) Alyson reveals her social experiment and confronts her friends' taunting while at a party.
   a. What sort of stigma is attached to being overweight/obese in this country?

b. What are your personal biases regarding obese individuals and how can that impact the quality of care that is provided?

c. What are the statistics for becoming an overweight/ obese adult if so as a child or adolescent?

d. What might be some reasons for "emotional eating"?

Impact of Stigma on the Individual and Family

1 (0:41:06–0:44:07) Ramona recounts to Alyson her experience of the emotional impact of being overweight.

2 (1:21:12–1:23:18) Alyson tells her mother how she was affected years ago by her mother's hospitalization for weight-induced health issues (i.e. diabetes).

3 (1:23:30–1:25:00) Alyson and Ramona share their feelings about the impact of being overweight.

a. What is your understanding of some of the psychosocial factors contributing to overweight/obesity and its maintenance?

b. What comorbid conditions (emotional/physical) are associated with overweight/obesity?

c. As a health-care professional, how can you support your overweight/obese client's/patient's emotional needs?

Overweight/Obesity and Understanding Stigma in Adults

What's Eating Gilbert Grape? (1993): This movie stars Johnny Depp (as Gilbert Grape), Leonardo DiCaprio (as Arnie Grape), and Juliette Lewis (as Becky). Gilbert Grape is a young man struggling to find his place in the world. He works as a stock boy in a local market in a small town named Endora. When Gilbert is not working, he takes care of his mentally handicapped brother, Arnie, and his morbidly obese mother, who has not left the house in 7 years. The sudden appearance of Becky, a new girl in town, helps awaken Gilbert, putting him on his path to self-discovery.

1 (0:17:31–0:18:29) Local kids come to stare at Mama through the windows of her house.

2 (1:05:15–1:09:06) Mama leaves her house to get Arnie out of jail and draws a crowd.

a. What sort of stigma is attached to being overweight/obese in this country?

b. What are your personal biases regarding obese individuals? Does it differ if they are clients/patients?

c. What are the health risks associated with being overweight/obese?

d. Given the stigma attached to being overweight/obese, it can be a difficult experience for such patients to go to their doctor. What accommodations can you make in your office to assist patients to maintain regular appointments?

e. As a health-care professional, where do you begin in assisting an over-weight/obese client/patient with nutrition and weight loss?

f. How can you help facilitate continued motivation for proper nutrition and weight loss in overweight/obese patients?

g. How do you handle a client/patient who, despite experiencing health issues, is resistant to making changes in their nutrition and weight?

h. What are your attitudes toward bariatric intervention? What does the research show in comparing the lap band procedure versus gastric by-pass surgery?

Emotional Impact on Patient and Family

1 (1:29:17–1:30:40) Gilbert shares his feelings about his mother with Becky.
2 (1:35:56–1:38:30) Gilbert and his mother share their feelings with each other.
3 (1:39:35–1:40:56) Mama meets Becky for the first time.
  a. What are the psychosocial factors contributing to overweight/obesity and its maintenance?
  b. What comorbid conditions (emotional/physical) are associated with overweight/obesity?
  c. How, as a health-care professional, can you support your overweight/obese client's/patient's emotional needs?
  d. How can you help facilitate family members' involvement in nutrition and weight changes?
  e. Given the rise in pediatric obesity rates, how can you educate parents about providing proper nutrition for their children? How does this change if the parents of your client/patient are overweight/obese?

(Note: The film clips from *Soul Food* listed later in this chapter under "Diabetes, Food, and Culture" can also be used to discuss the emotional impact of over-weight/obesity on the patient and family.)

Food Choices and Levels of Restriction

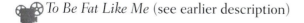 *To Be Fat Like Me* (see earlier description)

1 (0:7:15–0:8:05) Alyson, who is very strict with her food choices, and her mother debate the practice of indulging periodically versus depriving oneself completely of less healthy choices.
  a. How would you counsel a young patient in need of losing weight? What are your recommendations for diet and exercise?

    b. What are some indicators that a patient is engaging in too restrictive/
      unhealthy dieting behaviors? How do you work with such an individual?

    c. What are the long-term health risks associated with unhealthy (excessive/
      restrictive) eating behaviors?

    d. How, as a health-care provider, can you engage family members in promot-
      ing healthy eating habits for younger patients?

What's Cooking? (2000): This movie stars Mercedes Ruehl (as Lizzy Avila), Alfre Woodard (as Audrey Williams), Joan Chen (as Trinh Nguyen), and Lainie Kazan (as Ruth Seelig). A multicultural comedy, this film is about four different households from four different cultures, all celebrating Thanksgiving Day. The film is not as much about food traditions and their meanings as it is about family stressors and secrets that all begin to get exposed around the various dinner tables.

1 (1:25:00–1:27:09) This scene shows the Williams family having a meal together.

2 (1:29:29–1:32:44) This scene shows the Avila family having a meal together.

    a. These two scenes depict two different marriages in two different famil-
      ies that are in crisis. The women handle their emotions very differently.
      Compare, contrast, and discuss the responses of the women in these two
      scenes.

    b. Equate "stuffing" emotions with "stuffing" food.

    c. As a health-care provider, how might you assist a client/patient in identify-
      ing emotional eating?

    d. What is the role of anger management, stress reduction, and/or cognitive
      behavioral therapy in emotional eating?

    e. Are you familiar with Overeaters Anonymous and Recovery International?
      What are their basic tenets?

    f. In reference to dinner table conversations, is it a typical time for families
      to discuss difficult or emotional issues? What are the pros and cons of
      this practice?

    g. What were your own family dinner conversation experiences? Was culture
      a factor in what was discussed or how things were discussed?

Diabetes, Food, and Culture

Soul Food (see earlier description): The following scenes demonstrate the importance of proper nutrition for minimizing diabetic complications.

1 (0:12:25–0:13:05) Big Mama burns her arm, and her daughters address her noncompliance with her diabetic regimen.

2 (0:21:28–0:22:10) The family discusses Big Mama's need for an amputation.

3 (0:31:50–0:34:34) we see Big Mama's surgery and subsequent deterioration.

4 (0:37:35–0:39:37) Big Mama's hospitalization takes a toll on the family.

a. Discuss the role of food as medicine.
b. Discuss the impact on family when a loved one does not take care of his or her health.
c. How would you motivate a patient with strong food traditions to alter their dietary behavior?
d. What resources are available to educate and encourage patients to follow a healthy diet?
e. What is your familiarity with programs such as Weight Watchers?
f. What are some of the culinary traditions and significance of such in other cultures with which you have come in contact as a health-care provider?
g. Do you know how collard greens are traditionally prepared? Have you ever had chit'lins?

Alternative Views and Practices

Food Matters (2008; David Wolfe, authority on raw foods and superfoods; Ian Brighthope, professor of nutritional and environmental medicine; Andrew Saul, therapeutic nutrition specialist; Dan Rogers; Jerome Burne, medical journalist and author; Victor Zeines, holistic dentist and nutritionist; Philip Day, investigative journalist and author; Charlotte Gerson, founder of the Gerson Institute; Patrick Holford, founder of the Institute for Optimum Nutrition; Dr. Gert Schuitemaker, founder of the Ortho Europe Institute; Arnaud Apoteker, biologist and organic food specialist): This is a controversial documentary that features interviews with nutritionists, scientists, physicians, medical journalists, and naturopaths who present their opinions regarding the use of food and supplements for disease prevention, treatment, and overall well-being. Also discussed is the relationship between nutrition and the medical industry.

Patients sometimes share nutritional information with which providers are either unfamiliar or in disagreement. It is important for providers to have some understanding of alternative nutritional views as well as an understanding of their own emotional reactions to these views and practices. This documentary is best viewed in its entirety in order to gain a more complete understanding of the issues covered. Despite some of the questionable information and, at times, contentious format, this film offers an opportunity for good discussion.

1 (0:00:13–0:02:02) This clip introduces the film and offers a glimpse of the issues to be discussed.
   a. What does the quote, "let thy food be thy medicine" mean to you?
   b. What kind of information on nutrition did you receive in your training as a health-care professional?
   c. How do you feel about the term "sickness industry" that is used in the film?
   d. From where do you think the quoted health and health industry statistics came? Do you think they are presented accurately or in a skewed fashion for media entertainment?

e. Discuss the statement, "good health makes a lot of sense, but it doesn't make a lot of dollars."
f. What is the best way to respond to a client's/patient's use of complementary and alternative nutritional practices?

Are You What You Eat?

1 (0:02:05–0:06:48) This section reviews the agricultural, commercial processing, and cooking practices that affect the health and nutritional value of our food.
2 (00:06:48–00:12:14) Superfoods and raw foods are discussed in this clip.
   a. How can you research and evaluate the information presented?
   b. If the presented views are of value to you, how would you present such information to your patients?
   c. How would you advise a client/patient who wants to explore the use of dietary measures to treat a disease condition? How about for disease prevention?
   d. How do you encourage clients/patients to engage in "mindful" nutrition?
   e. How can you assist clients/patients in finding a balance between what is beneficial and what is practical?
   f. How costly or accessible are superfoods in the community in which you practice? Is there a farmer's market or a community garden?

Nutrition as a Prevention Strategy

1 (01:02:46–01:05:11) The concept of nutritional therapy (orthomolecular medicine) is presented in this clip.
2 (01:05:11–01:07:55) This scene presents nutrition as a prevention strategy in a disease care system.
3 (01:07:55–01:14:04) This scene emphasizes individual education, making choices, and taking responsibility.
   a. Is there any evidence for using therapeutic nutrition (high dose vitamin supplements) in reversing disease states? Which journals would you research?
   b. How do you proceed when you have a client/patient who utilizes high dose supplements to treat his/her illness? Describe your feelings about such clients/patients.
   c. What steps would you encourage clients/patients to take in researching the credibility of documentaries such as this, its contributors or any other information on alternative treatment to which they've been exposed?
   d. How would you discuss a client's/patient's nutritional belief system without alienating him/her?

e. Describe information in the documentary that you believe to be useful.

f. What are the philosophical commonalities between nutritionists, naturo-paths and traditional health-care practitioners? What are the differences?

g. How do you encourage clients/patients to take responsibility for their nutritional health?

References

1 Bidlack WR. Interrelationships of food, nutrition, diet and health: the National Association of State Universities and Land Grant Colleges White Paper. *J Am Coll Nutr.* 1996; **15**(5): 422–33.

2 Recommended Curriculum Guidelines for Family Medicine Residents. Nutrition. AAFP Reprint No. 275. Available at: www.aafp.org/online/en/home/aboutus/specialty/rpsolutions/eduguide.html (accessed May 22, 2011).

3 Bower AL, editor. *African American Foodways: explorations of history and culture.* Urbana: University of Illinois Press; 2009.

4 Hark L, Deen D, Jr. Taking a nutrition history: a practical approach for family physicians. *Am Fam Physician.* 1999; **59**(6): 1521–8.

Additional Reading

● Conan N. *The Importance of Soul Food: a Black History Month celebration of Southern cooking.* NPR; February 4, 2003. Available at: www.npr.org/templates/story/story.php?storyId=971241 (last accessed 12/01/11)

● NPR. *A Soul Food Journey from Africa to America.* NPR; October 20, 2008. Available at: www.npr.org/templates/story/story.php?storyId=95907586 (last accessed 12/01/11)

● Prochaska JO, DiClemente CC. Stages and processes of self-change in smoking: toward an integrative model of change. *J Consult Clin Psychol.* 1983; **51**(3): 390–5.

37

Nine to Five (and Then Some): Occupational Medicine

Lawrence Raymond

OCCUPATIONAL AND ENVIRONMENTAL MEDICINE (OEM) IS A SUB-specialty within the field of preventive medicine. Its scope is the recognition, prevention, and treatment of illness and injury due to chemical and physical agents, including trauma. Traumatic events may include slips, trips, and falls; damage to unprotected eyes from foreign bodies; lacerations from sharp objects; and musculoskeletal strains often related to lifting while twisting or bending. The ill effects of toxic or allergenic chemicals, noise, ionizing radiation, or thermal extremes causing heat stress or hypothermia are less common but no less significant safety issues.

When health and well-being are threatened by workplace conditions, the issues are considered the purview of occupational medicine. Many of the same toxic chemicals and damaging physical agents that pose threats on the job can, however, also inflict harm on the general public or subsets of community inhabitants. In such cases, the purview is that of environmental medicine.

OEM also involves administrative issues such as evaluating the worker's medical fitness for duty, with possible waivers for impaired workers. Collaboration with human resources is often a key interface as when racial discrimination in the workplace is masqueraded as a work-ability issue.

Although there are many films that depict issues relevant to OEM, two have been chosen here as a focus – these will be used to illustrate salient issues in the field.

Workplace Health, Safety, and Interpersonal Issues

Men of Honor (2001; Robert De Niro, Cuba Gooding, Jr.): Based on the true story of Carl Brashear (Gooding), the first African-American to become a US Navy diver, this film is rich in examples of OEM, mostly occupational. Brashear initially came into the Navy as a cook, the usual job for black enlistees in the United States of the mid-1900s, before becoming a Navy diver. While this film covers many issues germane to occupational medicine, it doesn't address the more usual health aspects of deep diving, such as painful limbs during decompression ("the bends"), paralysis from spinal cord "bends," nitrogen narcosis ("raptures of the deep"), and oxygen toxicity to the lungs or nervous system.

Occupational Racism

1 (Ch 5, 0:21:00–0:27:45) Racist attitudes are revealed as soon as Brashear arrives at diving school as the student-diver barracks empties out amid the echo, "I don't bunk with niggers."
   a. What increased risks might Brashear face given the racism being displayed?
   b. How might racial bias such as this be overcome in the workplace?
   c. What other forms of occupational bias (i.e. gender; sexual orientation) were overcome in the twentieth century? Have these been fully addressed?
   d. What recourse does a worker have in present-day America when he or she perceives discrimination in employment matters?
2 (Ch 11, 1:04:30–1:18:10) Racist overtones continue as master diver Billy Sunday (De Niro) colludes with his deranged commanding officer to expose Brashear to severe underwater hypothermia, aimed at getting him to drop out of the program. Despite this harrowing experience, Brashear completes the difficult assembly task, thus successfully completing his diving course.
   a. The master diver says, "Give it up, Cookie, ya go into shock down there, ya may not wake up!" (1:15:30). Do you think the master diver had second thoughts about letting his student diver continue to suffer from the cold?
   b. Can hypothermia lead to unconsciousness or just severe shivering? Could it be fatal?
   c. For extra credit: Do you recall what happened to Jack London's protagonist in the film *To Build a Fire* (2003)?

Dysbarism

1 (Ch 12, 1:24:20–1:29:00) We soon see Brashear in action, diving off of the USS *Hoist* in search of a lost nuclear device off the coast of Spain. A passing Russian sub fouls his line and he is tossed high off the seabed and exposed to rapid changes in pressure that cause him to lose consciousness. Such pressure changes can produce a host of ill effects, none of which usually reverse as quickly as what plays out in this cinematic version.
   a. What sort of chest damage would likely have occurred if Brashear held his breath while suddenly being yanked up 50 feet from the seabed?
      i. A broken rib or two?
      ii. A collapsed lung (maybe both)?
      iii. Acute pneumonia?
      iv. Pulmonary embolus (clot going from leg to lung)?

    b. Would the condition have resolved by itself? What might have happened to Brashear's eardrums?

(Explanation: None of the choices (i–iv) would have cleared up as quickly as in this film, but the most likely choice is a collapsed lung from sudden expansion of the gas trapped in his lungs by breath-holding. In reality, it would not have resolved on its own; however, in Hollywood, the rules of physics – and physiology – are sometimes suspended. One more thought: the rapid change in pressure on Brashear's suit might also have ruptured one or both of his eardrums.)

Accidents/Severe Trauma

1   (Ch 14, 1:28:50–1:29:25) Back on the deck of the *Hoist*, Brashear is caught when a thick hauling line breaks, whipping across his leg and nearly cutting it off. Shipmates keep him from bleeding to death.

2   (Ch 15, 1:31:05–1:38:20) Brashear's leg is so badly damaged that he chooses amputation rather than a future of infirmity. A weak leg would be the end of his navy diving career but he learns of aviators who were returned to duty postamputation. (In the less dramatic instances of today's steel industry, for example, some supervisors may favor completing an amputation of a finger or toe so as to avoid the cost and protracted healing of a plastic surgery repair.)

    a. What types of emotional trauma might Brashear experience as a result of his accident? How might witnessing this accident impact the other workers/divers? What are the best treatment approaches to help heal the residual emotional scars of severe trauma such as this?

    b. What are a company's liabilities in workplace accidents? How can occupational medicine physicians make sure that workers' health interests are not compromised by financial factors? Is this their responsibility?

Rehabilitation Therapy

1   (Ch 15, 1:41:20–1:59:00) Brashear begins the rigors of recovering the stamina needed for diving while also adapting to his new prosthetic leg. He has a surprise visitor, his former archenemy master diver Sunday (De Niro), who suggests a way for him to outwit Captain Wilks, the senior naval officer who wants Brashear declared unfit for any future active duty. Wilks convenes a board of medical review, angling for Brashear's forced retirement.

    a. Is there a mechanism for making an exception to a job requirement when a person's impairment seems incompatible with that job demand? [Answer: A waiver can be granted.]

    b. In civilian life, can a truck driver whose lower leg is amputated become medically qualified to drive again? Where would you look to find out? [Answer: The Federal Motor Carrier Safety Administration can grant a waiver if the amputee passes its Skill Performance Evaluation.]

Community Health Issues

Erin Brockovich (2000; Julia Roberts, Albert Finney): Based on a true story, this film offers examples of both occupational and environmental concerns. Erin (Roberts) is an unemployed, twice-divorced single parent with three children and she receives only meager child support. During the course of the film, she exposes unhealthy practices of a major industry in the town of Hinkley, California, and becomes an advocate for the Jensen family who are suffering health effects. Although not all agree with the validity of the claims of Ms. Brockovich, the movie is well done and thought-provoking.

Maintaining Professional Standards

1 (Ch 1, 0:1:00–0:2:00) Brockovich fails to impress the doctor who interviews her for a laboratory technician job. Her smooth talk does not hide her lack of any medical knowledge or the required skills and so her hunt for work continues.

2 (Ch 7, 0:12:30–0:13:30) Brockovich exclaims: "Don't make me beg ... if it doesn't work out, fire me."

   a. How is the public protected from unqualified persons working in health care? [Answer: In most jurisdictions, credentials are needed for medical laboratories and for the technicians who staff them.]

Environmental Noise

1 (Ch 8, 0:15:40–0:16:20) Brockovich finds the noise of her neighbor's revving of a motorcycle engine unbearable as she tucks her kids in bed.

   a. Can less dramatic loud neighborhood noises have adverse health effects? [Answer: Epidemiologic studies have identified associations between neighborhood traffic or airport noise and heart problems in adults and learning difficulties in children.]

   b. What recourse do individuals have in addressing high levels of environmental noise in their neighborhoods?

Workplace Dress Code

1 (Ch 7, 0:13:45–0:13:50; ch 9, 0:17:30–0:18:30) Brockovich's skimpy dress and full-busted endowment may have helped her get hired, but soon complaints arise from other women in the law firm who are less well endowed.

   a. What are common standards for work dress? Do such standards change with geographical region, societal mores, and administrative bias? How can employers most effectively address violations of workplace dress code?

Pollution

1 (Ch 11, 0:27:00–0:28:30) Soon after being hired as a file clerk, Brockovich gets permission to check out a possible link between water pollution by a major utility, Pacific Gas and Electric (PG&E) and a cluster of unusual serious illnesses including birth defects.

2 (Ch 12, 0:29:00–0:30:50; ch 13, 0:31:00–0:32:30) Brockovich visits a family whose home PG&E has offered to buy after the family's illnesses were described to a local doctor in the employ of PG&E. Suspicions are stoked when the wife mentions chromium. Brockovich next visits a university campus where a friendly toxicologist recites a list of bad things chromium can do: "chronic headaches, nosebleeds, reproductive failure, bone and organ deterioration, respiratory diseases, any type of cancer, liver failure and heart failure."

a. What variables are important to consider in determining the possible ill effects of a given chemical? [Answer: As Paracelsus (aka Philippus Aureolus, the German chemist and physician) first said, "It is the dose which makes the poison." But also important are:

  i. route of exposure, inhaled vs. swallowed vs. skin contact

  ii. duration of exposure

  iii. specific chemical form, i.e. hexavalent chromium (Cr-VI) is much more toxic than trivalent chromium (Cr-III) or metallic chromium (Cr-0)

  iv. the species exposed, rodent vs. subhuman primate vs. human.

In the case of contaminated well water serving the town of Hinkley, the route of exposure to Cr-VI was mainly ingestion, a less toxic route than inhalation of chromium particles, which can cause respiratory cancers in overexposed humans.

Industry Obfuscation

1 (Ch 17, 0:47:00–0:48:00) Her husband ill with Hodgkin's disease and herself in and out of the hospital, Donna Jensen tells Brockovich, "They held a seminar on chromium-III telling them how good it is, when all the time they're using chromium-VI." By taking advantage of the fact that Cr-III is an essential trace element in human nutrition, and is sometimes used to improve a diabetic patient's response to insulin, PG&E is playing on the public's ignorance so as to disguise the toxic nature of the form of chromium they used in their facility.

a. How widespread is the industry/government practice of playing on people's ignorance to hide serious environmental issues?

b. What is the responsibility of a community-based physician to try to improve the knowledge base of the public when it comes to environmental health issues?

c. We learn near the end of the film (2:05:30) that the settlement awarded to the plaintiffs in the case of Hinkley vs. PG&E was the largest in a direct-action lawsuit in United States history. However, the State of California (Morgan JW) conducted three separate studies that showed that the number of cancers in the community of Hinkley between 1996 and 2008 were actually fewer than expected number – 196 vs. 224. Given this information, why do you believe that PG&E agreed to pay this huge sum? Is it possible that the company's conduct in the entire matter might have left it vulnerable to even greater liability?[1]

Illness Clusters

1   (Ch 34, 1:35:20–1:38:10) In her new law office, Brockovich, though lacking in formal medical education, displays a dazzling grasp of the details of plaintiffs' illnesses. In one family, for example, she notes: (1) the daughter Annabelle is in need of radiation for a brain stem tumor; (2) Annabelle's father, Ted, is being treated for recent onset of Crohn's disease; and (3) Annabelle's mother, Rita, has chronic headaches and nausea and needed a hysterectomy at age 32. Brockovich points out that this family "lived on the plume" since Annabelle was born, referring to the aquifer serving the town's well-water supply, which is polluted with the toxic form of chromium.

   a. Does the variety of these medical conditions strengthen or weaken the argument as to cause-and-effect relationship of the putative chemical exposure? [Answer: It weakens the link. "Biological plausibility" is strongest when a single disease is consistently associated with a specific chemical, as when prolonged inhalation of hexavalent chromium is associated with an increased risk of respiratory ailments such as lung cancer and erosion of the nasal septum, often causing perforation.]

Reference

1   Wiles R., Environmental Working Group, Washington DC 20009 and Oakland CA 94612. Letter to Dr. J.A. Popp, president, Society of Toxicology. July 18, 2006. www.ewg.org/node/21951 (last accessed 4/16/2012)

Further Reading

● Blot WJ, Fryzek JP, Henderson BE, *et al.* A cohort mortality study among gas generator utility workers. *J Occup Environ Med.* 2000; **42**(2): 194–9. (No evidence that occupational exposures at PG&E resulted in lung cancer or any other cause of death. Could this be the result of the "health worker effect"?)
● Brockovich E, Praglin GA. 'Erin Brockovich' affirmed. *Wall Street Journal.* April 6, 2000.
● Fumento M. 'Erin Brockovich' exposed. *Wall Street Journal.* March 28, 2000.
● Kolata G. A hit movie is rated 'F' in science. *New York Times.* April 11, 2000.
● Morgan JW. Unpublished data on cancer incidence in Hinkley, CA. Desert Sierra Cancer Surveillance Program. (see Sahagun L, Fewer cancers found in Hinkley than expected. *LA Times.* December 13, 2010).

PART VII

Compassion and Medicine

38

Easing the Pain:
Palliative Care

Dawn Joosten, Amy E. Cassidy, Greg Dahlquist,
Patricia Lenahan & Anna Pavlov

DEATH IS A UNIVERSAL EXPERIENCE THAT IMPACTS ALL INDIVIDUALS. Yet it is difficult to find North American movies which realistically depict end-of-life in the hospital or death in the home. Hollywood often depicts death in a gratuitous fashion, often bloody and realistic during scenes of crime and war. Is Hollywood concerned there is no market for movies that accurately reflect end-of-life issues, or is it our culture that has no interest in this topic? Interestingly, there is not a paucity of films tackling this topic in other countries. Some of the classic movies in this area are from France, Spain, and Japan (See appendix of movies).

The Federal Uniform Determination of Death Act of 1981 mandates that states define death as the loss of all brain function.[1] Death, or the end of life, is defined differently by health-care providers specializing in geriatrics: "The end-of-life is that period in the life cycle where the person can expect a future of loss and diminishment on the physical and/or cognitive level."[2] Physicians trained in the medical model prevalent in Western society focus on diagnosis, prognosis, and a treatment plan that may involve options to either prolong life and death through life sustaining technology, surgery, and/or aggressive treatments and medications. In contrast, the treatment plan may focus on pain and symptom management available through palliative care.

Alternatively, when aggressive treatments are perceived as futile and/or there is no hope for cure then patients may be referred to hospice programs. For some patients, the expected physical loss may occur within minutes, hours, days, or weeks. For others with life-threatening or chronic illnesses the expectation of physical and/or cognitive loss can occur over months or years. Additionally, end-of-life care can be needed at any time across the lifespan from birth to old age.

The palliative care movement in the United States has brought to light the benefits of palliation and interventions employing an interdisciplinary team comprised of physicians, nurses, social workers, and chaplains in working with the atient/family dyad using a biopsychosocial/spiritual perspective. For the dividual the context of daily life includes: "coping with the physical, financial, psychological, and spiritual challenges of illness; maintaining relationships in light of change, conflict, and potential growth; and experiencing suffering, loss, spiritual growth, reconciliation, uncertainty, and physical discomfort."[3] The context for the family often involves balancing the tasks of physical care and accessing ancillary home and community-based services for their dying loved one along with managing their own self-care and psychological, emotional, spiritual, and physical responses.

In end-of-life care, the interdisciplinary team shares pertinent patient information through collaboration, communication, and shared decision making based on a foundation of respect[4] and commitment among team members to respond holistically to the biopsychosocial/spiritual needs of the patient/family dyad. The term "respectful death" refers to a process for exploring the values, goals, and meanings of the dying individual's "lived experience" by understanding stories of the dying individual, the family, and significant others.[5] For the social worker involved in end-of-life care, the story is appreciated for the power it holds for the dying individual and family members.[2]

With expertise in diversity and advocacy, crisis intervention, and brief therapy, the social worker plays a key role in identifying the specific end-of-life care wishes and preferences of the dying patients through the use of a biopsychosocial/ spiritual perspective. The social worker works collaboratively with the team to create an environment in which the patient feels safe to explore their journey with death, meeting the patient and family where they are, so that they can "deal with the pain, discomfort, anxiety, fear, and depression that can further degrade the quality of their remaining time."[4] In addressing the spiritual needs of patients, social workers, using a strengths perspective place the patients as the expert of their life circumstances and explore "questions that provide definition to thematic life strengths and values that constitute a person's sense of self in the world."[5] The interdisciplinary team promotes a respectful death for the dying individual as demonstrated when "the care provided closely supports the authorship of the dying patient and family, with the clinician acting as editor rather than author in the process."[2]

Addressing Death and Dying

Tuesdays with Morrie (1999) is based on the true story of Morrie Schwartz, a Brandeis University professor, played by Jack Lemmon, who is diagnosed with Lou Gehrig's disease or amyotrophic lateral sclerosis (ALS). The film illustrates the gradual destruction to the nerve cells in Morrie's body and his subsequent loss in functional health. Yet it highlights his remarkable resilience while approaching death, as demonstrated by his passion, wit, and love for life, family, friends, and society. Dedicated to sharing his "lessons on living," Morrie

(Lemmon) appears on an ABC News special with Ted Koppel. It is during one of the interviews that one of Morrie's former students, Mitch Albom (Hank Azaria), a sports commentator and journalist, sees Morrie on television and decides to record Morrie's "lessons on living."

1 (Ch 7, 0:41:38–0:49:25) In an interview with Mitch, Morrie recalls his childhood and talks about his first experience of death, that of his mother, as a child. He becomes tearful as he recounts the time when he "thought if I ignored her illness it would just go away." He describes his father, a Russian immigrant, as one who never showed how he felt. Morrie recalls how his father never came in the house after the death of his mother instead reading a newspaper outside by a tree. Morrie says, "What was he feeling, I never knew. Was he in pain, was he suffering? All I knew was I needed his love. I needed him to hold me so I would not be afraid." A year later Morrie reflects on the love he was able to get from his new stepmother. He shifts his focus again back to his father stating, "My father was afraid of love, he couldn't give it, didn't receive it." Morrie experiences shortness of breath and Mitch attempts to give him oxygen calling out to the nurse for assistance. The nurse transfers Morrie from the wheelchair to his reclining chair. He looks to Mitch and states, "don't look so sad, Mitch, because I'm gonna die, everyone's gonna die, but most people don't believe it. They should have a bird on their shoulder, that's what the Buddhists do, and look at the little bird and ask it, 'Is this the day I'm going to die?' 'Am I leading the life I should?' 'Am I the person I want to be?' If we can accept the fact that we are going to die at any time then we would lead our lives differently." The scene then turns to Morrie lying in bed crying on a dark night and reaching for a pen and paper that he cannot hold onto.

   a. Apply the biopsychosocial/spiritual perspective to assess the end-of-life care needs and responses of Morrie and significant others in his life in this scene.
   b. How would an interdisciplinary team respond to the end-of-life care needs of Morrie?
   c. What role would you anticipate each member of the interdisciplinary team having?
   d. How should information be shared across team members?
   e. Would you recommend palliative care or hospice care, why or why not?
   f. What values, goals, and meaning can one assume that Morrie holds surrounding his own death?
   g. What life strengths does Morrie appear to possess?
   h. Does Morrie achieve a respectful death? Why or why not?

The Role of Nurses in End-of-Life Care/Dying

The English Patient (1996; Ralph Fiennes, Juliette Binoche, Willem Dafoe): A complex plot is developed using a series of flashbacks. Count László de Almásy (Ralph Fiennes) has been extensively burned during the war and is dependent on the care of his nurse, Hana (Juliette Binoche). They shelter in a heavily damaged Italian monastery, where she provides care for him and initiates a romance with a British demolitions expert. Although the nurse is caring for the patient at the end of World War II, the patient's life is chronicled through a series of flashbacks. The flashbacks reveal that the patient was involved in a very complicated love affair that ultimately turned fateful.

1   (0:25:00–0:26:13) The nurse, Hana (Juliette Binoche), has given the patient morphine, changed his bed, and repositioned him.
    a. In what ways has nursing practice changed since the 1940s?
    b. In what ways has it stayed the same?
    c. What changes would you like to see in nursing practice for the future?

2   (1:59:29–2:00:15) The patient (Ralph Fiennes) is being granted a dying wish. He had spent many of his recent years in Africa and stated in an earlier scene that he would like to feel rain on his face. The nurse has her houseguests aid her in running the patient around the courtyard in the rain to fulfill his wish.
    a. To what lengths should health-care professionals go to adhere to the patient's final wishes?
    b. Does the health-care professional have an obligation to the patient to be involved in the planning of such activities, or should that mainly be the responsibility of the patient's family?
    c. With the term, "bucket list" becoming more mainstream in today's society, what are some things on your bucket list?

3   (2:28:59–2:33:52) It is clear that the Count (Fiennes) receives morphine on a regular basis for pain associated with his extensive burns. He is about to receive his standard dose but, as Hana draws up the dose, the Count gives her additional vials, making it clear he wants an overdose and death. She agrees with his unspoken request and administers the lethal dose. Hana then reads to him a part of his journal that he chose for her to read. As she is reading the journal, the patient dies.
    a. Take a quiet moment to reflect on this scene. What would you do as the patient's nurse or physician?
    b. How do you feel about the nurse's actions?
    c. How should health-care workers respond if a patient or their family requests an intentional overdose?
    d. Are there situations in which assisting suicide is appropriate for a health-care worker? What about active euthanasia, as depicted in this scene?
    e. In the few states (Oregon, Washington, and Montana) where physician-assisted suicide is legal, what safeguards are implemented to reduce abuse?
    f. Oregon legalized physician-assisted suicide in 1994. How many patients have made use of this statute?

The Sea Inside (*El Mar Adentro*) (2004; Javier Bardem, Belen Rueda): This film is based on the true story of Ramon Sampedro (Bardem), who was left quadriplegic after a diving accident fractured his neck at the age of 24. Over several decades it is Ramon's sister-in-law who is his main daily provider of care. Prior to the injury, Ramon travelled the world as a ship's mechanic. He uses these skills to adapt a number of inventions to make him slightly more independent, even though he is confined to bed.

1 (1:53:23–1:56:00) Ramon does not feel life is worth living as a quadriplegic and wants to end his life, but he would require the assistance of others to commit suicide. He unsuccessfully appealed to the Spanish courts to provide his euthanasia. His attorney, Julia (Rueda) suffers from a chronic neurologic syndrome and loses her physical and mental abilities as the movie progresses. Eventually, he is able to persuade family members and a trusted friend to provide him with a dose of potassium cyanide to end his life.

   a. How does Ramon value his quality of life as a quadriplegic?
   b. What is the appropriate standard to apply in judging quality of life?
   c. What other factors enter into this value judgment (besides the quadriplegia itself)?
   d. How do the values of loved ones, family, religion, or society enter into decisions regarding quality of life?

You Don't Know Jack (2010; Al Pacino): This HBO movie is based on the true story of Jack Kevorkian (played by Al Pacino), a Michigan pathologist who specializes in "death counseling," a discipline he developed to provide physician-assisted suicide. Dr. Kevorkian assists 130 individuals commit suicide, but in all cases he provides the mechanism of death, and the patient has to initiate the delivery of the toxic gas or medication. He is tried three times for providing physician-assisted suicide and is acquitted three times.

1 (1:47:32–151:26) Dr. Kevorkian wants to provoke a national discussion about euthanasia. As a result, he performs the injection himself for a patient with amyotrophic lateral sclerosis. He then brings the tape to a local reporter to request that the TV show *60 Minutes* play the videotape of this act on national TV. This leads to his arrest and conviction for homicide, partly because he decides to represent himself in court.

   a. What are the ethical and legal differences between physician-assisted suicide and active euthanasia?
   b. Kevorkian is known to have provided physician-assisted suicide for patients without a terminal illness or uncontrollable pain, what do you think of this?
   c. What did Kevorkian contribute to the national debate on physician-assisted suicide?

Southern Comfort (2001): This Sundance Film Festival award winner is the story of Robert Eads, a terminally ill 52-year-old female-to-male transgendered man living in rural Georgia. The film follows Robert with his "chosen family" of friends and family of origin during the last year of his life.

1   (Ch 7, 0:44:04–0:46:25) Robert is sharing that he thinks "it" (death) is getting close. He adds: "they have increased the morphine again, I bump into doorways and hospice finally said that I couldn't stay here by myself." They told him that he needed someone "24/7." Robert says that his girlfriend, Lola, said, "you are moving in with me." The scene shifts to Lola and Robert sitting at a table as Lola fills Robert's daily pill containers. Robert says, "this is a whole new role for Lola."

   a.   How would you discuss transitions in care with a patient and loved ones?

   b.   What does this loss of independence mean to Robert?

   c.   Robert acknowledges the new role Lola is about to assume? How does the added responsibility of being a caregiver affect a couple's relationship?

2   (Ch 8, 0:51:15–0:53:20) Robert's friend Tom brings Robert back to the mobile home in order to pick up some things in preparation for the Southern Comfort conference and Robert's speech. Robert is walking with a cane, and a wheelchair is seen outside. At one point, Robert almost falls. He looks and sounds quite weak and frail. Tom adds that it will be a "miracle" if Robert can give that speech.

   a.   What significance does the Southern Comfort conference hold for Robert? How important is it for him to "hold on" until then?

3   (Ch 8, 0:54:01–0:54:35) Robert's friends are sitting around and showing pictures from Easter. They comment about how "skinny" Robert looks then and how much thinner he is now.

   a.   What purpose does this reflective process serve for Robert's friends?

   b.   Will this mutual sharing enable them to cope better with Robert's death?

The Final Stage: Entering In-Patient Hospice

1   (Ch 11, 1:18:45–1:19:50) Robert has entered the in-patient hospice facility. He is seen sitting in a wheelchair and is having his temperature taken. Robert begins talking and shares: "the tumor is the size of a softball … to them I'm expendable."

   a.   How would you respond to his statement that he is expendable? In view of his situation and experiences, would you understand or concur with his beliefs?

   b.   What comfort or solace could you offer him?

   c.   How can health-care professionals demonstrate respect and individual worth?

2   (Ch 11, 1:22:05–1:25:12) Robert's friends are visiting him. It is Christmas time and they are wearing festive holiday hats. His room has a small Christmas tree. Robert's friends, his "chosen family," maintain a cheerful façade. Robert continues this façade by turning to Cass and telling him that they are going to

go fishing before the lake freezes over. The scene then pans the faces of his friends and focuses on photos of better days. The scene shifts again to Lola lying in the bed beside Robert. Lola shares: "As the end grew near, I noticed a change in his breathing. I gathered him in my arms, told him how much I loved him, and he left."

    a. What purpose did Robert's talking about going fishing serve? Did he believe that would happen? Did any of his friends believe he would be alive and healthy enough to engage in this activity?

    b. What types of services are offered to grieving friends and family?

    c. How might Robert's chosen family respond to the idea of engaging in those services, based on Robert's experiences in help-seeking?

Dementia-Related Decline

Barney's Version (2010; Paul Giamatti, Rosamund Pike, Minnie Driver, Anna Hopkins, Jake Hoffman): Barney Panofsky, a Jewish Canadian television producer, reflects in flashbacks on 3 decades of his life with three wives in this adaptation of Mordecai Richler's acclaimed novel. Barney develops a dementing illness and is cared for by his adult children.

1   (T1C4, 1:48:10–1:51:00) Barney (Giamatti) becomes enraged and verbally abusive to a coworker for no apparent reason. Male coworkers who witness the incident confront him. When he is asked what is wrong, he tells them that his friend just died. Barney is then told by his stunned coworker that his longtime friend died a year ago and he was a pallbearer. The scene shifts to Barney at his physician's office. Barney is doing poorly on a mental status exam. He cannot remember what kind of car he drives.

    a. The physician prefaces his questions for the mental status exam by stating "there are no right or wrong answers." How accurate is this? Why would a health-care provider choose to state this?

    b. What types of reactions/apprehensions do patients, especially individuals in the early stages of dementia, have regarding mental status testing?

    c. What is the purpose of a mental status exam? What does it measure?

2   (T1C14, 1:51:53–1:59:08) Barney reflects back on the day he met his wife and remembers her face on their wedding day. With the telephone in his hand, he becomes enraged and smashes picture frames and other objects in the living room. His daughter, Kate (Anna Hopkins), rushes in, pleads with him to stop, and asks him what is wrong. Barney replies, "I can't remember your mother's phone number."

    a. Discuss personality changes that can occur with dementing illnesses.

    b. What activities may trigger a catastrophic reaction?

3   (T1C14, 1:53:06–1:59:08) Please note: This scene can be divided into sections and paused, to allow for discussion of one section at a time. In the first section, Barney meets his ex-wife, Miriam (Rosamund Pike), for lunch. He

says he has his "crib notes" with his address and phone numbers and the numbers of their children with him in case he gets lost. He jokes that a dog collar might be better. She tells him that they are always doing new trials. Barney cuts her off by saying: "We all know where this is headed, right?" In the second section, as Miriam is savoring a first taste of the dessert, she realizes that Barney doesn't know how to eat the cake and she hands him the fork. When she leaves the table and enters the restroom, we see her release her emotional reaction to the situation. When she returns to the table, Barney is missing. She goes to find him. When Miriam locates Barney, it is as if he has been transported to an earlier time. He behaves as though their children were still young. Miriam says she thought she lost him.

a. What is the frequency of wandering among individuals with dementia? How can this behavior be monitored and lessened?

b. When Barney says he has his "crib notes," what feelings are aroused in him and in Miriam?

c. What recommendations would you make for a family regarding engaging in social activities in new locations with their family members with a dementing illness.

d. How would you interpret Barney's statement that "we all know where this is headed"?

4 (T1C16, 2:00:09–2:03:10) Barney's two adult children, Kate (Anna Hopkins) and Michael (Jake Hoffman), are reviewing their father's will while Barney is seated outside. One of Barney's wishes is that their mother, Barney's ex-wife, Miriam (who has remarried), be buried alongside him. Michael feels this is unfair since his mother is remarried. Michael goes outside to find his father having trouble peeling a banana and so he gives him a cigar instead. Michael reminisces with his father about his childhood.

a. What advice would you give to family members dealing with final wishes?

b. What was Michael's intent when he went outside to talk with his father? Did that change when he saw the difficulties his father was having?

c. What is the impact of dementing illness and loss on adult children? Is this a form of "living death"?

Discussions of Last Wishes and Funerals
• •

The Bucket List (2007; Jack Nicholson, Morgan Freeman): A movie about Edward Cole (Nicholson) and Carter Chambers (Freeman), two men from very different worlds who meet in a hospital and discover that they have one thing in common: a terminal cancer diagnosis. Together, they survive treatment and develop a plan for coping with the end-of-life process.

1 (Ch 7, 0:29:32–0:30:45) Thomas (Sean Hayes), Edward's assistant, arrives at the hospital. He says "rise and shine." Edward responds by making an obscene gesture. Thomas handles that in stride and goes about cleaning things up. He

says that he doesn't want to seem indelicate, but asks how he should handle Edward's death. Edward replies: "Like it was your own."

2   (Ch 21, 1:26:26–1:29:00) Carter is being wheeled away for surgery. His wife is seen waiting in the hospital while Edward is seen waiting outside in his car. He opens the letter from Carter. Viewers hear Carter's voice as Edward reads. Carter urges Edward to find the joy in his life. Carter dies during the procedure.

   a.   Edward and Carter knew each other for a short period of time, yet clearly they had become friends. How does terminal disease facilitate this type of bonding experience?

3   (Ch 22, 1:29:20–1:32:05) In the first part of this scene, Edward (Nicholson) is speaking at Carter's funeral. He is visibly affected and says: "The last months of his life were the best months of mine." The scene shifts to Thomas (Sean Hayes), Edward's assistant, climbing a mountain. Edward had died and Thomas is carrying his ashes up the mountain. He places the ashes next to Carter's.

   a.   What purpose do funerals serve for friends and family?
   b.   How would you describe Edward's emotional state?
   c.   Edward shares a terminal prognosis. What is the impact of speaking at his friend's funeral?
   d.   Thomas is fulfilling Edward's wishes to return his ashes to a place that he and Carter had visited. How does a dying person assure that his wishes will be followed?

References

1   Ferrini AF, Ferrini RL. *Health in the Later Years*. 4th ed. New York, NY: McGraw Hill; 2008.

2   Farber S, Egnew E, Farber A. What is a respectful death? In: Berzoff J, Silverman P, editors. *Living with Dying: a handbook for end-of-life healthcare practitioners*. New York, NY: Columbia University Press; 2004. pp. 102–27.

3   Corlee IB, Nicholas PK. The interdisciplinary team: an oxymoron? In: Berzoff J, Silverman P, editors. *Living with Dying: a handbook for end-of-life healthcare practitioners*. New York, NY: Columbia University Press; 2004. pp. 161–9.

4   Stein G, Esralew L. Palliative care for people with disabilities. In: Berzoff J, Silverman P, editors. *Living with Dying: a handbook for end-of-life healthcare practitioners*. New York, NY: Columbia University Press; 2004. pp. 499–507.

5   Jacobs C. Spirituality and end-of-life practice for social workers. In: Berzoff J, Silverman P, editors. *Living with Dying: a handbook for end-of-life healthcare practitioners*. New York, NY: Columbia University Press; 2004. pp. 188–205.

39

On the Outside Looking In: Health Disparities and Marginalized Populations

Anna Pavlov, Patricia Lenahan & Jeffrey M. Ring

> *Of all the forms of inequality, injustice in health care is the most shocking and inhumane.*
>
> —Martin Luther King, Jr.

It is incumbent upon health-care providers to deliver health-care services that are culturally responsive and patient centered,[1] particularly given the devastating health inequities in the United States.[2,3] Comprehensive patient-centered health care takes into account the psychosocial context in which patients live and develop health problems. Health-care and medical curricula must challenge learners to enhance empathy and self-reflection capacities, deepen their knowledge base of socioeconomic factors in health inequities, and broaden the scope of communication and negotiation skills that will improve the potency of the doctor-patient relationship.

Poverty and racism, educational level, and institutional barriers to care must all be considered when negotiating an ultimately successful treatment plan for patients/clients from underserved communities. Furthermore, health-care providers must actively engage in behaviors and communications that contribute to the development of trust, especially with patients who differ demographically, socioeconomically, by language and/or by religion and worldview.

Access to Health Care with and without Health Insurance

Sicko (2007): In this Oscar-nominated documentary, Michael Moore indicts the health-care industry by presenting stories he has solicited from Americans who have been denied health care and experienced life altering losses. Moore points out, "in the world's richest country, 45 million people have no health insurance, while HMOs [health maintenance organizations] grow in size and wealth."

1 (Ch 1, 0:03:46–0:07:50) Moore narrates that Larry and Donna Smith are forced to leave their home to move to Denver, Colorado, where they will have a room in their daughter's home (her storage room). They both had good jobs with health insurance but Larry had multiple heart attacks and then Donna was diagnosed with cancer. The co-payments and deductibles soon added up. As a couple in their 50s, they never expected to have to reach out to their twenty-something daughter.

2 (Ch 7, 0:41:40–0:43:48) Adrian Campbell, a 22-year-old single mother, drives in downtown Detroit. She explains that she was diagnosed with cervical cancer and was denied care by her insurance company, purportedly because, "you should not be having cervical cancer. You are too young." To get the care she needs, Adrian goes to Canada. We see her at the border.

3 (Ch 12, 1:27:53–1:32:54) A spotlight is shined on the practice of some hospitals of discharging the uninsured and homeless patients, putting them in a taxi, and then dropping them off in places like Skid Row in downtown Los Angeles. We see a taxi pull up and drop off a female patient, Carol. She is confused and does not know where she is. Time-lapse video shows her roaming the nearby street with heavy traffic passing by her. A union rescue staff member meets Carol and escorts her inside the building. It is noted that "at their shelter alone, over 50 people have been dumped off."

   a. What is your reaction to these profiles? Have you ever heard or known of anyone similarly affected?

   b. Discuss your experience of caring for the uninsured and underinsured in the setting you practice in. What are the health-care disparities you observe?

Yesterday (2005): This is set in the KwaZulu-Natal province of South Africa, an area that has been disproportionately affected by HIV/AIDS. The story focuses on one family coping with HIV: Yesterday (Leleti Khumalo), her daughter, Beauty (Lihle Mvelase), and her husband, John (Kenneth Kambule).

1 (0:6:15–0:8:33; 0:16:07–0:17:58) Yesterday (Leleti Khumalo) and her daughter, Beauty (Lihle Mvelase), have walked over two hours to the medical clinic in another village. Yesterday has been coughing persistently and arrives at the clinic to see a very long line. The woman in front of her has been there since 7am. Yesterday seems worried and asks if they will be seen by the doctor.

Later, a clinic assistant tells everyone beyond a certain point that they will have to return next week. In the second scene, Yesterday and Beauty arrive at the clinic very early, only to see another long line. The clinic worker comes out and counts the people who will be seen, ending at the person in front of Yesterday.

   a. What are the barriers to health care for people in the community you serve?

   b. What is the state of disease prevention in underserved communities and countries?

   c. How can health care be improved in these areas, especially in areas where a disease is prevalent?

   d. How could community workers be utilized in these situations?

   e. What are the overall costs associated with health disparities?

Physical, Emotional, and Sexual Abuse/Unwanted Pregnancy and Poverty

Precious (2009): This film is based on the novel *Push* by Sapphire,[4] and provides a number of opportunities for learners to consider and discuss the challenges of delivering excellent health care to marginalized patients. The emotionally powerful film follows the life of a young woman who carries the psychological burdens of incest rape, physical and emotional abuse, poverty, and limited educational opportunities as well as unwanted pregnancies.

1 (Ch 5, 0:18:40–0:20:41) The scene shows the main character, Precious, walking through her Harlem, New York, neighborhood. The scene depicts the poverty, environmental pollution, and harassment she faces along the way.

   a. What observations can be made about Precious's emotional state?

   b. What are the potential environmental factors contributing to her suffering?

2 (Ch 6; 0:23:10–0:25:07) On her way to school, Precious steals food from a local fast food restaurant.

   a. What are the relationships between eating and emotional distress?

   b. What are the challenges of making healthful food choices for low-income patients living in impoverished neighborhoods?

3 (Ch 9; 0:35:29–0:38:17) This scene depicts a private tutoring session between Precious and her instructor.

   a. What are the impacts of trauma on information processing? What are the implications for the delivery of health care?

   b. In the order to reach marginalized individuals such as Precious, what are the qualities that make for a remarkable teacher? An outstanding health-care practitioner?

4 (Ch 12; 0:43:49–0:45:37) This scene depicts a meeting between Precious and her social worker.

a. What communication strategies does the social worker use to attempt to build a relationship with Precious?

b. What is the role for social services in integrated, comprehensive, culturally responsive health care?

c. How can practitioners effectively navigate the emotional challenges of providing care to marginalized patients with an enormous list of problems, medical and otherwise?

d. How does one take care of one's own emotional well-being when working with extremely challenging patients and communities?

e. How would a patient-centered medical home benefit an individual like Precious?

Sexual Health and HIV Education for Minority Adolescents

All of Us (2008): This documentary focuses on Mehret Mandefro, an Ethiopian-American internal medicine resident at Montefiore Hospital in New York who treats many HIV-positive African-American women. Dr. Mandefro wants to understand why so many women of color are affected and develops a research project on HIV and minority women. The movie focuses on Dr. Mandefro and her interactions with two of her patients.

1 (1:12:20–1:16:34) Dr. Mandefro sits in on a high school sex education class for African-American girls and asks Chevelle to participate. She asks the students what percentage of the US population comprises African-Americans and then shows the disparity in the prevalence of HIV infections. The girls discuss dating and communication about sexuality and drugs. Dr. Mandefro tells the girls that they need to get tested and their partners need to be tested and show them their results before beginning a sexual relationship. She also discusses the link between abuse and violence and HIV status. Chevelle shares her story of abuse and being pressured into using crack at age 17. Dr. Mandefro says: "We're dying and no one's really talking about it."

a. What is the impact of the graphs showing health disparities?

b. How do the girls respond to this information?

c. How do personal empowerment and communications skills contribute to safer sexual practices?

d. What are the barriers to increasing assertiveness communication skills?

e. How would you interpret Dr. Mandefro's comment: "We're dying and no one's really talking about it"?

Homelessness
••••••••••••••••••••

📽️*Resurrecting the Champ* (2007; Samuel L. Jackson, Josh Harnett, Kathryn Morris, Alan Alda): This film is the story of a reporter, Erik Kirnan (Josh Harnett), who is facing being fired when he meets "Champ," a homeless man who is a former heavyweight boxer. The reporter sees a "story" in Champ that he hopes will revitalize his career. He pursues Champ and persuades him to tell his story.

1 (0:32:08–0:34:00) Erik (Josh Harnett) meets Champ at a free soup kitchen at lunch time. Erik asks Champ if he's afraid that someone will steal his shopping cart that he left outside. Champ (Samuel L. Jackson) looks at the reporter and simply says: "We have a homeless code of honor."

    a. Discuss the ethical issues involved in the reporter writing a story about Champ.

    b. Discuss the validity of Champ's claim that there is a "homeless code of honor."

    c. Have you ever volunteered in a free food program or shelter? Discuss any experiences of providing medical and/or mental health care to the homeless.

Mental Illness and Homelessness
••

📽️*The Soloist* (2009; Robert Downey, Jr., Jamie Foxx): This film is based on the true story and book written by *Los Angeles Times* newspaper reporter, Steve Lopez. It chronicles his unlikely friendship with Nathaniel Ayers, a homeless and schizophrenic musical genius.

1 (Ch 2, 0:08:00–0:10:48) Lopez hears music emanating near a bronze statue of Beethoven. As he walks closer to the music, we see a violinist (Nathaniel) playing a violin with two strings. A conversation occurs between the two men. Nathaniel demonstrates rapid and tangential speech. In one segment he says, "You have to treat a violin like a child. You have to protect it." He then apologizes for his appearance saying, "I've had a few setbacks."

    a. What is your reaction to this scene?

    b. How would you interpret Nathaniel's statement that "You have to treat a violin like a child. You have to protect it."

    c. What do you make of Ayers's apologizing for his appearance? Does this surprise you? Why? Does it reflect a level of insight?

    d. What are common reactions to realizing that an individual has a thought disorder?

    e. How do you develop rapport, interview and interact with such an individual?

    f. What factors may interfere with health-care providers' inability to develop rapport and obtain history from an individual like Nathaniel?

2 (Ch 4, 0:16:48–0:19:57) Steve spots Nathaniel on a freeway shoulder playing the violin. The shopping cart full of his possessions is nearby. Initially,

Nathaniel ignores Steve's attempts to engage him but then recites Steve's full name and workplace in a telegraphic manner. Nathaniel talks rapidly and disjointedly about various musical works composed by Beethoven. Steve informs Nathaniel that he wants to write a story about him, about "how a guy like him ends up on the freeway." Steve asks Nathaniel if there is anyone he can contact, any family.

    a. What ethical issues exist with Steve's plan to write a story about Nathaniel?

    b. Can Steve obtain "true consent"?

    c. In your setting, how would you consent such an individual for treatment, either medical and/or psychological?

    d. What personal and systemic barriers exist in helping someone like Nathaniel?

3 (Ch 7, 0:34:26–0:36:15) A cello is donated by a newspaper reader who is moved in response to one of Steve's newspaper stories in which it is mentioned that Nathaniel's first instrument was a cello, not a violin. Steve locates Nathaniel on the freeway curb deeply involved in his music. When he is presented with the cello, Nathaniel is awed and Steve allows him to play the instrument for a few moments but makes a deal with him that he can only play the cello at LAMP, a local agency. A struggle ensues as Steve takes the cello for safekeeping and drives off, hoping to meet up with Nathaniel later at LAMP.

    a. What is Steve hoping to accomplish by arranging for Nathaniel to play the cello at LAMP? Do you think Nathaniel will go to the social agency?

    b. What could be some reasons why he would be reluctant to go?

    c. What reactions do you have when you see people sitting/standing or soliciting for work or money on the street?

4 (Ch 10, 0:52:20–0:55:07) Steve is talking with Nathaniel and takes in the gritty and dangerous street environment. Almost as if he can read Steve's mind, Nathaniel says, "The children of God are going to be OK tonight." Two people are on the ground fighting. A woman is throwing a trash can. Nathaniel says, "They're going to sleep and dream as humans do." The scene concludes with Nathaniel reciting the Our Father prayer as the conditions on the street are surveyed. Steve narrates what we have seen.

    a. What is your reaction to the conditions observed?

    b. Have you ever been to such a location?

    c. How would you interpret Nathaniel's statement that "The children of God are going to be OK tonight"?

    d. How about his second comment that "They're going to sleep and dream as humans do"?

5 (Ch 13; 1:09:30–1:10:25) Nathaniel is in an apartment that Steve secured for him. Nathaniel paces wildly and has trouble coping with being in an enclosed space, and has auditory hallucinations that he will be protected.

    a. What theories do you have about why Nathaniel has such an intense reaction to his new apartment?

    b. What supportive measures might have eased his adjustment?

Incarceration
· · · · · · · · · · · · · · · · · · ·

Trouble the Water (2008): This is an Oscar-nominated documentary that focuses on a couple, Scott and Kimberly Roberts, and their extended family, as they cope with the events in their lives following Hurricane Katrina in New Orleans.

1 (Ch 9, 1:09:59–0:12:50) Kim has bailed her brother out of jail just in time for him to attend their grandmother's funeral. He had been incarcerated for a petty crime. He recounts his experiences immediately after Hurricane Katrina and says that the guards didn't tell them anything and they didn't know a hurricane was coming. The deputies all had left the jail. He adds that the inmates had no food or potable water. Some of the men were jumping out of windows.

   a. What reactions do you have when you learn that client/patient has been incarcerated?

   b. What do you think about individuals being incarcerated for petty crimes?

   c. Have you ever visited a jail or prison? If you have, what were your experiences? If you haven't, would you ever want to? Why/why not?

The Undocumented Labor Force
· ·

A Day Without a Mexican (2004; Caroline Aaron, Melinda Allen, Frankie J. Allison, Yareli Arizmendi): In this satirical comedy, California wakes up one morning to find that one-third of its population – the Hispanic third – has disappeared. A strange pink fog envelops the state, and communication outside its boundaries is completely cut off. The economic, political, and social implications of this disaster threaten California's way of life.

1 (T1C2, 0:16:57–0:17:43) Mexicans are mysteriously disappearing from California. A newscaster announces that "we are going live to Stockton," where a reporter interviews a fruit farmer who is without 70–80 workers. He says that they are going to lose the entire crop without the workers to pick it. He states that the Immigration and Naturalization Service is making it harder for people to come here and stay here. He adds that, "California depends on these people to make these fields work."

   a. What is the current US Immigration Policy?

   b. Why is immigration such a contentious issue, when the US was founded by immigrants?

   c. Discuss what you know about your immigrant roots.

   d. What health observations have been made about migrant farm workers?

2 (T1C3, 0:27:46–0:28:37) Who are these people we have taken for granted? A reporter reviews the various Latino groups that comprise the populations of California. He reminds the audience that they are first and foremost people and have helped make the California economy the fifth largest in the world.

    a. What Latino or other ethnic groups populate the region you live in?

    b. What are the similarities and differences between various Latino populations?

    c. Differentiate between use of the terms "Hispanic" and "Latino."

3 (T1C4, 0:28:57–0:29:32) A character portraying a "university authority" compares the absence of Mexicans with the "big one," referring to California's next major earthquake. He states that undocumented individuals working the fields 12 hours a day picked 90% of the crops in this state.

4 (T1C8, 0:54:57–0:55:29) The "university authority" addresses misinformation that Latinos use $3 billion of social services and do not pay any taxes. He adds that the Latino undocumented contribute $100 billion to the state of California. He concludes by saying that people want to exaggerate when it turns out that "these statistics are a lie."

    a. What stereotypes exist about undocumented and immigrant populations? Do they differ between Latino, Asian, Middle Eastern peoples? How do these stereotypes get created? Why?

    b. Is there validity to the statement that undocumented workers take jobs others would not want or will take?

Undocumented Individuals and Family Separation

Under the Same Moon (2007): Rosario (Kate del Castillo) is an undocumented woman who has been working in Los Angeles for 4 years to support her son, Carlitos (Adrian Alonso), who lives with her mother in Mexico. Carlitos longs to see his mother and on his ninth birthday he decides to join her by stowing away in a van. Things go awry when Carlitos is separated from his smugglers (America Ferrera and Jose Garcia) at the border.

1 (Ch 1, 0:06:00–0:8:15) Rosario calls Carlitos the same time every week. It's his ninth birthday. He tells his mother that he is ready to come to Los Angeles. Rosario tells her son that it's hard to get papers, adding that the last attorney robbed her of her money. Carlitos persists and tells her that 4 years is too long and suggests that if he can't come to Los Angeles, then she should return to Mexico.

    a. What dilemmas are presented in this scene?

    b. If someone like Rosario were your client/patient, how would you counsel her?

    c. What advice would you give her about how to respond to her son?

    d. What techniques and suggestions might you give her?

    e. What are the various ideas that have been proposed to reform the US immigration policy?

2 (Ch 4, 0:17:58–0:18:37) Under the guise of working in a dress shop, Dona Carmen operates a smuggling ring that helps people cross the border. Carlitos works for her and looks at an identification card. Three men nervously sit

across from Dona Carmen. She tells them that a truck is leaving that night and that the fee is $2000, and $2400 if they want a job contact. The men seem hesitant and respond that they were not prepared to leave so soon. Dona Carmen tells them they have two options: take the van or swim.

    a. What risks are present for individuals who attempt to smuggle people into another country? What are the risks to the individuals who utilize these services?

    b. Why do individuals take such serious risks?

3 (Ch 4, 0:18:58–0:19:55) Martha (America Ferrera) and her brother, David (Jesse Garcia) enter Dona Carmen's shop. They tell her they are legal residents of the United States and they can take "babies" across the border. They try to give Dona Carmen their card, but she tells them to leave.

    a. Why do you think Dona Carmen reacts this way?

    b. What risks exist in smuggling rings?

4 (Ch 6, 0:27:25–0:29:35) Carlitos has contacted Martha and David and is crossing the border with them. They stop the van when they approach a sign that says US border in 2 kilometers. They ask Carlitos for his money and instruct him to lie in a cut-out under the back seat. It is a very small space with little air. David says: "Are you kidding me? They are going to check this." He adds that he has a bad feeling about this. Martha responds to David that it's his choice: does he want tuition money or does he want to drop out of school? They proceed to the border crossing.

    a. What insights does this scene provide?

    b. How has Carlitos obtained the money to pay the smugglers?

Health Care and Sexual Minorities: The Transgendered Individual

Southern Comfort (2001): This is a docudrama that focuses on the last year in the life of 52-year-old Robert Eads, who is terminally ill with ovarian cancer. The film follows Robert, a female-to-male transgendered person and his adopted "family," a community of other transgendered individuals living in rural Georgia.

1 (Ch 3, 0:13:21–0:15:31) Robert says that over a year ago he was diagnosed with cancer in the cervix, ovaries and uterus. He says that he wanted a hysterectomy when he transitioned, but the doctors said he was menopausal so there was no need for the surgery. Robert says that he spent 3 weeks calling doctors, asking to be seen and he was turned down. The scene shifts to Robert's friends, Tom and Debbie. Robert was visiting them when he woke up in a pool of blood. They recount their experiences in calling doctors and hospitals to get help for Robert. They explain that he had no insurance and were told that was not a problem. However, when they shared that Robert was a transgendered male, they were turned down. According to Tom and Debbie, more than 20 doctors and countless hospitals refused to see Robert.

Some doctors said they "had no experience in the area" and Debbie asks what gynecologist doesn't know how to treat female issues? Other doctors said that to treat Robert would embarrass their other patients.

a. What is your reaction to physicians' refusal to treat Robert? What are the ethical considerations involved in refusing care?
b. Is there any reality to the stated reason to refuse treatment because other patients will be affected?
c. If you saw a colleague respond this way, how would you react?
d. What do you think is really at the core of the physicians' refusal to see Robert?
e. If you were on a disciplinary or patient relations committee and it was your task to investigate a formal patient complaint by Robert, what remediation would you consider for the physician(s) involved?

Support Groups

1 (Ch 9, 1:05:55–1:06:59) Maxwell, one of Robert's friends is giving a talk at "SoCo," Southern Comfort, an annual meeting for transgendered persons in Atlanta. Maxwell is showing slides of his mastectomy. He says: "the best doctors can have a bad day and the worst doctors can do a good job. Be prepared." The scene shifts to Cass who talks about his mastectomy and shows his scars. He shares that the doctor left a "gaping hole" where you could see the muscle "like you were looking at a side of beef or something."

a. What factors should be considered for individuals who undergo gender re-assignment surgery?
b. How would you interpret Maxwell's and Cass's comments about the quality of medical care they received?
c. What Lesbian Gay Bisexual Transgendered (LGBT) resources are available in your community?
d. Why are support services so critical for this population?

2 (Ch 11, 1:19:18–1:19:40) Robert is terminally ill and shares his thoughts with the group. He says: "I've got a tumor in me the size of a softball." He then recounts his experiences in trying to obtain medical care by mimicking what he has been told: "Oh, I'm sorry, we're not taking new patients. I'm sorry. To have you here in the office would be an embarrassment to my other patients. To them, I'm expendable."

a. How would Robert's group likely respond to his account of being refused treatment? What are the ethical considerations involved in refusing care?
b. What are some therapeutic re-frames to Robert's sense of being abandoned by the medical community? How would you assist a client/patient who appeared stuck in negativity?
c. If you saw a colleague refuse to care for a transgendered patient, how would you react?

d. How would you respond to meeting a transgendered patient/client coming to see you?

Health Literacy in an HIV Community

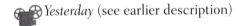*Yesterday* (see earlier description)

1 (0:29:30–0:33:30) Yesterday is in the clinic exam room where the female physician (Camilla Walker) examines her and asks about the cough. The doctor acknowledges the delay in treatment, stating that more than one doctor is needed here, but there isn't money to hire another one. The doctor looks pensive as she listens to Yesterday's lungs. Yesterday asks if there is something wrong. The doctor tells her that she wants to do a blood test to see if everything is OK. She explains that Yesterday will have to read the form and sign the consent. The doctor gives Yesterday a lab slip with the ICD (International Classification of Disease) codes on it. Reluctantly, Yesterday tells the doctor that she has never gone to school and that she cannot read or write. The doctor tells her it doesn't matter as long as Yesterday wants the test. Yesterday asks if it will hurt, but never gets an answer to that question. The doctor puts on the tourniquet and begins to draw the blood.
   a. What was the impact of the doctor's nonverbal expressions of concern on Yesterday and her fears?
   b. What ethical issues exist here? How does a physician provide informed consent in a culturally sensitive manner?
   c. What is the impact of literacy and health literacy in disease prevention and adherence to a medical regimen? What can health-care providers do to engage illiterate patients and to provide informed consent?

References

1 Ring J, Nyquist J, Mitchell S, *et al*. *Curriculum for Culturally Responsive Health Care: the step-by-step guide for cultural competence training*. Oxford: Radcliffe Publishing; 2008.
2 Satcher D, Pamies R, editors. *Multicultural Medicine and Health Disparities*. New York, NY: McGraw-Hill; 2006.
3 Smedley B, Stith A, Nelson A, editors. *Unequal Treatment: confronting racial and ethnic disparities in health care*. Washington DC: Institute of Medicine, 2003.
4 Sapphire. *Push*. New York, NY: Vintage Books; 1996.

Recommended Reading and Websites

- Agency for Healthcare Research and Quality, U.S. Department of Health and Human Services. *2010 National Healthcare Disparities Report*. Rockville, MD: AHRQ Publication

No. 11-0005, March 2011. Available at: www.ahrq.gov/qual/qrdr10.htm (last accessed 12/1/11)

- Birn AE, Pillay Y, Holtz TH. *Textbook of International Health: global health in a dynamic world*. Oxford: Oxford University Press; 2009.
- Chu C, Selwyn P. Complications of HIV infection: a systems-based approach. *Am Fam Physician*. 2011; **83**(4): 395–406.
- Eckstein B. Primary care for refugees. *Am Fam Physician*. 2011; **83**(4): 429–36.
- *Health Literacy: help your patients understand* [20-minute instructional CD-ROM]. American Medical Association and American Medical Association Foundation; 2003.
- Peterson P, Shetterly S, Clarke C, *et al*. Health literacy and outcomes among patients with heart failure. *JAMA*. 2011; **305**(16): 1695–700.
- Powers B, Trinh J, Bosworth H. Can this patient read and understand written health information? *JAMA*. 2010; **304**(1): 76–84.
- resource@xculture.org
- Thompson M. Challenges to improving adherence to HIV therapy. *Am Fam Physician*. 2011; **83**(4): 375, 379.
- Weiss BD. *Health Literacy: a manual for clinicians*. American Medical Association and American Medical Association Foundation; 2003.
- www.aafp.org/online/en/home/membership/ruralcommunity/governmentandnongovern mentresources (Links to national resources for family physicians who provide health and mental care to the underserved population in rural and urban areas from the American Academy of Family Physicians.)
- www.aafp.org/online/en/home/policy/policies/h/homelessness.html31k (The American Academy of Family Physicians supports legislation and programs that develop social and health-related resources for the homeless population in America.)
- www.xculture.org

40

The Humanitarian Physician: International Medical Missions

Silvia Quadrelli & Henri Colt

Humanitarian Medicine
• ••

HUMANITARIAN ACTIONS* ARE USUALLY DEFINED AS A SET OF ACTIONS destined to help victims of natural and man-made disasters, armed conflict, or individuals suffering from societal exclusion because of economic, ethnic, or social discrimination. Actions are performed in order to ease suffering and pain, guarantee basic subsistence, protect fundamental human rights, defend personal dignity, and slow destructive socioeconomic processes in preparation for future natural or man-made disasters or conflicts. In addition to those performed by local groups, volunteers, and faith-based organizations, many actions are performed by nonprofit national or international nongovernmental organizations (NGOs), that adhere to principles of nonengagement, independence, impartiality, and neutrality. These organizations usually insist on having access to vulnerable populations in order to proceed with impartial needs assessments and wish to maintain a free choice of methods used to address those needs. Of course, the true neutrality of humanitarian actions is debatable. Some perspectives depend on societal and individual value statements and those thoughts, feelings, and responsibilities that individual health-care providers may or may not share when they work in zones of conflict or natural disaster.

The terms humanitarian action, humanitarian aid, and humanitarian assistance

---

* This is completely different from a term more recently coined as "humanitarian intervention." While there is no standard definition of humanitarian intervention; it includes the threat and use of military force to enforce humanitarian objectives, and thus entails interfering in the internal affairs of a state by sending military forces into the territory or airspace of a sovereign state that has not necessarily committed an act of aggression against another state.

are often used interchangeably but, in reality, have different connotations. Humanitarian assistance, or emergency assistance, corresponds to an emergency response to catastrophic situations such as natural disasters (cyclones, floods, earthquakes, tsunamis, droughts), and social or political events (economic disaster, internal conflicts, civil war, population migrations, and refugee-related issues) for which consequences such as epidemics, violence, or famine create suffering and danger. Immediate action to save lives and reduce suffering is usually given priority over future developmental aid. Humanitarian aid encompasses a larger construct, including, for example, prolonged interventions to secure the safety and well-being of refugees and internally displaced persons during the aftermath of a conflict or natural disaster. These actions are not limited to immediate assistance, and are destined to assure a long-term presence that will reduce or prevent further economic and social degradation, and create a foundation for growth and development. Humanitarian action encompasses all of the above, and additionally includes assistance, protection, the development of long-term projects to assure education, sustenance, health and well-being, and advocacy in defense of human rights, individual and societal freedoms, and giving voice to witnesses and victims of abuse or injustice of any kind.

This chapter focuses on these various concepts as they pertain to medical work with remote or foreign populations in high-risk situations. It also portrays some of the challenges faced by humanitarian health-care providers who must work with respect for cultures and customs different from their own.

The Concept of Humanitarian Action

The Nun's Story (1959; Audrey Hepburn, Peter Finch, Edith Evans): In *The Nun's Story*, Audrey Hepburn portrays Sister Luke, a nun whose life journey leads her to a much-desired position as a nurse in a Belgian Congo missionary hospital. After she returns to her native Belgium, World War II breaks out and she finds her commitment seriously tested – torn between the pull of the Resistance and the Church's neutrality. Her arduous soul-searching results in her decision to leave the Holy Order, realizing that she is spiritually unsuited to the discipline imposed by it. The film shows the various stages through which she must pass before taking her final vows and how deeply her personal and private tug-of-war is, between her wish to respect the ingrained discipline and her spirit to rebel. Then, in the Congo she suffers from tuberculosis and is sent back to Belgium. Denied from serving as a nurse with the Belgian underground in World War II, she finds herself unable to endure the discipline of her order, and in the end, is granted her wish to be released.

1 (1:19:08–1:20:19) In this scene, Sister Luke (Audrey Hepburn) has just arrived in Africa. The Mother Superior is showing her the work of the nuns. One of them is teaching a group of African mothers how to wash a baby. Sister Luke expresses how happy she will be working with the natives. The Mother

Superior, however, notifies her that orders from central headquarters demand that she work in another hospital, not with the natives, but with Europeans.

2 (1:23:58–1:24:40) In this scene, Sister Luke meets Dr. Fortunati (Peter Finch), the European surgeon of both hospitals. He explains that she will have to assist him during surgeries, beginning very early in the morning, which means that she will miss early morning mass. Sister Luke replies that she should ask for permission from the Mother Superior, but Dr. Fortunati insists that Mother Superior has no authority in his government hospital, that her salary is paid by the Belgium government, and that he, not Mother Superior is responsible for Sister Luke's work.

   a. Is Sister Luke a humanitarian aid worker?

   b. How might faith-based humanitarian actions differ from those performed by NGOs? How might they be similar?

   c. Are faith-based workers such as Sister Luke and the Mother Superior protected by international law? Do you know of any circumstances when faith-based workers were killed in their attempts to assist an oppressed population?

   d. In providing humanitarian aid, is there a difference if working in a government hospital, NGO-sponsored health-care unit, or combatant group?

Triage (2009; Colin Farrell, Jamie Sives, Branko Djuric; France-Spain-Ireland): Two expert war photographers, Mark and David, are working in war torn Kurdistan. They live and film the terrifying realities that shock them both. They not only witness killings and landmine explosion deaths, they also watch how the camp's doctor triages the wounded, deciding who can survive care and who will die anyway. He marks these victims to be "executed" later (by himself) in a compassionate gesture that ends their awful and hopeless suffering. Mark returns home with deep wounds and despite hospitalizations and medical care, continues to deteriorate. His colleague and friend, David, does not return. No one knows what happened to him. Psychotherapy helps Mark slowly discover and reinvestigate the truths about the incidents he witnessed, in a war for which he had blamed himself, as well as the circumstances of David's disappearance.

1 (0:04:55–0:07:38) In this scene the two photographers arrive in a Kurdish camp clinic in the middle of the mountains. There, Mark (Colin Farrell) and David (Jamie Sives) meet the physician in charge who allows them to take photographs under certain rules and conditions. The clinic has little by way of medication, has inadequate ventilation and is far from being able to guarantee clean work areas. A group of wounded men has just arrived and the two photographers see how Dr. Talzani (Branko Djuric) performs an initial triage, deciding who may survive care and who are so near death that they are set aside.

   a. Should Dr. Talzani be considered a humanitarian worker?

   b. What are the practical and ethical differences between working among high-risk populations, government hospitals, a combatant group or an NGO?

c. Is the work Dr. Talzani does the same sort of work an NGO humanitarian worker does?

d. What is the moral foundation of the work of Dr Talzani as a part of a military group? How might it differ from that of Sister Luke in The Nun's Story, who was part of a confessional organization, or of a humanitarian aid worker who is part of an international NGO?

e. Do all of these individuals have the same rights, and are they protected by the same international laws?

Motivations to Become Involved in Humanitarian Action

Live and Become (2005; Moshe Abebe, Surak M. Sabahat; France-Belgium-Israel): The story begins in 1985, when a 9-year-old boy is living with his mother in a refugee camp in the Sudan. Because the black Falashas in Ethiopia were recognized as genuine Jews, they were being brought secretly to Israel. The day before a scheduled transport, the son of a Jewish mother dies. The mother takes a Christian boy in his place and uses her dead son's name (Schlomo). This boy is warned to never reveal his true identity in order to remain safe and avoid being deported. Soon after arriving in Israel, this "false mother" dies from tuberculosis and a liberal French-Israeli couple adopt the boy (Moshe Abebe). It isn't until years later that he realizes his true mother's rejection was his salvation and not a punishment. Finally, when the boy grows older and reaches adulthood, he moves to Paris and becomes a humanitarian physician.

1 (2:01:14–2:02.12) In this scene, Schlomo (Surak M Sabahat) is working as a doctor for the Israeli Army. In the middle of an urban battle, he sees a Palestinian young boy become injured and runs to assist him. The father of the boy takes him away, using a gun to threaten others, and orders to not touch his son. In Schlomo's group, his military superior shouts furiously that he must not assist the enemy but instead help only his own colleagues in arms. "Don't you understand that?" he asks. Schlomo looks at him strangely, and suddenly wounded answers "No, I do not understand that."

a. When Schlomo worked as a military doctor, also caring for people in great danger, he did not understand that he should not take care of the enemies: what were his reasons?

b. During armed conflicts is there a difference between caring for military and civilian victims? Would you triage them the same way? How would you prioritize your allocation of scarce resources?

3 (2:14:11–2:14:39) Schlomo has returned to the Sudan as a doctor working for Médecins sans Frontières. This scene shows a huge camp where Schlomo, working now in the middle of nowhere, receives a phone call from his wife and listens to his very young son on the phone. While talking with his family over the phone, he sees a refugee woman and instantly recognizes his birth mother.

a. Are personal motivations improper or unethical justifications to decide on embarking on a life with a humanitarian aid organization?

b. Do you envision yourself participating in humanitarian work? If so, how and why?

c. Working in difficult conditions or in other countries may seem exotic and fulfilling. Why not offer your services instead (or as well) in a clinic or hospital for the underserved and marginalized in or near the community where you live?

The Last King of Scotland (2006; Forrest Whitaker, James McAvoy, Gillian Anderson, Adam Kotz; UK): In 1970, the just-graduated doctor Nicholas Garrigan moves to Uganda to seek adventure by taking up a position in a Ugandan missionary clinic. He arrives after the coup-d'état that overthrew the former government. Shortly thereafter, he meets the new President, Idi Amin, who has been injured in an automobile accident. Amin is impressed by the young doctor and asks him to become his personal physician. Accepting the offer, Garrigan assumes his position, eventually accepting gifts, such as a Mercedes Benz, having an affair with one of the dictator's wives, and becoming responsible for many violent deaths. When members of the cabinet start disappearing, Garrigan has reason to fear for his own safety, and is only able to escape the country thanks to the personal sacrifice of a colleague.

1 (0:08:31–0:09:47) Upon arrival at the Ugandan missionary clinic, the wife of the lead doctor there tells Dr. Garrigan (James McAvoy) that he seems to be a very unlikely candidate for the job. Garrigan replies that he wants to make a difference through his work, but that he is also looking forward to having fun and adventure.

a. What do you think should be the major motivating factor for choosing to risk one's life and work in the humanitarian world, especially for providing care to some of the most vulnerable populations, while potentially endangering one's own life?

b. Do you perceive differences in the motivations of Schlomo (protagonist of *Live and Become*) and Nicholas Garrigan for getting involved in the care of the most underserved?

The Daily Work of Doctors Working in the Field of Humanitarian Action

Beyond Borders (2002; Angelina Jolie, Clive Owen; US): Sarah Jordan (Angelina Jolie) is a wealthy American married to a British industrialist. At a fundraiser to support relief efforts, Sarah is moved by the intervention of Dr. Nick Callahan (Clive Owen) appearing with a suffering child and claiming lack of money for support of his program from the sponsoring charity in England. Sarah is moved by the doctor's speech, and decides to donate her savings and time to famine relief. Subsequently, she begins work for the United Nations and over the course of the next dozen or so years, meets up with Dr. Callahan in various war environments. Eventually Sarah develops a long-term romance with him. The film is an unrealistic melodramatic love story set against the backdrop of various humanitarian aid projects filled with unbelievable and fallacious vignettes.

1   (0.33:12–0.35.03) During this scene Dr. Callahan (Clive Owen) and his whole team are having their daily debriefing session. They discuss the results of the work of the day, their major difficulties and their plans for the next day. Their different attitudes before the extreme difficulties they face to achieve their objectives are seen in the various characters: optimism and hope, anger, resignation, and cynicism.

   a.   The members of the team Dr. Callahan leads are not all health-care workers and are discussing issues that are not strictly related to health care. What are the usual components of a humanitarian health organization team on the field?

   b.   What aspects of care are essential to be included in a health-care project? How do you think various jobs are shared among humanitarian aid workers?

   c.   What kind of training is necessary for a health-care provider wishing to work for a humanitarian organization?

The Last King of Scotland (see earlier description)

1   (0:08:31–0:09:47) This scene describes the work of lead doctor, Dr. Merrit (Adam Kotz), and his more junior assistant, Dr. Garrigan, in the Ugandan clinic. Resources are scarce. Nearby, a witch doctor is treating a patient.

   a.   What differences do you foresee for health-care providers working in a regular clinic, a refugee camp, or in any setting serving extremely vulnerable populations?

   b.   Scarce resources, difficulties understanding local customs and practices, and achieving only limited results are common problems encountered in the humanitarian field: should NGOs leave their work in the hands of larger structures like government or multi-government agencies?

Live and Become (see earlier description)

1   (0:03:13–0:06:12) This scene shows a huge refugee camp in Sudan. In the tent of a humanitarian NGO, a doctor is providing care to a very sick child lying in the arms of her mother. The child is dying and finally dies. The doctor closes his eyes. The mother cries in silence and takes the hand of the doctor. He comforts her in silence and with obvious moral suffering.

   a.   Health-care providers working among underserved and disaster stricken populations are constantly faced with the discouraging reality that they can make just a small difference. What is the emotional impact of working in often desperate conditions for humanitarian workers?

b. Does the philosophy of the organization a health-care worker is joining affect the sort of work he or she does?

c. Much of a physician's work may be providing comfort to patients. In fact, humanitarian NGOs have been accused of simply covering problems with bandages without providing long-term solutions. What is the position of the different NGOs about that topic?

Triage: Dr. James Orbinski's Humanitarian Dilemma (2008): This film describes the work of James Orbinski, past international president of Médecins Sans Frontières/Doctors Without Borders, who accepted the Nobel Peace Prize for MSF in 1999. Previously a family doctor in Canada, Orbinski worked in Peru, Somalia, The Democratic Republic of Congo, Rwanda, Afghanistan, and Zaire. He was a frequent witness to famine, suffering, and civil war. While this film focuses on one man's work, depicting his thoughts and feelings as he returns to Africa to visit sites where he had once worked, it raises many questions pertaining to the interplay of humanitarian action and politics, the meaning of life and service, and what we as individuals must and can do to help relieve suffering and combat evil.

1 (0:17:20–0:18:34) This scene shot in a camp for internally displaced persons in Somalia in 1992 shows MSF's efforts to provide food and medical care to 150 000 people sitting silently waiting for food. In subsequent scenes the film depicts how, to assure that at least some resources are delivered to the population, NGOs must work with local warlords who enrich themselves by trading food for weapons, money, and power.

a. Do you think NGOs are compromising themselves by negotiating with local warlords or politicians, or military leaders to help assure that at least some resources actually are delivered to target populations?

b. Do you think that funding agencies and individual donors should be told details of financial considerations and resource allocation when it comes to humanitarian aid considerations in areas that require emergency assistance?

c. Famine strikes many parts of the world each year. Do you think you have an individual responsibility to help relieve hunger, and if so, when and how do you or would you assume that responsibility.

d. Would you qualify the work portrayed in this film as humanitarian? In which circumstances would you classify it as assistance, aide, action, intervention, or something else?

Security Issues in Humanitarian Work

The Last King of Scotland (see earlier description)

1 (0:16:17–0:18:41) Idi Amin (Forrest Whitaker) has had a car accident and

his soldiers look for a physician. Since Dr. Merrit is out of the area, Garrigan is called and he assists Amin to fix a wounded hand. His car has hit a cow and the poor animal is screaming in pain while everybody is talking. Garrigan (while taking care of Amin's hand) asks that someone ends the animal's suffering, but no one pays attention to him. Suddenly Garrigan takes a gun and shoots the animal. Every single soldier points his weapon at him and Amin notices him and asks him who he is.

a. Garrigan was moved by the compassion when shooting the injured cow: was his action appropriate?
b. What could have been the consequences of Garrigan's action?
c. Working as they do in extremely risky environments, should humanitarian aid workers have weapons for their protection? What are the reasons for and against the possession of weapons by them?
d. Who decides on security norms for a working team in the field?
e. What are the most important elements concerning security when working in a war zone?

Relationship between Humanitarian Workers and Local Populations

1   (0:12:22–0:15:15) The new president, Idi Amin, is going to come to the village. Garrigan is excited about seeing him, but Dr. Merrit's wife (Gillian Anderson) is reluctant. Finally they both go to the demonstration. Their attitudes during the meeting are very different. Garrigan is enthusiastic and joins the village population in their hurrahs and shouts of greeting. Dr. Merrit's wife is obviously uncomfortable, and views the scene from a distance. Finally, she insists on leaving the demonstration.

a. What are the differences between the attitudes of Garrigan and Dr. Merrit's wife?
b. Is it appropriate or desirable that humanitarian workers get involved in political issues of the country in which they are assigned?
c. Viewing Garrigan's attitude, what is the difference between being aware of and fully knowing and understanding political context and its ramifications
d. Humanitarian workers usually work with a local team. How should they behave in regards to voicing their own opinions about local political issues when sharing daily life with those local partners?

Relationships of Humanitarian Workers with Military Personnel

Tears of the Sun (2003; Bruce Willis, Monica Bellucci; US): A. K. Waters, a veteran officer of a Navy SEAL unit, received orders to lead his extraction team to evacuate Dr. Kendricks, an American medical doctor, and some foreign missionaries from a mission station in the east of Nigeria. A military coup has occurred, and there is civil war in that area of West Africa. The doctor insists that she will only go with them if they also agree to rescue 70 refugees. Waters calls his Captain, and not having a definite answer, concedes to taking those refugees able to walk. Kendricks begins to assemble those able to deal with a long walk, and is ready to leave a priest and a few nuns behind to care for the more severely injured. Serious trouble begins when Waters faces the dilemma of following orders or doing what is right, and finally decides to try to save all of the Nigerian patients.

1   (0:08:43–0:10:10) In this scene Lieutenant Waters (Bruce Willis) and his team arrive at the village of Dr. Kendricks's (Monica Bellucci) clinic. They enter the small, precarious clinic and see Dr. Kendricks and her team operating on a patient. Waters orders the doctor, kindly but firmly, to get ready to depart immediately as they have orders to begin the evacuation. The team reacts somewhat vehemently and Dr. Kendricks tells Waters to immediately remove his men and their guns from her operating room.
   a. Should be the relationship of humanitarian workers with their own country's army be different from that with other military personnel?
   b. In an armed conflict, is there a difference for humanitarian workers between neutral armed forces and those of the belligerent sides?

The Last King of Scotland (see earlier description)

1   (0:18:49–0:20:02) Idi Amin is happy knowing Garrigan is Scottish, as he declares himself a fan of the Scottish people. They start talking in a friendly fashion, and Idi Amin asks Garrigan to give him his Scotland T-shirt. In exchange, Amin gives him his military jacket. He laughs, as Garrigan now appears to be a General. Garrigan makes fun by giving Amin a military salute.
   a. What are the differences between the attitude of Dr. Kendricks and Dr. Garrigan in their relationship with military personnel?
   b. What are the risks of coming into close contact with military personnel as Garrigan does?
   c. Who sets the rules about relationships between humanitarian workers and military personnel?

Moral Duties of a Humanitarian Worker

The Constant Gardener (2005; Ralph Fiennes, Rachel Weisz; US): Justin Quayle was married to Tessa, a dedicated political activist, who was killed recently while traveling in a jeep along a lonely stretch of highway in the company of a Kenyan doctor. The official cause of death is a bandit raid, but Justin suspects a cover-up. Tessa had secretly uncovered proof of a diabolical conspiracy to allow illegal research by a powerful pharmaceutical company. In order to protect British financial interests, the mandate of the British High Commission in Nairobi is to ignore any potentially dangerous information about the drug Dypraxa, which has not yet been approved in the West and is being investigated with little or no protection of research subjects in Africa. Justin travels to the UK and Germany, where he obtains crucial information. He returns to Kenya to confront the people he has concluded were most directly responsible for Tessa's death, and behind the business of using African people as guinea pigs without rights.

1 (1:49:25–1:51:50) Justin Quayle (Fiennes) meets Dr. Lerbeer. On their way to the clinic, the doctor says he only gives food to women because they build homes while men only build alcohol and war.

2 (1:49:25–1:51:50) A violent attack from another tribe takes place. People run for their lives. Quayle and Dr. Lerbeer run to catch the UN plane that is waiting for them to evacuate foreigners to a safe place. A little girl very close to the doctor joins them in the run. They reach the plane but on seeing the girl the pilot firmly refuses to take her with them. Justin Quayle argues with him and even tries to bribe him. The pilot refuses the money, answering that he will not make an exception, and that there are thousands of natives outside the plane and that he cannot take them all.

   a. The UN pilot responds that he cannot save one and leave thousands behind: what can be the moral reasoning behind this response?

Tears of The Sun (see earlier description)

1 (0:10:29–0:11:55) In this scene Lieutenant Waters tells the doctor she must get ready immediately. She states that she is in charge of 70 people, many of them severely injured and will not depart without them. Waters says he has clear orders about evacuating only the foreigners, as the natives are not his responsibility. Dr. Kendricks answers that he is right, it is not his responsibility but it is hers and she will not abandon them.

   a. Is it the duty of humanitarian workers to help local people escape in cases of high risk?

   b. Is it the duty of a physician to risk his/her own life to remain with their patients in case of danger?

   c. Is there a limit between protecting civilians and taking part in differences between two armed sides? How does your opinion affect your beliefs pertaining to a physician's role and social responsibilities?

2 (1:49:25–1:51:50) After much violence, and many deaths, including the loss of most of the Navy Seals, Dr. Kendricks and the evacuated natives reach the border and are safe. A helicopter is waiting for Dr. Kendricks and the few remaining military personnel to fly away from the area. The native people bid a teary farewell to the doctor, telling her how much they love her. Dr. Kendricks departs in the helicopter.

   a. Foreigners (including humanitarian workers) almost always have better resources to protect themselves or escape if situations become critical: how far should they go in protecting the local population?

The English Surgeon (2007): This documentary, directed and produced by Geoffrey Smith, depicts the work of English neurosurgeon Henry Marsh, who, for more than 15 years, has returned repeatedly to the Ukraine to assist in the performance of complex operations in a hospital serving many unfortunate and impoverished patients. The films shows highlights of his association with a Soviet neurosurgical colleague, delivery of surgical instruments that Marsh brings legally into the country in his suitcase, the experiences of a patient undergoing awake craniotomy for resection of a tumor causing epileptic seizures, grief and difficulties related to delivering bad news to patients. The film also provides a vehicle for Marsh's thoughts and philosophies regarding hope, futility, his profession, and the meaning of life.

1 (0:21:00–0:22:20) Dr. Marsh seems haunted by the memory of a young girl who had been told she had advanced inoperable disease from a benign tumor that would ultimately kill her. Explaining his philosophy that "whatever the risk, whatever the costs, we've got to do something," because "hope is more important than anything else in life," we learn that the girl was brought to England where she underwent surgery unsuccessfully. "Because of my operation," Marsh says, "she had a terrible last 2 years of life. It really couldn't have been much worse."

   a. Do you agree that whatever the risk, whatever the cost, we've got to do something? Do you think that such a philosophy might cause an unwarranted financial burden on society? How might such a philosophy affect decisions pertaining to the fair (or unfair) allocation of health-care resources?

   b. Do you agree that hope is more important than anything else in life? If one of your patients has an ultimately fatal illness, would you tell the truth, and if so, how would you deliver the news? How might you still provide hope?

   c. Is there a difference between hope, faith, and miracle-seeking? How would you respond if a patient tells you that their hope is in God and asks you to pray with them for a miracle?

   d. Do you think that under the guise of providing humanitarian aid, especially in underdeveloped and developing nations, physicians might be inclined to do things they would not normally do in their own medical environments, including extending indications for operating on patients or using unproven medical or surgical treatments? Do you think this practice is ethical? What dilemmas might you foresee?

   e. As a humanitarian aid health-care provider working in an underserved, disaster zone, or impoverished area, do you think it is appropriate to single out individuals for special care? If so, how should it be done? If not, why not? What might be some of the moral and psychological consequences of your decision?

f. How would you deal with the sadness, sense of guilt, and sense of power-lessness that often accompanies the act of losing a patient to illness or environmental circumstances? If a medical error had been committed, would your feelings be different? How would you behave if you felt the loss was related to social injustice?

The Ethics of Working in Conditions of Extreme Vulnerability

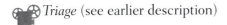 *Triage* (see earlier description)

1 (0:09:12–0:10:15) In this scene Mark sees how the Kurd soldiers transport their mates who have been marked as "code blue" (those desperately ill and unlikely to survive), who are made to lie on the ground in the mountains. In a seriously circumspect act, carefully performed as a sort of ceremony, Dr. Talzani shoots one patient after the other in the head. Afterwards, he prays for them and goes back to work.

  a. Dr. Talzani's behavior can be considered a quite brutal form of active euthanasia. What are your feelings regarding active euthanasia in ordinary conditions? Is such a behavior acceptable in the desperate war context portrayed in the film? Is there any circumstance in which you feel active euthanasia might be acceptable.

The Constant Gardener (see earlier description)

1 (1:49:25–1:51:50) Dr. Lerbeer shows Justin Quayle boxes of medicines that have just arrived by donation from some pharmaceutical companies. Many of the medications are already expired. Apparently, companies prefer to donate them, hence taking advantage of tax savings, rather than assuming the high cost of destroying them. Lerbeer says that this is common practice, as Africa deserves only low-quality medicines for low-quality people.

  a. Working in extreme situations may force one to make difficult decisions that might be different from those made "back home": is the use of expired medicines or low-quality medical care acceptable in such conditions?

Beyond Borders (see earlier description)

1 (0:25:29–0:26:27) Dr. Callahan is shown a desperately ill boy and his severely injured mother. He quickly assesses them and declares they are both too sick to survive and that no care should be provided to them.

  a. Dr. Callahan's performance of triage means some subjects will not receive any care: is this an acceptable ethical position? What are the reasons behind such a decision?

    b. Should the ethical norms that form the basis of ordinary medical care differ from those applied during work in extreme conditions? If so, which ones and why?

🎥 *Triage: Dr. James Orbinski's Humanitarian Dilemma* (see earlier description)

1   (0:29:50–0:31:10) In this scene Dr. Orbinski relates how he was asked, at gunpoint, to cease operating on a child in order to provide care instead to a wounded soldier. He goes on to say that humanitarian assistance, including working in a war zone, creates risks that are inherent to the profession, and recalls with sadness the brutal murder of Dr. Ricardo Marques on June 21, 1997.

    a. Would you risk your life to help unknown others in another part of the world?

    b. Sometimes, NGO workers have been killed while doing their work saving lives and relieving suffering in disaster areas, war zones and the like. When this occurs as a result of malicious and evil human behaviors, do you think an NGO should voluntarily remove all of its personnel from the area, or should this be regarded as part of the risk of doing business?

    c. Do you think NGO workers warrant special protection and assistance to prevent them from being harmed? How might this be affected by the principle of impartiality and neutrality manifested by many NGOs?

Funding Humanitarian Action

🎥 *Beyond Borders* (see earlier description)

1   (0:35:33–0:36:22) In this scene Dr. Callahan is discussing the desperate condition of their current funding with his logistician. They discuss the different agencies of whom they have asked money but have had had no results. Dr. Callahan suggests they could get some money from a local political group. The team logistician refuses, strongly arguing that that is not, and never will be, the way they work.

    a. What are the different agencies they are talking about? Are all organizations the same or are they different?

    b. What is the usual source of funding for humanitarian organizations?

    c. Are there any differences about the source of funds accepted by different types of organizations?

    d. Why is the logistician refusing so strongly to receive money from a political group? Is it a matter of security or a matter of philosophy?

    e. If refusing funds means having a shortage of resources and delivering less efficient or even poor care to those underserved populations, is it ethical?

Should humanitarian teams accept any sort of funds in order to deliver the best possible care to their target populations?

f. Who sets the rules for funding an organization?

g. What is the relationship between different humanitarian organizations and the United Nations?

Humanitarian Action or Volunteer Professional Service?

 The English Surgeon (see earlier description)

1 (0:05:40–0:06:40) In this scene, a bankrupt Soviet medical system in and around Kiev is described. Marsh explains that during one of his first trips there in 1992, he felt a need to help, but was told by officials that doing so would be "a waste of time. Anything you do is a drop in the ocean – the whole system would have to change."

a. Have you ever felt this way about medical care in your own hospital? What might you do about it?

b. Do physicians have a moral and social responsibility to advocate for their patients? Is this responsibility different from that of non-physician health-care providers?

c. From an ethics and individual behavioral perspective, do physicians serve their individual patients or society as a whole? Can you envision conflicts between these two roles? How would you handle such conflict in your own practice?

d. Speaking "truth to power" can be a dangerous undertaking, especially when authorities directly discourage one's desires or actions to help. Can you think of any times when you stood idly by because you felt or were told that doing otherwise is just a waste of time or that anything you do is just a drop in the ocean? How did you feel about that? Is there anything you would do differently in the future?

e. Would you qualify the work portrayed in this film as humanitarian? Would you classify it as assistance, aide, action, intervention, or something else?

Further Reading

- Colt HG, Quadrelli S, Friedman L, editors. *The Picture of Health: medical ethics and the movies*. New York, NY: Oxford University Press; 2011.
- Code of Conduct for the International Red Cross and Red Crescent Movement and NGOs. In: *Disaster Relief in SHERE Handbook*. Oxford: Oxfam; 2000. Article 1, pp. 312–22.
- Damieson J. Duties to the distant aid, assistance and intervention in the developing world. *J Ethics*. 2005; **9**(1–2): 151–70.

Cinemeducation

- Holmes D, Perron A. Violating ethics: unlawful combatants, national security and health professionals. *J Med Ethics*. 2007; **33**(1): 143–5.
- Jayasinghe S. Faith-based NGOs and healthcare in poor countries: a preliminary exploration of ethical issues. *J Med Ethics*. 2007; **33**(1): 623–6.
- Luck EC. The humanitarian imperative. *UN Security Council*. 2006; **1**(4): 81–92.
- Slim H. Claiming a humanitarian imperative: NGOs and the cultivation of humanitarian duty. *Refugee Survey Q*. 2002; **21**(3): 113–25.
- Sphere Project. *Humanitarian Charter and Minimum Standards in Disaster Response*. Oxford: Oxfam; 2000.

41

When Nature Becomes the Enemy: Disaster Medicine

Renee Hickson, LaTasha K. Crawford,
Leslie Wind & Patricia Lenahan

GLOBALLY, CATASTROPHIC NATURAL DISASTERS APPEAR TO BE occurring with greater frequency. Television and social media sites bring these devastating events into our homes: tsunamis in Indonesia and Japan, earthquakes in China, Haiti, Chile, and Japan, wildfires in Australia and the United States, flooding in Europe, tornados in the United States, and hurricanes like Katrina, can dominate the news. Such disastrous events are an inevitable part of life. Many of us observe the loss of life and property from a safe distance, while others will serve as volunteers to provide medical, mental health, and veterinary assistance to these affected areas, and others will send financial assistance to aid in the recovery. The prospect of reconstructing lives and communities often is difficult to comprehend. Individuals who are economically and socially disadvantaged may be at greater risk for developing health and mental health problems as a result of these events.

The films used in this chapter all focus on Hurricane Katrina, but they are applicable to discussions of coping with the health and public health interventions for natural disasters in general. The chapter focuses only on natural disasters and not events related to war or terrorism.

This chapter departs from the usual format in that it includes Dr. Renee Hickson's brief introduction and personal account of Hurricane Katrina and her work following the disaster.

Dr. Hickson writes:

> The list of psychosocial stressors that can induce mental illness includes loss of home or property, death of spouse or loved one or pet, change or loss of employment/career status. Most of the people of New Orleans experienced all of these in a matter of days following Hurricane Katrina. Ironically, it wasn't the hurricane itself that caused us so much hurt and pain. It was the failure of

our levee system, infrastructures and our local, state, and federal government. It was being called "refugee" in your own country, where you and your ancestors fought, worked, bled, and died for the life you lived. Only to be treated like a foreigner looking for a handout. Many people asked whether New Orleans was "worth it" to rebuild, adding to our sense of frustration. The city where so many tourists find an escape from their own lives for a weekend of "lassiz le bon temp rouler," happens to be our home.

Just like our funeral processions depict a "first line" of loss and pain and sorrow, our "second line" is one of celebration and perseverance and hope for the future – the afterlife. We gather our faith, hope, defiance, and love – the greatest of these – and we show the world why New Orleans matters.

It matters because we are a spiritual people – people of great faith. We worship our God (Catholics, Jews, Protestants), or gods (food, alcohol, music), and our saints (who dats, yats, Indians, voodoo dolls). We respect our differences, but come together to do the work required to rebuild our neighborhoods and to maintain our traditions. We are a close-knit family that got scattered, shattered and bent – but not broken. We picked up the ties that bind us – our culture, our music, our food, and our Saints – and created a bond that can never be severed.

As doctors, by definition we are the healers. We came back, and stayed to do the work we love. Not only to provide comfort and relieve disease and illness, but to give and receive love, hope, compassion, and patience. To let people know they aren't crazy, or alone or stupid, for returning home. To let one another know that we are here for each other. As much as we had to renew, we also needed some things to remain constant.

The importance of the role of the family doctor became huge after the storm. There was no denying how much our communities needed us. We knew the people needed us, which makes it hard to leave. This was never more evident than at the massive health fairs set up around the city after the storm, where hundreds of people came to seek care.

It was a humbling honor to have patients "find me" and come to see me no matter what part of the city I practiced. Some patients still lived out of town, but would schedule appointments when they came to check on their homes. These were long visits, as they had to share their storm story, hear what happened to me, and then finally address their medical needs.

Everyone has a story. Each one having common elements of suffering and pain, the kindness and meanness of human beings, the struggle to get back home and the triumph of making it.

Advance Preparations for Disasters

Music in Exile (2008): This documentary takes an unusual look at post-Katrina New Orleans: a focus on the musicians of the city and the losses and experiences they faced.

1 (0:12:03–0:13:37) A woman is talking about her reactions to the predictions of "doom" related to the arrival of Hurricane Katrina. She shares that if you live in New Orleans for a long time, you never think a hurricane will hit the city. She adds: "We've heard the doomsday scenarios for years." Later she says that she evacuated to Baton Rouge where her sister lived. They were watching TV and couldn't believe what they saw. They had no Internet and worried if everyone was safe.

   a. How would you assess this woman's reactions? Is this a typical response in areas that are prone to specific kinds of natural disasters?
   b. What is the impact of being displaced and being unable to contact loved ones?
   c. How dependent are we on the Internet as a source of communication?
   d. What types of interventions would be helpful in addressing pre-warning systems?
   e. Who do you rely on for accurate information regarding the safety of your environment/surroundings? Government? Friends/Family? TV/media/Internet?
   f. Do you think our systems accurately count the morbidity and mortality associated with disasters?

Trouble the Water (2008): This is an Oscar-nominated documentary by film-makers Tia Lessin and Carl Deal. The film chronicles the people and the events of New Orleans following Hurricane Katrina, following a couple (Scott and Kimberly Roberts) from the Ninth Ward.

1 (Ch 1, 0:1:15–0:3:40) Scott and Kim are talking about trying to get out. They have food, their cat and dog. The scene shows the National Guard trucks with footage taken both before and after Katrina.

   a. What level of preparedness is evident here?
   b. What are the priorities of this family?
   c. What factors contribute to vicarious trauma for first responders?
   d. Should first responders undergo mandatory counseling before/during/after disasters?
   e. Do you think first responders should be given laxity regarding rules/regulations during disasters?
   f. What preparations and accommodations are made for families with pets?

The Initial Aftermath

1   (0:14:55–0:17:15; 0:19:00–0:20:16) Legendary singer Irma Thomas, takes the videographer on a tour of what is left of her place, The Lion's Den Lounge. She discusses the smells, the mold concerns, and explains the "X's" on the walls. She continues by taking the filmmaker on a tour of what is left of her home.
    a. What things in your home are invaluable to you? Who determines what is salvageable?
    b. What is an appropriate emotional response to the loss of one's business or home?
    c. Do you think people should reside in areas prone to natural disasters?
    d. Does insurance adequately cover your losses?

Disasters and First Responders

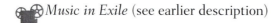*Music in Exile* (see earlier description)

1   (0:20:20–0:21:05) Irma Thomas greets the National Guardsmen outside. She says most of them are from the area. She speaks with the commander who states that 75% of the company suffered loss of homes destroyed or damaged and their families were displaced.
    a. What is the impact of natural disasters on first responders who also may be victims of the disaster?
    b. How would you counsel a first responder who is coping with personal losses?
    c. What are the potential long-term sequelae of being a first responder?
    d. How can first responders balance their community commitment with the needs of their own families?

Devastation, Discomfort, and Disbelief

1   (0:32:04z-0:33:09) David Freeman, WWOZ radio, is talking about Katrina. He says that if you leave the French Quarter, the devastation is apparent. He states that people don't want to live at the level of discomfort in New Orleans at present: no phone, no water, no electricity, no mail and curfews. He adds: "New Orleans is an amputee with phantom memory."
    a. How would you respond to a patient/client who describes the city as an amputee with phantom memory? What feelings does that statement evoke?
    b. What is empathic strain? How would it apply to therapists working with victims of natural disasters?

    c. Do you think modern conveniences have made us more detached or more connected to one another?

    d. Which parts of your life are necessities vs. conveniences? Where does Internet access fall?

    e. How can you help him envision a healing community?

2 (Ch 1, 0:4:38–0:5:40) Kim is talking to some children in the neighborhood and asks them if they are afraid of hurricanes. The children say they aren't scared. Kim adds: "hurricanes are nothing, but water, who's scared of water?" Again the children say they aren't afraid.

    a. What are the mental health concerns for children following a natural disaster?

    b. Is it "normal" for children to react to threats of disasters without fear?

    c. To what extent should the government aid people who choose not to evacuate during predicted disasters?

    d. Should resources be extended to families with pets?

    e. Do you think it's reasonable to not evacuate because of lack of accommodations for pets?

    f. Should schools provide counseling to children following disasters? Can you think of effective ways to provide counseling for adults?

    g. Are children or adults who are victims of natural disasters at increased risk to develop mental or behavioral disorders?

    h. What can you say to help children acknowledge their concerns?

    i. What role can parents and teachers play in addressing children's fears?

3 (Ch 1, 0:13:40–0:14:53; ch 5, 0:30:17–0:32–38) It is 2 weeks since Katrina struck the city and the Roberts's return. Kim says: "This can't be real; it's horrible. This is my neighborhood, I know everybody." She talks about the various people in the neighborhood. In the second scene, Kim shares that the area still hadn't been checked two weeks after the hurricane. Her Uncle Nat, whom she tried to coax into accompanying her, was found dead in the front room.

    a. How are the dead and missing accounted for after a disaster?

    b. Are people adequately trained for search and rescue when they are traumatized themselves?

    c. Who holds the final responsibility for the accuracy of mortality numbers after disasters?

    d. How do you feel about the term "storm-related" as it applies to people who die soon after disasters? What about the same term applied to your homeowners insurance? How long should it apply?

4 (Ch 5, 0:33:420:36:40) Kim and Scott are talking about the lack of transportation and how the government let them down. They began walking to a decommissioned U.S. Naval Base in New Orleans. Kim and Scott pondered why the facility couldn't be used for emergency housing. They were greeted by a guard who ordered them off "our property," adding "or we'll shoot."

    a. How do you feel about the distinct separation of the "military" from "civilians"? It's rather alarming when you see them in your neighborhood with large guns. Who are those bullets for? Will they receive orders to shoot their fellow Americans? I always thought they only aimed at foreign threats.

   b. Why does the military protect us, but have to "wait for orders" to help us in times of disaster?

   c. Would a soldier shoot a civilian for trespassing?

   d. Why is the threat of violence necessary for enforcement?

5 (Ch 6, 0:42:45–0:45:03; 0:45:50–0:46:45) The first scene occurs 2 weeks after the levees failed and pans well-known footage of the convention center and onto a montage of people of various ages, races, injuries, and disabilities lined up along the highway.

   a. How did our government/we allow people to end up like this?

   b. What can be done to identify people who need assistance *before* disasters occur? What systems have been put in place since Hurricane Katrina that have been demonstrated to be beneficial in New Orleans or other communities?

   c. Should we be obligated to help people who are unwilling or unable to heed warnings to evacuate?

6 (Ch 6, 0:48:32–0:51:00) Kim and Scott have evacuated to Alexandria (Louisiana) to stay with relatives. They share that everything they did, they did as a family. They also brought one older woman with them who had no family and was going to be re-located to an unknown area.

   a. What impact do disasters have on the now broken family unit?

   b. How does the loss of family and community structure impact people personally, socially, financially?

   c. How would you feel when you can no longer go to Sunday dinner at your mom's house? Make a quick stop at Wal-Mart? Go to your favorite bar for a drink? Attend the place of worship you've gone to your whole life?

   d. How would you decide who stays with the elderly or physically impaired that cannot travel? What about pets?

7 (Ch 6, 0:51:55–0:52:38) Kim talks about her grandmother who had been hospitalized when Katrina struck. She was told the hospital evacuated, but adds, "they never did." The scene pans an area with multiple dead bodies. Kim adds that it's been 2 weeks and we still don't have a body. They left my grandmother behind."

   a. What are current standards for evacuating hospitals and nursing homes? (few/none in place prior to storm)

   b. What responsibility do family/caregivers have regarding evacuation of loved ones from these facilities? Is it fair to put it all on the institution?

   c. Should the inherent risks involved in caring for patients during disasters alter the "standard of care"?

   d. How are we identified in life and after death? What are the "bar codes" on us that say who we are?

    e. Should institutionalized persons be "tagged"? Or "linked" to next of kin/a responsible party?

    f. What additional services may be needed for elderly individuals?

8 (Ch 7, 0:55:25–0:57:13) Scott and Kim go to a FEMA disaster recovery center. The scene pans the myriad people waiting for assistance. One woman says: "we're still waiting."

    a. How are the needs of the displaced determined?

    b. What are basic necessities to you?

    c. How long should the government (fellow taxpayers) provide these needs after disasters? Have you paid enough taxes for your upkeep?

9 (Ch 8, 0:59:20–1:03:31; 1:04:31–1:05:27) In the first scene, Kim and Scott have packed a truck and are on the road to Memphis after Hurricane Rita hit New Orleans. Kim says: "we're displaced again." The second scene shows Kim and her cousin talking. Kim says she's still in shock and maybe she'll start crying in a couple of weeks. Her cousin says she's been crying the whole time. The cousin talks about what she has seen on TV, adding that what happened in New Orleans looks like what happens in a Third World country.

    a. What are the stages of grief/loss?

    b. Are there any responses to profound or repeated loss that should be considered abnormal? How long should this response persist before it's considered abnormal?

    c. How many Americans live one disaster away from "Third World" status?

10 (Ch 11, 1:19:36–1:21:55) It is ten months since Hurricane Katrina struck the city and Kim and Scott return to their house in the Ninth Ward. They see an eviction notice on the door. Scott said he returned to New Orleans for work and Kim said it was too hard to start all over in a strange place, adding, "New Orleans is home."

    a. Are we obligated to return people "home"?

    b. Should people be forced into areas where the most assistance (job opportunities, education, housing) is available?

    c. Should existing laws, regulations, and practices regarding housing rights be adhered to after disasters? How long should leniency be considered?

11 (Ch 11, 1:22:25–1:23:20) The scene takes place at the New Orleans tourist office where a representative says that people want to come to the city on vacation. She states: "They don't want to be reminded of devastation when they are on vacation."

    a. Does our socioeconomic system foster the idea that our need for pleasure outweighs the burden of recovery?

    b. How often do we supplant individual needs for that of the "greater good"?

    c. Do you think about how the residents of your favorite "vacation cities" live? Have you ever been off the beaten path to their neighborhoods?

12 (Ch 11, 1:23:50–1:25:00) This scene provides an overview of the Ninth Ward 1 year after Katrina. Much of the area remains devastated. Kim says the "hood's" always going to be the last place to be fixed.

   a. Do disasters birth poverty? Can this be prevented?

   b. Can disasters ever improve the pre-disaster condition of the poor?

   c. Is it the "natural order" that the poor be helped last?

   d. What can we do to change this?

Coping with Loss and Change

The Axe in the Attic (2007): This documentary is the work of filmmakers Lucia Small and Ed Pincus who travel from their New England homes to chronicle the impact of Hurricane Katrina on the lives of the evacuees they meet en route to New Orleans and in the city itself.

1 (Ch 3, 0:8:50–0:10:50) Victoria Elfer, a single mother, has been evacuated from Chalmette to Cincinnati with her two teenagers. She is staying with her sister. She is seen trying to dry out family photographs and says this is what hurts the most. "You can replace other stuff, but you can't replace family photos." Victoria adds that she wants her children to be settled. Her son, Colton, says the teachers in New Orleans had a sense of humor, and while they are nice here, they are more focused on academics. His sister, Tori, is sitting in her aunt's lap and shares her dreams about having a plantation of her own. She says she is going back.

   a. What is the significance of family photographs?

   b. How would you interpret Colton's statement about the New Orleans teachers having a sense of humor, but that the teachers here are more focused on academics?

   c. How realistic are Tori's dreams?

   d. What are the effects of loss and trauma on adolescents?

Music in Exile (see earlier description)

1 (1:40:29–1:41:45) Voodoo priestess, Sally Ann Glassman, is seen performing the "Raising the Dead" Ceremony for New Orleans.

   a. What is your response to this scene? Are you surprised by the heterogeneity of the participants?

   b. What role/purpose does this have culturally in healing?

Mine (2009): This documentary looks at several perspectives surrounding the plight of the domestic animals that belonged to those people that were forced to evacuate due to the Katrina disaster. Several pet owners and their advocates tried to locate their animals after being forced to leave them because shelters and Red Cross rescue missions would not allow families to bring their pets. Humane society workers and volunteers worked tirelessly to search for pets in the rubble of destroyed homes, provided veterinary care, and found new families to adopt the thousands of animals that were left without owners.

We also see the conflict that arises when the original dog owners that were displaced by Katrina search for their pets that have now been adopted by new families.

1   (0:0:36–0:0:1:36; 0:31:20–0:32:30) Melvin Cavalier is an 89-year-old widower and a self-described "full-blooded Creole." He is talking about his dog, Bandit, and showing viewers his yard and Bandit's leash. Melvin says that he used to take Bandit for a walk at night and that Bandit would sit by him. Melvin says that he loved Bandit, adding, "I never thought I'd lose Bandit the way I did." In the second scene, Melvin has returned to New Orleans after 5 months in Houston. He has his FEMA trailer. He says his own home wouldn't be done for a year, but he built a doghouse for Bandit, hopeful that he would be able to find his dog. Melvin shares that he and Bandit grew closer after his wife died in 2003.

   a.   What is the impact of pet loss on Melvin? How do older adults cope with loss and accumulated losses?
   b.   Melvin shares that he and Bandit grew closer after his wife died. How can animals help people cope/adjust to other losses?

2   (0:18:35–0:20:45; 0:25:30–0:28:00) The first scene introduces Gloria, a retired nurse, who said she had reassured her Labrador retriever, Murphy, that she wouldn't leave him. Gloria says I would have stayed, but the National Guard forced me to leave. She says she was put on a bus with other people and they didn't know where they were going. The second scene finds that Gloria had been sent to an evacuation facility in St. Louis. Her daughter and volunteers are working to try to find Murphy for her. Gloria says: "dogs and their loved ones have a connection."

   a.   What actions could be taken to allow evacuees and their pets remain together?
   b.   How is the impact of re-location on older adults?
   c.   How would you respond to Gloria's statement that dogs and their loved ones have a connection?

Health and Mental Health Effects of Disaster Evacuees

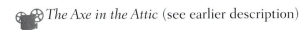 *The Axe in the Attic* (see earlier description)

1   (Ch 1, 0:4:17–0:7:40) The filmmakers meet Laurel Turner who was evacuated to Pittsburg. Laurel is experiencing winter and snow for the first time. She says they don't know how to feel. She is on unemployment and still waiting for FEMA to help pay the rent. Laurel says we were warned about the hurricanes 5 or 6 years ago … the same old levee system. The scene shifts to Laurel's brother, a pastor who helped them relocate. He talks about the hurricanes in the 1960s. He clearly is quite affected.

  a. How might Laurel and her family view responsibility for their current circumstances?
  b. What meaning might Laurel and her brother attach to having been "warned"?
  c. How might religious beliefs and values impact psychological outcomes?
  d. Consider the effect of repeated exposure to hurricanes. What would you want to know about previous exposures? How might previous exposure relate to current psychological outcomes?

2 (Ch 4, 0:12:30–0:16:11) In Murray, Kentucky, viewers are introduced to Tara Jackson, who was a full-time student at the University of New Orleans prior to Katrina. She is a single mother of five children who all evacuated with her. Tara says that the memories she has "would make you cringe." She talks about being sent to the convention center where all she saw was death. She related an incident where her neighbor's brother "lost it" and jumped out in front of a police car. Tara says: "one shot to the heart … they were going to kill us all. His body was 2 feet away from me." When she arrived in Murray she was told to take off her clothes because they were contaminated. She said she tried to wash them and it was then that she discovered she had "his blood" on them.
  a. What symptoms would you look for related to Tara Jackson's direct exposure to others' deaths?
  b. How might being a single mother of five children and a full-time student, now evacuated to Kentucky, impact psychological functioning when faced with disasters and death?
  c. Tara faced the potential death of her children and herself. What do you want to know about her thoughts and behaviors during her time at the convention center?
  d. How could Tara Jackson's previous experiences with the police have impacted her response to rescue efforts?

3 (Ch 5, 0:18:00–0:19:15) The filmmakers have arrived in a FEMA trailer encampment in northern Alabama where they meet Donna and Julius Thompson, an interracial couple. Julius is a 10-year army veteran. He says that the FEMA official asked him if he needed counseling to which he responded, "no … God is my counselor. All I'm asking for is housing so I can get a job."
  a. How might Julius Thompson's experience in the military affect his willingness to engage in counseling?
  b. What do you want to know about this couple's spirituality in relation to coping with disaster and relocation?
  c. What potential barriers to utilizing services might be explored based on status as an interracial couple?
  d. The only assistance Julius Thompson wants is housing so he can obtain a job. Would you open the discussion of resources needed beyond housing? If so, how? Could the Veteran's Administration be a resource for this couple?

4 (Ch 5, 0:22:58–0:23:28) Olivia Reed and her husband Daryl are living at the same encampment. Olivia shows the filmmakers the "sores" on her arms. She says she was told that they are the result of "having been in the water." Daryl is heard off camera saying, "they don't know what it is and are going to do tests." Olivia says "All my life, they've got me on Zoloft for depression. I don't know what that is, but it ain't working."

   a. What impact might not knowing what the "sores" are have on Olivia's chronic depression?
   b. How could you act as an advocate for this couple?
   c. Considering the potential health issues, how might others in the encampment react to the sores on Olivia's arms? How could their response impact recovery?
   d. What information about Olivia's early history of depression would you want to know as a foundation for assisting her?

5 (Ch 5, 0:23:49–0:29:30) Susan Cross and her husband, Ray, are interviewed. They recently had sold their home in the upper Ninth Ward and had purchased a home in Chalmet. The Crosses are visibly shaken during this interview. Ray and his older son, Wes, went to protect the new house while Susan and their younger son stayed with her parents in the upper Ninth Ward. Ray says the water began to rise and when it was up to his neck, he and his son went to the roof. Eventually the water rose up to 23 feet and Ray told his son they would have to swim. Susan adds that she didn't have any contact with Ray or Wes for 2 days and she was sure her family was gone. She smiled as she recounted seeing Wes walking down the street with his arms open and saying "I'm home." Susan said those were the sweetest words she ever heard.

   a. How would you incorporate spirituality into crisis response for this couple?
   b. As an interracial couple, how might discrimination play a role in the availability of resources? How might ethnic differences in coping impact their adaptation?
   c. Julius is a 10-year army veteran. Does his identity as a veteran and possible previous experience with war and/or disasters affect his psychological response to this disaster?
   d. What effect might stigma regarding mental health support have on asking for help? Consider the ethnic context for help-seeking as well.

6 (Chs 7–8, 0:35:20–0:38:51) Jimmy Brown, Laurel's brother, stayed in the New Orleans area because he still had a job. He is seen with his wife, Lisa, taking the filmmakers on a tour of their old house and Laurel's as well. Lisa says: "our normal little house, a normal little life, now everything is abnormal."

   a. In spite of still having a job, how could the loss of normalcy affect Jimmy and Lisa Brown's recovery?
   b. How would you address the multiple losses being experienced by this couple (e.g. home, lifestyle, family support)?
   c. How could your interventions vary across phases of recovery?
   d. How might use of different modalities benefit this couple?

7   (Ch 10, 0:56:50–0:58:30) Hurricane Katrina has displaced Reverend Charles Jackson. He says that he wants "a helping hand, not a hand out." He is staying in a FEMA trailer in Baker, Louisiana. Reverend Jackson says: "If it wasn't for God, I'd jump off the Mississippi River Bridge. I'm tired and I need help. I don't know what to do."

   a. How might Reverend Jackson's spiritual beliefs contribute to his ability to cope?

   b. Are you concerned about suicidality?

   c. What is the difference between a "handout" and a "helping hand"? How can you help Reverend Jackson define a "helping hand" as a foundation to offering desired assistance?

   d. How do your own beliefs about receiving help and dependence on God influence how you approach helping this individual?

Veterinary Issues in Disaster Response

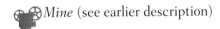*Mine* (see earlier description)

1   (0:06:45–0:10:03) These scenes feature testimony of volunteers that supplemented the humane society efforts to rescue pets following Katrina. For disasters of this magnitude, the normal avenues of rescue efforts proved to be overwhelmed and far from adequate.

   a. What are key elements of triage in a patient population following a natural disaster such as the floods that followed Katrina?

   b. What types of infectious disease and other medical conditions should be higher on your radar when examining a shelter population of animals compared with a typical companion animal population?

   c. What additional challenges do shelters pose for veterinarians that are not faced by veterinarians that work with kennels or animal hospitals?

   d. What are some approaches used in shelter medicine to prevent infectious disease outbreaks?

2   (0:18:15–0:21:00) In these scenes we hear testimony from owners that had to leave their pets behind during the mandatory evacuations in Louisiana.

   a. What lessons can you extrapolate from the aftermath of Katrina to help prepare pet owners in your communities for other types of natural disasters? For more common events such as earthquakes or house fires? For everyday emergencies?

   b. What resources can you suggest to your clients when discussing a family disaster plan that incorporates their pets?

   c. What are the benefits of using ID tags and microchips? What are the potential oversights that can make microchips less useful?

   d. What new mechanisms were recently put in place by the federal government to include pets in disaster plans and evacuations?

3 (0:32:31–0:36:40) A potential conflict can arise when animals are presumed abandoned and are thus adopted out, with the new owners unaware that the original owners are searching for their pet. These scenes illustrate the perspective of the both the original owner, Victor, and the new owners, Tiffany and Jeremy.

4 (0:37:06–0:39:40) In these scenes we hear the tale of a woman who is helping to reunite one owner, Melvin, with his dog Bandit. She and Melvin encountered an array of hurdles when trying to locate Bandit, including those who believed that some displaced owners did not deserve to be reunited with their pets.

    a. What can shelters do to prevent the problems highlighted in these scenes?

    b. What are the potential benefits of placing displaced or abandoned animals in foster homes following a disaster, in lieu of adoptive homes? What are the potential drawbacks?

    c. What are some of the prejudices that may hinder reuniting an evacuee with their pet?

The Humane Society has a useful online resource for a disaster plan for family pets, with links to pages that address horses and livestock (www.humanesociety. org/news/news/2011/03/disaster_planning_2011.html).

Further Reading

- Abramson D, Stehling-Ariza T, Garfield R, *et al*. Prevalence and predictors of mental health distress post-Katrina: findings from the Gulf Coast Child and Family Health Study. *Disaster Medicine Public Health Prep*. 2008; **2**(2): 77–86.
- Chen AC, Keith VM, Leong KJ, *et al*. Hurricane Katrina: prior trauma, poverty and health among Vietnamese-American survivors. *Intern Nurs Rev*. 2007; **54**(4): 324–31.
- DeSalvo KB, Hyre AD, Ompad DC, *et al*. Symptoms of posttraumatic stress disorder in a New Orleans workforce following Hurricane Katrina. *J Urban Health*. 2007; **84**(2): 142–52.
- Glandon DM, Miller J, Almedon NM. Resilience in post-Katrina New Orleans, Louisiana: a preliminary study. *Afi Health Sci*. 2008; **8**(Suppl. 1): 321–7.
- Gold JI, Montano Z, Shields S, *et al*. Pediatric disaster preparedness in the medical setting: integrating mental health. *Am J Disaster Med*. 2009; **4**(3): 137–46.
- Hawkins RL, Mauerer K. Bonding, bridging and linking: how social capital operated in New Orleans following Hurricane Katrina. *Br J Soc Work*. 2010; **40**(6): 1777–93.
- Park Y, Miller J. The social ecology of Hurricane Katrina: re-writing the discourse of "natural" disasters. *Smith College School of Social Work*. 2006; **76**(3): 9–24.
- Rhodes J, Chan C, Paxson C, *et al*. The impact of Hurricane Katrina on the mental and physical health of low-income parents in New Orleans. *Am J Orthopsychiatry*. 2010; **80**(2): 237–47.
- Rowe CL, Liddie HA. When the levee breaks: treating adolescents and families in the aftermath of Hurricane Katrina. *J Marital Ther*. 2008; **34**(2): 132–48.

42

Crocks and Docs: Disruptive Patients/Disruptive Providers

*Patricia Lenahan, Dael Waxman, Edward Thibodeau,
Lauren M. Consonni, LaTasha K. Crawford, Gurvinder Kalra,
Dinesh Bhugra, Snezana Begovic, David Stanley & Amy E. Cassidy*

IN RECENT YEARS, A GREAT DEAL OF ATTENTION HAS BEEN PAID TO the issue of disruptive and/or impaired providers. Studies indicate that nurses and physicians are equally as "disruptive." Disruptive behaviors may include impairment from substances, inappropriate displays of anger toward patients, and seductive interactions – either between health-care professionals and their patients or between health-care professionals themselves, e.g. doctor to doctor and doctor to nurse. The impact of unprofessional behaviors such as verbal and sexual harassment, dismissive attitudes, and confusion regarding medical orders may have a significant impact on patient care and outcomes, including increases in adverse or sentinel events.

As a result, various programs have been developed to specifically enhance the communication between doctors and nurses. Communication difficulties – such as abrasive comments, curt responses, and language discordant issues – between doctors and nurses have been explored extensively in the literature. A series of articles, beginning with Stein's article, "The doctor-nurse game,"[1] have described ways in which doctors and nurses communicate with one another.

Recent efforts to address communication difficulties include the development of SBAR (Situation, Background, Assessment and Recommendation), a tool developed by Kaiser. SBAR was developed to foster teamwork and to help enhance the communication between physicians and nurses by identifying a focused means of discussing an individual patient's care needs, especially when a change in the patient's condition may occur. The SBAR allows doctors and nurses to share information in a concise, efficient manner. It also is an effective tool used to transmit information during "handoffs."[2,3] Another program, similar in intent to the SBAR, has been developed for use in military facilities.

Cinematically, perhaps the best personifications of the disruptive provider (whose disruptive behaviors impact both patient care and interaction with other health-care providers) include Nurse Ratchet in *One Flew Over the Cuckoo's Nest* (1975) and George C. Scott's portrayal of the depressed, suicidal, and rage-filled physician in *The Hospital* (1971). Television portrayals of impaired or disruptive physicians include John Becker (Ted Danson), the cynical, abrasive internist in the series *Becker*, and the quintessential example of the impaired practitioner, Gregory House (Hugh Laurie) on the series *House*. The influence of this particular television show is reflected in the fact that there are websites (www. housemd-guide.com) devoted to "everything House" including "House-isms" such as: "I don't ask why patients lie, I just assume they all do."

Another challenge for health-care providers is the disruptive patient. Through the ages, physicians have been taught that part of their responsibility as a healer is to "know all, love all, and cure all." While most physicians will acknowledge that it is impossible to "cure all," many providers may succumb to the belief that they "should" be able to work well with all patients, thus denying their own humanity, frailties, personal values and attitudes. The seminal article by Groves,[4] "Taking care of the hateful patient," was one of the first attempts to codify behaviors, actions, and personalities of patients who are difficult to treat. The subtypes in Groves's article have been illustrated in a chapter in Volume 1 of *Cinemeducation*[5] but have been expanded since Groves's initial publication. Current types of difficult patients include drug-seeking patients, chronic pain patients, and Internet surfers who challenge their health-care providers with the latest information on the Web.

This chapter will provide an overview of a variety of health-care providers – physicians, nurses, dentists, veterinarians, and ancillary personnel – who are disruptive and/or impaired.[6,7] Some of the films cited in this chapter are older (classic) films that provide excellent representations of problematic behaviors. The chapter also will address examples of the various types of patients who inspire fear and dread in the practitioner. In some instances, individual contributors have added brief and specific introductions to their sections.

The Patients Are the Problem

The Disruptive Patient: Seductive and Litigious

Reign Over Me (2007; Don Cheadle, Adam Sandler): This film explores the relationship between successful Manhattan dentist Alan Johnson (Cheadle) and his former dental school roommate, Charlie Fineman (Sandler). Charlie lost his family during the 9/11 attacks. The storyline revolves around Dr. Johnson's attempt to help his old friend deal with depression and emotional instability while facing his personal self-doubts and career problems.

1   (0:17:58–0:20:48) This scene begins with Dr. Johnson being propositioned by an attractive but troubled patient, Donna Remar (Saffron Burrows), and ends by showing us how he and his staff initially deal with the unwelcome encounter.

  a. From a malpractice perspective, are there situations in which it may be inappropriate to be alone with a dental patient behind closed doors? Are there risks associated with this type of interaction?
  b. Is Dr. Johnson's reaction to Ms. Remar's advances appropriate? Why or why not? How could he have handled the situation differently?
  c. Discuss the importance of Dr. Johnson documenting this encounter with Ms. Remar in the patient record.
  d. What could motivate patients to behave inappropriately toward their health-care provider? Could conscious or subconscious actions on the part of the health-care provider encourage such patient behavior?
  e. Were the actions of the receptionist appropriate to the situation? How should she have handled Dr. Johnson's request to no longer see Ms. Remar? Could there be any legal ramifications of the receptionist's actions?
  f. From a legal perspective, are there patient abandonment issues with the way Dr. Johnson's office handled Ms. Remar?
2 (0:27:47–0:29:10) In this next scene, we learn that Ms. Remar has threatened to sue Dr. Johnson for sexual harassment.
  a. Were ethics, finances or practice reputation the primary concerns of Dr. Johnson's partners?
  b. In confronting Dr. Johnson, did the partners give him the opportunity to explain his perspective on the encounter with Ms. Remar?
  c. Was the partner's providing good advice when he recommended that they make the problem disappear by any means necessary?
  d. Does it appear from this clip that Dr. Johnson has a history of inappropriate patient interactions? Is this pattern a liability from a practice management perspective? If so, how should it be handled?

Dressed to Kill (1980; Michael Caine, Angie Dickinson, Nancy Allen): This movie is about Kate Miller (Dickinson), a middle-aged housewife who gets killed by a blonde lady. A call girl, Liz Blake (Allen) is the only witness to this murder of Kate. Kate's psychiatrist Dr. Robert Elliott is also involved in the story's plot, adding another dimension to the suspense.
1 (0:10:24–0:12:13) This clip shows Kate (Dickinson) having a consultation with her psychiatrist Dr. Elliott (Caine) and talking about her relations with her husband Mike (Keith Gordon). At one point she asks Dr. Elliott if he finds her attractive. To this Dr. Elliott replies "Of course." Later, when she asks if he would want to sleep with her, he replies in the affirmative.
2 (1:19:39–1:23:31) This clip shows Liz Blake going in for consultation to Dr. Elliott where the talk gradually slips into a sexual talk and Liz directly asks Dr. Elliott if he would like to have sex with her. Even though Dr. Elliott refuses initially, he does not mind Liz getting undressed in front of him in his consultation room and challenging both his "personal and professional ethics."

a. What transference and counter-transference issues are portrayed in the clips?

b. How can you handle personal questions from the clients regarding your marital status, or you as a therapist finding them attractive?

Just Like Heaven (2005): Reese Witherspoon stars as an emergency department resident, Dr. Elizabeth Martinson, who is vying for a position as an attending physician by working long hours.

1   (Ch 1, 0:1:56–0:5:20) In these series of scenes, Dr. Martinson (Witherspoon) meets Mr. Clark, an older gentleman who asks her to marry him, telling her that he has his own bus pass. She encounters him later walking in the hall, pulling his IV with him and wearing only a hospital gown. Mr. Clark again asks Elizabeth to marry him. She agrees once again. Dr. Martinson also encounters another resident being hit by a young male patient who had been licking the wall. To protect her colleague, she matter-of-factly obtains an injectable medication and inserts it in the man's buttocks, thereby averting any further injury to her colleague.

a. How would you assess Dr. Martinson's handling of the seductive older patient? Are female medical students and residents more likely to encounter seductive patients than male physicians? If so, why?

b. Dr. Martinson has been working for over 24 hours. What impact might fatigue have on her ability to cope with these situations?

c. What are the risks of intervening with a patient who is under the influence of drugs or who has a severe mental disturbance?

Gift-Giving and Patients

Analyze This (1999; Robert De Niro, Billy Crystal, Lisa Kudrow): This movie is about a psychiatrist, Dr. Ben Sobel, who is slowly losing interest in his practice because none of the problems presented to him by his patients are challenging enough. But his life is turned upside down when the Mafia Don, Paul Vitti (Robert De Niro) comes to him seeking help for his "panic attacks."

1   (0:48:05–0:50:35) In this clip, Dr. Ben comes home with his fiancé (Lisa Kudrow) and son and finds that his high profile patient, Vitti, has sent him a huge fountain as a wedding gift that has already been installed at his house entrance. Later when they enter their house, they find FBI agents waiting for them to question about Ben's link with the mafia don, Paul Vitti. When the agents question him about the fountain-gift, he mentions that he routinely gets gifts from his patients and that his television set was actually a gift from a kleptomaniac patient.

2   (0:53:29–0:54:05) This clip shows Dr. Ben talking to Vitti, his patient about not sending him gifts anymore, since it represents a "boundary issue."

a. Why is the professional distance between a mental health professional (or any other health professional) and client important?

b. What about gifts? Are there circumstances in which receiving gifts from a patient is acceptable?

c. How does the issue of gifts affect the professional relationship?

d. What are the basic principles of professional ethics as they pertain to gifts?

Unethical and Illegal Behaviors: Deceptive Patients

Where the Money Is (2000; Paul Newman, Linda Fiorentino, Dermot Mulrone): An elderly prisoner (Paul Newman) fakes a stroke to be admitted to a residential facility so that he can escape. A nurse (Fiorentino) recognizes the con and pressures him into helping her get rich by robbing a bank.

1 (0:09:50–0:33:40). Carol, realizing that Henry is not as severely affected by his "stroke" as he makes out to be, undertakes a series of "tests" culminating in her pushing him into a canal in order to ascertain whether or not he is faking. Henry is shown to be conning everyone, but Carol colludes with the ruse in order to personally profit from her discovery. Henry is more deceptive than disruptive, but he does seek revenge on a male nurse who has been stealing from him and other patients, by cutting the brake fluid cable on his bike causing him to crash.

a. The script does stretch belief, but was Carol right to use such extreme measures to discover Henry's ruse? Did it matter that she was proved right?

b. What else could Carole have done to deal with Henry's deception?

c. Henry was shown to be hardly incapacitated at all, but was he right to seek revenge the way he did? Why?

d. How can nurses deal with patients who seek to cause trouble, threaten or harm health-care staff?

e. What responsibility do employers have when nurses are threatened or harmed in the course of their work?

Burnout and Health Professionals

Burnout is a syndrome of emotional exhaustion and depersonalization that leads to decreased effectiveness at work.[8] Common symptoms of burnout include treating patients as objects rather than human beings and becoming emotionally depleted.[9] Burnout is also associated with poor physician health. Sleep disturbances, headaches, marital difficulties, hypertension, anxiety, depression, alcoholism, and other health issues have all been described by those that affected. Burnout can influence physicians' satisfaction with their work and the quality of medical care.[10–12] Studies have revealed that as physician burnout decreases, patient adherence to recommendations, degree of trust/confidence patients have in their physician, and patient satisfaction with their care increases.[8,13] Using the Maslach Burnout Inventory,[14] the research standard for studying burnout, the incidence of physician burnout ranges from 25% to 60%.[15]

With the high incidence of professional burnout and its effects on physicians and their patients, attention to this impairment is paramount. This section will be divided by the three components of burnout: emotional exhaustion (losing enthusiasm for work), depersonalization (treating people as if they were objects), and low personal accomplishment (having a sense that one is ineffective as a clinician).

Emotional Exhaustion

The Hospital (1971): This is a dark comedy that juxtaposes the midlife crisis of Dr. Bock (George C. Scott) with 2 days in the life of a Manhattan hospital in which incompetence, political protests, and mysterious in-house murders are taking place.

1 (0:08:39–0:09:50) In this clip, the executive director of the hospital confronts Dr. Bock about his recent behavior.
   a. What are Dr. Bock's verbal and nonverbal responses to the executive director's questions?
   b. What are your thoughts about how the executive director goes about inquiring about Dr. Bock's behavior? Setting? Tone?
   c. What signs and symptoms of burnout or associated health issues are raised in this clip?
2 (0:16:17–0:20:08) In this scene, Dr. Bock spontaneously seeks counsel from a staff member.
   a. What signs of burnout does Dr. Bock display?
   b. What are some personal issues/personality traits that physicians often possess that could lead to burnout? Which ones are prominent in Dr. Bock?
   c. What is the psychiatrist's role in this situation (Dr. Bock did not set up an appointment)? What should it be?
   d. How might you express concern to a colleague about their burnout?
   e. The literature states that burnout can lead to depression (but not necessarily the other way around). What features of major depression are present in Dr. Bock?
3 (0:50:00–0:53:00) In this powerful scene, Dr. Bock, who is at the height of dysfunction, begins to develop an intimate relationship with the daughter of one of his patients. A discussion of his sexual impotence with her leads to a revelation of his perceived professional impotence.
   a. This film takes place in 1971. What themes illustrated in this clip are still relevant today?
   b. How does the practice of medicine itself contribute to the advent of burnout?
   c. What are some examples of dysfunctional behavior that result from burnout? In this clip? In other medical settings?

     d. How might you recognize burnout in yourself? What would you do about it?

Depersonalization

The House of God (1984): This is a film adaptation of the classic medical house staff coming-of-age book by Samuel Shem, MD. The story centers on the experiences of seven recent medical school graduates during their internship year at a hospital in Boston. This is a humorous, gritty, yet somewhat realistic, though often seen as exaggerated by non-medical viewers, portrayal of the life of house officers. One theme is a primary survival tactic of medical students; namely, depersonalization of certain types of patients (gomers – acronym for "get out of my emergency room") that frequent the hospital but seemingly cannot be helped by medical science.

In the following three scenes, the Fat Man (Charles Haid), a resident who has just completed his intern year, introduces the newly hired house staff to the laws of "gomers." A mentor in the "how" of being a house officer, the Fat Man demonstrates the cynical, crass, and impersonal attitude that physicians can develop in response to the harsh, hazing experience that internship can potentially become. As the incidence of burnout in house staff is higher among interns than practicing physicians, the depersonalization depicted here is a slightly exaggerated portrayal of this component of burnout.

The educator may choose to show all three clips in sequence or one at time. The discussion questions can be used for the independent clips or after all have been viewed.

1. (0:10:35–0:13:25) In this clip, the Fat Man begins his introduction to "gomers" using a patient that is to be admitted to illustrate some of the seemingly immutable laws that apply to them.
2. (0:16:30–0:19:29) The Fat Man, teaching via patient rounds, reinforces the laws of "gomers" while almost totally ignoring the human responses that the house officers display.
3. (0:36:56–0:38:48) Taking depersonalization to the extreme, the Fat Man demonstrates how to accomplish a permanent transfer of a "gomer" off the inpatient service.
   a. How does the Fat Man depersonalize patients?
   b. What are your hypotheses about how the Fat Man developed this attitude?
   c. Discuss times in which you have been a witness to patient depersonalization. How did you handle it?
   d. Discuss times in which you depersonalized patients. What were the circumstances?
   e. What are other examples of depersonalization in hospitalized settings? How do nursing staff, attendings and other house staff treat each other at your institution?

Low Personal Accomplishment

A common experience for physicians is feeling ineffective as a clinician. The medical education milieu is steeped in a long tradition of focusing on what the learner does not know or does not execute well rather than what is done or executed well. As a result, physicians introject a self-critic whose voice, if not tempered, results in persistent feelings of incompetence and lack of clinical efficacy. There is a fine line between psychologically healthy self-feedback and unhealthy self-criticism. A physician's professional life commonly involves walking back and forth across this line.

The following clips illustrate the effect self-criticism has on the physician's psyche.

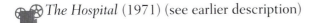 *The Hospital* (1971) (see earlier description)

1 (0:50:00–0:53:00) In this scene, which is also illustrative of emotional exhaustion (as previously mentioned), Dr. Bock reveals his sense of personal ineffectiveness as a clinician and the collective lack of efficacy of the healthcare system.
   a. How does Dr. Bock illustrate his sense of low personal accomplishment?
   b. In other parts of the film, Dr. Bock's excellent clinical and diagnostic skills are displayed. What causes the gap between how one is perceived by others and how one perceives oneself?
   c. How do you react internally when a colleague reveals their feeling of clinical ineffectiveness?
   d. How do you handle your own feelings of low sense of accomplishment?

The House of God (see earlier description)

1 (1:04:10–1:07:59) This clip contains two scenes that involve patients of Dr. Potts (Wayne Sacks). In the first scene, one of Dr. Potts's patients dies. Soon after, the chief resident (Joe Piscopo) falsely displays concern while insinuating that Potts may be partially responsible for the patient death. In the same conversation, the chief resident admonishes Potts for not starting steroids sooner on another patient. Potts had already been reprimanded about this shortcoming several times. The following scene concerns the death of the second patient.
   a. What are the subtle and obvious ways in which Dr. Potts's competence is questioned?
   b. How might Dr. Potts describe his effectiveness as a clinician?
   c. A few minutes later in the film, Dr. Potts unexpectedly commits suicide. How might this have been prevented?
   d. What do you do when you are feeling clinically ineffective or have made a medical error?

    e. How can supervisory physicians give honest feedback without engendering feelings of low self-esteem in their learners?

    f. What can supervisory physicians do when they recognize low self-confidence in their learners?

The Impaired Professional: Alcohol, Drugs, and other Substances

Little Shop of Horrors (1986; Rick Moranis, Steve Martin): This campy B-rated cult musical features Seymour Krelborn (Moranis) and his co-worker Audrey (Ellen Greene) as employees at a struggling flower shop. Dr. Orin Scrivello (Martin) is a sadistic dentist, as well as Audrey's abusive boyfriend.

1   (0:49:10–0:52:30) In this scene Seymour, enraged by Dr. Scrivello's treatment of Audrey, has decided to murder the dentist and feed him to his flesh-eating plant. Posing as a patient, Seymour visits Dr. Scrivello's office armed with a pistol. Prior to treating Seymour, the dentist dons his "personal" nitrous oxide delivery system to enhance his pleasure at inducing pain.

    a. What are some factors that predispose dentists to become addicted to legal and illegal substances?

    b. Would you expect addiction rates to be higher in dentists as compared with other health-care professionals? Why or why not?

    c. What substances or drugs do dental professionals have access to in their offices?

    d. What is your obligation if you know of an impaired colleague? Are there support organizations or groups that deal with impaired health-care professionals?

Intoxicating (2003): This is the story of up-and-coming heart surgeon, Dorian Shanley (Kirk Harris) who works long hours, deals with his father's (John Savage) dementia, and copes with all of the various demands using alcohol and cocaine. He steals drugs from the hospital to trade for his cocaine.

1   (Ch 4, 0:16:32–0:16:42 and 0:18:50–0:19:03) Dorian is driving his Corvette and smoking. He reaches into the glove compartment for a vial of pills. In the second scene, viewers notice injectable medications here, as well.

2   (Ch 6, 0:25:14–0:27:40) Dorian is back in the pharmacy, taking more medications. While driving to his dealer's house with the medications, Dorian takes a few. When Dorian arrives there, he tells the dealer the vial contains "pharmaceutical grade" meds and that he won't get in trouble for having it. Dorian snorts two lines of cocaine and drives back to the hospital. He's also drinking coffee and his hands are shaking. Finally we witness him also taking several more vials of medication.

3   (Ch 10, 0:54:01–0:55:40). Dorian is in surgery. Everything seems to be occurring in slow motion. A nurse asks him if he is OK. Things blur and Dorian

passes out. The scene shifts to Dorian grabbing pills in the pharmacy and walking the hospital corridor in a daze.

4   (Chs 15–16, 1:28:01–1:30:25) Dorian is drinking at a bar. He begins sparring with another man there. They hit each other once and Dorian buys him a drink. They continue sparring, but Dorian loses control and pummels the man who doesn't get up. The bartender calls the police. The scene shifts to Dorian sitting in a holding cell and demanding his phone call. The guard says: "not very becoming of a doctor, mister."

5   (Ch 17, 1:36:00–1:37:33; 1:37:50–1:39:42) In the first scene, Dorian arrives at his dealer's house. The dealer says that Dorian looks like a man in need of a pick-me-up. Dorian tells him that he's there to settle up. The dealer says he can keep paying him back in pharmaceuticals. Dorian replies that he's probably not a doctor anymore and hands his dealer the keys to his Corvette to settle his debt. In the second scene, Dorian goes to the hospital to meet with his chief, Dr. Preminger (Joanne Baron). She acknowledges that Dorian has been working hard to get his life in order, but says the Board asked her to dismiss him. Dr. Preminger says, "that's not enough." She's arranged for him to work in the emergency department at the county hospital. She adds: "If saving lives isn't enough for you, Dorian, I hope you find something that is."

a.   Comment on these scenes? Are the depictions of Dorian's drug use an exaggeration? How is drug addiction among health-care professionals handled at your worksite?

Disruptive and Unethical Behaviors in Nurses

Angels in America (2003; Patrick Wilson, Al Pacino, Meryl Streep, Emma Thompson, Mary-Louise Parker, Justin Kirk, Jeffrey Wright, Ben Shenkman): Described as a TV miniseries, this epic movie revolves around a group of individuals as they deal with the HIV/AIDS crisis in the mid to late 1980s in New York.

1   (Disk 2, 0:07:50–0:18:00) A doctor approaches the nursing station to inform an African-American, openly homosexual male nurse, Belize (Jeffery Wright) that a new patient is to be admitted. This patient's chart states that he has "liver cancer" but in fact he has AIDS. The scene shows the dialogue between the doctor and nurse and then the nurse and patient, Roy Cohen (Pacino). Roy is hostile, prejudiced and belligerent, but Belize talks honestly and explains the risks of taking part in a research trial. Belize also undertakes a cannulation on Roy and in the process he implies he can do it well or make it more painful for the patient.

a.   The doctor is put off by the fact that Belize is not wearing a "standard" uniform. Does it matter what the nurse is wearing?

b.   What is the place of uniforms in the health service and why might this doctor be so upset by Belize's attitude and responses?

c.   Belize is quite frank and confrontational at times both with the doctor and patient. Is this type of communication approach appropriate in these circumstances or could he have dealt with both the doctor and patient differently?

   d. Have you ever encountered a patient who was this hostile and offensive? How have you dealt with them?

   e. How can you address issues of racism in patient care situations?

   f. Should the behavior by the doctor and patient be tolerated and if so, under what circumstances or why?

   g. Roy is clearly abusive and offensive, but does this justify Belize's threat to harm him when he cannulates him?

   h. Do health professionals have to tolerate this type of behavior? What other options are there?

   i. To what extent does Belize's sexuality influence how he deals with Roy?

   j. To what extend does Roy's condition influence how he behaves with Belize?

2 (Disk 2, 0:46:30–0:53:10) In these scenes Belize, a male nurse, brings in medications to the new patient, Roy Cohen. Roy is hostile and abusive and reveals that he has a personal supply of azidothymidine. The drug is new, expensive and rare and Belize asks for some of the drugs for his friend who has none. After a verbal dispute with Roy, Belize takes a number of bottles of the drug from Roy's large supply.

   a. Is Belize justified in taking some of Roy's azidothymidine?

   b. What might be an effective way to deal with Roy? Is there a way to support and care for patients who are this hostile without engaging in conflict?

   c. Should health care be only for those who can pay or pull the right strings? How are health-care resources dealt with in other countries?

3 (Disk 2, 1:41:30–01:47:10) In this scene the patient, Roy Cohen (Pacino), comes from his room with a drip, in a state of confusion induced by the morphine infusion. The male nurse, Belize mischievously plays along with Roy's delusion before a female nurse leads him back to bed.

   a. What does the research say about supporting a patient who is delusional?

   b. Was Belize correct to play along with Roy's delusion in such a mischievous and potentially distressing way?

   c. What impact have their previous conversations and interactions had on Belize and how might these have impacted his dialogue?

   d. Do you think Roy might be seen as a "difficult patient" and if so what does this mean for his expectations of care or the nurses' attitude toward him?

The English Patient (1996; Ralph Fiennes, Juliette Binoche, Willem Dafoe): This is about a nurse who cares for a severely burned man at the end of his life. Although the nurse is caring for him at the end of World War II, the patient's life is chronicled through a series of flashbacks. The flashbacks reveal that the patient was involved in a very complicated love affair that ultimately turned fateful and tragic.

1   (2:28:59–2:33:52) In this clip, the patient (Fiennes) uses his hand to imply that he wants the nurse to give him a lethal dose of morphine. The nurse agrees with the patient's unspoken request and administers the lethal dose. She then reads to him a part of his journal that he chose for her to read. As she is reading, the patient dies.

    a. Take a quiet moment to reflect on this scene. What would you do as the patient's nurse or physician? Is her action unethical or merciful?

    b. What legal ramifications may ensue?

    c. How do you feel about the nurse's actions?

Ancillary Staff and Unprofessional Behaviors

Juno (2007; Ellen Page, Michael Cera, Jennifer Garner): This movie addresses the impact of a teen's unplanned pregnancy, her emotional changes, and her decision regarding her unborn child. It also depicts health-care professionals who can improve their care of teen moms.

1   (0:39:20–0:41:20) Juno is having an ultrasound examination with her family by her side. They are all excited about the images of the baby. The ultrasound technician makes comments that upset them all.

    a. What do you think of the ultrasound technician's behavior? If you were supervising the technician, what feedback would you give her?

    b. Was the comment by the ultrasound technician appropriate? How should she have behaved? How should medical professionals manage their bias about teen pregnancies?

Disruptive Clients and Disruptive Veterinarians

Dark Horse (1992; Ed Begley, Jr., Mimi Rogers, Ari Meyers): Allison (Meyers) is the new girl in town having a tough time fitting in to her new high school. She starts to hang out with the wrong crowd and gets into trouble. After she is arrested, she is sentenced to community service at a horse ranch owned by Dr. Susan Hadley, an equine veterinarian. While there, Allison finds a connection with Jet, a troublesome horse who, like herself, has been misunderstood. Through her budding relationship with Jet and the handicapped children that visit the ranch, we see a vivid portrayal of the mutual benefit of the human–animal bond. We also see some of the challenges Dr. Hadley faces as the owner of an equine veterinary practice.

1   (0:21:10–0:22:52) Dr. Hadley (Rogers) arrives at her ranch to find that Jet, a patient who is still healing from injury, is being ridden without her approval. While galloping, Jet falls down as a consequence of a worsened leg injury. Dr. Hadley becomes angry that the client, Jack (Begley, Jr.) has not heeded her instructions to limit Jet's activity and the client storms off. He consequently

removes Jet from Dr. Hadley's care without paying for services rendered with the intention of taking Jet to another veterinarian.

   a. What would you do if a client becomes angry and threatens to leave without paying for services rendered?

   b. Discuss Dr. Hadley's approach to the noncompliant client. What could she have done differently to improve the outcome?

   c. What are some strategies you can use when the client does not agree with your diagnosis or your treatment plan?

2 (0:33:51–0:37:44) In this scene, Jet and his owner return to Dr. Hadley's ranch to seek treatment once again. Dr. Hadley agrees to admit Jet, but only on three conditions: that the client pay off some of his bill, that the client yield to her treatment and training plan, and that the client reveal the other equine vets that have seen Jet since he left her care. The client begrudgingly agrees and writes a check for part of his outstanding bill. Jet proves to be unruly when he is unloaded from the trailer and the client deals with him harshly. Dr. Hadley has a more calm approach as she leads Jet inside and begins to treat his leg injury.

   a. As a veterinarian, would you continue to treat a patient whose owner has proven to be disruptive in the past?

   b. How would you address a client whom you feel is excessively harsh in his or her handling of his or her pet?

   c. Critique the methods that are used to manage the unruly client. What are some techniques you can use when approaching a client that has been disruptive in the past? It is a little confusing when you use the terms client and patient as these are identical in mental health for the most part.

Beethoven (1992; Charles Grodin, Bonnie Hunt, Dean Jones): George Newton's (Grodin) family is changed for the better when a mischievous St. Bernard puppy named Beethoven enters their world. However an evil veterinarian is kidnapping dogs to use in illegal experiments and he has his eyes set on Beethoven. Some of the challenges of raising a giant breed puppy are illustrated in this comedic tale that also depicts a deceitful veterinarian and a disruptive yet lovable canine patient.

1 (0:58:05–1:01:30) In this scene, Beethoven's veterinarian (Jones) makes a house-call to the Newton family under the pretext of a check-up following a vaccination. He stages an attack, ripping his own clothes and pouring fake blood on his arm and on Beethoven's face. He then strikes Beethoven several times to incite aggressive behavior. The vet then lies to George, telling him that the law states that Beethoven needs to be turned over to the vet or else the vet will press charges.

   a. Discuss the negative repercussions of this portrayal of a veterinarian.

   b. What are the laws and local regulations surrounding dog bites? How might this differ for owned dogs compared to stray dogs? How might the situation vary, depending on whether the dog has been vaccinated for rabies?

    c. What are the risks for families with children if their dog has bitten someone?

    d. What resources are available to pet owners if they believe that a vet has acted in neglect or has abused their pet?

2 (0:49:18–0:53:37) In this scene, George's potential business partners have been invited to George's home for a barbecue dinner. The business partners try to persuade George to sign a contract without reading all the terms and try to distract his wife so that she remains unaware of their duplicity. Finally, they try to distract George and his wife by interacting with Beethoven. The female business partner, Brie (Patricia Heaton) approaches Beethoven as he rests across the yard, removes his leash from the tether, and leads him over to the dinner table. Calamity ensues as Beethoven seemingly seeks revenge for the unfriendly comments the business partners have said in the family's absence.

    a. What should owners do when guests try to interact with a disruptive pet that is poorly trained or that has behavioral problems?

    b. What solutions can you suggest to clients whose pets are beyond their control in the vet's office or at home?

    c. As a veterinarian, how can you protect yourself and your staff from disruptive or potentially dangerous patients?

References

1 Stein LI. The doctor-nurse game. *Arch Gen Psychiatry*, 1967; **16**(6): 699–703.
2 Haig KM, Sutton S, Whittington J. SBAR: A shared mental model for improving communication between clinicians. *Jt Comm J Qual Patient Saf*. 2006; **32**(3): 167–75.
3 Velji K, Baker GR, Fawcott C, *et al*. Effectiveness of an adapted SBAR communication tool for a rehabilitation setting. *Healthc Q*. 2008; **11**(3): 72–9.
4 Groves JE. Taking care of the hateful patient. *N Engl J Med*. 1978; **298**(16): 883–7.
5 Alexander M, Williams JC. The difficult patient. In: Alexander M, Lenahan P, Pavlov A, editors. *Cinemeducation: a comprehensive guide to using film in medical education*. Oxford: Radcliffe Publishing; 2005. pp. 137–40.
6 Kelley JL. *Psychiatric Malpractice: stories of patients, psychiatrists, and the law*. New Brunswick, NJ: Rutgers University Press; 1996.
7 Rowe MM, Sherlock H. Stress and verbal abuse in nursing: do burned out nurses eat their young? *J Nurs Manag*. 2005; **13**(3): 242–8.
8 Maslach C, Jackson S, Leiter M. *Maslach Burnout Inventory Manual*. 3rd ed. Palo Alto, CA: Consulting Psychologists Press; 1996.
9 Shanafelt TD, Balch CM, Bechamps GJ, *et al*. Burnout and career satisfaction among American surgeons. *Ann Surg*. 2009; **250**(3): 463–71.
10 Shanafelt TD, Bradley KA, Wipf JE, *et al*. Burnout and self-reported patient care in an internal medicine residency program. *Ann Intern Med*. 2002; **136**(5): 358–67.
11 West CP, Huschka MM, Novotny PJ, *et al*. Association of perceived medical errors with resident distress and empathy: a prospective longitudinal study. *JAMA*. 2006; **296**(9): 1071–8.

12 Firth-Cozens J, Greenhalgh J. Doctors' perceptions of the links between stress and low-ered clinical care. *Soc Sci Med*. 1997; **44**(7): 1017–22.

13 Shanafelt TD. Enhancing meaning in work. *JAMA*. 2009; **302**(12): 1338–40.

14 Maslach C, Jackson S. The measurement of experienced burnout. *J Occup Behav*. 1981; **2**: 99–113.

15 Wallace J, Lemaire J, Ghali W. Physician wellness: a missing quality indicator. *Lancet*. 2009; **374**(9702): 1714–21.

43

Right, Wrong, and In-Between: Medical Ethics

Henri Colt & Silvia Quadrelli

WHAT BETTER WAY IS THERE THAN TO USE FILM IN ORDER TO PORTRAY the physician encounter and reflect on what the viewer might perceive as right, wrong, and in-between behaviors? Judgments about right and wrong reflect a society's perspective of what ought to be done in certain circumstances, and for the basis for what constitutes normative behaviors subject to the effects of diversity, culture, time, and moral reasoning. However, a principle-based approach to resolving ethical dilemmas is subject to criticism; not the least of it is that without the benefit of a single irrefutable principle, moral conflicts will always be encountered among competing principles, and that generally accepted principles might reflect the social and historical context from which they arose.

Despite these possible shortcomings, we believe that thinking along the lines of moral principles can be a starting point for reflection on medical ethics and resolving ethical dilemmas. For this reason, we have chosen to select a handful of films from which scenes may be analyzed from the perspective of the four principles approach to health-care ethics developed by Beauchamp and Childress[1] more than 3 decades ago. These are Beneficence (the obligation to provide benefits and balance benefits against risks), Nonmaleficence (the obligation to avoid the causation of harm), Respect for autonomy (the obligation to respect the decision-making capacity of autonomous persons), and Justice (obligations of fairness in the distribution of benefits and risks).

While using the four principles for a medical ethics case analysis may be justified from a historical perspective, much recent work has expanded on the principle-based approach, adding elaborate discussions of rules, rights, and virtues to the context from which we may frame moral guidelines. Furthermore, moral principles do not necessarily dictate to us how to lead our lives, and must be embedded into context, reflected in medical ethics by the importance of casuistry and case-based reasoning. Casuistry is defined in the *Oxford English Dictionary* as "that part of ethics which resolves cases of conscience, applying general rules of religion and morality to particular instances in which circumstances alter cases or in which there appears to be a conflict of duties."[2]

The purpose of this section is to present a few case scenarios, represented by scenes from a select number of films that portray, for the most part, certain physician behaviors that might be viewed as right, wrong, or in-between. We have grouped these scenes under this principle heading; we encourage the reader to reflect upon this heading when answering the questions accompanying each description, but we also encourage the reader to examine the issue from within their own social or medical environment. We remain cognizant of the fact that a single principle or practice model may not always have priority over another (e.g. whether autonomy should always trump beneficence), and that sometimes, even a combination of principles and models may not suffice to resolve the complex dilemmas so frequently linked to issues of social justice, that are encountered by health-care providers.

Beneficence and Truth-Telling

Wit (2001): Emma Thompson plays Vivian Bearing, a middle-aged English professor and literary scholar whose expertise resides in the metaphysical poetry of John Donne. She is prickly, precise, and intensely rational. Her intelligence and biting wit frequently alienate her students. When Vivian learns that she has advanced ovarian cancer and has only a short time to live, she undergoes an experimental regime of high-dose chemotherapy proposed by medical researcher, Dr Kelekian (Christopher Lloyd). As she suffers through the various side effects (such as fever, chills, vomiting, and abdominal pain), she learns that compassion is of greater importance than intellectual wit.

1 (1.12:52–1.14:12) In this scene, Vivian is in excruciating pain. A nurse administers analgesics and advises her to ask for a self-administered analgesic system that would allow her to self-treat as needed. However, Dr. Kelekian insists that she needs respite from her pain, and prescribes high doses of morphine that render Vivian unconscious. The nurse tries unsuccessfully to convince the physician that Vivian may have preferred to make the decision herself regarding pain control and level of consciousness.

   a. The principle of beneficence is often used to justify actions, and reinforce the legitimate desire of health-care workers to avoid unnecessary suffering in their patients: do you think it imposes one's own will on a patient?

   b. How is beneficence different from nonmaleficence (to avoid doing harm)? Do you think these two principles that guide physician actions are mutually exclusive?

Dark Victory (1939): A young socialite-heiress named Judith Traherne (Bette Davis), is diagnosed with a brain tumor. After a surgery that was unsuccessful in removing the tumor in its entirety, her physician, Dr. Frederick

Steele (George Brent) knows she has less than a year to live. He opts to keep the diagnosis a secret and assures Judith and her friend Ann that the surgery was a success. He and Judith fall in love, and both Steel and Ann hide the truth about the prognosis from Judith, who eventually uncovers the secret and flies into a rage at the treachery, breaking off her wedding engagement with Steele. Ultimately she resigns herself to her fate, marries the doctor, and spends her final days with him.

1   (0:33:00–0:34:37) In this scene, the doctors discuss Judith's diagnosis with the pathologist in the physician locker room and then proceed to the patient's bedside. They choose to hide the diagnosis, feign good cheer, and lie about the patient's status.

   a. Do you think it is right to withhold the truth from a patient? Is there a difference between telling a lie, and avoiding the truth? Physicians often practice paternalism, and, in their attempts to protect patients from pain or depression might withhold information, avoid sharing statistics, or color the facts in such a way as to provide hope. What do you think might be positive and negative consequences of such actions?

   b. Can you cite reasons why one should tell the truth to patients even in life-threatening conditions? Are there exceptions that you think justify a physician to not to tell the truth?

   c. In this film, Dr. Steele is in love with his patient? Although he does marry her, what are your thoughts about emotional attachments between physician and patient? Had Steele not married Judith, and they had simply had a sexual relationship, would you think differently?

Nonmaleficience (Do No Harm)

The Death of Mr. Lazarescu (2005). Ion Fiscuteanu, Luminata Gheorghiu, Gabriel Spahiu. In this Romanian film, 60-year-old Mr. Lazarescu lives alone with his cats in a small, gloomy Bucharest apartment. Headaches and stomach pains prompt him to call for an ambulance. When it arrives, a very unsuccessful search for a hospital begins. The rest of the film depicts how Mr. Lazarescu's physical and mental suffering is for the most part left untreated as he becomes victim to depersonalized medical care, and inhumane behaviors that finally contribute to his demise.

1   (1:00:17–1:06:26) This scene takes place in an emergency department where Lazarescu is roughly told to sign an informed consent form that will allow surgeons to operate on him, even at the risk of paralysis. Little is shown by way of consideration, kindness, humility, or respect for Lazarescu's dignity and ability to function as a human being.

   a. We often view nonmaleficence as one's ability to avoid doing harm to a patient. This pertains to more than hurting someone though invasive procedures, medical error, or nonindicated treatments. What behaviors might physicians adopt that can be more hurtful than harmful to their patients?

   b. How is the principle of nonmaleficence different from that of beneficence?

   c. What preventive measure do you foresee to help you prevent maleficence during the course of your career?

🎬 *The Elephant Man* (1980): This is the true story of Joseph Merrick (called John in the film), a British man horribly deformed by a congenital disease (neurofibromatosis or Proteus syndrome). Dr. Frederick Treves (Anthony Hopkins) is a surgeon at the Royal London Hospital in the late nineteenth century. One day, while at a fair, he sees a freak known as "The Elephant Man" (John Hurt). The freak is just too disgusting and upsets everyone who sees him. Treves rescues John from his abusive sideshow entrepreneur to bring him to his hospital so that he can inspect him. Merrick turns out to be a very intelligent, refined, and sensitive person. He becomes a celebrity, but Treves becomes uncomfortable, feeling he is just one of the many people taking advantage of the man he originally set out to save.

1 (0.16:40–0.18.34) In this scene, Dr. Treves is lecturing in front of his colleagues to show them the amazing "Elephant Man." He describes in detail, coldly and scientifically all the deformities that characterize John Merrick's physical aspect while the poor man stands there, being naked in front of everybody, as a mere object.
   a. What do you think about the practice of describing a patient, in full earshot of the patient, during medical rounds? What would you do to avoid hurting a patient's feelings, or to preserve the patient's dignity?
   b. Do you think Treves's behaviors were maleficent? If patients are harmed by our behaviors or actions, is there a different whether the harm is intentional or unintentional?

🎬 *Wit* (see earlier description)

1 (0.14:16–0.20:42) In this scene, a young doctor is taking Vivian's clinical history. Vivian is an extremely intelligent woman, but the treatment she receives is cold, slightly depreciative and without any care for her feelings and concerns. The doctor becomes impatient when Vivian does not describe her symptoms with the precision he understands she should. Then, the doctor leaves her for several minutes, feet up in stirrups in the gynecological position because he must find a female nurse to be present during the pelvic examination.
   a. Sometimes doctors need to see four to six patients an hour in order to comply with productivity measures in their institutions and practices. What can they do to help patients feel more at ease and respected, even if seen for only a short time?
   b. It was obviously not "right" of this doctor to leave Vivian hanging in the gynecological position, but was it "wrong" of Vivian to accept being treated in this way? What would you have done? Do you think being ill changes how people behave towards their doctor?

c. Medicine is a "service" profession, increasingly dependent on technology for diagnosis and treatment. If doctors use technology well and are able to cure disease and effectively relieve symptoms, does it matter whether they have a warm bedside manner? Do you expect the same warmth and understanding from a dermatologist, radiologist, ophthalmologist, orthopedic surgeon, or cancer specialist? If yes, why? If not, why not?

2   (0.31:38–0.34:49) In this scene, Dr. Kelekian is doing rounds with some students. They talk about Vivian's disease openly in front of her and perform some of the physical examination, showing her uncovered in front of the whole group. In front of her, they loudly discuss the potential side effects of the medications she is receiving.

a. Do patients have the right to be treated with respect and consideration? How can patients, who are very vulnerable because of their disease and hospitalization, exercise that right? How should health-care providers behave in order to assure that patients are in fact treated with respect and consideration, no matter the circumstances?

b. Should patients bear the burden of medical student learning? Do patients have a moral duty towards society and the medical profession at large to subject themselves to learning?

c. Is the dilemma between making patients uncomfortable and allowing students learn inevitable?

d. What are the moral obligations of students and doctors to patients serving as learning material? Can maleficence be avoided?

e. How can the teaching process and the involvement of students at the bedside actually be beneficial for patients? Can you give some examples?

Autonomy and Self-Determination

Dying Young (1991): Hilary (Julia Roberts) is a young working-class woman from Oakland, California, who answers a classified ad that calls for a young and attractive woman with some nursing experience. Victor Geddes (Campbell Scott), a shy young man with leukemia, needs someone to help him get through his next course of chemotherapy and he hires her for the job. At first, Hilary wants to flee from this man with a terminal illness but, progressively, she becomes actively involved with helping him get well. When his health improves, they rent a house near the ocean and enjoy his remission. Their growing friendship quietly grows into a deep and powerful romance that must ultimately face Victor's impending death.

1   (1.09:37–1:13:50) In this scene, Hilary realizes that Victor has been lying to her and that he is sick again. She tells him they must go to the hospital immediately. However, his plan was to never return to the hospital. He wants to go his cottage and wait for death in Hilary's company. He cannot bear more treatment, and no longer wants to suffer the side effects of chemotherapy,

which he has received repeatedly for the past 10 years. Hilary is furious. She feels betrayed and believes that he has made decisions without involving her. She refuses to just watch him die without a fight, so she leaves the house, calls his father and, against Victor's will, tells his father that he is very sick again and so that his father might come to persuade him to enter the hospital.

a. Victor refuses to receive treatment: Does he have the right to do that? Is he obliged to explain or justify his decision?

b. Victor's fiancée Hilary, who is devotedly caring for him, is against his decision to refuse treatment. If Victor does enter the hospital, and is still refusing treatment, should the doctors listen to her and treat him against his wishes? What if Victor's father also requests that his son be treated? Should the doctors' actions be different if Hilary were married to Victor?

c. Victor appears to have made an autonomous choice to no longer pursue medical treatment with chemotherapy. Perhaps this is because he is tired of being ill from side effects. Perhaps he is simply depressed. What might the health-care team do to persuade Victor to undergo further treatment? Is it appropriate for them to attempt to persuade him to do so? How might coercion be viewed in the health-care setting? Have you ever persuaded someone to do something they did not originally want to do, and see them thank you for it at a later time?

My Life without Me (2003): Ann (Sarah Polley) is a hard-working 23-year-old mother with two small daughters, a husband (Scott Speedman) who spends time on and off work, a mother (Deborah Harry) who sees her life as a failure, and a father who is in prison. She and her mostly unemployed husband live in a trailer in the backyard of her mother's house on the outskirts of Vancouver and most of their money comes from her job as a night janitor. When an emergency hospital exam reveals terminal cancer and a shy and clearly pained doctor tells her she has only a few months to live, Ann decides to keep the news to herself and makes a list of "things to do before I die" that include tape-recording annual birthday greetings for each of her children until they reach the age of 18, having an affair, and visiting her dad in jail.

1 (0.57:16–0.59:43) Ann has kept her doctor appointments. They find her and ask her to come in for new studies, but she refuses. She knows she cannot be cured, and she does not want to spend more time than is absolutely necessary at the hospital. Her doctor suggests that she at least come in to get some pain medication, and she agrees.

a. What should a doctor do when a patient refuses treatment that the doctor knows can be useful and may prolong or improve the patient's life?

b. What does it mean to make an autonomous decision? What factors might influence one's decisions? For example, family life, finances, personality, and physician behaviors. Can you name several others?

c. When one is ill, one's physical, emotional, and psychological well-being is substantially altered. One may not think or behave as one would have before the illness. How might this be taken into account during the medical decision-making process?

Mar Adentro (2004): This Spanish film is based on the true story of Ramón Sampedro (Javier Bardem), who, following a diving accident as a young man, has been a quadriplegic for the last 26 years, He is now 54, with an enviably rich emotional life, a worldly wisdom and wit, but being a cultivated autodidact, he must depend on his family to survive. His loving relatives care for him. While grateful to his family and friends for their help, Ramón had in his youth been an active person, and as the years wear on, he has come to see his life as frustrating and pointless. The basic functions of a private existence – eating, bathing, and using the bathroom – are denied him. He wishes to die. He contacts the Die with Dignity foundation to take on his case, for in Spain, at that time, any form of assisted suicide or euthanasia was illegal. He will finally get help from a friend, Rosa, allowing Ramón to record his quiet passing on video as a brave document of his death.

1   (1.46:14–1.52:29) Rosa has decided to help Ramón bring an end to his life. They have left his home and gone to a hotel with a beautiful view of the ocean, according to Ramón's wishes. They watch the sunset together, and Ramón, very firmly and convincingly says that he is not afraid of dying. He lies in bed and Rosa has prepared the video camera to register his death. He explains to the camera that he is doing this of his own free will and that many anonymous hands have helped.

   a. The scenes in this chapter have been used to help illustrate what might be judged as right or wrong behaviors. In this scene, Ramon wants to protect his friend from legal action since Spanish law prevents Ramon from taking his own life with assistance. Is Ramon right? What about his friend Rosa? Is she wrong to remain present?

   b. Today, many people document moments of their lives using video, even posting videos on YouTube or MySpace. Would it be wrong for Ramón and his friends to post his death on YouTube? Would his documenting a death be any different from documenting a birth or another moment in a person's life?

   c. Do you know the meaning of the terms physician-assisted death, euthanasia, physician-assisted suicide, and palliative sedation? Can you describe how these terms are used in various settings?

The Bone Collector (1999): Lincoln Rhyme (Denzel Washington) is a renowned expert in forensics and author of numerous books on crime theory. He is bed-ridden from a near-fatal accident he had 4 years earlier, and has only the use of one finger and anything above the shoulders. His intellect and his expert eye for forensics remain sharp, but he is absolutely dependent on his full-time nurse. Repeated neurological crises make him suffer very much and create a risk of deteriorating his intellectual abilities. Although bedridden, Rhyme is called upon to help solve a mysterious murder. Unable to work the crime scenes in the field, he calls on Amelia Donaghy (Angelina Jolie), a headstrong beat cop who assists him with the investigation, uncovering puzzling evidence that had been planted at the crime scene by the killer. More murders are committed and it becomes a race against time to try to save the next victim, who might be identified from clues at the site of the previous murder.

1   (0.07.30–0.11.32) In this scene Rhyme, the quadriplegic homicide detective, is arranging for his doctor to give him medicines to help him die because he is worried that he will become a vegetable. His repeated seizures will one day leave him as a "vegetable." Not wishing to die in such a manner, he is trying to secure his doctor's promise to end his life. He is absolutely lucid and he says he wants to pass that "transition" in his own manner. The doctor, who has been extremely distressed by the request, finally accepts to help him. They arrange to end his life when the doctor returns from a medical conference. Rhyme has only a week to live as the following Sunday he will be dead.

The English Patient (1996): The opening sequence of this film takes place during World War II. It shows a British plane being shot down over the North African desert. The pilot, Count László de Almásy (Ralph Fiennes), fails to die despite his terrible burns, and is instead rescued by passing Bedouin. He is unable to recall anything of his past (except that he's not German). With so little to go on, he is named the "English Patient" and winds up in the care of a Canadian medical unit stationed in Italy. Although his outward injuries have healed, leaving his features scarred beyond recognition, he is dying. One of the nurses, Hana (Juliette Binoche), realizing that her charge hasn't long to live takes special care of him and takes him to an isolated, abandoned monastery to allow him to die in peace. There, injecting him with morphine and reading to him from his beloved volume of Herodotus, Hana seeks to stimulate his memories. In the end de Almásy remembers his whole sad story and relives the sorrow of discovering what he has lost when it is already gone. In great physical and emotional pain, he considers himself already dead.

1   (2.28.58–2.33.44) In this scene Hana comes into the patient's room carrying flowers and sets them down on the table next to several vials of morphine. She picks up the syringe to prepare his injection. She takes a vial. At that moment the patient, who can hardly move, reaches out and pushes two more vials toward her. Their eyes meet, and then he shovels another, then all of them towards her. She looks at him knowing he is asking her to administer a massive, lethal dose. She starts to prepare the injection, her eyes filling with tears. The patient nods, smiles, whispers and finally says, tenderly and calmly "Thank you. Thank you." She kisses him, gently on the mouth. He closes his eyes, and asks her to read to him the final letter his dead lover had left him. Recalling those final memories he peacefully passes away.

a. In each of the films cited above, a patient has decided to die with dignity. Does a person have such a right?

b. What are the differences between assisted suicide and euthanasia? What is the legal status for each? What moral considerations come into play in the assisted suicide-euthanasia debate?

c. Should a physician or any health-care provider help a patient to die if that is what is being asked? How would you respond to such a request if you were the patient's doctor? How would you respond if you were the patient's friend, lover, or spouse?

d. Is active euthanasia equivalent to murder? What is the difference, if any, between active euthanasia and passive euthanasia

Wit (see earlier description)

1 (0.00:38–0.04:15) In this scene, Dr. Kelekian tells Vivian very directly that she has advanced ovarian cancer. He also tells her that there is no other hope than accepting a very difficult experimental treatment. He anticipates that she will have to be very courageous to tolerate the treatment, but without giving additional details, asks her to sign the informed consent document allowing them to begin the treatment.

a. In order to help patients make an autonomous decision regarding treatment, doctors obtain what is known as informed consent. What do you think are the necessary elements that should be part of the informed consent process?

b. In this scene, the doctor requests permission to proceed with treatment at the same time as he informs Vivian of the bad news about her diagnosis. What do you think about the way Vivian's doctors communicates the bad news? Is there anything you would do differently?

c. Do you think there is a right and wrong way to deliver bad news? What might you do to learn to deliver bad news in a more empathic, sympathetic, and caring manner?

2 (1.03:00–1.08:50) In this scene, a nurse is talking to Vivian about end-of-life decisions. She mentions the option of a "do not resuscitate order" (DNR), realizing that the doctors have not explained to Vivian her various options, in case her heart should stop: full treatment with chest compressions and ventilatory support, medications, or DNR (do not resuscitate). Vivian makes a decision and requests to be made DNR.

3 (1.17:44–1.33:07) A few minutes later in the film, Vivian has a cardiac arrest. A young doctor calls the emergency cardiopulmonary team who promptly begin resuscitation. The nurse becomes very angry, shouting that Vivian had requested to be DNR. Resuscitation continues in spite of the nurse's claims. Vivian is completely naked on her bed, victim to the resuscitation maneuvers. Finally her doctor understands what he is doing and admits that he has made a mistake, and tells everyone that the patient was DNR. The team members stop their maneuvers, obviously angry for having been called with no purpose. They abandon Vivian, naked and dead, lying like an object on the bed. The

nurse covers her and tends to her dead body with gentle attention.

   a. Advanced directives allow patients to identify what interventions they prefer to undergo should they lose the ability to make decisions for themselves. What is the moral foundation on which the concept of advanced directives is based?

   b. Should advanced directives always be respected? Are advanced directives only valid if they are in writing and signed by both patient and witnesses?

   c. Are there any valid reasons why a doctor might refuse to respect a patient's advanced directives?

   d. What is the role of health-care providers in helping patients make end-of-life decisions?

   e. What should a physician say in case of opposition between a patient's wish and the wish of their families regarding what to do in emergency or near-death situations?

Justice

Dirty Pretty Things (2002): Okwe (Chiwetel Ejiofor) is a Nigerian doctor who drives a taxicab during the day and watches the front desk of a hotel by night. It turns out that the hotel is being used as an underground organ-donor ring where immigrants in need of money subject themselves to backroom operating tables to donate their kidneys in exchange for cash and a passport. Okwe is soon pressured to become a black market surgeon.

1   (0.33:17–0.38:05) In this scene, Okwe goes to a hospital, pretending to be a cleaner, he is able to enter the pharmacy to steal medication he needs to treat a seriously ill man who refuses to go to the hospital because he is an illegal immigrant and will be taken by the immigration authorities.

   a. Is it appropriate for health-care institutions to denounce illegal persons?

   b. Okwe is obviously doing something illegal (stealing). Do you consider this immoral? Is there any justification for a person to break the law if he/she is denied access to health care because of his or her social or legal immigration situation?

John Q (2002): John (Denzel Washington) and his wife Denise (Kimberly Elise) are devastated when they learn that their son needs a heart transplantation that costs $250 000. John's insurance plan has recently changed to a health maintenance organization and the maximum catastrophic coverage payout limit is only $20 000. Desperate and unable to pay for the transplant, he takes an emergency ward hostage until his son's name is put on the transplant list, finally persuading doctors to perform the operation, and asking two of his hostages to bear witness to a will stating his last request, as John holds a gun to his own head and prepares to end his own life.

1   (0.21.07–0.23:31) In this scene John Q. and his wife learn that a transplant

will cost $250 000. John's wife breaks into tears saying that she cannot believe her son is dying and they are talking about money. The hospital director answers that it takes money to provide health service and that with other options available, they are not obliged to cover a procedure this costly, and that regardless, a down payment of 30% would be required before their son's name could be added on the transplant list.

a. Is resource allocation just? In the setting of scarce financial resources, who should benefit from costly procedures?

b. John Q. is obviously doing something illegal that will put him in jail (hostage taking, threatening people with a gun). Is what he did a crime? Is there any justification for a person to break the law if he/she is denied access to health care because of his or her social economic status?

c. Marginalized populations are often perceived to be marginalized because of race, gender or social context, but financial situation is also a predominate cause, contributing to lower health status, health illiteracy, and lesser opportunities for education. Is John Q right in "speaking truth to power," and revolting against what he feels is a social injustice, or is he simply acting selfishly to find resources necessary for his son's survival?

d. Is health care a right or a privilege? Do your best to justify your response.

e. What are the responsibilities of government to assure the health of people living in their own country? Are those responsibilities different and dependent upon whether they are citizens, legal residents, or illegal immigrants?

Outbreak (1995): The annihilation of an entire village in Zaire's Motaba River Valley in 1967 was ordered by two army officers (Donald Sutherland and Morgan Freeman) because it was the only way to contain a deadly virus. Twenty-five years later, the virus resurfaces in Africa again, spreads to the United States, and mutates into an even more deadly strain prompting the quarantine of the town of Cedar Creek.

1 (1:18:30–1.21:23) In this scene officers argue that it is necessary to kill 2600 people in Cedar Creek in order to save the whole country and perhaps the whole world.

a. When it comes public health, are individual rights naturally trumped by concerns for public safety?

b. In what cases might individual freedoms be sacrificed in the name of social justice?

c. What would be the moral reasoning behind making an extreme decision to kill some people in order to save a larger number of people?

References
•••••••••••••••

1 Beauchamp TL, Childress JF. *Principles of Biomedical Ethics*. New York, NY: Oxford University Press; 2001.
2 www.oxfordictionaries.com/definitions/casuistry (last accessed 4/15/12)
3 Battin MP, Francis LP, Jacobson JA, *et al*. Pandemic planning: what is ethically justified. In: *The Patient as Victim and Vector: ethics and infectious disease*. New York: Oxford University Press; 2009. pp. 329–58.

Further Reading
••••••••••••••••••••••

● Colt HG, Quadrelli S, Friedman L, editors. *The Picture of Health: medical ethics and the movies*. New York, NY: Oxford University Press; 2011.
● Fallowfield LJ, Jenkins VA, Beveridge HA. Truth may hurt but deceit hurts more: communication in palliative care. *Palliat Med*. 2002; **16**(4): 297–302.
● Hancock K, Clayton JM, Parker SM, *et al*. Truth-telling in discussion of prognosis in advanced life-limiting illnesses: a systematic review. *Palliat Med*. 2007; **21**(6): 507–17.
● Jonsen AR, Toulmins S. *The Abuse of Casuistry*. Los Angeles: University of California Press; 1988.

44

I Feel Your Pain:
Empathy in Medicine

Pablo González Blasco & Graziela Moreto

WE LIVE IN AN ERA WHERE OUTCOMES, GUIDELINES, AND CLINICAL trials are at the forefront of medical training. However, "to care" implies having an understanding of the human being and the human condition, and for this endeavor, humanities and the arts help in building a humanistic perspective of doctoring. Through these means, doctors are able to understand patients in their whole context. The humanities and arts provide a source of insight and understanding for proper doctoring and, as such, they should be as much a part of medical education, as training in differential diagnosis or medical decision making. Teaching how to effectively take care of people requires creating educational methods that address the human aspects of medicine.

Because people's emotions play a specific role in learning attitudes and behavior, educators cannot afford to ignore the student's affective domain. Although technical knowledge and skills can be acquired through training with little reflective process, it is impossible to refine attitudes, acquire virtues, and incorporate values without reflection. The challenge here is to understand how to effectively provoke the student's reflective process.

Learning through aesthetics – in which cinema is included – stimulates a reflective attitude in the learner. The first step in humanizing medical education is to keep in mind that students are reflective beings who need an environment that supports and encourages this activity. Because emotions and images are ubiquitous in the many forms of media that saturate modern life, popular culture should be the front door in the student's learning process about feelings. In fact, when systematically incorporated into the educational process, and allowed to flow freely in the educational setting, emotions make learning both more memorable and more pleasurable for students.

Complexity comes mostly from patients, not from diseases. While technical knowledge helps in solving disease-based problems, the patient affected by these diseases remains a real challenge for the practicing doctor. To care implies having an understanding of the human being. Arts and humanities, because they enhance the understanding of the human condition, are useful resources when incorporated into the educational process and help in building a humanistic perspective of doctoring.[1]

The Soft Edges of Empathy

Empathy, from the Greek *empatheia*, means understanding someone else's feelings. In the English vocabulary, empathy was used initially to describe the observers' feeling when interfacing with artistic expression. Afterwards, the term was related to understanding people, and in 1918, Southard incorporated the word empathy into the doctor-patient relationship, as a resource for facilitating diagnosis and therapeutics.[2]

Whether empathy is mainly an affective or a cognitive condition, or indeed both, is a broad discussion that brings us to another dilemma, an educational issue: could empathy be taught or is it a trace of personality?

The majority of the authors with an affective-oriented approach presuppose that, during the empathic event, there is something that can be characterized as a partial identification of the observer with the observed. This aspect also becomes clear especially in Carl Rogers's[3] definition, which describes empathy as being the ability "to sense the client's private world as if it were your own, but without losing the 'as if' quality." According to this definition, the differentiation between one's own experience and the experience of another is the decisive criterion for defining effective empathy. Other authors[3] stress the importance of making a distinction that has significant implications for the relationship between patients and clinicians because joining with the patient's emotions can impede clinical outcomes. Moreover, a clinician who is merely sympathetic in the clinical encounter can interfere with clinical objectivity and profession effectiveness. The sympathetic doctor cares about quantity and intensity of the patient's suffering, while the empathetic doctor cares about understanding the quality of the patient's experience.[4] These authors' general conclusion is therefore that sympathy must be restrained in clinical situations, whereas empathy does not required a restrictive boundary.[5]

It is not easy to separate in practice (herein meaning in action) the affective from the cognitive domain. Thus, some other authors explain that empathy, rather than continuing to focus on "feeling into" the experiences of another, has more to do with the understanding of the other's feelings than the sharing of them.[6] Following the "symbolic interactionism" and Piaget's theory of cognitive development, Mead[7] articulates the term "role taking," a process of understanding and anticipating the actions and reactions of another individual. Role-playing implies that an individual produces the perspectives of another person within himself: "The immediate effect of such role taking lies in the control which the individual is able to exercise over his own response ... It is the ability of the person to put himself in other people's places that gives him his cues as to what he is to do in a given situation."[7]

Two conclusions might be drawn from our discussion of definitions and our questions regarding the right location (affective, cognitive, or both) in which empathy occurs. First is that a prerequisite for both affective and cognitive empathy is that an individual should not be overly preoccupied with himself and his own concern, because, if the experience is to a greater extent focused on the individual himself, then the willingness to help the other person decreases.[8] Only through self-awareness is it possible to see the behavior of the observed person as an expression of his emotional state and to make a mental distinction between oneself and the "other self." The second conclusion is that empathy could bridge the provider gap between patient-centered medicine and evidence-based medicine therefore representing a profound therapeutic potential.

And here we come to the education issue. Can empathy be taught? Is it possible to establish a learning process for empathy?

Teaching the Non-Teachable Issues

A classic study published 25 years ago comes to mind.[9] This study was mainly designed to help medical school admission committees best select college students for medical school. The authors of the study emphasized that it is probably more important to select college students who will be superior physicians than to select those who will be excellent medical students. Based on a previous publication, subjects were asked to rank order a list of 87 characteristics of a superior physician, considering the importance of each characteristic and how easily it could be taught. Those ratings were validated by high correlations across several subgroups. The importance and the teachability ratings were combined into a non-teachable-important index (NTII) that provides a rank order of traits that are important but cannot be taught easily.

This study aimed to determinate the important qualities of a superior physician that cannot easily be taught in medical school or later training. The authors proposed to select college students for medical school not only on the basis of academic achievement, but also on the basis of characteristics identifiable in the college student that predict excellence in the physician who many years later will emerge from the educational system.

The NTII generated by this study gives equal weight to importance and to non-teachability. The top of the list comprises qualities closely related to empathy: understanding people; sustaining genuine concern for patients, motivated primarily by idealism, compassion and service; oriented more toward helping people than making income; enthusiasm for medicine and dedication to his work; ability to get to the heart of a problem; to separate important points from details and, finally, adaptability. All those qualities score high in the NTII index, which means that the most important qualities to be a good doctor are the most challenging to teach.

Neurophysiological studies bring some clues on how to teach something that is difficult to teach.[10,11] Even though empathy is a nontraditional teaching content, it might be promoted through examples and role taking through which the neurophysiological indicators of empathy could be activated. There are some neurons in the brain that can control certain actions (e.g. behavior or emotion) in the body and can even be activated if the same action is observed in another person. Known as "mirror neurons," these nerve cells respond spontaneously, involuntarily, and even without thinking.[12] Mirror neurons use the neurobiological inventory of the observer in order to make him feel what is taking place in the person that he/she is observing by way of inner simulation. Various experiments conducted by the so-called "social neurosciences" document the functioning of the mirror neurons with regard to the empathic perception of the other person.[13,14] The functioning of mirror neurons is, therefore, an essential prerequisite for empathy.[15]

Another question arises in this mirroring role model theory: is a subsequently learned empathic ability authentic or does it give a patient the impression that it is an artificial and superficial behavior (i.e. a routine checklist of empathic actions that a clinician is simply required to go through)? Do clinicians need to have previous experience being patients themselves or to witness their family/friends being patients in order to be more empathic? These questions can have great implications for medical education and medical care considering that empathy seems to be a determinant of quality in medical care because it enables the clinician to fulfill key medical tasks more accurately, thereby leading to enhanced health outcomes.

Those who are involved in medical education know that a broad range of biographical experiences and situational factors influence the development and promotion of empathy. Part of these experiences could be the role model teaching scenario, in which students and young doctors are inspired by the teacher's attitudes in dealing with patients. The tag-along model (or shadowing model) allows medical students to incorporate attitudes, behaviors, and approaches to real patients and identify emerging issues useful for their professional future.[16]

Beside tag-alongs, some authors emphasize the importance of art, literature, cinema, and reflecting on one's own life in developing empathy.[17] Literature certainly has plenty of examples. In A Fortunate Man,[18] a classic book about the story of a country doctor, there is a broad description of empathy, here called Recognition. "The task of the doctor is to recognize the man. [...] A good doctor is acknowledged because he meets the deep but unformulated expectation of the sick for a sense of fraternity. He recognizes them. Sometimes he fails, but there is about him the constant will of a man trying to recognize."

Using Movies to Foster Reflection, Not for Lecturing Empathy
•••••••••••••

Opportunities for teaching with cinema are well suited to the learners' environment and they stimulate learner reflection. In life, important attitudes, values, and actions are taught using role modeling, a process that impacts the learner's emotions. Since feelings exist before concepts, the affective path is a critical shortcut to the rational process of learning. While technical knowledge and skills can be acquired through training with little reflection, reflection is required to refine attitudes and acquire/incorporate values.

As other educators have discovered cinema is useful in teaching because it is familiar and evocative. Movies provide a quick and direct teaching scenario in which specific scenes point out important issues, emotions are presented in accessible ways where they are easy to identify, and learners are able to understand and recognize them immediately. In addition, learners have the opportunity to "translate" movie life histories into their own lives, and into a medical context, even when the movie addresses a non-medical subject. Movie experiences act like emotional memories for developing attitudes and keeping them as reflective reference in the daily activities.

Cinema is the audiovisual version of storytelling. Life stories and narratives enhance emotions, and therefore set up the foundation for conveying concepts. Movies provide a narrative model framed in emotions and images that are also grounded in the everyday universe. As in the clinical setting, the patients' life histories are a powerful resource in teaching. When the goal is promoting reflection – including both cognitive and emotional components – life histories derived from the movies are well matched with the learner's desires and expectations.[19] The purpose is not to show the audience how to incorporate a particular attitude, but rather to promote their reflection and to provide a forum for discussion.

The experiences we, the authors of this chapter, have with cinematic teaching span more than a decade.[20-25] Our experience affirms the effectiveness of using the movie-clip methodology in which multiple movie clips are shown in rapid sequence, along with facilitator comments while the clips were going on. Teaching with clips in which several, rapid scenes, taken from different movies, are all put together, works better than viewing the whole movie. Nowadays, we live in a dynamic and fast-paced environment of rapid information acquisitions and high emotion impact.

The value of instructor commentary during the viewing of clips is a conclusion based on our own experience. Although the sudden changing of scenes in the clips effectively evokes the participant's individual concerns, and fosters reflection in them, making comments while the clip is playing acts as a valuable amplifier to the whole process. Because learners are involved in their personal reflective process, they may at times disagree with the facilitator's comments and form their own conclusions. This may, in fact, be desirable. Participants note that divergent comments are particularly useful to facilitate the reflecting process. A quote from one medical student elucidates this point: "Don't keep quiet, please. You must make your comments while the movie is going on …. Do you ask if I agree with you? No, I don't agree at all …. But your comments push me to reflect … so please, go on."

The effect is a rich generation of perspectives and points of view, which in turn trigger multiple, often contradictory, emotions and thoughts in the viewers. In this context, learners have an intensely felt need for reflection about what they have just seen. American movies are particularly useful, since they tend to tell stories in a straightforward and uncomplicated manner. Although European or Asian movies often stimulate deep meditation on human values, they demand more time and attention on the part of learners.

The last part of the movie clip teaching methodology is the most important and constructive. There may be a temptation on the part of both audience and instructor to feel satisfied with the emotions (and often tears) appearing by the end of the clip. In fact, this is where the real work starts. People need to share, and further consider, their thoughts and feelings in light of the comments and responses of their peers. This final discussion is absolutely necessary to put into coherent perspective the emotions, insights, dreams, and fears that the film clips evoked.

Fostering reflection post viewing often stimulates conversations about the interaction of health and illness within the breadth of human experience and can elicit profound conflicts and concerns from students about their future professional roles and themselves as human beings. Students identify easily with film characters and movie "realities," and through a reflective attitude gain new insights into many important aspects of life and human relationships. The educational benefit also is expanded by the phenomenon of the student "carrying forward" into his or her daily life the insights and emotions initially generated in response to the movie clips. Students report that the movie clip training acts like "an alarm" to make them more aware when similar issues and situations occur in their daily lives.

Participants understand that the purpose of the film-clip methodology is not only to evoke emotions but also to help the audience reflect on these emotions and figure out how to translate what they learn into attitudes and action. Reflection is the necessary bridge to move from emotions to behavior. The goal is to move beyond a specific medical solution to reach a human attitude in life that requires integrity and wholeness. The purpose is to move from technical responses to deep reflection on how to call forth the best learners have inside themselves. The specific translational process is intentionally left up to learners as they encounter their own lives as doctors and as people.

In our experience, the topics that emerge in these discussions are critical to understanding the human condition. Thus, the importance of dialogue and respect for the opinions and perspectives of others, caring about little things in life (which makes a difference when dealing with people), promoting compassion, empathy, and commitment are all invaluable.

For teaching the human matters of doctoring, which implies refining attitudes, acquiring virtues, and incorporating values, one can employ the purely rational method favored by ethics lectures and deontology courses. But movies offer another path: exposing learners to particular examples with strong emotional consequences to either follow or reject. Movie clips serve to reconnect learners with their original idealistic aspirations and motivations as physicians by eliciting strong emotions and then allowing students to reflect upon their own emotional make-up.

In addition, emotions are a universal language that help people to bridge cultural differences and achieve agreed upon interpretations and mutual understanding. At this point, we can envision why those "intangible" issues, difficult to teach and to assess, in which empathy, compassion and commitment are included, could be reinforced through the cinema education methodology.

Action! Let Movies Go On

Because of the soft edges of empathy, and because empathy is more related to the response we expect from the audience rather than something we are putting in them, making a list of empathetic films is quite a challenge. All we can do is to grasp a group of movies – mostly scenes for building clips – that in our experience have evoked empathic reactions in the audience. If learners suggest some other scenes, from their own viewing, as a kind of answer, you can be sure there is an empathic climax going on and that the methodology is indeed working.

In keeping with our methodology, scenes are described in this chapter and examples of the educator's responses while the clip is playing are shown. In some scenes, no responses are offered and educators are encouraged to articulate their own responses. Clips under each subheading are run together as a unit with all the clips having been put onto one disk. Of course clips may be used individually.

Listening

The Spitfire Grill (1996; Alison Elliot, Ellen Burstyn, Marcia Gay Harden)

1 (01:31:36–1:35:05) Consider how we need to listen to peoples' stories, with a kind of watchfulness. While Percy tells her tragic story (rape, miscarriage), her friend just listens, and at the end places her hand on Percy's shoulder without saying a word.
   a. Are we able to just listen to the patients' stories without interrupting? How long?

Dead Man Walking (1995; Tim Robbins, Susan Sarandon, Sean Penn)

1 (1:36:00–1:37:30) The murderer is about to be executed. The nun listens

to his story with a watchful attitude: "I don't know what love is. I have never been loved. I need to die to discover what love is."

    a. Just the nun is listening to him, showing full understanding. Listening is a kind of wonderful endurance and support.

The Prince of Tides (1991; Barbara Streisand, Nick Nolte, Blythe Danner)

1 (1:32:00–1:34:10) The psychiatrist listens to the brother of one of her patients. The psychiatrist is able to read between lines. She just puts the question out there and waits. "You really learned how to cover your pain, haven't you? I can feel your pain." There is a tremendous explosion of emotions, and she can manage it because she knows how to listen, she is ready for every unexpected reaction.

One True Thing (1998; Meryl Streep, Renée Zellweger, William Hurt)

1 (1:39:00–1:40:20) Professor Gulden is missing at home. His daughter thinks he is having an affair with some other woman. Her mother, Gulden's wife, has cancer. She goes out looking for his father and finds him in a bar, depressed, alone. Here is the real reason why he returns late to home every day. "The first time I saw your mother she was so full of light. She lightened everything around her, even me. I can't imagine that light coming out."

    a. Attunement through listening is about understanding others' reasons, and not setting previous judgments on them before listening carefully.

Momo (2001; Diego Abatantuono, Peter Dollinger, Victoria Frenz)

1 (0:38:40–0:40:15) Momo is the little girl who knows how to listen (the movie is from Michael End's book). In this scene, one of the gray men from the bank comes to her with a lot of dolls. He is trying to bribe her because her attitude brings trouble for the gray men in the bank. Momo realizes that the gray man has no love, and never has been loved and so she puts her hand on his face. The gray man is confused by this unexpected gesture.

Who are They? Understanding People

The Legend of 1900 (1998; Tim Roth, Pruitt Taylor Vince, Bill Nunn)

1 (0:50:00–0:52:40) In this scene the pianist explains to his friend the origin of his inspiration: observing people. His music does not come from the musical notation but from the people he observes.

    a. Doctoring is all about a creative art. Do we care about schedules and guidelines, even about the right diagnosis, before observing carefully patients' needs, their stories, and realizing who they are?

Amistad (1997; Morgan Freeman, Djimon Hounsou, Matthew McConaughey, Anthony Hopkins)

1 (1:03:00–1:04:35) "What is their story? You know they are Africans. But you don't know their story. You are not just a man from Georgia. You are an ex-slave and now devoted to the cause of abolition slavery. This is your story. So, you need to know their story."

   a. Maybe, by putting a quick diagnosis on the patient – even correct – the physician is led to miss the patient's whole story. Are we really intrigued by the patient's story?

Blood Diamond (2006; Leonardo DiCaprio, Djimon Hounsou, Jennifer Connelly)

1 (1:56:51–1:58:35) The young boy has become a guerrilla fighter who doesn't recognize his father, even his own roots and family. In this scene, the boy's father faces his own son, pointing an arm toward him, and slowly starts reminding him about family, about good memories, showing compassion and understanding for the devilish process in which the young boy has been immersed. "You are a good boy, who loves soccer and school. Your mother loves you so much. She waits by the fire making plantains with your sister. And the new baby. The cows wait for you, and Babu, the wild dogs who minds no one but you. I know they made you do bad things, but you are not a bad boy. I am your father who loves you, and you will come home with me and be my boy again."

Nurse Betty (2000; Renée Zellweger, Morgan Freeman, Chris Rock)

1 (1:40:30–1:41:25) Morgan Freeman talks to Renée Zellweger, fostering confidence in her. "You don't need that doctor. You don't need any man. You know why? Because you've got yourself."

   a. One of the great challenges in doctoring is to help patients and people look inside, reflect and find who they really are. Helping people be rid of self-delusion is immensely therapeutic, a process which requires expertise and previous understanding of the human being with whom we are dealing.

Meeting People's Needs

Marvin's Room (1996; Meryl Streep, Leonardo DiCaprio, Diane Keaton)

1 (1:33:00–1:34:00) In this wonderful scene, Lee (Meryl Streep) realizes the meaning of caring. Bessie (Diane Keaton) calms down her ill father, Marvin, while playing with a little mirror. To care implies, very often, not only technical support but also, and mainly, an absolute dedication.

Patch Adams (1998; Robin Williams, Daniel London, Monica Potter)
   This is a classic movie for medical education. There are two scenes focused on meeting people's needs.

1   (0:12:33–0:16:30) Patch helps patients to shoot "imaginary squirrels" during night time. After that, he realizes that his time in the hospital is done, realizing that what he wants to do is to help people by using his gift of knowing how to talk to them.

2   (1:35:31–1:36:28) In this pasta swimming-pool scene, Patch finds a way to help one patient self-nourish.

A Beautiful Mind (2001; Russell Crowe, Ed Harris, Jennifer Connelly)

1   (1:43:42–1:45:15) Alicia explains to her husband, John Nash, what is real through touching him and letting him touch her face and heart. "Do you want to know what is real? This is real. Maybe the answer is not in here" (in the brain) "but in here" (touching his heart).

Analyze This (1999; Robert De Niro, Billy Crystal, Lisa Kudrow)

1   (0:19:50–0:22:30) Robert De Niro plays a Mafia Godfather. He visits a psychiatrist, and tells a story of a friend with psychological troubles. Billy Crystal, the psychiatrist, realizes that the Mafia boss is talking about himself, and takes the risk of pointing this out. The results are fantastic, and he gains the gangster's confidence and compliance.

Scent of a Woman (1992; Al Pacino, Chris O'Donnell, James Rebhorn)

1   (2:00:00–2:00:39) "Give me one reason to not kill myself. I will give you two: You dance tango and drive a Ferrari as no one else." You can complete this scene, going back in the movie to the Ferrari scene (1:42:30–1:43:10) and the tango scene (1:26:00–1:27:15), and put it all together in a clip. The whole picture is inspiring.

Limelight (1952; Charles Chaplin, Claire Bloom)

1   (0:59:28–1:00:43) This scene in Chaplin's classic movie points out the superb results you can get when instead of focusing on your own problems, you care about people. This is how Teresa recovers from her illness because she is worried about Calvero, who is depressed, and she tries to help him.

Understanding Another One's Suffering

Shadowlands (1993; Anthony Hopkins, Debra Winger, Julian Fellowes)

1   (1:45:50–1:48:1) Joy Gresham asks CS Lewis what will happen to him when

she has died. She has Ewing sarcoma, and the end is quite close. Lewis avoids the topic, but Joy insists: "The pain you will feel then, is part of the happiness you are feeling right now."

a. To understand others' suffering implies a broad perspective in which happiness and suffering are mixed together in life. Maybe this scene can bring some inspiration to brighten people's suffering.

My Life (1993; Michael Keaton, Nicole Kidman, Bradley Whitford)

1 (0:20:50–0:22:40; 0:23:10–0:23:40) Bob Jones (Keaton) has a terminal disease. The attending doctor says there is nothing more that could be done. Bob gets out of the office but suddenly he comes back: "You took away my hope. This is the only thing I still have and you have no right to deprive me of it."

a. Telling bad news: how you can be honest, and at the same time keep hope alive. How can we deal with other's suffering without depressing them?

Dead Man Walking (1995; Tim Robbins, Susan Sarandon, Sean Penn)

1 (1:41:49–1:42:09) "Look at me. I will be the face of love for you while they do it." To be the face of love is the essence of sharing suffering and supporting those who are in pain. How can we perform the face of love when seeing patients?

In the Name of the Father (1993; Daniel Day-Lewis, Pete Postlethwaite, Alison Crosbie)

1 (0:47:10–0:48:18) Daniel Day-Lewis is imprisoned along with his father. The young man thinks his father is weak and pusillanimous and argues with him. At this moment his father calms him down with kind gestures since he realizes his son's suffering.

The Story of Us (1999; Bruce Willis, Michelle Pfeiffer, Colleen Rennison)

1 (1:15:40–1:16:52) "Today, I saw myself through your eyes and I am sorry." This couple (Willis and Pfeiffer) has frequent arguments. But they reflect and find their own responsibilities instead of blaming each other.

Bicentennial Man (1999; Robin Williams, Embeth Davidtz, Sam Neill)

1 (1:24:40–1:25:20) "It is cruel to see you cry and I cannot. This terrible pain I cannot express. Does every human being that I care for just leave?" Understanding other's suffering sometimes implies a willingness to share, and even demonstrate it. Is it possible to share without expressing those feelings?

La Mome (The story of singer Edith Piaf) (2007; Marion Cotillard, Sylvie Testud, Pascal Greggory)

1 (1:52:00–1:54: 21) Edith Piaf is depressed and has already given up singing. Her friends don't know how to encourage her. In this context, a young composer brings her a new song: "Non, Je Ne Regrette Rien" – that is, I don't regret of anything I did in my life. The music cheers up Edith: "I love this. This is me, you grasped my entire life." The scene portrays how little things well adapted to those who are suffering can make a tremendous difference. In the next scene, Edith is singing again on the stage (2:07:15–2:09:19).

Empathy on Command: Teachers and Leaders

In this session, the list of scenes provided has a common ground: How empathy is useful for those in command of others. Empathetic teachers and leaders are real facilitators. They push people they lead to perform their best. And they are always inspiring role models. We can find multiple examples in the movies. These scenes are some of our favorites: we have used them several times and they score high in their empathy impact.

Searching for Bobby Fischer (1993; Joe Mantegna, Ben Kingsley, Max Pomeranc)

1 (0:35:00–0:37:00) The chess master asks the boy to think about the next four moves without moving the pieces. "I can think without moving them." And the master: "I will make it easier for you" (the teacher throws the chess pieces to the floor, clearing the chessboard).

Music of the Heart (1999; Meryl Streep, Cloris Leachman, Henry Dinhofer)

1 (0:28:00–0:29:00) The violin teacher helps the disabled girl who cannot stand up to play the violin. What really matters is to get strength inside.

2 (1:48:00–1:49:00) "Don't look at the audience, look at me. And play from the heart." These are the encouraging words to the young members of the violin orchestra before the performance.

Mr. Holland's Opus (1995; Richard Dreyfus, Glenne Headly, Jay Thomas)

1 (0:33:28–0:34:39) The girl can't play the clarinet properly. She is worried and can't succeed. Mr. Holland finds the right advice for getting her to relax and perform well. "Just play the sunset!"

Men of Honor (2000; Cuba Gooding, Jr., Robert De Niro, Charlize Theron)

1 (1:57:21–1:59:37) The disabled man is required to walk 12 steps to prove he can be a navy diver. He is able to perform the task because of the great mentoring of his coach. Mentoring is essential to bring out the best in people.

We Were Soldiers (2002; Mel Gibson, Madeleine Stowe, Greg Kinnear)

1   (0:34:00–0:35:00) "I will be the first to set foot on the battle and the last to step off. I will leave no one behind." The story of the Lt. Col. Hal Moore and his leadership in the Vietnam War.

Spartacus (1960; Kirk Douglas, Laurence Olivier, Jean Simmons)

1   (II Part, 0:49:30–0:50:50) This is a great scene from Kubrick's classic movie about empathy in a team. "Slaves you were, and slaves you remain. But you will be spared of the terrible penalty of the crucifixion on the single condition that you identify the body or the living person of the slave called Spartacus." And then, here and there, men stand up shouting "I am Spartacus, I am Spartacus." Everyone is Spartacus. More than a person, it is an idea.

K-19: The Widowmaker (2002; Harrison Ford, Liam Neeson, Sam Spruell, Peter Stebbings)

1   (1:45:30–1:47:45) The Soviet nuclear submarine is in a great trouble. The Captain has to decide how to save the boat and prevent a nuclear disaster. At this point, one of the officers (Liam Neeson) gives a different suggestion to engage all the crew: "Don't give orders to the men. Just ask them." The captain explains the situation and stands by waiting for the responses. And they come, one by one, addressing the consensus and the strength of teamwork.

Her Majesty, Mrs. Brown (1997; Judi Dench, Billy Connolly, Geoffrey Palmer)

1   (1:06:10–1:08:20) Empathy and leadership often come from those who, theoretically, are not in command. This is an elegant movie about Queen Victoria's horseman and how he helps the Queen to recover from depression after the death of Prince Albert. In this scene the servant asks to resign his duty, but the Queen forbids him. "I need you to be what I must be. Without you I cannot find the strength to accomplish my obligations."

The King's Speech (2010; Colin Firth, Geoffrey Rush, Helena Bonham Carter). The story of George VI and his fight against stammering, helped by the speech therapist who is a real teacher and leader backstage.

1   (1:23:46–1:28:10) The king is told that the therapist has no credentials or qualifications. "I have the experience. I helped those boys who came from the war, and that war was a real experience." In this scene, the therapist provokes the King and gets from him the best response: a strong voice!

2   (1:42:20–1:48:15) The second movement of Beethoven's Symphony no. 7 in A major frames *The King's Speech*. The King talks through the radio microphone to all the country, and overseas, while the therapist is "conducting"

the speech and, seemingly, the symphony at the same time. A touching scene with a highly empathic score.

References

1 Blasco PG. Literature and movies from medical students. *Fam Med*. 2001; **33**(6): 426–8.
2 Hojat M. *Empathy in Patient Care, Antecedents, Development, Measurement and Outcomes*. New York, NY: Springer; 2007.
3 Neumann M, Bensing J, Mercer S, *et al*. Analyzing the 'nature' and 'specific effectiveness' of clinical empathy: a theoretical overview and contribution towards a theory-based research agenda. *Patient Educ Couns*. 2009; **74**(3): 339–46.
4 Hojat M, Vergare MJ, Maxwell K, *et al*. The devil is in the third year: a longitudinal study of erosion of empathy in medical school. *Acad Med*. 2009; **84**(9): 1182–91.
5 Hojat M, Gonnella JS, Mantione S, *et al*. Physician empathy in medical education and practice: experience with the Jefferson scale of physician empathy. *Semin Integr Med*. 2003; **1**: 25–41.
6 Kohler W. *Gestalt Psychology*. Oxford: Liveright; 1929.
7 Mead GH. *Mind, Self, and Society*. Chicago: University of Chicago Press; 1934.
8 Aderman D, Berkowitz L. Self-concern and the unwillingness to be helpful. *Soc Psychol Q*. 1983; **46**: 293–301.
9 Sade R, Stroud M, Levine J, *et al*. Criteria for selection of future physicians. *Ann Surg*. 1985; **201**(2): 225–30.
10 Decety J, Jackson P. A social-neuroscience perspective on empathy. *Curr Dir Psychol Sci*. 2006; **15**: 54–8.
11 Gallese V. The roots of empathy: the shared manifold hypothesis and the neural basis of intersubjectivity. *Psychopathology*. 2003; **36**(4): 171–80.
12 Rizzolatti G, Sinigaglia C. *So quel che fai. Il cervello che agisce e i neuroni specchio*. Milano: Raffaello Cortina editore & publisher; 2006.
13 Decty J, Jackson PL. The functional architecture of human empathy. *Behav Cogn Neurosci Rev*. 2004; **3**: 71–100.
14 Wicker b, Keysers C, Plailly J, *et al*. Both of us are disgusted in my insula: the common neural basis of seeing and seeking disgust. *Neuron*. 2003; 40: 644–55.
15 Bauer J. *Warum ich fühlst: Intuitive Kommunikation und das Geheimnis der Spiegelneurone* [Why I feel what you feel: Intuitive communication and the mystery of mirror neurons]. Hamburg Hoffmand & Campe; 2005.
16 Blasco PG, Ronocolett AFT, Moreto G, *et al*. Accompanying physicians in their family practice: a primary care model for medical students' learning in Brazil. *Fam Med*. 2006; **38**(9): 619–21.
17 Larson EB, Yao X. Clinical empathy as emotional labor in the patient-physician relationship. *JAMA*. 2005; **293**(9): 1100–6.
18 Berger J, Mohr J. *A Fortunate Man: the history of a country doctor*. London: Penguin Press; 1967.
19 Blasco PG. *Medicina de Família & Cinema: Refursos Humanísticos na Educação Médica*. São Paulo: Casa do Psicólogo; 2002.
20 Blasco PG, Moreto G, Ronocoletta AFT, *et al*. Using movie clips to foster learners' reflection: improving education in the affective domain. *Fam Med*. 2006; **38**(2): 94–6.

21 Blasco PG, Mônaco CF, Benedetto MAC, *et al.* Teaching through movies in a multicultural scenario: overcoming cultural barriers through emotions and reflection. *Fam Med.* 2010; **42**(1): 22–4.

22 Blasco PG, Pinheiro TRP, Ulloa-Rodriguez M, *et al.* El Cine en la Formación Ética de Medico: Un recurso pedagógico que facilita el aprendizaje. *Persona Bioética.* 2009; **13**: 114–27.

23 Blasco PG, Benedetto MAC, Garcia DSO, *et al.* Cinema for educating global doctors: from emotions to reflection, approaching the complexity of the human being. *Prim Care.* 2010; **10**: 45–7.

24 González-Blasco M, Levites MR, Moreto G, *et al.* Cineam y Educación: Cómo mejorar las habilidades pedagógico de los profesores y fomenter la reflexión de profesores y alumnus. *Arch Fam Med.* 2010; **12**: 137–49.

25 Blasco PG. *Humanizando a Medcina: Uma Metodologia como Cinema.* São Paulo: Centro Universitário São Comilo; 2011.

PART VIII

Alternative Formats

45

Too Reel for Comfort:
Reality TV

Patricia Lenahan

REALITY TV HAS EMERGED AS A FORMIDABLE MEDIA GENRE, SURPASSING many more conventional television dramas and comedies as viewers' choices. A 2001 study commissioned by American Demographics indicated that more than 45% of Americans watch reality television. In addition, American Demographics found that more than 25% of these viewers also post messages or read posts on reality TV websites while 70% of self-described "avid fans" go to show-related websites.

The rapid growth and proliferation of reality TV formats is staggering, from food (*Cupcake Wars*, *Iron Chef*), fashion (*Project Runway*, *America's Next Top Model*), family issues (*Supernanny*, *Wife Swap*, *Teen Mom*), relationships (*The Real Housewives*, *Jersey Shore*) to the dating-related series (*The Bachelor*, *The Bachelorette*), adventure (*The Amazing Race*), law enforcement (*Cops*, *Police Women of Broward County*) and numerous others that can become character studies in themselves (such as *Big Brother* and *Survivor*). This television format has proliferated so greatly that the Emmy Awards now includes two categories for reality TV.

Another aspect of reality television is the health-related series. Some of the current offerings appear to be a hybrid between documentary and reality-based series. These shows frequently address aspects of health (physical and psychiatric) and/or disease and may influence the general public in many ways, including their perceptions of health-care providers and hospitals. Additionally, these series may influence the ideas, beliefs, and behaviors of patients or even serve to escalate their anxieties and fears regarding a symptom they may be experiencing. Patients also may expect or request a specific type of treatment or surgical intervention based on what they have observed on TV.

The concept of reality television is not new. It was introduced to American viewers more than 50 years ago with the debut of Allen Funt's *Candid Camera* in 1959 (*Candid Camera*, 1959–67) and the various court-based dramas that followed. However, it may be that our current obsession with reality TV began in 1989 when ABC first aired *America's Funniest Home Videos*. The videotapes, taken and submitted by "average" television viewers who were willing to make fun of themselves (and others) resonated with the television audience. The series is currently in its twenty-first year and still garners a large audience.

The reality TV genre has exploded and morphed in the last decade. Various hypotheses have been suggested for this trend: the rise in social media, the impact of the digital age and Gen Y'ers. (American Demographics found that this genre is extremely popular among the younger generations.) A more sociological perspective espouses the concept that reality TV makes it easier for the viewer to identify with these "real people" who have "real problems" than it is to identify with the fictionalized characters, heroes, and villains, seen in the more mainstream television series. Often viewers also feel a greater tie-in to these "characters" and shows by using the social media to post comments on Facebook and Twitter as well as to watch additional footage on YouTube. Director James Cameron reportedly has referred to the reality TV phenomenon and its fans as a "surveillance culture."

Needless to say, reality television provides a plethora of teachable moments for the cinemeducator. This chapter will provide a brief overview of several series that have merit for health and graduate educators. Although it is not possible to include the typical trigger question format for each series since the topics addressed vary from week to week, several examples will be illustrated. The appendix also will provide other examples of reality TV.

How to Access and Use Reality TV

Reality series can be found both on the traditional network stations and on the cable networks such as TLC, Lifetime, Animal Planet, The Food Channel and more. Many of the full episodes also may be found on the particular channel's website or the show's website, while excerpts often are found on YouTube. The show's websites often include synopses of the episodes. Reality TV series vary greatly as to their utility in the educational arena. Some of the more popular series also have produced DVDs.

Ethical Dilemmas

What Would You Do? (ABC)

This ABC series hosted by John Quinones is, in many respects, a modern version of Candid Camera – but with a twist. The series stages scenarios designed to test the reactions of everyday individuals and to present ethical decision-making for these unsuspecting onlookers. The question is: will they respond to the situation or will they ignore what is occurring around them. The individuals who have been filmed eventually are informed that what they observed had been staged. The host focuses on people who reacted the strongest to the scenarios. They are interviewed about their feelings and what prompted their reactions.

A recent episode focused on individuals who were feigning disabilities and asking for money, observing a very rude customer in a diner and watching a waiter question, demean, and harass a dad about his child who appeared to be of a different race. The dad was African-American and the child was Caucasian. Eventually, his Caucasian wife entered the restaurant and joined the family. Other episodes have addressed store clerks "evicting" potential customers whom they didn't view as desirable, dating violence in a restaurant, public drunkenness among teenagers, and petty theft.

1 What are your immediate thoughts when you see an individual on the street asking for assistance?
2 Do you genuinely believe this person is in need or are you skeptical? Why?
3 Have you had any experience in donating food or money to a homeless person?
4 What would your reaction be if you saw an adult and child together who were racially different?
5 Would you assume there was something wrong?
6 What motivated the reaction of the waiter?
7 How would you respond if you saw someone treating a fellow diner in this manner?
8 What would you do?
9 What is the value of airing TV segments such as these?
10 What do they say about American culture and society?

Another episode addressed the perceptions of what was appropriate behavior for soldiers in uniform. In the first series of scenes, a male soldier is seated at a diner when his male partner, also in uniform, enters the diner. The two soldiers are meeting each other since separated during a deployment. As they greet each other with hugs and then continue to caress one another, the camera focuses on other patrons in the diner. Some of the patrons appear clearly offended while others seem supportive. However, when the scenario changes to female soldiers engaged in the same behavior, the reactions of the diners intensifies, eventually leading to the women being asked to leave the diner.

1 What factors contribute to the differing responses of the patrons?
2 What are the public's expectations for the behavior of soldiers in uniform?
3 How might the "don't ask, don't tell" policy have affected individual attitudes?
4 Some of the patrons interviewed regarding their reactions had served in the military? Were you surprised by their reactions? Were there any generational patterns observed?
5 What message do scenes like these give to LGBT soldiers?

Substance Use and Other Dependencies
• •

Addicted (TLC)

Each episode of *Addicted* follows one individual who is struggling with some form of addiction/dependency. The episodes take a broad look at who the person is and how the substance use affects the individual in terms of both professional and personal relationships.

Intervention (A & E)

Participants initially believe they are being filmed for a documentary about their addictions/problems, however, this is all in preparation for an intervention with family and/or friends. The individual is confronted with the concerns and fears of their loved ones and presented with an option: get help or face the consequences. The consequences could involve loss of jobs or loss of marriages and loved ones. Those participants who agree to accept treatment are offered a 90-day in-patient program.

Celebrity Rehab with Dr. Drew (VH1)

This series offers a view of "celebrities" who are being treated for their addictions. At times, it appears as if these "patients" are acting and at other times sheer petulance and self-centeredness emerges.

Celebrity Rehab Presents Sober House (VH1)

This spinoff of *Celebrity Rehab with Dr. Drew* looks at several former celebrities who are now participating in a thirty-day sober living environment in a "Beverly Hills mansion." The series follows them as they attempt to maintain their sobriety, to transition back into society in a drug-free state, and to relaunch their careers.

Sex Rehab with Dr. Drew (VH1)

Another spinoff, *Sex Rehab* utilizes the same format as the other shows, but focuses on individuals who are experiencing various forms of sexual addiction.

Obesity and Eating Disorders
• •

The Biggest Loser (NBC)

Perhaps one of the most widely watched shows in the reality television genre focusing on obesity and weight loss is *The Biggest Loser*. Here contestants vie against one another to lose the greatest percentage of weight in order to stay on the ranch and to win the $250 000 prize for being the biggest loser. Contestants are seen in the gym, discussing the hows and whys of their obesity and seen with the show's physician reviewing their initial and ongoing state of health. Although the show provides a caveat about not beginning a strenuous exercise program without medical clearance, contestants are seen engaging in hours of exercise from their first day on the "ranch." It is clear that many of these contestants have not participated in any type of aerobic exercise in quite a while and the show presents an unrealistic and potentially dangerous expectation regarding the extent of exercise done initially.

1 What are the risks associated with heavy exercise for formerly sedentary (and obese) individuals?
2 What factors have the participants identified, if any, that they associate with their weight gain?
3 How has obesity affected their lives? Their relationships?
4 What is the role of childhood trauma in the development of obesity?
5 What triggers have been identified that contribute to overeating?
6 How does *The Biggest Loser* address relapse prevention?

One Big Happy Family (TLC)

This series follows a morbidly obese family from Charlotte, North Carolina. The parents each weigh over 340 lbs, while their 16-year-old daughter also weighs over 340 lbs and their 14-year-old son weighs over 300 lbs. Viewers observe the day-to-day struggles of the family as they try to lose weight.

Thintervention (Bravo)

This series is hosted by a work-out reality star. Unlike *The Biggest Loser* where contestants strive to stay on the ranch, *Thintervention* participants are seen living in their own everyday worlds and coping with the personal and professional stressors.

Heavy (A & E)

This series follows 22 people, two individuals per episode, during a 6-month period. Each individual, like Tom, who weighs over 625 lbs. and is seen in the first episode, confront the life-threatening consequences of morbid obesity. Unlike *The Biggest Loser*, *Heavy* takes a more realistic and perhaps healthier view of initiating an exercise program.

What's Eating You? (E!)

This series follows two individuals per 60-minute episode and focuses on the identified patient, family, and a team of health-care professionals (physician, psychotherapist, and dietitian). One episode featured a 22-year-old male with obsessive-compulsive disorder and an eating disorder who described his "restricting" days and his "binging" days. The "patient's" family history revealed childhood trauma (parental divorce at age 3) and death of his mother due to an eating disorder and use of methamphetamines. The other individual seen in this episode was a 38-year-old married former model who stated that her life was based on "trying to be perfect" and that if she couldn't be perfect, then she didn't want to live. Her family history also was significant: she described gaining weight during pubescence and the disapproving attitudes, comments, and behaviors of her mother who mourned the loss of her perfect daughter. The individual approaches taken by professional team members appear questionable at times.

Families

Sixteen and Pregnant (MTV)
    This is the original series that followed the lives of teens who discovered they were pregnant. Most of the girls were in their second trimester when they were filmed initially.

Teen Mom (MTV)
    This series is a spinoff of *Sixteen and Pregnant*. It follows four of the original teens from that show as they try to forge lives for themselves and their infants. Teen parents are seen having to forego spending time with their peers, inability to engage in "typical" teen activities, missing the prom, and assuming greater responsibility than their peers.
1 How do other teens respond to this series? For example, does the "reality" of being a teen parent serve as a deterrent to engage in sexual behavior by other teens?
2 What is the incidence of unplanned pregnancies among teenagers? STIs?
3 How could health-care providers effectively engage in risk reduction behaviors for this population? How would you address abstinence and birth control?
4 What is the role of the parent?
5 What childhood factors contribute to an early sexual debut?
6 What is the role of peer pressure? Alcohol or drug use?

Supernanny (ABC)
    This series provides a good source of family dynamics in action as a British "supernanny" is called to action when families are experiencing difficulty in disciplining and managing their children.

Wife Swap (ABC)
    This series also provides a glimpse into the varied worlds of "family," roles, responsibilities, and child-rearing practices and beliefs. Often the couples featured in an episode display attitudes and beliefs that are polar opposites of the other family.

Raising Sextuplets (WE TV) and *Ouch! Sextuplets* (UK)
    This series began as a 1-hour special in 2008. It focused on a couple, Jenny and Bryan, who met via email when Bryan was serving in the military in the Middle East. They subsequently married and began their family with sextuplets. Jenny became pregnant as a result of IVF. They are seen coping with

the day-to-day demands of rearing six children. The series began its second year in June, 2010. However, Bryan was arrested for intimate partner violence in September, 2010 and Jenny later filed for separation.

It's Me or the Dog (Animal Planet)

This may seem like an odd entry in this category; however, it is clear that communication, discipline, and family issues raised in trainer Victoria Stillwell's interventions with owners of unruly dogs, often applies to their relationships among themselves and other members of the family. The show also has featured episodes that address hoarding.

But the Sex is Good (HBO)

This series focused on couples who were having significant relationship difficulties but who stayed together because, as the title suggests, the sex was good.

Little People, Big World (TLC)

This series aired for six seasons and followed a family at their Oregon farm. Both parents and one son had a form of dwarfism, while another son and a daughter were of normal height.

Little Couple (TLC)

Neonatologist Jennifer Arnold and her husband, businessman Bill Klein, both are short-statured, standing less than 4 feet. This series follows the couple as they date, marry, and plan both families and careers while coping with some of the challenges associated with being "little people." Jennifer is frequently seen at work in the hospital where accommodations are made for her height when treating patients. One of the issues the couple faces is fertility.

1 What are the reactions of Jennifer's patients to her?
2 What are some of the common health-care issues faced by little people?
3 What environmental issues do they face (e.g. the height of appliances and so forth)?
4 How do they cope with being "little" in a "bigger" world?

Amish in the City

This half-hour series followed Amish teenagers during Rumspringa, the time they are able to leave their families and explore life outside their communities before deciding to be baptized into the Amish faith.

Diagnostic and Statistical Manual of Mental Disorders

Obsessed

Each episode of this series follows two individuals who manifest symptoms of an obsessive-compulsive disorder that impairs their lives personally and professionally. Therapists provide the intervention for them utilizing cognitive behavioral therapy techniques. During one episode, a woman cleaned constantly (more than 8 hours a day) and was unable to meet any of her obligations. The second individual seen in that episode counted (everything) constantly, also had a drinking problem and was disengaged from his family and adult children. The "patients" or "clients" are seen learning and practicing the techniques, addressing their overarching problems and finding varying degrees of success in coping with their problems.

The OCD Project (VH1)

While *Obsessed* shows individuals in their own environments, The *OCD Project* follows six individuals with a diagnosis of obsessive-compulsive disorder who live communally in a treatment facility for several weeks. They are observed in both individual and group therapy sessions. Some of the fears identified in an episode include a fear of causing a child to develop cancer and fear of contracting HIV. Dr. David Tolin treats the patients with exposure and response prevention therapy.

My Strange Addiction (TLC)

This series focuses on a variety of behaviors including individuals with pica (a man who eats Kleenex), an individual who wears a fur suit, and a woman who collects dolls and stuffed animals.

Hoarders (A & E)

Each 1-hour episode follows two people who are compulsive hoarders, possessed by their possessions. The lives of the individuals are exposed as family and friends share their frustrations and attempts to help. Therapists and professional organizers are seen as they try to intervene before even more dire consequences occur.

Hoarders: Buried Alive (TLC)

This series also focuses on the growing problem of hoarding, showing some more severe examples and the consequences of this behavior. Each episode focuses on two individuals and their friends and/or families. Clinical therapists who specialize in treating hoarders and professional organizers are seen interacting with the individuals and/or families. One episode introduced viewers to two hoarders: Debbie and Jeff.

Debbie, age 41, is a self-described "obsessive." She says she spends 75% of her day in performing her rituals that include reading the labels of everything she buys so she can "understand" them thoroughly. Another ritual related to her purchases while shopping. Debbie said: "I buy things. I need to check them off on the receipt." Debbie also was seen washing the pop-top lids of dog food cans, plastic take-out coffee cups endlessly. She does not want to get rid of things that can be recycled or have another use, including the wads of cotton found in over-the-counter medications. However, since she spends so much time engaging in these rituals, Debbie says she becomes too tired to get rid of these things. She states: "My OCD has led to my hoarding." As a result, Debbie has filled her three-level home in suburban Maryland with trash, clothing, plastic bags of purchases she has never unpacked, and so forth. The couple lives with two dogs and three cats and Debbie acknowledges that hoarding has affected their ability to start their own family. Her husband, Mike, describes the situation in this way: "Living with a hoarder is a constant battle with chaos." Debbie fears that Mike will leave her. Family members have not been allowed to visit them and are not aware of the extent of the problem.

Jeff, a man in his 50s, lives in suburban Illinois and works as a bus driver. His hoarding has pushed away the people he loves most during the past four years. The behaviors appear to have developed and/or escalated after Jeff suffered a heart attack followed by a quadruple bypass and subsequent second heart attack. His wife left him during this time. The hoarding also has affected his relationship with his three adult children who seldom visit him. Jeff states: "I am coping with isolation." Jeff saves newspapers and clips out articles that he wants to save for historical reasons. He acknowledges that he is "burying myself in my own layers of paper" and that the stove hasn't been used in four years. Jeff adds: "I sleep, eat, and live here in the living room … in this little area." Jeff's three children, two daughters and one son, state that they miss being able to share activities, such as game night, with their Dad. They arrange to have a clinical psychologist visit Jeff. Dr. Moran is seen arriving at Jeff's house. He tells Jeff that he can call him DJ. Dr. Moran quickly assesses the situation and says that Jeff wants control and wants to keep what he can. When Dr. Moran brings in the professional organizer, Jeff greets her by saying: "This is where the pain begins … you conspiracy theorist you." The organizer brings a computer and scanner and tries to encourage Jeff to scan one article. Jeff resists, chastises the organizer for folding an article and, while he eventually agrees to scan one page, he frequently asserts that he will not be getting rid of anything that day.

Debbie is seen 1 month after the therapist and organizer made their first visit. She and Mike are going through some files and articles in the living room. While it looks less cluttered, it is far from clean. However, the kitchen is spotless. Debbie acknowledges that the difficulty will be to keep from cluttering again.

Jeff is seen 2 months after he promised his children that he would clean up the house. He insisted on cleaning the house on his own, resisting the aid of the therapist and the organizer, adding: "she (organizer) rubbed me the wrong way from the first." The children are anxious when they arrive and are pleasantly surprised to see how clean things are. His daughter tells him: "Dad, it looks like our old kitchen." Jeff and his children quickly settle into playing a game while sitting around the dining room table.

1 What is the impact of hoarding on family relationships?
2 What are the potential health consequences of hoarding?
3 What types of psychological factors or childhood experiences/trauma might contribute to hoarding?

4 What is the impact of loss in re: the onset of hoarding behaviors?

5 What does hoarding "do" for the hoarder?

6 What types of interventions have been successful in addressing hoarding behaviors?

7 How can the family become a catalyst for change?

8 What are the public health implications for hoarding?

9 How do the behaviors of animal hoarders or animal collectors differ from Debbie and Jeff?

10 What role does building trust have in working with hoarders?

11 What is the impact of clutter on an individual's abilities to perform ADLs?

12 How would you respond to potential/actual health code violations?

13 What clinical disorders contribute to hoarding? What comorbid disorders are common?

14 What are the different types of hoarding? How do saving/acquisition hoarders differ from clutterer/disorganized hoarders? What is the effect of acquisition exposure therapy?

15 What contributes to an individual's motivation to change?

Confessions: Animal Hoarding (Animal Planet)

This series focuses on a very specific type of hoarding: animal hoarding and collecting. Veterinarians, animal control officers and community workers often confront the problems exposed in this series.

Animal Cops (Animal Planet)

Animal Cops initially followed four individuals in New York City who were charged with investigating allegations of abuse, neglect, abandonment, fighting, and other issues involving animal welfare. This series has expanded to include animal cops in Miami, Houston, Detroit, and Philadelphia. The variety of situations addressed in these shows includes the effects of violence and abuse, poverty and homelessness, neglect, dog-fighting, cock-fighting, and hoarding. The investigators are seen working with the pet owners to try to find a healthier solution for both pets and the people. Poignant examples include helping an elderly owner find the resources to properly care for her dog's health or mobilizing other agency resources to assist with problems associated with hoarding and collecting.

Animal Cops also provides an intensive look at the investigators, veterinarians, technicians, animal behaviorists, volunteers, and shelter care staff who are charged with caring for the sick and wounded animals. Compassion fatigue, something most health professionals will address, is quite evident at times.

Pit Boss (Animal Planet)

Little person, Shorty, and his staff of three other little people, operate a pit bull rescue. Shorty intervenes to save dogs from fighting rings, abandoned homes, and situations involving abuse and neglect. Shorty, as an "ex-con," also intervenes to help teens from "taking the wrong path." The show has a dual focus:

rescuing pit bulls and highlighting some of the difficulties faced by little people in their day-to-day lives, such as dating. One episode finds Shorty experiencing severe back pain, which he acknowledges is a common ailment among little people. He fears that he will become disabled like his father.

Medically Related Reality Television

Dr. 90210

No discussion of reality television would be complete without mention of *Dr. 90210*. The title comes from the upscale Beverly Hills zip code made famous in another television series. *Dr. 90210* follows plastic surgeon, Dr. Robert Rey, as he consults with patients regarding plastic and reconstructive surgeries. Some graphic scenes of surgeries are shown.

Hopkins 24/7 (ABC)

This brief, six-part series aired on ABC in 2008. It followed hospital staff in their day-to-day work and explored the lives of these individuals as well. One episode focused on a neurosurgeon, who climbed over a fence at the Mexican-US border as a youth to work as a migrant laborer in the fields. Other episodes focused on a resident who was having marital difficulties and the issues faced by a female urologist.

Untold Stories of the ER

One episode recounted the appearance of a gunman in the ER whose barrage of bullets struck one of the physicians in the head and neck, requiring heroic and dangerous efforts by other hospital staff to save his life. Both the physician who was shot and the surgeon were seen in subsequent interviews, describing the events. In the same episode, a physician is seen treating a construction worker who self-diagnosed and treated an ankle fracture by making a cement cast. It was also revealed that this inventive man also had sutured a gash in his side using brass wiring.

1   What is the impact of workplace violence?
2   How can health-care providers identify potentially violent individuals?
3   How would you respond to an individual who self-treats?
4   What are your immediate reactions to seeing the gentleman who diagnosed and treated himself?
5   What patient education techniques might be useful to address this patient's behavior?

One Born Every Minute (Lifetime)

This is one of the newest additions to the genre, with the first episode airing on Lifetime on February 1, 2011. The series focuses on the obstetrics patients and staff of Riverside Methodist Hospital in Columbus, Ohio. The hospital is described as one of the busiest in terms of deliveries, citing more than 6500 deliveries per year. The theme of the first episode was "medications or no medications" and followed three women of various ages and races who were about to go into labor. It was stated at the outset of the show that the epidural rate was 90% and that few women were opting for natural childbirth anymore.

The first woman, Melissa, was a 40-year-old woman who was having her second child in 12 months. She was a self-described "late starter" in the marriage and pregnancy arena. Melissa was clear that she wanted an epidural: "You wouldn't go to the dentist and get a tooth pulled without medication. Why deliver a baby without an epidural? I never wanted a baby without an epidural." Melissa is seen interacting with the nurses, anesthesiologist, and physician. She and her husband appeared to have developed a good and trusting relationship with the health-care team.

The second patient was 26-year-old Tasha, an obese African-American woman who was accompanied by her mother. This was her second pregnancy. Tasha experienced some difficulties with her prior pregnancy because of the size of the baby: 9.7 lbs. While her doctor had discussed a C-section, Tasha was adamant that she did not want to be "cut." The baby's father believed that C-sections were dangerous. Unlike the first patient who had a good rapport with the nurses, Tasha's first nurse appeared somewhat disapproving (Tasha shared that she was told that she was "two centimeters and a finger" and the nurse said that it didn't make sense). The nurse also used language that seemed discordant with the patient's level of understanding. Tasha also was afraid of the epidural. One of the nurses empathized, sharing that many women have heard horror stories about epidurals and the size of the needles. Eventually a C-section was needed (a nurse is heard on the phone: "I've got tones down"). The nurses were seen in the delivery room encouraging Mom and Dad and fostering bonding between Dad and his son.

The third couple, Susan and Steven, self-described "hippies" arrived at the hospital when Susan was 2 weeks overdue. This was their first baby and Steven presented the nurse with a copy of their lengthy birth plan. The nurse commented to the camera that when birth plans were that long then they tended to be rigid. Susan and Steven had a nurse midwife who would deliver the baby and they also had hired a doula to be with them. They requested no medication and Susan was seen taking multiple showers and chanting to ease the pain. Susan's labor did not progress (21 hours) and she finally agreed to Pitocin. Conflicts between the couple and the nurse were evident with the nurse stating that she respected individuals' rights to have a delivery plan but she reiterated that "different ways of delivery can cause conflict." This was evident when the nurse expressed concern about the fetal heart rate and suggested internal fetal monitoring. Steven was heard saying not to listen to the nurse and turned to her saying "if you would keep things positive ..." The nurse midwife is informed and along with the doula, encourages Susan to agree to the fetal monitor.

1   How would you respond to these varying situations?

2   Which type of situation are you most comfortable with?
3   What is the impact of literacy/health literacy on communication between patient and health-care provider?
4   What are the effects of obesity and pregnancy?
5   How would you counsel a patient who is fearful?
6   What is the role of complementary-alternative approaches to delivery? How can discordant attitudes/beliefs affect the quality of the relationship with the obstetrics staff?
7   How would you interpret the nurse's comment about the link between the thickness of the birth plan and parental rigidity? What types of communication issues might result in this situation?

Veterinary Medicine

The Bionic Vet
    This British, BBC series aired in the spring of 2010. While considered a documentary, it should be mentioned here. The show follows Dr. Noel Fitzpatrick and his staff who operate a state-of-the-art veterinary practice. The veterinarians attempt pioneering surgeries including providing a bionic knee for a border collie, as well as addressing trauma-related services (a puppy trampled by a horse) and consultations for a Gatwick airport detection dog. The veterinarians also are seen dealing with situations involving communications and decision making with difficult owners.

Emergency Vets (Animal Planet)
    This series followed the day-to-day practices of a group of veterinarians at the twenty-four-hour emergency veterinary hospital, Alameda East Animal Hospital in Denver, Colorado. Drs. Kevin Fitzgerald, Holly Knor, Robert Taylor and others faced a variety of issues: animals hit by cars, a rescued turtle with a hole in its carapace, tumors in zoo animals, as well as communication difficulties with the animals' owners. The doctors also were seen mentoring veterinary interns who were coping with new challenges.

Further Reading

● Andrevijevic M. *Reality TV: the work of being watched*. New York, NY: Rowman & Littlefield; 2004.
● Bach J. How teachers negotiate the use of reality television in their pedagogy. *Pedagogies*. 2011; **6**(2): 144–53.
● Essany M. *Reality Check*. London: Focal Press; 2008.
● Gambles R. Supernanny, parenting and a pedagogical state. *Citizenship Studies*. 2010; **14**(6): 697–709.
● Gardyn R. The tribe has spoken: reality TV is here to stay. *American Demographics*.

September 5, 2001. Available at: www2.realitytvfans.com/newspub/story.cfm?id=3335 (last accessed 12/1/11).

- Lewis T. *Changing Rooms, Biggest Losers and Backyard Blitzes: a history of makeover television in the United Kingdom, the United States and Australia*. London: Routledge Press; 2009.
- Ouellette L, Murray S. *Reality TV: remaking television culture*. New York, NY: NYU Press; 2008.

46

The Small Screen: Television, Medicine, and Teaching

*Tracy R. Juliao, Roger Y. Wong, Rohit Pai, Anna Pavlov,
Patricia Lenahan & Gary Fontan*

Television and Medicine: A Historical Review

Marshall McLuhan[1] predicted in his book *Understanding Media: the extension of man*, that medical dramas would be successful additions to the television line up because "this genre creates an obsession with bodily welfare." The public's interests in medicine as media can be traced back to its popularity in early radio shows and movies such as *Dr. Christian* and *Dr. Kildare*. The advent of television gave this genre a new viewing vehicle and a new, expanded audience.

The medically themed program seems almost synonymous with the origins of television itself, with the first TV drama in this genre appearing in the early 1950s: *City Hospital* on CBS (1951–53) and *The Doctor* on NBC.

Medic appeared in 1954 (NBC, 1954–56) and introduced viewers to Dr. Konrad Styner (Richard Boone) who served as narrator and periodic participant in the episodes. TV Guide described this series as "telling the story of the medical profession without pulling any punches." *Medic* often offered controversial content: ECT for a middle-aged man suddenly displaying bizarre behavior, a young woman diagnosed with breast cancer 1 week prior to her wedding, the life of a busy family physician (general practitioner in that era) who was trying to balance family needs with those of his patients, and parents of a 10-year-old boy, comatose as the result of an auto accident, trying to cope with their guilt and myriad emotions.

Medic worked closely with the Los Angeles County Medical Association (LACMA) and received permission to film in area hospitals and clinics, often including real physicians and nurses as part of the cast. As a result of this relationship, *Medic* gave LACMA control over the medical accuracy of the scripts, many of which involved real case histories. LACMA also was concerned with the image of the doctors portrayed in this series, insisting that the image "fit organized medicine's ideal image."[2] This "image" extended to the types of cars the doctor drove, how he dressed and his idioms of speech, i.e. the absence of the use of contractions or slang terminology.

Medic strove to achieve clinical accuracy in its scripts and even filmed a live birth. The show raised the ire of Cardinal Spellman of New York when he successfully lobbied NBC to prevent the airing of an episode that planned to film a C-section. (Full episodes of *Medic* are available on DVD and synopses of episodes can be found on YouTube.)

The medical dramas in the 1950s and 1960s used these medical consultants to achieve a degree of accuracy in programming content. The American Medical Association (AMA) created The Physicians Advisory Committee for Radio, TV, and Motion Pictures in 1955. Producers of TV series sought this "AMA seal of approval," giving the AMA veto power over scripts so they could display this seal at the end of each episode. The Physicians Advisory Committee subsequently disbanded in the early 1990s.

The early 1960s gave rise to multiple medical series including the very popular series *Dr. Kildare* (1961) and *Ben Casey* (1961–66) with its signature opening: "man, woman, birth, death, infinity." These series focused on the lives of resident physicians, James Kildare, an internist and Ben Casey, a neurosurgeon and their relationships with their chiefs, mentors, and patients. *The Eleventh Hour* (1962–64) gave voice to the lives and issues faced by psychiatrists who were also featured in the short-lived series, *Birdland* (January to April 1994). *Birdland* also introduced viewers to the impaired professional: the series chief of staff, portrayed by Brian Dennehy, was a compulsive gambler.

Dr. Kildare and *Ben Casey* drew large audiences and set the stage for future medical dramas including *Marcus Welby, MD*; *Medical Center*; *St. Elsewhere*; *Chicago Hope*; *Trapper John, MD*; *ER*; *Grey's Anatomy*; and more.

The Nurses (CBS, 1962–65) became *The Doctors and the Nurses* in its second season. This series later became a half-hour daytime soap opera on ABC (1965–67) and should not be confused with a situation comedy titled *Nurses* that appeared on TV from 1991–94. This series, set at a large metropolitan hospital, focused on two nurses: the older head nurse and the young "naïve" student nurse. *The Nurses* addressed controversial issues such as a young physician providing morphine to an addicted patient, another physician (described as a "maverick") who decided to run a clinic in a slum area and to provide care for the poor, as well as the moral and ethical dilemmas that the nurses encountered in their day-to-day work. *Julia*, *M*A*S*H*, *China Beach*, *ER*, *Mercy*, *HawthoRNe*, and *Nurse Jackie* also focus on the role of nurses in health care.

The "kindly family or country doctor" was introduced to viewers in the United Kingdom with the advent of *Dr. Finlay's Casebook* (BBC, 1962–71), Australia's *A Country Practice* (1981–93), and the United States' *Marcus Welby, MD* (1969–76). These series focused on the doctor-patient relationship and the role of the doctor within his/her community. Contrast, if you will, the communication styles and professionalism displayed in *Marcus Welby, MD* with those seen in *House*. This could prompt a lengthy discussion!

Viewers as Patients and Patients as Viewers

It is clear that the medical genre garners a large market share of the TV-watching audience. It isn't a far reach to suggest that viewers (patients) may identify with some of the characters seen on these series and present to the physician's office with concerns based on what they have seen on TV. A 2001 study published in Health Affairs[3] found that 15% of survey respondents indicated that they had contacted a physician based on what they had seen on *ER*.[3]

The Advent of the New Doctors in Television

ER is perhaps one of the most influential medical TV series. It upped the ante in terms of presenting doctors and nurses in a more realistic light, the use of medical jargon, the demonstration of various coping skills and differing communication styles, and the hierarchy of medical practice. In fact, medical educators have used episodes and excerpts from *ER* in a quasi-tutorial fashion to examine case histories and to test students' clinical reasoning skills. Goodman[4] cites the advantage of the medical dramas as teaching tools because of their ability to engage the medical students: "They [medical dramas] contextualize illness and disease with narrative arcs structured by rich characterization, emotional and psychological depth and story-line intrigue." Goodman also stresses how these shows demonstrate the effects of health and illness on the patients: "allow medical students to engage at an intellectual and emotional level with other people's experiences of socially significant health issues such as poverty, domestic violence, substance use disorders and chronic and critical illness."[4] Dr. Ellen Rothman[5] underscored these thoughts in talking about her experiences of watching *ER* as a medical student at Harvard: "my appreciation of the show broadened as my understanding of the clinical issues and the dynamics of the doctor-patient relationship deepened."

House presents another side of medicine and its practitioners. House may be famous as the doctor who epitomizes many less than admirable characteristics such as his own pain pill addiction and his "unique" communication style ("all patients lie"). However, *House* also has upped the ante in addressing many of the legal and financial issues of running a hospital and the costs of medical care. Viewers were first introduced to this theme in *Chicago Hope* where a hospital administrator played a key role in the series.

One of the newest and most short-lived series, *Off the Map*, focused on a group of seven physicians, who traveled to a remote area of South America to provide medical care. The humanitarian physician is a role rarely seen in a television series. This group also qualified as "human" since each of them appears to have frailties (recovering addict, cardiac conditions, history of losses, crises of confidence, and so forth).

Combat Hospital (ABC, 2011), a Canadian series, focuses on the professional and personal lives of a multi-national (United States, Canada, Australia, Germany, United Kingdom) group of physicians and nurses who work in a combat hospital in Afghanistan. The series lacks the comedic qualities of *M*A*S*H*, but offers viewers a glimpse into the daily lives and pressures experienced by the men and women in war-torn areas. It offers a current day approach to emergency medicine in war zones.

A Note about the Comedic View of Medicine

While *M*A*S*H* combined comedy with drama in the lives of surgeons and nurses providing care in the combat theatre, comedy reigned supreme in two series: *Becker* and *Scrubs*. These half-hour comedies introduced viewers to a surly internist in private practice (*Becker*) and a group of residents and nurses (*Scrubs*). "Teachable moments" can be found in both series. For example, *Becker* offers an excellent example of how to take a sexual history while a variety of topics (including how to take a pain history and to use the FACES pain scales) can be found on *Scrubs*. Both series are available on DVD and many clips from *Scrubs* can be found on YouTube.

Many of the other TV series are available on DVD as well or online at the websites for the shows themselves. Synopses and episode guides for many of these shows are available online (www.tv.com).

Use of Television Medical Dramas for Teaching

In recent years there has been increasing interest in the development and delivery of competency-based curriculum within medical education at both the undergraduate and postgraduate levels.[1,2] Some of these competencies, such as communication skills, collaboration skills, and professionalism, are difficult to teach by traditional didactic methods. Innovative teaching methodologies such as cinemeducation can be helpful in teaching these competencies. While previous efforts have focused on using scenes from movie films, it has been demonstrated that scenes from contemporary and popular television shows can be effectively arranged to teach communication skills to internal medicine residents.[3]

From the medical education perspective, there are no substantial differences between using television and movie films at least in terms of their content, accessibility (both forms are now readily available on DVD and on the Internet), technological features (high definition digital signal is the industry standard, with advances such as three-dimensional viewing), and costs. Television is a part of the popular culture of our medical learners. Using scenes from television that may be familiar to our learners and part of their social norm, increases interest level in the delivery of the medical curriculum. Newer forms of social mass media such as YouTube, Dailymotion, Sevenload, Viddler, Vimeo, and Metacafe, may also be used in much the same way.

House (2005; Hugh Laurie, Omar Epps, Jesse Spencer, Jennifer Morrison): This popular American medical drama follows Dr. House (Hugh Laurie) and his team of staff – including Dr. Eric Foreman (Omar Epps), Dr. Robert Chase (Jesse Spencer), and Dr. Allison Cameron (Jennifer Morrison) – as they attempt to solve various medical mysteries. Dr. House is known for his unconventional and often controversial approach to medical diagnosis and treatment.

Do Not Resuscitate Order

1   (Season 1, ch 9, 0:06:05–0:07:32) Dr. Foreman discusses the likelihood that the patient's underlying respiratory condition is related to an incurable illness, amyotrophic lateral sclerosis. During the discussion, the patient requests a DNR (do not resuscitate) order, which surprises Dr. Foreman. It is apparent that he is hesitant to make the patient a DNR although the patient is competent to make this decision and it is therefore granted.
    a. Why do you think Dr. Foreman reacts to the patient's DNR request in the way that is portrayed in the scene?
    b. How well do you think the patient in the scene understands the elements of a DNR order? What and how much information do you think a physician needs to convey during a DNR discussion?
    c. How well do you feel physicians are trained in managing "end of life" issues?
2   (Scene 2, season 1, ch 9, 0:10:30–0:12:07) The medical team finds the same patient from the previous scene in hypoxemic respiratory failure following an infusion of intravenous immunoglobulin. They attempt initial resuscitation only to discover the patient is DNR. Dr. House does not agree with the patient's decision and decides to take matters into his own hands.
    a. How well do you think the team is informed of the patient's DNR status? What are some ways to improve the information flow?
    b. Do you think Dr. House's actions are appropriate? Why or why not? Are there circumstances where reversing a DNR order is reasonable?

Grey's Anatomy (2005; Ellen Pompeo, Chandra Wilson, Sandra Oh): This medical drama follows the professional and personal lives of a diverse group of interns, residents, and staff physicians at the fictional Seattle Grace Mercy West Hospital in Seattle, Washington. The show has a diverse cast and demonstrates the complex interplay between the social and professional lives of the characters.

Patient Privacy and Conflict among Physicians

1   (Season 2, ch 7, 0:14:00–0:15:05) Various physicians are assessing a male patient who is admitted to the hospital because of an intra-abdominal mass resulting in a distended abdomen and making him appear as if he is pregnant. Dr. Meredith Grey (Ellen Pompeo) is disturbed by the team's handling of the situation, especially their posing for photographs with the patient. There is also a conflict of interest, as Dr. Miranda Bailey (Chandra Wilson) tells her resident, Dr. Cristina Yang (Sandra Oh), to "not ignore her pager." She uses this as an opportunity to gain more media publicity with the patient.

   a. What are your concerns about patient respect in this situation? What can be done differently to address the concerns in this situation?
   b. How would you interpret Dr. Meredith Grey's thoughts in this scene? How well does she communicate her concerns to the health team members?
   c. What are your thoughts on Dr. Miranda Bailey's management of the situation? What would you recommend doing differently in this situation?

Scrubs (2001; Zac Braff, Sarah Chalke, Donald Faison, Ken Jenkins, John C. McGinley): This popular medical comedy-drama follows the perspective of main character Dr. Michael "JD" Dorian as he progresses through medical training in a teaching hospital. Dr. Dorian's character is well known for comedic monologues often exaggerating the reality of scenarios faced during medical training.

Breaking Bad News

1   (Season 8, ch 5, 0:06:08–0:06:43; 0:15:55–0:17:25) Dr. Michael "JD" Dorian (Braff) and his medical student have to tell a patient and his wife that he has a recurrence of cancer with pulmonary metastases. The patient is initially in denial and the medical team rescinds their initial comments, revising the diagnosis as pneumonia.

   a. Why do you think the medical team behaves in the way portrayed in the scene, which is to change the medical diagnosis in response to the patient's reaction?
   b. How would you describe Dr. Dorian's way of delivering the bad news? How is it different from the medical student's approach?
   c. What are the key elements to breaking bad news in a patient-sensitive manner?

2   (Season 4, ch 23; 0:06:40–0:07:21) Dr. Michael "JD" Dorian has to tell a patient that she has a severe respiratory illness, and is unlikely to be discharged from hospital. The shift of care towards comfort is discussed with the patient and a friend, as no next of kin is found.

   a. How would you describe Dr. Dorian's approach to end-of-life goals of care?

b. Dr. Dorian has an interesting reflection on "comfort care." What does "comfort care" mean to you? And how would you explain this concept to the patient?

3 (Season 4, ch 23, 0:11:10–0:11:30; 0:18:17–0:19:16) This scene is the extension of the previous one. Unbeknownst to Dr. Dorian, the patient's brother, who is a lawyer, appears disturbed by the decision to switch the goals of care to comfort care. He threatens to sue the patient's young friend who is actually a neighbor. The friend stands up against the brother, declaring that a change in the goals of care is in accordance with the patient's wishes. The brother realizes this is appropriate as he sees his sister's clinical status decline.

a. How would you describe the appropriateness of the role played by the young friend of the patient as opposed to her brother? How would you approach the goals of care of the patient when the next of kin is not available?

b. What are the legal implications of the friend's action in deciding that the patient's care be switched to comfort care?

c. What would you do differently in this situation?

Private Practice, Seasons 1–3 (2007–10): This television series is a spin-off from *Grey's Anatomy*, in which Dr. Addison Montgomery (Kate Walsh), a double-board certified neonatal surgeon and obstetrician/gynecologist, relocates from Seattle to Los Angeles to join a multidisciplinary private practice of physicians, Oceanside Wellness. The practice group includes her best friend, Dr. Naomi Bennett (Audra McDonald), a fertility specialist; Naomi's ex-husband, Dr. Sam Bennett (Taye Diggs), who specializes in internal medicine; Dr. Cooper Freedman (Paul Adelstein), a pediatrician; Dr. Violet Turner (Amy Brenneman), a psychiatrist; and Dr. Peter Wilder (Tim Daly), who specializes in complementary and alternative medicine. Dell Parker (Chris Lowell) is the receptionist at Oceanside Wellness and is also studying to become a midwife.

Delivering Bad News of a Fatal Pediatric Genetic Disease
• • • • • • • • • • • •

1 (Season 1, episode 2, ch 2, 0:09:36–0:10:42) Dr. Freedman asks Dr. Montgomery for a second opinion regarding laboratory test results, which leads to both physicians speaking with the parents of a child with a fatal genetic disease.

a. How would you approach informing patients of news like this?

b. What did you like/dislike about how Dr. Montgomery provided the news? How might you have approached this discussion differently, if at all?

c. Once the parents realized that the disease was genetic, the mother asked about genetic testing for herself, her husband, and other family members.

How would you manage a discussion with patients regarding genetic diseases, a sense of responsibility that may be experienced regarding passing on a disease to one's children, and the need for testing?

Uncovering Genetic Incompatibility between a Pediatric Patient and the Parents

1 (Season 1, episode 2, chs 2–3, 0:11:30–0:12:38) In these successive scenes, Drs. Naomi Bennett, Freedman, and Montgomery compare the results of the parental genetic tests with the pediatric patient's genetic tests and conclude that the child is not the parents' biological child. The three physicians then sit with the parents and deliver this shocking news. The last scene in this series concludes with Dr. Freedman expressing his concern regarding the father's lack of emotional reaction to the two sets of bad news he has received within the same day (first that his child has a terminal illness and second that the child is not his biological child and may have been switched with another baby at birth).

   a. How would you approach delivering news such as this to your patient(s)? Would you deliver this news via phone or insist that the patient(s) meet you for a face-to-face meeting? Why?

   b. How would you help prepare the family for the sense of confusion and emotional distress they are likely to experience at learning news such as this?

   c. How would you anticipate and prepare to answer the many questions they might have?

   d. What do you think of Dr. Freedman's reaction to his patient's lack of emotional response to the devastating news he received? How might you respond to a patient who appears to lack emotional expression in the face of surprising and overwhelming news? What sources of support or resources might you offer, if any?

Adolescent Sexuality, HIV Status, and Duty to Warn

1 (Season 2, episode 1, ch 2, 0:10:41–0:11:35) Dr. Freedman talks with his adolescent male patient about the patient's decision to have sex for the first time. It is clear that there is an established relationship between the two.

   a. What did you think about Dr. Freedman's approach to discussing sex with his patient?

   b. How would you have approached a similar conversation with an adolescent patient who is known to you?

   c. How would you have approached a similar conversation with an adolescent patient who is new to you?

2   (Season 2, ch 2, 0:12:57–0:13:25) Dr. Freedman discusses with his colleagues, Drs. Bennett and Wilder, his concern for his 14-year-old HIV-positive patient, who has just revealed that he plans to have sex with his girlfriend. A larger part of the discussion centers on the fact that the patient's parents have not told him that he is HIV-positive. Dr. Freedman decided to accept and treat him as a patient when he was 5 years old under the condition that the patient remain blind to his condition.

    a. Would you agree to accept a minor patient who has not been told about his/her chronic, possibly terminal, and known to be communicable, medical condition? Why or why not?

    b. If you agreed to treat a minor patient who was unaware of his/her medical condition, how would you establish the rules of treatment and how they might change over time with the patient's parents?

    c. Beyond the risk of undisclosed sexual activity, what are other risks associated with treating a minor HIV-positive patient who has not been told of his/her condition?

3   (Season 2, ch 2, 0:13:26–0:14:08) This scene is an immediate continuation of the prior scene. It focuses on Dr. Freedman's struggle of whether or not to break confidentiality to the patient (reveal to him that he is HIV positive) and/or his parents (reveal to them that their son plans to have sex). Further, the discussion occurs between the three physicians while walking a dog along a path near the beach.

    a. What would you do if you were in Dr. Freedman's position?

    b. If you were Dr. Freedman, would you have let the patient and/or his parents leave the office when you learned that the patient plans to have sex with his girlfriend without further discussion with the patient and/or his parents? If you would have kept them in the office, what would you have done/said?

    c. If you were Dr. Freedman, would you contact the patient's parents and reveal that their son plans to have sex? Why or why not?

    d. If you were Dr. Freedman, would you contact the patient to inform him of his HIV-positive status? Why or why not?

    e. If you were Dr. Freedman, would you contact the patient's girlfriend to warn her of potential harm? Why or why not? What are the ethical/legal issues involved in your decision?

    f. Even without mention of identifying information, is this an appropriate discussion for an open area, such as a path along the beach? How about a hallway within a hospital? Why or why not?

Agenda Setting and Ethical Issues Related to Genetic Selection in Pregnancy
••••••••••••••••••••••••••••••••

1 (Season 2, episode 1, ch 1, 0:07:07–0:08:04) Dr. Montgomery is covering for her colleague, Dr. Naomi Bennett, and meets with a pregnant patient (27 weeks) and her husband for the first time. During the encounter, the couple asks her to deliver their baby prematurely in order to save their dying 7-year-old son, who has acute lymphoblastic leukemia and requires their newborn baby's cord blood in order to save his life.
   a. What did you notice about how Dr. Montgomery began this medical encounter? What did you like? What would you do differently? How do you think agenda setting might have influenced the flow and communication that occurred within this encounter?
   b. How would you respond to the couple?
   c. What would you be willing to do if faced with this type of life and death dilemma? Why?
2 (Season 2, episode 1, ch 2, 0:08:37–0:09:50) Dr. Montgomery and Dr. Naomi Bennett discuss the case from the previous scene. Dr. Bennett practiced selective in vitro fertilization (IVF) by implanting an embryo that is a genetic match for her patients' dying son. The 7-year-old son will die within a week if Dr. Montgomery does not agree to deliver the 27-week-old fetus.
   a. Dr. Montgomery tells Dr. Bennett that selective IVF, implanting an embryo that is a genetic match to its sibling, is entering a slippery slope morally and ethically, and that in this case, the parents are not "growing a child," but rather "growing organs" (cord blood) for their sick son. Do you agree with Dr. Montgomery's assessment? Why/why not?
   b. Given the new information garnered from this scene, would you respond to the couple's request any differently than you indicated previously? Why/why not?
   c. When attempting to make a decision, what concerns (medical and psychological) do you have for the unborn baby? The 7-year-old son? The parents of both children?

Medical Decision Making and End-of-Life Issues in a Minor Patient
•••••••••••••••••••

1 (Season 2, episode 2, ch 1, 0:08:47–0:10:05) A 17-year-old male with bronchiolitis of the larynx is in the hospital and intubated after being found unconscious and in respiratory arrest in Dr. Sam Bennett's outpatient office (earlier scene). As the scene opens, Dr. Bennett and the patient's father are talking about the progression of the patient's disease. When the patient awakens, he removes the respirator tube himself to the dismay of his father. The patient's father immediately asks Dr. Bennett to intubate his son again,

while the patient pleads with his father and Dr. Bennett, telling them both that he does not want to be on a ventilator, or for that matter, continue invasive treatments.

a. If you were in Dr. Bennett's position, how would you respond in-the-moment?

b. Given the luxury of time that this scene did not afford, is it possible that you might approach the same situation in a different manner? While the laws differ from state-to-state regarding the age at which a minor can speak for him/herself in medical decision making, it is likely that you will be faced with many situations in which a minor child who is approaching the age to legally be able to make decisions for him/herself wants something different in terms of medical treatment than his/her parent(s). Would you try to facilitate a family meeting to discuss all points of view? If so, how would you approach such a meeting? Would an ethics consult be helpful?

c. If you do not agree with the choices that the patient and/or his/her family is making regarding available medical care, how would your opinion influence your interactions with the patient/family? How would you reconcile treating a patient when the decision for medical treatment, or withdrawal of medical treatment, is contrary to your personal value system?

Cultural Competence and Sensitivity, Ethical Issues, Whole Person Care, and Professional Consultation

1 (Season 2, episode 4, ch 3, 0:14:29–0:15:44) Dr. Montgomery meets with a young female patient individually for a follow-up visit to discuss her lab results and her request for surgical repair of her hymen. In a prior scene, the patient and her mother met with Dr. Montgomery together and the patient's mother told Dr. Montgomery that the patient was raped and that within their culture, the patient will never be respected or find a suitable marital partner if she is not a virgin. The mother indicates that this is an even more pressing issue as the patient is about to enter into an arranged marriage to a man that will not accept her if she is not a virgin. In the current scene, the patient reveals that she was not raped as reported previously, but instead that she has an American boyfriend with whom she is in love. However, for the financial well-being and social standing of her parents and herself, it is important that she go through with the arranged marriage that her parents set up for her. She notes, "This is the only way that we can be happy … I want them to be happy."

a. How would you respond to this patient in a manner that would be culturally sensitive?

b. What ethical issues might arise if a patient presents with a request such as this?

c. What are the emotional implications that the patient might not be considering for herself when pursuing this type of surgical intervention as a means toward a goal that appears to put the desires/needs of others over her own?

d. If you are not in agreement with this patient's decision, how would you proceed? What factors would influence you?

e. If you agreed to perform the procedure that the patient is requesting, would you seek outside consultation for yourself and/or your patient? If so, whom would you consult (which discipline) and why?

Duty to Warn: The Legal and Ethical Issues

1 (Season 2, episode 7, ch 4, 0:23:20–0:25:29) In this scene, the patient, a known sex offender, in the context of discussing his own history of being sexually abused when he was a child, reveals to Dr. Turner that he thinks about a specific young girl frequently and envisions himself going to her house, talking to her, followed by the girl getting into the car with him and "I take her." He denies wanting to do anything other than talk to the young girl, but it is clear that Dr. Turner doesn't believe him. In fact, she responds to him at one point saying, "Hal, you want to do more than just talk to Jody …"

a. Although the patient denies a desire to harm the young girl, his body language and tone of voice lead Dr. Turner to be distrustful of his words. If you were in Dr. Turner's position, what would you do?

b. What does the law say about what you should do? Is it clear in this case?

c. How would you document this encounter regardless of how you decide to handle the information you learned/suspect?

d. Clearly, this scene brings up the duty to warn. What are the factors that must be present when you are required to warn an individual of possible harm?

2 (Season 2, Episode 7, ch 5, 0:28:14–0:28:39) In this scene, which occurs shortly after the one above, Dr. Turner reveals to her colleague, Dell, that she is unsure whether the thoughts that the patient has discussed with her "is a plan or just something that's going to stay in his head." Dell tells her that she has to do something and she responds, "It's not a crime to think bad things" and notes that the patient wants to get better. Dell asks, "Is that enough?"

a. Given what you know about this patient, his history, and his current mental state, do you agree with Dell or Dr. Turner? Why?

Use of Complementary and Alternative Medicine, Treating a Fellow Physician, Giving Bad News, and Assisted Suicide
••••••••••••••••••••••

1 (Season 2, episode 13, ch 3, 0:07:59–0:09:43) This scene opens with Dr. Wilder providing acupuncture treatment to a patient for the pain associated with pancreatic cancer. The patient is a doctor who is older than Dr. Wilder. Within their discussion, the patient contemplates his choice of specialty in his younger years, noting interest and intrigue regarding complementary and alternative medicine. As the treatment and discussion continue, Dr. Sam Bennett enters the room and informs the patient that his most recent chemotherapy treatment was not successful and that there are no remaining treatment options for the patient. The patient expresses his understanding of his prognosis and elaborates regarding what he can expect in his final weeks/days. Drs. Wilder and Bennett demonstrate compassion and promise to help the patient manage his pain through his final days, with Dr. Bennett stating, "Whatever we need to do to help." The scene ends with the patient stating, "I'm going to need your help. I want you to help me die."

a. This is an instance where the laws in various states are different. However, regardless of the law, typically there are ethical and moral issues related to requests for assisted suicide. What are those issues?

b. How would you respond to a patient who requests your involvement in assisted suicide? What would be involved in the conversation? Would you want others involved in that conversation, such as family members of the patient and/or your colleagues? Why/why not?

c. This scene highlights the difficulty experienced by both patients and physicians when physicians give bad news to patients. What did you like about how this discussion was handled? What didn't you like? Why?

d. When you are delivering bad news to patients, how do you prepare? What are things that you must consider in order to insure the best possible discussion?

e. As was noted above, treating a physician as a patient may differ from treating a non-physician. How so? In what ways might you alter the way in which you interact? Do you think that the doctor-patient relationship would be easier or harder to develop and maintain? Why? What factors would influence the doctor-patient relationship?

f. Acupuncture is being utilized as a legitimate method of medical intervention in this scene. How familiar are you with acupuncture and would/do you refer patients for acupuncture and/or other complementary and alternative medicine treatments?

g. Do you regularly ask your patients whether they are participating in any treatments outside of traditional Western medicine? Do you ask about the use of supplements and/or herbal remedies? What are the legal ramifications for neglecting to ask these types of questions?

The Postpartum Mother
•••••••••••••••••••••••••••••

1   (Season 2, episode 16, ch 1, 0:04:53–0:05:47) Dr. Freedman is examining an infant and talking with the infant's mother about the details of an accident that occurred leading to the mother bringing the infant in for this visit.
  a. What do you notice about the mother as she interacts with Dr. Freedman? What behaviors appear out of the norm?
  b. Given your observations of the mother within this medical encounter, what do you suspect might be going on for her? What questions would you like to ask to gain a clearer understanding of the mother's presentation?
  c. While the infant is the primary patient in this encounter, it is clear that the mother may need to be evaluated as well. What psychiatric diagnoses would you like to rule out while assessing the mother during this visit?
  d. What are some subtle cues that postpartum mothers might give during a typical infant medical visit that would lead you to inquire in more detail about the mother's well-being?
2   (Season 2, episode 16, ch 2, 0:17:19–0:18:29) In this scene, which occurs in the common area of the practice where other patients are present, it becomes clear that the postpartum mother intentionally tried to harm her infant.
  a. What would you do if your patient revealed such information to you? What would you do in the moment (interventions, logistics, and so forth)?
  b. Assuming that this mother is your patient, how would you manage the patient's care on a longer-term basis once the immediate crisis is addressed?
  c. What would you do if you found yourself in a public setting with a patient who is in emotional distress like this postpartum mother? Would you have handled the interaction differently than the staff of Oceanside Wellness did in this scene? If so, how? Do you think that if the staff had been able to remove the postpartum mother from the common area that she would have revealed the same information? Why/why not?

Domestic Violence and Personal Values Clashing with Patient Behaviors
•••••••••••••••••••••••••••

1   (Season 3, episode 2, ch 1, 0:05:59–0:08:00) In this compilation of scenes, Dr. Freedman responds to an emergency call to learn that a family for whom he is the pediatrician is in the emergency room. All members of the family present with wounds related to an apparent domestic violence incident. Dr. Freedman calls for his colleagues, Drs. Sam Bennett and Montgomery, as they are the treating physicians for the parents. The scenes continue showing interactions between various family members and the medical staff. (You may wish to stop the clip at 0:06:42 and ask the first discussion question).
  a. What do you notice about the interaction among the family members

when Dr. Freedman first encounters them? What do you observe in their interaction with Dr. Freedman? Based on your observations for just this short period of time, what questions do you have? What do you want to know more about?

b. What did you like about Dr. Freedman's interaction with the daughter when he was wrapping the injury on her arm? What didn't you like? Why? How would you have interacted with her differently? Why?

c. What did you notice about Dr. Bennett's interaction with the father? How would you have interacted differently with him?

d. How would you assess for domestic violence in an instance such as this? Would your questioning differ depending upon which member of the family you are speaking to? If so, why?

e. How do you assess for domestic violence in the office setting? Does it differ from an acute care setting such as the emergency room? If so, how?

f. When you encounter patients for whom you don't approve of their apparent or real behaviors, what do you do to enable yourself to remain professional in your interactions with them?

Language Usage, Informed Consent, and Withdrawal of Treatment
· · · · · · · · · · · · · · · · · ·

1 (Season 3, episode 15, ch 1, 0:06:33–0:08:09) Dr. Montgomery, along with Drs. Naomi Bennett and Wilder, inform new parents of the many medical issues that their premature newborn faces and offer them the choice of treatment including several surgical interventions, suffering, and "no real chance of a normal life" or "ending his life." During the conversation, Dr. Montgomery uses medical terminology that the parents don't understand. All three of the physicians use language that is reflective of their advanced education.

a. How would you approach a difficult discussion with a family such as the one observed in this scene? What would you do differently than Dr. Montgomery? Why?

b. While surgery requires formal written informed consent, the discussion that the physicians are having with the family in this scene constitutes verbal informed consent regarding treatment options for their child. How would you insure that the parents truly understand the information that is being presented to them so that they can make informed decisions regarding the treatment options?

c. Some would argue that withdrawal of treatment is no different than assisted suicide. In this instance, the option to withdraw treatment is offered as a means of preventing suffering. While the goal of assisted suicide is also to prevent suffering, how does the option of withdrawing treatment differ in this instance or others similar to it?

d. When Dr. Montgomery uses medical terminology that is not familiar to the parents, the mother asks her to clarify. Oftentimes, patients do not ask for clarification of unknown terminology. How often do you think patients do not follow treatment recommendations or take the wrong medication due to lack of understanding of what physicians have said to them? What efforts can you make to insure that your patients understand what you have said, even if you don't use medical terminology and/or high-level vocabulary when talking with them?

e. How important is health literacy in situations such as this?

Prescription Drug Addiction

Nurse Jackie (2009–10): The characters are Edie Falco (Jackie Peyton), Paul Schulze (Eddie Walzer, a pharmacist with whom Jackie is having an affair), Eve Best (Dr. Eleanor O'Hara, a British doctor and Jackie's best friend at work), Merritt Wever (Zoey, a jubilant but inexperienced new nurse), Peter Facinelli (Dr. Cooper), Haaz Sleiman (male nurse, Mo-Mo), Dominic Fumusa (Jackie's bar-owner husband, Kevin) and Jackie's daughters played by Ruby Jerins (Grace) and Daisy Tahan (Fiona in season 1). This Showtime series is a medical drama based on an experienced and highly respected emergency room nurse, Jackie Peyton, who works in a hectic New York City hospital. Jackie has chronic back pain and is addicted to prescription pain medications. The series chronicles Jackie's professional career as a nurse and her secret struggle with pain medication. It is a realistic portrayal of the lengths to which an addict will go to in order to hide an addiction and still attempt to be fully functional in a workplace where pain medications can be accessed easily.

1 (Season 1, episode 1; 0:09:51–0:11:20) Jackie has intercourse with a pharmacist colleague while at work. She complains of back pain and asks him for "Oxy's" (Oxycontin).

2 (0:24:40–0:25:35) The Pharmacist, Eddie Walzer tells Jackie, "I brought you something for your back," showing her a soda and a snack. Jackie replies, "I was thinking about Vicodin." Eddie gives her some pain medication and Jackie replies, "I love you."

   a. What moral obligations do health-care professionals have to keep their sexual relationships out of the workplace?

   b. Is Jackie using her relationship with the pharmacist to get pain medications illegally?

   c. How do chronic medical conditions contribute to drug addiction?

   d. What measures can be instituted to prevent pain patients from becoming addicted to opioid medications?

3 (0:22:40–0:23:51) Jackie is having a conversation with a senior nurse and being complimented for a job well done while she is under the influence of drugs. The next scene shows Jackie in the emergency room with a patient.

She makes a medication error with an intravenous medicine. Jackie admits out loud that she almost killed the patient.

   a. What are some of the myriad ways in which addiction can interfere with an individual's work performance?

   b. How could a medical professional like Jackie rationalize, minimize, or deny that he/she is putting others at risk from personal drug use?

   c. For those in medicine, what is the procedure in your facility for reporting a medication error?

   d. If you were a colleague of Jackie's and knew of her addiction and use at work, what would you do?

4 (0:25:58–0:27:13) Jackie comes home to her two small daughters and husband after her long shift. She rushes to discretely put back on her wedding ring and says hello to her husband.

5 (Episode 2, 0:03:15–0:04:15) While making lunch at home for her children, Jackie crushes up a Percocet pill and then pours it into an open sugar packet and glues the packet together to be used later in the day.

   a. What is your reaction to such ingenuity by an addict?

   b. Is Jackie putting her children at risk? How do you think she would respond to the notion that she is?

6 (0:07:45–0:08:26) Working in the emergency room, Jackie is hit by an angry patient. In response to this event, Jackie opens up her previously prepared packet of drugs and pours it into her coffee at the nurse's station.

   a. What is your reaction to seeing this? How would a non-addicted person respond to being hit by an angry patient? Why do you suppose Jackie doesn't respond similarly?

   b. What does the research demonstrate about health professionals in various specialties and their risk of addiction?

7 (0:25:00–0:26:19) Jackie leaves the emergency room at the end of her shift and encounters a taxi driver with chest pain lying out in the street. She gives the driver one of her pain medications to relieve his pain until help can arrive.

   a. What is your reaction to Jackie's behavior? In what way has her judgment been impaired?

   b. While one could say that Jackie had the patient's best interest in mind, what was problematic with her action? Was that a rational decision?

8 (Episode 3, 0:02:00–0:03:05) While Jackie is getting ready for work, she begins to search for hidden drugs on top of the medicine cabinet. When she is startled by her husband, one pill falls down the sink. Jackie uses a piece of gum on a pencil to retrieve the pill.

   a. What is your reaction to this scene? Does the ingenuity of the addict to get the drug surprise you?

   b. What personal and professional risks is Jackie taking?

9 (Episode 7, 0:13:54–0:15:57) Dr. Eleanor O'Hara, an ER physician, is in her office taking prescription Xanax with Nurse Jackie by her side. Dr. O'Hara offers Jackie one of her pills and Jackie cautiously accepts it. While Jackie at

first glance appears to take only one pill from the bottle, she secretly steals extra pills.

  a. Allowing another person to use prescription medications is illegal. How is the emergency room physician enabling Jackie?

  b. How is Jackie using her friendship with the physician to continue her addiction?

  c. What would you say to a client/patient who told you that they gave a friend or family members some of their medication?

  d. What treatment resources are available for individuals with pill addictions?

Mental Illness, Dissociative Identity Disorder, and its Impact on the Family

The United States of Tara (season 1, disk 1, 2009; Toni Collette, John Corbett, Keir Gilchrist, Brie Larson): This ShowTime Series follows Tara (Collette), an artist, wife, and mother suffering from dissociative identity disorder (DID). As she wrestles with multiple personalities, Tara works to keep her family from falling apart. Tara's husband (Corbett) is very supportive and tolerant, while their two children, Kate (Larson) and Marshall (Gilchrist), have additional challenges as adolescents.

1 (Episode 1, Pilot T3C1; 0:06:20–0:8:24) Tara's sister, Charmaine walks into her kitchen where the family is gathered and states, "Something tells me my sister is not here tonight. I cannot remember what this one is called." Charmaine asks to talk privately with Max. She then ventilates about her sister and says, "It's about her. It's really hard for me to see my sister like this. Why can't she just stop?" Max responds, "We're all angry at the crazy. I have been married to her for 17 years." Charmaine concludes, "It's not a real diagnosis."

  a. What is DID?

  b. Review the DSM-IV-TR criteria.

  c. Are there skeptics of the diagnosis in the psychiatric community? How about in the lay public?

  d. What is at the source of this skepticism?

2 (Episode 1; T3 C2; 0:14:30–0:15:40) Tara walks into her son, Marshall's, room. She apologizes to him, referring to her earlier appearance and behavior. She thanks him for being such a "supportive kid." Marshall responds, "We're lucky mom. Because of you, we get to be interesting."

  a. Discuss any experiences you have had with DID patients/clients.

  b. What is your reaction to Marshall's response to his mother?

3 (Episode 1, T3 C2–C3, 0:18:01–0:23:43) Tara witnesses her daughter being pushed by her boyfriend on school grounds. She gets out of the car to defend her daughter. She is upset and is triggered. She closes her eyes and assumes a different identity. Her behavior changes as she drives off fast and becomes

"Buck," an aggressive male alter who likes to go to the shooting range. At the house, her husband confronts her about not attending their daughter's recital.
a. Would others be afraid of someone like Tara? Would you? Why/why not?
b. Do alters typically take on such extreme changes in their physical personas?

4 (Episode 1, T4 C1; 0:02:00–0:03:53) Tara, who keeps a video record of her thoughts and feelings, speaks about "cleaning up after" her alters. She states, "Having multiples is like a kegger in your brain while you're trashed out." The scene shifts to a family meeting where Tara reconstructs lost time to remember what happened when she was in another state.
a. Why do you think Tara keeps a video diary? Is that something you would suggest to a client/patient?
b. What do you think of these family meetings? What benefits do they serve for each family member?

5 (Episode 1, 0:04:00–0:04:19) Tara's husband, Max, states that they knew when went she off her meds, that the whole gang would resurface – the multiple personality tour.
a. Why would an individual like Tara decide to discontinue her medications?
b. Does this appear to be a good decision? How would you discuss this with a patient/client?

6 (Episode 2: Aftermath, T4 C1–2, 0:09:18–0:10:56) Tara is shopping with her sister, Charmaine, and is aware that she embarrasses her family. Her sister asks her, "Why do you care if Marshall doesn't want you to talk to his teacher?" Tara shares that her 14-year-old son, Marshall, wet the bed. Charmaine suggests that it is in response to trauma, to Tara's "schizophrenia situation." Tara explains the difference between schizophrenia and dissociative identity disorder. Charmaine suggests all Tara needs is "Mood Booster Remix," a product she sells and wants Tara to purchase.
a. What is your reaction to Charmaine's attitude toward Tara and her disorder?
b. What do you think of Tara's response to her sister?
c. What is the state of stigma and mental illness?

7 (Episode 3: Inspiration, T6 C1–2, 0:09:00–0:10:53) Tara is in a therapy session. She is excited to be developing a friendship with Tiffany who she has been commissioned to do a mural for. The therapist talks about the impact of trauma. Although Tara is unaware of the source of her trauma, her therapist adds that Tara's alters know the source and that is why the system was created to protect her. Tara asks if her recent progress qualifies as a breakthrough.
a. Why does dissociation occur? How is it protective of an individual?
b. What are the clinical guidelines in approaching an individual with dissociative identity disorder?
c. Why would periodic clinical consultation be indicated?

8 (Episode 5: Revolution, T7 C3, 0:22:24–0:24:03) The stress of a mother with DID takes a toll on Marshall who yells at the alter referred to as "T." He tells her to, "Shut up. Haven't you caused enough trouble?" His parents missed

his open house and other events and he blames T. Marshall asks, "Are you my mother? Then why are you inside my mother?" "I want my real mother and only my real mother and not one of you other freaks. Just her – Everyone else go away." Marshall's father than comforts him.

a. What psychotherapeutic supports could assist Marshall in coping with his mother's illness and often chaotic family life?

b. Could having a mother with DID offer have any developmental benefits? What might they be?

c. What evidence is available on the adjustment of the children of mothers with mental illness? Is there any research available specifically on the adjustment of children of mothers with DID?

References

1 McLuhan M. *Understanding Media: the extension of man*. New York: McGraw-Hill; 1964.

2 Turow J. *Playing Doctor: television, story-telling and medical power*. New York, NY: Oxford University Press; 1989.

3 Brodie M, Foehr U, Rideout V, *et al.* Communicating health information through the entertainment media. *Health Aff (Millwood)*. 2001; **20**(1): 192–9.

4 Goodman K. Imagining doctors: medical students and the TV medical drama. *Virtual Mentor*. 2007; **9**(3): 182–7.

5 Rothman EL. *White Coat: Becoming a Doctor at Harvard Medical School*. New York: Perennial Press; 2000.

Further Reading

● McNeilly DP, Wengel SP. The "ER" seminar: teaching psychotherapeutic techniques to medical students. *Acad Psychiatry*. 2001; **25**: 193–200.

● Midmer D. Cine-ed: using films to teach medical learners. *BMJ*. Careers, 2004; **329**: 140–1.

● Pavlov A, Dahlquist, G. Teaching communication and professionalism using a popular medical drama. *Family Medicine*. 2010; **42**(1); 25–7.

● Summers S, Summers HJ. *Saving Lives: why the media portrayal of nurses puts us all at risk*. New York: Kaplan Publishing; 2009.

Medical TV Shows

● *Julia* (1968–71)
● *Medical Center* (1969–76)
● *M*A*S*H* (1972–83)
● *Trapper John, M.D.* (1979–86)
● *St. Elsewhere* (1982–88)
● *China Beach* (1988–91)

- *Chicago Hope* (1994–2000)
- *ER* (1994–2009)
- *Becker* (1998–2004)
- *Providence* (1999–2002)
- *Strong Medicine* (2000–06)
- *Scrubs* (2001–09)
- *Presidio Med* (2002–03)
- *MDs* (2002–03)
- *Dr. Vegas* (2004)
- *House* (2004–present)
- *Medical Investigation* (2004–05)
- *Inconceivable* (2005)
- *Grey's Anatomy* (2005–present)
- *Private Practice* (2007–present)
- *Hopkins* (2008)
- *HawthoRNe* (2009–present)
- *Nurse Jackie* (2009–present)
- *Mercy* (2009–10)
- *Off the Map* (2010–present)

References for Use of Television Medical Dramas for Teaching

- Frank JR, editor. *The CanMEDS 2005 Physicians Competency Framework: Better Standards. Better Physicians. In Better Care*. Ottawa: Royal College of Physicians and Surgeons of Canada; 2005.
- ACGME Outcome Project General Competencies. Excerpted on July 10, 2008. Available at: www.acgme.org/outcome/comp/compFull.asp (last accessed 12/1/11)
- Wong RY, Saber SS, Ma I, Roberts JM. Using television shows to teach communication skills in an internal medicine residency. *BMC Med Educ*. 2009; **9**: 9.

47

Is Fact Better than Fiction? Documentaries

H. Russell Searight, Danielle Vanier & Kevin Krause

WHILE DOCUMENTARY FILMS HAVE AN EXTENSIVE HISTORY, THEY became increasingly popular in the early to mid-1990s. Several factors have contributed to the increase in their popularity and use. First, as costs for making traditional "Hollywood" films have soared, documentary films have remained relatively inexpensive to make. Second, the rise of cable television provided a ready outlet for films of this genre.

There are multiple approaches to making documentary film. These documentary "schools" vary according to the extent to which the filmmaker is trying to make a specific point, the organizational sequence of the film, the presence of narration, and more recently, the centrality of the filmmaker.[1] These three major approaches to documentary film include: Direct Cinema, Cinema Vérité, and the Cinematic Essay.

In Direct Cinema,[2] the filmmaker is often "a fly on the wall," with minimal or no narration and often without interviewing the subjects. The films of Frederick Wiseman, such as *Near Death* (1989) and *Domestic Violence* (2001) provide the viewer with a direct experience of "being there" without any narration or formal interviews. In Cinema Vérité, while often very similar to Direct Cinema, the role of the documentarian is more evident. However, the filmmaker's appearance in the film is a result of their subjects' reaction to them or because they inadvertently became involved while filming. The classic Cinema Vérité work, *Harlan County, USA* (1976) includes an attack on the film crew by the striking Kentucky coal miners who are the film's subject.

In the Essay documentary, the filmmaker is a much more central figure. Michael Moore best typifies this approach to documentaries. In films such as *Sicko*, in which he compares the United States health-care system to that of several other countries, Moore is the central character. In keeping with the essay approach, he organizes the film sequences and intersperses them with newsreel footage to make a particular point – namely, weaknesses of the US health-care system compared with other Western countries.

Below is a listing of the topics covered.

Topic	Film
Autism	*A Mother's Courage: Talking Back to Autism* (2009)
Childhood vaccination controversy	*The Vaccine War* (2010)
Childhood obesity	*Killer at Large* (2008)
Academic struggles	*Waiting for "Superman"* (2010)
School violence and handguns	*Bowling for Columbine* (2002)
Sexual identity/parental mental illness	*Tarnation* (2003)
Adolescents and the Internet	*Frontline: Growing Up Online* (2008)
Domestic violence	*Domestic Violence* (2001)
Substance abuse (heroin dependence)	*Methadonia* (2005)
HIV/AIDS	*The Age of AIDS* (2006)
Genetic testing (breast cancer risk)	*In the Family* (2008)
Suicide and the survivors	*The Bridge* (2006)
Logotherapy/existential perspectives	*Grizzly Man* (2005)
Posttraumatic stress disorder	*Prisoner of Her Past* (2010)
Obsessive-compulsive disorder (hoarding)	*My Mother's Garden* (2008)
Medical ethics: decision making at the end of life	*Near Death* (2004)
Medical ethics: physician-assisted suicide	*The Suicide Tourist* (2007)

References

1 Macdonald K, Cousins M, editors. *Imagining Reality: the Faber book of documentary.* London: Faber & Faber; 1996.
2 Vogels JB. *The Direct Cinema of David and Albert Maysles.* Carbondale, IL: Southern Illinois University Press; 2005.

Autism
• • • • • • • • • • •

Autism, a developmental disability characterized by severe language and social skill deficits, is being diagnosed with increasing frequency. Other features of the condition include rigid adherence to routines and rituals, restricted affect, and the inability to form peer relationships.[1] Often, children with this condition will exhibit normal development until their second year when functioning deteriorates. Historically, parenting style ("cold"/distant demeanor) was seen as an etiological factor while current evidence supports a neurological explanation for autism.[2] Some clinicians and investigators have argued that persons with autism can demonstrate sophisticated communication with letter boards guided by a facilitator. This approach, facilitated communication is controversial and has relatively little research support.[3]

A Mother's Courage: Talking Back to Autism (2010; Fridrik Thor Fridriksson; Frontier; approximately 1 hour 45 minutes): The film presents a family from Iceland comprised of mother, father, and three sons. One of the sons, Keli, is diagnosed with autism. The family is seeking intervention to help their son communicate. After interviewing multiple US experts on the condition, they bring Keli to the HALO Foundation, where a type of facilitated communication, rapid prompting, has been developed. Keli appears to respond to rapid prompting.

1 (0:05:30–0:08:29) Keli is seen in his school. It is noted that he is being trained on basic self-care skills. He then is seen on the soccer field with other "typical" children. While the other children are actively engaged in the game, Keli is with them, but not really participating and is carrying a tree branch.
   a. Which symptoms of autism does Keli exhibit?
   b. Keli is being mainstreamed (taught in a regular versus special education class) for some activities but in special classes for others. What are the advantages and disadvantages of mainstreaming for a child-like Keli?

2 (0:09:50–0:15:30) A family in Minnesota with three sons diagnosed with autism. One of the sons has yet to be formally diagnosed and the film follows the family as they take him to a specialty clinic for evaluation. Some of the testing procedures used for assessing and diagnosing possible autism are shown. Additionally, the mother's distress about having a son with autism is poignantly displayed.
   a. Which symptoms of autism do the children exhibit?
   b. How would you counsel the mother?
   c. There appears to be a significantly elevated risk of divorce among couples with a child diagnosed with autism. What types of suggestions might you give to improve the quality of the marital relationship among these couples?

3 (1:10:00–1:20:00) Keli's parents take him to a therapist who uses a form of facilitated communication, the rapid prompting method. Even though Keli does not know English, Soma, the therapist, indicates that he can communicate through her approach.
   a. What is your opinion regarding whether Keli is genuinely communicating through rapid prompting?
   b. Why do these techniques become popular in working with children with autism?
   c. What is your advice to parents of a child with autism about these techniques and whether their child should receive these forms of communication therapy?

References

1 American Psychiatric Association. *Diagnostic and Statistical Manual of Mental Disorders*. 4th ed. Washington, DC: 2000.
2 Wicks-Nelson R, Israel AC. *Abnormal Child and Adolescent Psychology*. 7th ed. Upper Saddle River, NJ: Pearson Prentice Hall; 2009.
3 Jacobson JW, Mulick JA, Schwartz AA. A history of facilitated communication: science, pseudoscience, and antiscience. *Am Psychol*. 1995; **50**: 750–5.

Childhood Vaccination Controversy

The measles, mumps, and rubella (MMR) and influenza vaccine have been the subject of recent controversy. In the popular media, the vaccines have been linked to neuromuscular conditions and developmental disabilities such as autism. While many of the positive associations have been based on case reports, larger scale epidemiological studies have not supported these conclusions. The rise in Internet use and social media appears to fuel much of the public perceptions that vaccinations are harmful and unnecessary.[1] A challenge for physicians is to be able to accurately convey the level of risk associated with vaccinations and educate parents and adult patients while countering popular, unsupported claims.

The Vaccine War (2010; PBS; approximately 1 hour): Many parents in the United States are choosing not to have their children receive recommended vaccinations. The controversy surrounding the role of childhood vaccines and autism pits medical science against celebrities and social media. There is concern about a renewed rise in childhood communicable diseases as a result of this publicity. Conversations with researchers, practicing physicians, celebrities, and antivaccine activists are included.

1 (0:04:55–0:08:50) In Ashland, Oregon, 28% of children are currently unvaccinated. A mother states that illness is "natural," while vaccination is not. There are concerns by public health officials about possible outbreaks of vaccine preventable disease.
   a. What is your reaction to the position that these vaccines are no longer needed?
   b. How would you respond to the mother depicted, who does not see it as necessary for children to be vaccinated?
   c. How does increasingly global travel impact susceptibility to infectious disease?
2 (0:09:00–0:11:00) In San Diego, parents can obtain a "personal belief exemption" so that their children do not have to be vaccinated when they enter school. There has been recent concern about increases in measles in nearby suburbs.
   a. From an ethical perspective, what is your opinion of the of personal belief

exemption for childhood vaccination? Which ethical principles are in conflict here?

b. Should these exemptions be legally permitted?

c. If you were a public health officer in San Diego, how would you address this issue?

3 (0:18:30–0:21:30) Scientists and physicians at the Centers for Disease Control and Prevention (CDC) are struggling with the issue about how to accurately convey risks of vaccines without seeming alarmist. The head of the National Vaccine Infant Information Center, a private organization, is critical of vaccinations and offers information about negative side effects.

a. Go to the CDC website on childhood vaccinations. What is your opinion about the balance of accurate information conveyed and whether the communication is responsible versus alarmist?

b. Go to the National Vaccine Information Center website. What is your assessment of the accuracy of the information presented here?

4 (0:31:00–0:38:20) Wakefield's paper[2] on the role of vaccines in autism is discussed, along with multiple larger scale epidemiological studies that have not found any difference between autism rates among those who received the MMR versus those who were not vaccinated. However, activists do not accept these findings and appear to rely heavily on anecdotal case reports.

a. Read the original Wakefield paper in the *Lancet*.[2] In your assessment of the report, are there flaws in the study that are apparent?

b. Read the retraction of Wakefield study in the *Lancet*. Were any of these issues apparent in your critique of the original article?

c. Despite the overwhelming evidence,[3] antivaccine activists still believe that there is a link between vaccination and autism. Why do you believe this to be the case?

d. Examine the report from Denmark. Apply Hill's criteria[4] for inferring causality to these reports. Do you believe that the reports effectively refute the autism vaccination link?

References

1 Offit PA, Coffin SE. Communicating science to the public: MMR vaccine and autism. *Vaccine*. 2003; **22**: 1–6.

2 Wakefield AJ, Murch SH, Anthony A. Ileal-lymphoid-nodular hyperplasia, non-specific colitis, and pervasive developmental disorder in children. *Lancet*. 1998; **351**: 637–41.

3 Madsen K, Hvid A, Vestergaard M, *et al*. A population-based study of measles, mumps and rubella vaccination and autism. *N Engl J Med*. 2002; **347**(19): 1477–82.

4 Hill AB. The environment and disease: association or causation? *Proc R Soc Med*. 1965; **58**: 295–300.

Childhood Obesity
••••••••••••••••••••••••

According to the US Department of Agriculture, only about 20% of young children's diets are classified as "good," meaning that they have no more than recommended levels of fat, cholesterol, and sodium and otherwise conform to the recommended "Food Pyramid."[1] Among adolescents, only 5% meet this standard. At present, approximately one in five American children are overweight.[1] Between 1982 and 1994, there was a 10-fold increase in type II diabetes among children.[2] It is estimated that 100 000 deaths per year are attributable to obesity including one-third of all cancer deaths. Beginning early in their development, there are strong social forces, including the media, that encourage and sustain children's loyalty to fast food and high sugar cereals.

Killer at Large: Why Obesity is America's Greatest Threat (2008; Shinebox Media; 1 hour 42 minutes): This documentary argues that obesity is a much greater threat to American society than terrorism. Brief interviews with former president Clinton and Senators Harkin and Brownback among others are interspersed with fast food and cereal ads directed toward children. Former surgeon general Cardona describes being "muzzled" on the issue of childhood obesity by the Bush Administration because of the influence of food companies.

1 (0:03:20–0:13:00) A liposuction procedure is performed on a 12-year-old girl. She is followed through the film while she regains the weight lost in the procedure. By the film's end, she and her parents are preparing to have the procedure performed again in Mexico.
   a. What is your reaction to a child of this age receiving liposuction?
   b. What are the risks of liposuction at this age?
   c. Why are patients who have had these procedures very likely to regain lost weight?
2 (0:47:00–0:58:24) Amidst multiple short clips of a typical high school cafeteria, physical education teachers, policymakers, and critics as well as politicians describe many of the factors associated with the rise in childhood obesity. The impact of US Department of Agriculture policy as well as No Child Left Behind legislation is also discussed.
   a. What are some recent Government policies that may be contributing to childhood and adolescent obesity?
   b. Several of those interviewed indicated that adolescents are engaging in far less physical activity today. Why do you believe this is the case?
   c. How would you counsel an obese adolescent?
3 (0:59:39–1:06:28) Discussions of how children develop habits of eating sweetened cereals and fast food are interspersed with television advertisements of these products directed toward children.
   a. Young children may not be able to make the distinction between a TV show and the commercials accompanying it. What impact do you believe this has on children as consumers?

b. What role do you believe parents should have in children's dietary habits? Why do you believe it is difficult for parents to overcome the unhealthy dietary choices that are advertised to children?

References

1 National Institute of Child Health and Human Development. *NICHD and other NIH Institutes Aim to Prevent Obesity and Overweight in Children.* Washington, DC: NICHD.

2 Koplan JP, Liverman CT, Kraak VI, editors. *Preventing Childhood Obesity: health in the balance.* Washington, DC: National Academies Press.

Academic Struggles

Waiting for "Superman" (2010; Davis Guggenheim; Electric Kinney Films; 111 minutes): Director Davis Guggenheim narrates a broad investigation of the American school system. Children and concerned parents from all over the country describe the failings of their public schools. The parents strive to get their children into chartered and private schools, but the huge demand from likeminded parents has led to a random lottery system, leaving most children with the less desired status quo. Experts such as Michelle Rhee, the Washington, DC, Chancellor of Public Schools, offer their perspective as they try to reform "drop-out factories" (schools that graduate 60% or less of their students). Guggenheim explores the difficulties of firing bad teachers because of tenure laws and the strong teachers' union. Through interviews with leaders at KIPP, SEED, and other successful charter schools, parents are given the chance to place their kids on more academically successful tracks. We follow the children as they put their hopes against the school lottery systems.

Academic Decline/Dropout

1 (0:18:49–0:22:25) Social activist Geoffrey Canada questions the mind-set children have when their grades drop over the years. What causes a "B" student to change to a "D" student in a couple of years, and how do they see themselves? In East Los Angeles, the parents of a fifth grader, Daisy, offer their own perspectives and reasons why they dropped out of high school.
   a. Though both of Daisy's parents dropped out of high school, Daisy states that she plans to go to either medical or veterinarian school, knowing how many years of higher education that requires. Describe a few social and cultural factors that contribute to the decision to drop out of school?
   b. What practical methods can teachers and counselors implement in their schools to help improve children's self-efficacy?
   c. Does the label of a "dropout factory" create a patterned way of thinking within the school? Practically, how can the patterned mind-set of "failure" be broken in a subculture such as a school?

Improving Public Education via Raising Teacher Standards

1   (1:22:40–1:26:05) Chancellor of the Washington, DC, Public Schools, Michelle Rhee, tries to implement sweeping changes to improve DC's inadequate school system. She tries to remove tenure laws by incentivizing good teaching with pay bonuses. Her proposal is denied by the teachers' union.

   a. Rhee tries to alter the mind-set of "teaching." Instead of seeing it as a "right," Rhee tries to make it a "privilege." How might reframing techniques be used in the workplace to increase productivity?

   b. What are a few psychological consequences of working in a system that is perceived to be unchangeable? What are some therapeutic methods to reduce stress and depression in fields where needed change is slow to take place?

   c. In one of the scenes, Rhee quickly asks a student in class what he thinks of his teacher. What are effective ways for school personnel to get students' input about what works?

School Violence and Handguns

Bowling for Columbine (2002; Michael Moore; Dog Eat Dog Films; 120 minutes): In this Academy Award–winning documentary, Michael Moore explores the roots of the obsession the United States has with guns and violence. This documentary is made following the 1999 Columbine High School massacre. After Moore investigates the motivations of the Columbine shooters, he expands his investigation onto the entire country. With interviews and statistics, Moore asks why the murder rate in the United States is significantly higher than other developed countries. He discovers that US culture has a disposition towards fear, bigotry, and violence that is perpetuated by the news media. Juxtaposing tragic imagery with sardonic humor, Moore confronts business and media leaders with the knowledge that they are contributing to the culture's problems.

1   (0:55:58–1:01:19) Moore narrates over a montage of fear mongering in the media. There are clips from the Y2K scare, killer bees, and terror threats from then president Bush. Author and sociologist Barry Glassner discusses the "culture of fear" that the media reinforces.

   a. What emotions do these images elicit, and how might they affect a person's perception? How might someone become addicted to fear-enforcing media?

   b. How might these media images affect US culture?

   c. Apart from fear, what other factors might affect a person's disposition towards violence?

2   (0:41:31–0:47:50) In a similar media montage, Moore explores the news stories that were popular immediately after the Columbine massacre, which

reflect and enhance the culture's fear of children and students. Then Moore interviews singer Marilyn Manson.

   a. In a few of the clips, teachers and school authorities react with aggressive suspicion to their students. How might procedures such as metal detector screening and zero-tolerance suspensions affect a developing mind?

   b. After a tragedy or act of violence in a school, how should teachers, counselors, and administrators respond?

   c. What effect do video games and music have on a person's disposition toward violence? Were people right to criticize musicians such as Marilyn Manson?

3 (1:04:15–1:06:52) In South Los Angeles, Moore interviews author and sociologist Barry Glassner, who discusses how news stories enhance bigotry in US culture.

   a. Glassner offers this statistic: After a 20% decrease in the murder rate, the media coverage of murder increased by 600%. What effect might disparities like this have on a community?

   b. Glassner believes the news media perpetuates racial bigotry in the United States. Is his argument valid? How might the news media and other forms of media perpetuate racial bigotry?

Sexual Identity/Parental Mental Illness

Tarnation (2003; Jonathon Caouette; Wellspring Media; 88 minutes): Told through home-videos, super-8 footage, and video diaries, this documentary is the autobiography of Jonathon Caouette. Starting in his childhood, Jonathon grows up with a mother who, in her youth, was incorrectly treated with electroshock therapy, resulting in schizophrenia. At a young age, Jonathon witnesses a man rape his mother, and he sees many of her psychotic episodes. With an absent father and mentally ill mother, Jonathon is placed in foster care, where he is beaten and emotionally abused by his foster parents. After a few years, Jonathon's caring grandparents gain custody of him while his mother lives in a mental hospital. Jonathon grows up surrounded by moments of turmoil, but he finds escape through films, acting, and playing with his camera. As he gets older, Jonathon comes out as gay and lives with his boyfriend in New York. Occasionally, his mother lives with them. Jonathon tries to find mental security, given his tumultuous upbringing and mentally ill mother.

Sexual Identity Development and Depersonalization Disorder

1 (0:22:23–0:27:20) Over home-video footage and fictional horror scenes, a young Jonathon reveals his homosexuality, memories of being molested, and his conflicting inner dialogue. We learn that Jonathon was wrongfully given PCP dipped in formaldehyde, resulting in his depersonalization disorder.

   a. At a young age, Jonathon expresses his confusion over his sexuality.

Drawing from the clip, can you describe typical issues in sexual identity development in adolescents?

b. A few of the symptoms of depersonalization disorder are described in the clip. What are all the symptoms, as described by the DSM-IV-TR criteria? Does Jonathon exhibit some of these symptoms?

c. As a health-care provider, how can you assist individuals with this disorder cope? In addition to having depersonalization disorder, what other disorders are also often present?

Parental Mental Illness/Overdose/Brain Damage

1 (1:09:55–1:18:41) In this difficult-to-watch segment, Jonathon learns that his mother has overdosed on lithium and is brain-damaged. He visits her and his grandfather and films her psychotic episodes.

a. If a brain-damaged person is to continue to live in a house, what structures and protections need to be present for the care of that person?

b. Depending on the origins of brain damage, the prognosis varies. Can you describe treatments used to help restore some brain function?

Anxiety about Inheriting Mental Illness

1 (1:20:53–1:25:26) An adult Jonathon locks himself in his apartment bathroom. He is currently living with his boyfriend and his brain-damaged mother. He confesses some of his anxieties about his future, given that he has a mentally ill mother.

a. What are a few of the concerns that Jonathon expresses, both directly and indirectly, about how his mother's mental illness affects him?

b. What are typical fears and anxieties that children of mentally ill parents face? How can they be educated and reassured?

c. Can you describe ways to help protect children from experiencing these fears in the future? What are a few protective therapies?

Adolescents and the Internet

While all physicians who treat children and adolescents often counsel patients and parents about violent television and video games, less attention has been paid to the impact of the Internet on development. Being aware of adolescents' online activity is particularly important, given that computers are the preferred media for 8- to 18-year-olds – far outweighing video games and television.[1] Among 14- to 18-year-olds, the average time spent on the Internet is 50 minutes per day. At least 20% of adolescents report receiving a sexual solicitation online.[2] There has also been growing concern about cyber "bullying" online with several publicized suicides associated with this practice. Approximately 20% of children and adolescents report being victims of cyber bullying while 10% reported being online bullies themselves.[3]

Frontline: Growing Up Online (2008; PBS; 56 minutes): The film describes how the Internet is affecting the current generation of adolescents. Parents share their concerns about potential consequences of having their children "grow up online." However, at the same time, there is considerable evidence that parents are unaware of their children's online activities. Several health risks associated with Internet use among adolescents are portrayed. These include cyber bullying and Internet sites supporting eating disordered behaviors such as purging.

1 (0:21:30–0:24:13) Jessica is an adolescent girl who developed an alternate online persona, including suggestive pictures. Eventually, her parents became aware of it and forced her to remove her suggestive website. Jessica describes how she often misses the notoriety associated with her alternate online identity.

    a. Is trying on different identities a problem in adolescence or a normal developmental process? What are some of the implications of the Internet for trying out various identities?

    b. Does Jessica appear to appreciate any of the risks involved in posting suggestive pictures of herself?

    c. Jessica's website had been up for some time before her father became aware of it through another adult. How should parents monitor adolescent activities?

2 (0:31:57–0:34:43) Sarah uses the Internet to find tips to maintain her eating disorder. There are online sites, including message boards, used primarily by young women to obtain advice on binging, purging, not eating, and losing weight.

    a. Does Sarah meet criteria for an eating disorder?

    b. What is the potential impact of Internet sites that are clearly "pro-eating disorder" and which promote this behavior?

3 (0:40:10–0:50:15) Ryan is a young man who committed suicide after being bullied online. His father is interviewed and describes how he found out about the online interactions that precipitated his son's suicide.

    a. What would difference are there between being bullied online from being bullied face to face?

    b. What are the risk factors that may predispose an adolescent to suicide?

    c. The parents in this documentary seem almost oblivious to their children's online activity. How would you counsel parents to monitor their children's Internet use?

    d. To what extent were you aware of the issues depicted in this documentary?

References

1 Hellenga K. Social space, the final frontier: adolescents on the Internet. In: Mortimer JT, Larson RW, editors. *The Changing Adolescent Experience: societal trends and the transition to adulthood*. New York, NY: Cambridge University Press; 2002. pp. 208–49.

2 Arnett JJ. *Adolescence and Emerging Adulthood*. 4th ed. Boston, MA: Prentice Hall; 2010.

3 Hinduja S, Patchin JW. *Cyberbullying Victimization*. Cyberbullying Research Center; 2010. Available at: www.cyberbullying.us/2010_charts/cyberbullying_victim_2010.jpg

The Reality of Domestic Violence

Approximately one in four women are victims of domestic violence.[1] Victims of domestic violence are commonly seen in primary care clinics, mental health settings, and emergency departments. In addition to presenting with injuries directly associated with abuse, victims of domestic violence appear to seek medical care more frequently for nonspecific symptoms.[1] Some useful questions for screening for domestic violence include "Do you feel safe at home?" "Are you ever afraid of your partner?" "How are things at home?"[1] For women continuing to reside with a batterer, developing a "safe plan" for possible future assaults is indicated.

Domestic Violence (2001; Fredrick Wiseman; Zipporah Films; 196 minutes): Wiseman films multiple aspects of domestic violence. These include police responding to incidents and talking with women about options for prosecution. Filming also occurs in a domestic violence shelter and includes counseling sessions, intake sessions, as well as a group therapy session with children. In a similar vein as his other films (see *Near Death*), Wiseman does not provide any narration and leaves it up to the viewer to interpret the film.

1 (0:17:00–0:22:27) The police arrive on the scene where a woman is covered in blood. The alleged perpetrator is not present. The police talk with a neighbor who provides some background information.

   a. This scene is somewhat disturbing. How you believe it affects police officers who frequently encounter these situations?

   b. What are some social factors depicted here that are often associated with domestic violence?

2 (0:23:35–0:32:10) We see a busy hotline at a women's domestic violence shelter. An older woman relates her history of abuse to one of the caseworkers during an intake interview.

   a. What is your reaction to the responses of the hotline workers?

   b. The client being seen for an intake interview indicates that she had previously obtained an order of protection. What is an order of protection? Why are they frequently ineffective?

3 (0:37:50–0:43:32) A shelter client undergoes screening assessment for different types of domestic abuse. The client indicates that she experienced multiple forms of emotional, physical, and sexual abuse. She indicates that she has left her partner at least 15 times.

   a. What are the different types of abuse that are part of the screening interview? Were you aware of the broad range of types of abuse?

    b. A pattern that often accompanies violence is that the perpetrator attempts to control their partner through psychological, social, and financial means. What types of coercion does the client report?

4 (0:44:00–0:48:05) A new client describes an incident occurring the previous day that led her to come to the shelter. She provides a graphic account of physical and psychological abuse as well as being threatened with murder.

    a. What is the role of substance use in domestic violence, as suggested by this incident?

    b. The client reports that she was sure that neighbors heard her screaming, but did nothing. Why do you believe this failure to respond occurs?

    c. A common sequela of domestic violence is posttraumatic stress disorder. How would an incident like the one described contribute to posttraumatic stress disorder?

5 (0:54:35–0:63:10) An attorney and client discussed possible prosecution of the woman's husband. Client indicates that she had recanted and withdrew charges in prior incidents of being assaulted by her husband. She also has apparently withheld details of a recent incident of abuse use from the prosecuting attorney

    a. What types of issues make it difficult to successfully prosecute perpetrators of domestic violence?

    b. Why do you believe that the victim is being protective of her husband?

6 (0:70:45–0:76:17) This clip shows a therapy group for children exposed to the violence. The therapist uses children's drawings to stimulate conversation.

    a. Which types of incidents do the children report witnessing?

    b. What is the likely impact of witnessing domestic violence on children?

    c. One of the children described being spanked. What do you believe about the appropriateness and effectiveness of spanking? What are your thoughts about the effectiveness of spanking in the households being described by the children?

Reference

1 Chadhi S, Rovi S, Vega A, et al. Intimate partner violence and cancer screening among urban minority women. J Am Board Fam Med. 2010; 23: 343–53.

Substance Abuse (Heroin Dependence)

Heroin and oxycodone are relatively commonly abused drugs. It is estimated that there are a quarter million people in the United States dependent on heroin.[1] Treating opiate addiction is particularly difficult because of the severity of withdrawal symptoms. These include nausea, vomiting, chills, muscle aches, diarrhea, and insomnia. For persons dependent on heroin, a controversial treatment has been substitution of methadone for heroin. These symptoms are particularly intense for 1–3 days and have disappeared in a week after last heroin use.[1] Methadone is a substitute opiate used to prevent heroin withdrawal. There is considerable evidence that methadone maintenance significantly reduces the likelihood of heroin relapse as well as related criminal activity.[2] In addition, because methadone is taken orally, there is a reduced risk of conditions such as HIV associated with injection drug use. However, there is concern that many former heroin addicts become dependent on methadone.

Methadonia (2005; Michel Negroponte; First Run Features; 88 minutes): This film depicts persons at various stages of methadone treatment for heroin addiction. The general tenor of the film is critical of methadone. While *Methadonia* presents heroin addiction's reality very effectively, there are two issues in using segments of the film for education. First, the film tends to jump back and forth between patient stories. Second, at multiple points during the film, the subjects being interviewed will abruptly begin to "nod" from heroin's effects.

1   The narrator notes that many former heroin users combined methadone with either Xanax or Clonazepam to produce a "high." Physicians should be aware that these minor tranquilizers are often used illicitly.
    a. What do you think of the use of methadone as a treatment for heroin addiction?
    b. Were you aware of the use of benzodiazepines to augment the effects of methadone? Would this alter your prescribing practices?
    c. Most of these patients have been using heroin and or methadone for at least a decade. How would you approach the patient like this in your own practice?

2   (0:45:28–0:50:09) Several patients on methadone maintenance are interviewed in some detail. Among them is a 38-year-old woman who is pregnant and whose husband is released from jail. She sees a physician for prenatal care and describes being on methadone, and likely benzodiazepines, through the pregnancy. She and her husband are shown at home.
    a. What are the risks to the fetus associated with opiate and benzodiazepine use during pregnancy?
    b. What would be the effects of opiate withdrawal during pregnancy?
    c. She describes having had other children who were removed from her custody. Do you believe that she and Eddie can parent effectively? Why or why not?

3   (1:13:26–1:15:59) Steve wants to get off of methadone. He talks with another methadone user who is pessimistic about Steve's ability to succeed "cold turkey." Steve stops methadone and has pronounced withdrawal symptoms. There is some discussion by the narrator about how methadone clinics, since they are private businesses, are often not very supportive of patients wishing to reduce their use of methadone, since it directly impacts on their finances.
    a. Which symptoms does Steve exhibit during withdrawal?
    b. Do you believe that withdrawal can occur on an outpatient basis or should only be done as an inpatient? Why?

References

1 American Psychiatric Association. *Diagnostic and Statistical Manual of Mental Disorders.* 4th ed. Washington, DC: APA; 2000.
2 Farrell M, Ward J, Mattick R, *et al.* Methadone maintenance treatment in opiate dependence: a review. *Br Med J.* 1994; **309**: 997–1001.

HIV/AIDS
• • • • • • • • • • • • • •

AIDS was initially described in 1983. Twenty years later, the virus had infected more than 60 million people – a third of these individuals have died.[1] As an emerging infection, the etiology of AIDS was determined through classic epidemiology as different segments of the population such as gay males, intravenous drug users, and recipients of blood donations, exhibited a higher incidence of the disease.[1] While AIDS became well known after the death of the actor Rock Hudson, there was still considerable public disparagement of those with the disease. Government policies were conflicted about issues such as open HIV prevention strategies and even research on the virus. Policies on HIV reduction strategies such as providing clean needles to heroin users are still controversial.

The Age of AIDS (2006; PBS; 4 hours): This documentary provides a detailed history of AIDS. The film does a particularly good job of describing the origins of the disease and the accompanying epidemiological research. The political and social aspects of AIDS are also highlighted.
1 (0:04:15–0:14:15) In the early 1980s, several unusual cases of young men with Karposi sarcoma were reported. Two California physicians describe these patients. The finding of the disease among gay male patients, recent African immigrants to Europe, and intravenous drug users is described.
   a. Which approach to epidemiological case identification is depicted?
   b. While today we know the population risk factors for HIV, these were not well known in the early 1980s. What are the issues that made it difficult to specify risk factors for the disease?
2 (0:26:06–0:28:05; 0:29:21–0:37:00) The scope of the illness expands with cases in the Congo, Haiti, and Europe and in heterosexual males as well as females. In the United States, bathhouses frequented by gay males are targeted.
   a. If you were an epidemiologist working on HIV at this point in time, how would you proceed in looking for causes of the disease?
   b. In the United States at this time, AIDS was generally characterized as a disease of gay males. Why did these other cases not involving gay males have little impact on this perception?
   c. If you were a public health officer in San Francisco at this time, how would you have handled the issue of bathhouses?

3 (0:58:00–0:61:47) Rock Hudson, the actor, is severely ill. Eventually, it is determined that he has AIDS, and he permits this to be publicly known. While gay activists have had difficulty engaging public attention around HIV/AIDS, Hudson's death from AIDS garners considerable public attention.

   a. What impact did Hudson's death have on public perceptions of HIV/AIDs?

   b. Can you think of other celebrities who have become associated with particular diseases? What impact does this have on public perception of the disease?

4 (1:01:24–1:04:20) While testing is strongly encouraged, there is also a public backlash when children with hemophilia are found to be HIV-positive because of blood transfusions. Parents openly protest sending their children to schools where an HIV-positive child is in attendance, analogizing it to "pointing a loaded gun at their own children."

   a. Are there infectious diseases today that have elicited a similar response?

   b. How would you counsel parents who are concerned about their children becoming infected as a result of attending school with an HIV-positive child?

5 (1:26:40–1:30:58) In England, a major route of transmission appears to be through intravenous drug use – particularly heroin. A needle exchange program is implemented. A similar program when initiated in the United States has far less governmental support. One of the leaders of the needle exchange program has been arrested multiple times for distributing clean syringes and needles.

   a. What is the public health rationale for needle exchange programs?

   b. What are the legal issues associated with these programs?

   c. In analyzing needle exchange programs from the perspective of Beauchamp and Childress',[2] four dimensions of principalism in medical ethics (autonomy, beneficence, nonmaleficence, justice) can be applied. Which dimensions are particularly salient?

References

1 Fauci A. HIV and AIDS: 20 years of science. *Nat Med.* 2003; **9**(7): 839–43.

2 Beauchamp TL, Childress JF. *Principles of Biomedical Ethics.* 6th ed. New York, NY: Oxford University Press; 2009.

Genetic Testing (Breast Cancer Risk)

The knowledge that some forms of breast and ovarian cancer have strong heritability has contributed to research on specific genes predisposing individuals to these conditions. The BRCA1/2 mutation is one of the best known and carries with it a 70%–90% risk of developing breast cancer. This raises a number of ethical issues, including whether these women should reproduce and then have a prophylactic mastectomy and hysterectomy. Because of the relatively early onset of breast cancer among those predisposed, this decision will have to typically be made in their 20s or 30s.

In the Family (2008; Joanna Rudnick; Kartemquin films; approximately 90 minutes): This is a film made by a 31-year-old woman who is at high risk for genetically determined breast cancer (BRCA1). It could be beneficial to view this film in its entirety. Joanna Rudnick intersperses her own decision making about whether to have a prophylactic mastectomy and hysterectomy with discussions between herself and her boyfriend, breast cancer support groups, multiple oncologists, and other women and family members at risk for breast cancer.

1   (0:05:24–0:11:05) Background information about BRCA1 and the high associated risk for breast and ovarian cancer is presented. Ms. Rudnick's physician sees her for surveillance. She is told that she has a 75%–90% risk for breast cancer and a 50% or 60% risk of ovarian cancer. She has her boyfriend present during the physician's counseling.
    a. Critique the physician's discussion of cancer risk with the patient.
    b. What issues are raised by the boyfriend's presence at the visit?
    c. Ms. Rudnick indicates that she wants to have children. How would you counsel her under these circumstances?

2   (0:11:06–0:12:03) Ms. Rudnick and her boyfriend talk about the information presented by the physician.
    a. What does he mean when he says he feels that he is being selfish?
    b. What are some of the issues with which Ms Rudnick and her boyfriend are struggling?

3   (0:27:50–0:29:15) A family of young women whose mother has breast cancer prepares to go for genetic counseling. The sisters have all been tested for the BRCA1 allele. A genetic counselor and physician deliver the results of the tests to the sisters, their significant others, and mother.
    a. During the car ride, it appears that the younger sister is at least ambivalent about being tested. Under the circumstances, do you believe that she experiences subtle coercion? Given the circumstances, do you believe that she should be tested? Why or why not?
    b. During the counseling session, the sister who does not carry the allele seems particularly distressed. Why do you believe that she is so upset?
    c. What is your opinion about how the results of the tests are given?
    d. Do you believe that the women should be informed individually instead of in a group?

4   (0:43:10–0:46:20) Ms. Rudnick visits a support group of African-American women who have or are at genetic risk for breast cancer. Rudnick attends a church service with some of the women.
    a. African-American women are four times less likely than women of white European background to receive genetic testing for breast cancer. What are some of the reasons for this disparity?

b. One of the women makes reference to the Tuskegee Study. Why is this historical study relevant to genetic testing?

c. One of the women explicitly states that she does not want to know her genetic risk status. She supports her position by stating that she has enough stress in her life as it is. Is her position reasonable? How would you respond to her?

Reference

1 Patenaude Farkas A. *Genetic Testing for Cancer: psychological approaches for helping patients and families*. Washington, DC: American Psychological Association; 2004.

Suicide and the Survivors

The Bridge (2006; Eric Steel; Koch Lorber Films; 93 minutes): In 2004, Eric Steel set up a camera below the Golden Gate Bridge and captured 23 of the 24 suicides that year. Steel interviews friends, families, bystanders, and survivors. He documents how the people left behind cope and make sense of the decision to commit suicide. The film depicts scenes of both suicide and rescue. At times, friends and family try to comprehend the reasons why their loved ones ended their lives. Many of the jumpers struggle with depression, mental illness, and substance abuse. More people commit suicide off the Golden Gate Bridge than any other place in the world. Steel explores why people choose this place instead of others.

1 (0:46:55–0:52:50) A suicide survivor, Kevin Hines, recounts his story. He describes what was going through his mind before and after his attempt.

a. Hines is later diagnosed with bipolar disorder. When he describes his thought process, what evidence of bipolar disorder do you see?

b. Apart from bipolar disorder, what other common warning signs do you see in Hines's life at the time?

c. After his suicide attempt, Hines describes how his friends and family treat him. After surviving a suicide attempt, what are positive ways for friends and family to interact with the survivor?

2 (1:01:42–1:04:52) Police prevent a crystal-meth addict's suicide. The man describes his thought process just before. A woman who survived describes her thought process and her possible motivation.

a. As depicted in the clip, what aspects of addiction potentially lead to suicide?

b. At the end of the second clip, the woman states that perhaps she hoped someone would tell her, "No, don't do it." How should one respond to a "cry for help" attempt without reinforcing the behavior in the future?

3 (0:26:50–0:28:16) Friends of Gene discuss a few of the warning signs that he exhibited before killing himself.

    a. In addition to the warning signs Gene exhibits, what are other common warning signs for suicide?

    b. What are common problems that the people left behind face after a suicide?

4 (1:07:13–1:12:03) Over images of suicide notes, friends and family describe what they thought the jumpers were like.

    a. What feelings and thought processes do the suicide notes express?

    b. There is an example of incorrect antidepressant use above. Please describe what should accompany the use of antidepressants.

    c. Director Eric Steel does not interfere with the jumpers and potential jumpers on the bridge. Does this film alter your perception on the idea of euthanasia? If so, how?

Logotherapy/Existential Perspectives

Grizzly Man (2005; Werner Herzog; Real Big Production; 2005): This film illuminates the life and death of Timothy Treadwell, an amateur grizzly bear expert and environmental activist. Treadwell spent 13 summers living inside of bear territories in Alaska. In 2003, a rogue bear, not from the territory, kills both Treadwell and his girlfriend, Amie Huguenard. Herzog interviews family, friends, and people who believe Treadwell's death was inevitable. With footage that Treadwell shot of himself, we see that Treadwell is a complicated person who has overcome depression and addiction with something he found meaningful.

1 (1:05:47–1:09:53) A friend of Treadwell describes his troubles with alcohol and drugs. She describes how Treadwell refused antidepressants because he wanted his emotional highs and lows. In Treadwell's footage, we see very emotive scenes.

    a. Without diagnosing Treadwell, the scene displays traits of bipolar disorder. What are common symptoms of bipolar? What are the risks of leaving it untreated?

    b. In the later scenes, Treadwell is experiencing extreme emotional highs. How can a health-care professional respond to a person with bipolar disorder who is afraid of losing the emotional highs?

2 (0:40:41–0:46:15) In a confessional moment with the camera, Treadwell describes how he once was an alcoholic at rock bottom. Now, he found what he describes as a miraculous feeling of purpose among the grizzly bears.

    a. Logotherapy is concerned with helping patients fill an existential vacuum with meaning. How might this clip be an example of redirecting inner turmoil onto the environment?

    b. In overcoming addiction and mental illness, how can the "will to have meaning" play a role in recovery? When is it appropriate to bring it up in therapy?

Posttraumatic Stress Disorder: Onset in Late Life

Posttraumatic stress disorder (PTSD) is a DSM-IV-TR anxiety disorder characterized by three symptom clusters following an event in which one was afraid of being seriously hurt or killed, or witnessed an event in which somebody else was harmed or threatened with harm: re-experiencing the trauma (nightmares and flashbacks), avoidance of situations associated with the trauma, and persistent symptoms of increased arousal (e.g. difficulty falling asleep).[1] While it is common for symptoms to occur relatively soon after the traumatic event, delayed onset of symptoms may occur when triggered by a present-day event. While delayed onset of symptoms in the absence of any previous PTSD symptoms is rare, exacerbation of previous symptoms is not – particularly among combat veterans.[2] Delayed exacerbations from childhood sexual abuse, and/or sexual assault may occur among adults. Given the high frequency of various types of sexual victimization, it is likely that health-care providers will see patients with either chronic or later life exacerbations of PTSD.

Prisoner of Her Past (2010; Howard Reich, Gordon Quinn, Jerry Blumenthal, Joanna Rudnick, Kartemquin Films; 70 minutes): This is based upon the same-titled book.[3] Howard Reich, a music critic for the *Chicago Tribune*, presents the story of his mother, a Holocaust survivor who develops pronounced posttraumatic stress disorder symptoms late in life. Reich's mother is shown throughout the film, which focuses on his efforts to understand his mother's past and her current distress. Reich travels to New York City as well as to the Ukraine to interview relatives and visit sites from his mother's childhood. The film concludes with Reich visiting a high school in New Orleans to interview students impacted by Hurricane Katrina. Additionally, he shows his mother the book, which served as the basis for the film.

1 (0:00:00–0:07:15) This shows brief clips of Sonia Reich with her son. A psychiatrist explains her symptoms in the context of her childhood experiences during the Holocaust. While many of the pronounced PTSD symptoms shown are of relatively recent onset, her son recalls some unusual behavior that she exhibited during his childhood such as being awake and "on guard" throughout the night.
   a. What are the DSM-IV symptoms of posttraumatic stress disorder?
   b. Which of these symptoms does Ms. Reich exhibit?
   c. Why do you think that these more severe symptoms have appeared only recently?

2 (0:12:15–0:18:56) Ms. Reich often says "I am not a whore; I am not a prostitute." A psychiatrist talks about the sexual abuse that many girls and women experienced during World War II. While asking a male family member questions about events he witnessed during the Holocaust, Reich is repeatedly interrupted by the man's wife who becomes visibly distressed during the conversation.

a. Sexual abuse is, sadly, a common traumatic event in the lives of girls and women, with up to 20% of American young adult women reporting a history of sexual victimization. Which factors are associated with severe forms of PTSD secondary to sexual abuse?

b. Why do you think that the psychiatrist interviewed suggests that Ms. Reich may have been sexually abused?

c. Which of the DSM-IV symptoms is suggested by the wife's agitation and request that Reich and her husband stop talking about the past?

3 (0:40:55–0:48:40) Ms Reich's cousin, Leon, comes to Chicago to visit. Leon visits Ms. Reich at the nursing facility. She initially refuses to acknowledge him and then, visibly distressed, repeatedly asks Leon to leave.

a. How does Ms. Reich respond to Leon's visit?

b. Why do you think that her behavior and verbalizations become particularly disorganized during his visit?

c. Why is she reacting this way to him?

d. The psychiatrist notes a parallel between being fearful of incarceration for being Jewish during the war and Ms. Reich's current situation "incarcerated" in a nursing home. What types of placement options are there for Ms. Reich?

4 (0:50:45–0:53:15) A psychiatrist joins Reich as he visits a high school in New Orleans and listens to adolescent girls describe their experiences during Hurricane Katrina. One of the students begins crying as she describes still having her bag packed in case she needs to leave again suddenly. Reich notes that his mother always had her bag packed as well.

a. While the Holocaust and Hurricane Katrina are obviously very different events, are there shared features that would contribute to PTSD symptoms?

b. Do you believe that the distressed teenager shown here should be formally assessed for PTSD? How would you approach her and evaluate her symptoms.

c. If the girl does meet criteria for PTSD, what types of treatment do you believe would be most helpful?

References

1 American Psychiatric Association. *Diagnostic and Statistical Manual of Mental Disorders.* 4th ed. Washington, DC: APA: 2000.

2 Andrews B, Brewin CR, Philpott R, *et al.* Late-onset posttraumatic stress disorder: a systematic review of the evidence. *Am J Psychiatry.* 2007; **164**: 1319–26.

3 Reich H. *The First and Final Nightmare of Sonia Reich: a son's memoir.* New York, NY: Public Affairs; 2006.

Obsessive-Compulsive Disorder (Hoarding)

Obsessive-compulsive disorder (OCD) is characterized by recurrent and persistent thoughts or images experienced as intrusive and outside of the patient's control. These experiences typically trigger anxiety, which may be reduced temporarily by engaging in some type of repetitive behavior – a compulsion. While the patient typically recognizes that this pattern of behavior is irrational, they do not experience the ability to control it. If they cannot engage in the compulsion, they experience an overwhelming sense of anxiety. To meet criteria for a formal psychiatric disorder, symptoms must occur for at least an hour a day and disrupt daily functioning.[1] Among compulsions, hoarding occurs in about 15% of patients with OCD. Often, patients with hoarding behavior have had their condition for many years before they come to attention. The average age of initiating treatment is approximately 50.[2] When confronted with the possibility of throwing something away, these patients experience intense anxiety and view items such as fast food wrappers as either having potential use or sentimental value. While hoarding often accompanies an obsessive-compulsive disorder, there is growing evidence that there may be a form of severe compulsive hoarding without other OCD symptoms. Approximately 25% of hoarders in a recent study had more severe symptoms in which they kept bizarre items and needed to perform extensive mental compulsions before they could throw anything away.[3]

My Mother's Garden (2009; Cynthia Lester; SeeThroughFilms; 70 minutes): Cindy Lester has made a documentary about her mother, who has severe obsessive-compulsive hoarding disorder. The film begins with the filmmaker and her brothers gathered at their mother's home because the dwelling has become a health hazard and is threatened with being demolished. Amidst considerable emotional distress, Ms. Lester is able to convince her mother to leave her home and join her in her apartment in New York City. However, the hoarding behavior continues, and becomes a source of conflict between mother and daughter. The elder Ms. Lester suddenly returns to her home in California, and is overwhelmed when she finds that her two sons have cleaned the home. She is hospitalized in a psychiatric facility for approximately 1 month, but cannot remain there because of insurance reasons. She then enters an assisted living facility.

1 (0:16:35–0:20:00) After a period of refusing to permit her children into her house, they finally enter. The house is filled with clutter and trash including rat feces.

2 (0:41:05–0:43:30) The house is being cleaned and many items thrown away by her sons. One of Ms. Lester's sons finds a dead rat.

   a. What are the causes of hoarding behavior?

   b. Recent research suggests that hoarding may be a unique condition distinct from obsessive-compulsive disorder. Is the mother's behavior consistent with OCD?

   c. What are the health risks associated with hoarding?

3   (0:44:00–0:46:30) While her house is being cleaned, Ms. Lester accompanies her daughter to New York City. Eventually, she begins rearranging her daughter's apartment and begins hoarding items there as well. After a major conflict with her daughter, Ms. Lester suddenly returns to California.
   a. How effective is moving out of the home as an intervention for hoarding?
   b. Why do you believe that Ms. Lester's boarding behavior is so intractable?
   c. Which symptoms of obsessive-compulsive disorder does Ms. Lester exhibit?

4   (0:50:30–0:55:10) Ms. Lester is taken to a mental health facility. Her daughter consults with a psychologist who briefly describes some of the diagnostic issues. The children are confronted with insurance and financial limitations in paying for their mother's continued care. After a month in an inpatient unit, she is then transferred to an assisted living facility. Her room soon becomes cluttered with new acquisitions.
   a. How effective does Ms. Lester's course of treatment appear to be?
   b. What is your reaction to the role that insurance and financial constraints play in limiting care?
   c. Do you believe that placement in an assisted care facility is warranted? Given the clinical and financial issues, are there other alternatives that might be better?

References

1 American Psychiatric Association. *Diagnostic and Statistical Manual of Mental Disorders*. 4th ed. Washington, DC: APA; 2000.

2 Barlow D, Durand VM. *Abnormal Psychology: an integrative approach*. 6th ed. Belmont, CA: Wadsworth; 2012.

3 Pertusa A, Fullana M, Singh S, *et al*. Compulsive hoarding: OCD symptom, distinct clinical syndrome, or both? *Am J Psychiatry*. 2008; **165**(10): 1289–98.

Medical Ethics: Decision Making at the End of Life

Because of medical technology, a growing number of elderly persons with chronic illnesses continue to survive with diminished functional capacity as well as diminished quality of life. Case law and federal regulations emphasize that patients have the right to self-determination regarding their medical care.[1] However, only about 20% of the overall US population has a written advance directive (living will or durable power of attorney). It is assumed that all competent patients can make their own medical decisions. However, there are suggestions that physicians' decisions are often inconsistent with the patient's advance directives.[2] This may be particularly true when family members are requesting a more aggressive level of treatment than the patient desires.

Near Death (1989; Frederick Wiseman, Zipporah Films): *Near Death* is a 6-hour black-and-white documentary focusing on the intensive care unit at Boston's Beth Israel Hospital. There is no commentary or narration. The film focuses on the processes of end-of-life decision making. Since Beth Israel is a teaching hospital, the daily activity on the unit includes residents and medical students as well as rounds directed by the intensive care unit attending. While the viewer has to provide the meaning of much of the film, the "micropolitics" of the unit is on display, with nurses and physicians talking about one another and whether they agree with their colleagues' clinical decisions. Ethical and psychological dilemmas of end-of life care as experienced by health-care professionals, patients, and their families are evident. However, the reality of addressing these issues in the context of caring for very ill patients is the major contribution of this film.

1 (Disk 2) This segment has been studied in detail by ethicists, linguists, and psychologists. Mrs. Factor, an elderly woman, has had a stroke and is being maintained on a ventilator. She has been reintubated five times in the past 6 months. A tracheotomy is being considered as well as weaning Mrs. Factor from the ventilator.

2 (0:00:49–0:07:25) Dr. Kirlin, her longtime physician, and Dr. Weiss, the intensive care unit attending, discuss aspects of Mrs. Factor's case with nursing staff and each other.
   a. What is the head nurse's view of aggressive treatment for Mrs. Factor?
   b. What is Dr. Kirlin's view?
   c. What is Dr. Weiss's view?
   d. From the perspective of the Beauchamp and Childress model of ethical decision making balancing autonomy, beneficence, and nonmaleficence, which of these dimensions are most important to Dr. Weiss? To Dr. Kirlin?

3 (0:08:35–0:15:00) The intensive care unit team, including students, residents, and nurses, directed by Dr. Weiss discuss Mrs. Factor's care in detail. Dr. Weiss emphasizes the balance between the patient, primary physician, consultants, and family when addressing end-of-life care. However, in this case, Mrs. Factor's wishes do not appear to be taken into account.
   a. Based on the discussion, what do you think Mrs. Factor's wishes would be about her care?
   b. Several members of the team state that the level of care currently being provided is against the patient's wishes. Does it appear that Mrs. Factor is competent to make decisions about her care?
   c. If Mrs. Factor has not wanted to be repeatedly intubated in the past 6 months, why did this level of care occur?

4 (0:23:45–0:29:30) Dr Kirlin explains the treatment options and consequences to Mrs. Factor. A nurse is present and reiterates the information and treatment options. Mrs. Factor does not indicate a clear choice.
   a. Does Mrs. Factor appear to understand the information being presented? Why? Why not?
   b. How would you evaluate Dr. Kirlin's presentation of the treatment options?
   c. Dr. Kirlin repeatedly tells Mrs. Factor that "we will abide by your wishes."

Based on the earlier discussion, do you believe that Dr. Kirlin will support Mrs. Factor's decision if she decides to stop the ventilator and refuses a tracheotomy?

d. Why is Mrs. Factor not verbalizing a decision?

e. How would you communicate the choices and their consequences to Mrs. Factor?

References

1 Searight HR, Gafford J. Cultural diversity at the end of life: issues and guidelines for family physicians. *Am Fam Physician.* 2005; **71**(3): 515–22.

2 Hardin SB, Yusufaly Y. Difficult end-of-life treatment decisions: do other factors trump advance directives? *Arch Intern Med.* 2004; **164**(14): 1531–3.

3 Budwig N. The conduit metaphor: language and informed consent. *Fam Syst Health.* 1991; **9**(4): 313–27.

Medical Ethics: Physician-Assisted Suicide

Physician-assisted suicide (PAS) remains a controversial issue in the United States. As of this writing, three states (Oregon, Washington, and Montana) have legalized the practice when conducted according to specific guidelines. Despite legalization, patients rarely choose this option. In Oregon, where the practice has been legal for a decade, significantly less than 1% of the state's deaths occur through PAS.[1] Of interest, when terminally ill Oregon patients meeting the criteria are given lethal prescriptions, only about 40%–50% actually use them.[2] This pattern suggests that having control over the circumstances of one's death alone may have palliative value. However, PAS has been used much more commonly in the Netherlands, with up to 5% of the nation's deaths in a year attributable to PAS. While inappropriate use of PAS does not appear to be common in the United States, reports from the Netherlands suggest that physicians directly or indirectly hastened death in about 6% of patients who expired.[3]

The Suicide Tourist (2010; PBS; approximately 50 minutes): *The Suicide Tourist* prompted considerable controversy when it was initially shown. It is worthwhile to view this film in its entirety. The film follows a US college professor with amyotrophic lateral sclerosis (ALS) living in England with his wife as they make the journey to Zurich to end his life. According to critics, Switzerland has become the home of "death tourism," since its laws are much more liberal than its European neighbors and also because Dignitas, a physician-headed organization for PAS is located there. The film shows Ewert with his wife and Dignitas volunteers as he ends his life.

1 (0:04:50–0:14:44) While his wife shaves him, Ewert describes his reasons for seeking PAS – both in general and in the context of his experience with ALS. The founder of Dignitas outlines the general process of PAS as conducted by the organization.

a. What do you think of Ewert's reasoning for supporting and requesting PAS?

b. How much of a difference does the diagnosis of ALS make in your reasoning?

c. Are there circumstances under which PAS is appropriate? If yes, what are they? If no, why do you see PAS as always inappropriate?

d. Patients have come to Switzerland for PAS from many countries. Given that PAS is illegal in most of the industrialized world, what is your opinion of "death tourism"?

2　(0:28:20–0:33:10) A physician working with Dignitas reviews Ewert's medical records, meets with him and his wife, and explains the process of PAS.

a. What is your opinion of the encounter between the physician and Ewert?

b. Do you believe that the evaluation of the appropriateness of PAS for Ewert, as depicted in the film, is adequate?

c. If not, what else would you see as necessary or beneficial?

3　(0:39:00–0:49:25) In a Zurich apartment, Ewert ends his life with his wife and Dignitas volunteers present. Ewert has to initiate a timing device that will terminate his oxygen supply in 45 minutes. In addition, he must directly ingest the sodium pentobarbital immediately after the Dignitas volunteer explicitly states: "If you drink this, you are going to die."

a. In the United States, most deaths occur in hospitals. How does the quality of Ewert's death compare with patients who die in a hospital or nursing home?

b. How is the context of Ewert's death the same or different than hospice care?

References

1　Sullivan AD, Hedberg K, Fleming DW. Legalized physician-assisted suicide in Oregon: the second year. *N Engl J Med*. 2000; **342**(8): 596–604.

2　Ganzini, L, Nelson H, Schmidt TA, *et al*. Physicians' experiences with the Oregon Death with Dignity Act. *N Engl J Med*. 2000; **342**(8): 557–63.

3　Ten Have HA, Welie J. Euthanasia: normal medical practice? *Hastings Cent Rep*. 1992; **22**(2); 34–8.

48

Me, You, and YouTube: Cutting-Edge Teaching

David Stanley, Patricia Lenahan, Edward Thibodeau,
Lauren M. Consonni & LaTasha K. Crawford

Anatomy of e-Sharing: YouTube Dissected

WORDS SUCH AS TWITTER, FACEBOOK, MYSPACE, LINKEDIN, YOUTUBE, Flickr, and Google are now an integral part of the lexicon of contemporary society and represent just a few of the core elements of the World Wide Web. The goals of facilitating communication, sharing information, and collaborating electronically are common to many of these tools and programs. YouTube was established in 2005 and acquired by Google in 2006.

YouTube is one of the most popular websites on the Internet, receiving more than 2 billion visits per day. YouTube allows users the opportunity to post, view, and comment on videos on virtually any topic. The program is based on a simple keyword, search term, or query format. Once a keyword(s) is entered into the search engine text box, any video in the database with the appropriate matching keyword either in its title, general description, or designated categories or tags will appear in a list on the screen. Search results can then be sorted by highest ranking, most views, most linked, or by relevance. Drawing one of the largest audiences on the Internet, YouTube has the potential to provide the health-care community with an important means for inexpensive communication, education, self-promotion, and entertainment. At the same time, patients and potential patients may receive information from sources that are not necessarily accurate or reliable since virtually anyone can post a video on YouTube. Health-care providers will need to assess the sources of the patient's information in order to correct any misinformation.

From an educational viewpoint, PowerPoint presentations often can benefit by having video excerpts embedded in the lecture. It gives educators a way to break up the monotony for their learners, as well as to "reach" the current generation of students who utilize YouTube frequently.

The following video clips provide examples of the use of YouTube in the various areas: public health, medical and dental issues, nursing, specific disease conditions, violence and abuse, veterinary medicine, and other aspects of health and wellness. Some specific examples are provided here, but these serve only as a brief introduction to what educators may find on YouTube.

Although substance abuse and mental health-related videos are not described in this chapter, YouTube abounds with examples of these. Additionally, several television series that relate to health and veterinary medicine have excerpts available on YouTube. Movie scenes that may be useful in addressing particular topics can be found as well.

Nurses on YouTube

YouTube offers insight into the contemporary image of the nurse. The study of nursing's identity is significant in that it offers a view into how the profession of nursing is perceived by nurses themselves, other professionals, and the public. The traditionally dominant mass media of cinema and TV are now being challenged by the emergence of the Internet and YouTube and it is through these mass media means that the public is developing its knowledge of and attitudes towards nurses.[1]

Little research exists which examines the image of nursing on the Internet. In 2007, Kalish *et al.*[2] examined the image of nursing on a sample of 144 websites in North America in 2001 and 152 sites in 2004. Their conclusions were that images were mainly positive in 2001, with nurses being shown to be skilled, accountable, trustworthy, respected, educated, intelligent, and competent. In 2004, the nurses were also shown to be innovative and powerful. However, reference to their being sexually promiscuous was also evident.

YouTube offers a democratizing format by which the nursing profession can be presented globally. Importantly, nurses themselves have recognized the global scope of YouTube and post the majority of videos identified under the term "nurse" to YouTube themselves. A wide range of topics are evident when viewing YouTube videos. Generally speaking, two broad themes appear evident: nurses or nursing that is shown to be either competent or incompetent and nurses that are shown to be a sexual object.

The Competent Nurse
The following video clips all offer positive insights, promoting nursing as fun, stimulating, and rewarding.
- ER promotional rap: a rap song from the University of Alabama at Birmingham. (Available at: www.youtube.com/watch?v=n5Zw4ZARvNg&feature=related)

- The Nurse's Story: from Harris Methodist Southwest Hospital. (Available at: www.youtube.com/watch?v=nKaqqzUGrRI&feature=related)
- "Go be a Nurse": a promotional music video about joining the nursing profession. (Available at: www.youtube.com/watch?v=5kVv2aqnEjs)
- "Footloose": another promotional video set to music. (Available at: www.youtube.com/watch?v=fU0f5bgj0s)
- UTA Nursing Song: another promotional rap song. (Available at: www.youtube.com/watch?v=sBs7nieDgsU)

The Incompetent Nurse

The following video clips use satire to show nurses who are "dumb" and incompetent.

- Mad TV Hospital Nurse: TV sitcom (Available at: www.youtube.com/watch?v=oq878U1WeWQ&feature=related)
- Two examples offered of computer-generated cartoon images (there are many of these on YouTube) (Available at: www.youtube.com/watch?v=vytuDdFv13w&feature=related; www.youtube.com/watch?v=-PVtNyeAy74&feature=related)
- Prick his boil: an excerpt from a UK comedy program (Available at: www.youtube.com/watch?v=5TdoklnKSQY)

The Nurse as a Sexual Object

The following YouTube images represent video clips that gratuitously show nurses as the object of male sexual fantasy and accomplice in the sexual titillation of male patients.

- The Young Turks: Internet TV news show. (Available at: www.youtube.com/watch?v=Ekaclt7GNdQ)
- Virgin Mobile: a video mobile phone advert (Available at: www.youtube.com/watch?v=iGGjjDHfO9k&feature=related)
- Naughty Nurse: a cartoon satire on nurse promiscuity (Available at: www.youtube.com/watch?v=fMzQk4N2aWc&feature=related)
- Sexy Nurse: American sitcom *Frasier* (Available at: www.youtube.com/watch?v=xR1mb8p5YbQ&feature=related)
- Typical Men: sexy nurse lingerie – a Belgian lingerie advertisement (Available at: www.youtube.com/watch?v=oZXaVwiqcis)

Music Videos: A Focus on Violence and Abuse

Violence and abuse has been a recurring theme in music, from opera to rap and virtually every other music genre. Rock music offers a multitude of songs that allude to violence: Mary Wells ("I Have Two Lovers"), The Crystals ("He Hit Me"), Tom Jones ("Delilah"), The Rolling Stones ("Under My Thumb"), Jimi Hendrix ("Hey, Joe"), The Police ("Every Breathe You Take"), and Pearl Jam ("Alive," "Better Man," "Daughter") are excellent examples of this. Country music also provides a plethora of material with Martina McBride ("Independence Day," "Concrete Angel," "A Broken Wing"), Johnny Cash ("Delia's Gone"), the Dixie Chicks ("Goodbye Earl"), Shania Twain's ("Black Eyes, Blue Tears"), and Jewell ("Daddy"). Virtually every genre has songs that address some aspect of violence and abuse from incest, sexual assault, child abuse, intimate partner violence, and bullying.

The synopses of music videos included in this chapter will give cinemeducators a sample of the extensive material available for teaching. Many of these music videos are available in DVD format from the musical artist while others are found on YouTube. It is important to note that the content on YouTube changes frequently as information is added and/or deleted. Also, many of the music videos cited have multiple versions available for viewing. Some of the titles listed here are not for the faint of heart: they are graphic in nature and may contain offensive lyrics. Others offer statistics about violence and abuse and national resources available to victims. Frequent viewing of these videos can lead to a sense of vicarious traumatization.

"Facedown" by Red Jumpsuit Apparatus (3:21)
There are multiple versions of this music video. A powerful rendition portrays intimate partner violence between a heterosexual African-American couple. The woman is seen looking at herself in the mirror and covering up bruises, telling herself it will never happen again. The chorus is very telling: "Do you feel like a man when you push her around? Do you feel better as she falls to the ground?" There is hope and a belief that she will leave in the words: "Face down in the dirt, she says it doesn't hurt. She says I've finally had enough."

"Love is Blind" by Eve (3:51)
This rap song video is very graphic, powerful and contains potentially offensive language that may not be suitable for all audiences. A friend of a woman who is the victim of intimate partner violence sings the song. She sings: "I don't know you, but I'd kill you myself." The video follows a young woman's life – and death – at the hands of her perpetrator husband. Scenes include abuse in the presence of her children as well as her attempts to hide the bruises with makeup. This video is dedicated to a victim of violence.

"Independence Day" by Martina McBride (3:55)
This powerful video alludes to substance-related violence and focuses on an 8-year-old girl who witnesses the abuse of her mother. She leaves the chaos at home and goes to town, seeking relief, and watches the Fourth of July parade. However, her fear and worry are apparent. She winces and ducks as the clowns are seen hitting each other. She runs home to find that her parents had fought and that her mother had set the house on fire. As she attempts to run up to what is left of the house, she is grabbed by a police officer. The song says she was "taken to the county home" demonstrating yet another devastating effect of violence.

"A Broken Wing" by Martina McBride (3:35)

This video demonstrates psychological abuse and power and control dynamics (lyrics: "he broke her spirit" and "he would give a little and take it back"). The woman's relationship with the perpetrator is described as "she loved him like he was the last man on earth." The video ends with the "hope" that she has been able to leave successfully: a note and an open bedroom window. However, the listener is left with the haunting lines: "only angels know how to fly."

"I'm OK" by Christina Aguilera (5:24)

Again, there are multiple versions of this music video. One example was made by the artist to raise awareness of intimate partner violence. It is full of scenes of abuse interspersed with descriptions of different types of violence, statistics and facts about violence and abuse. Another version shows a young woman looking at family photos and recounting her experiences: "Once upon a time there was a girl in her early years; she had to learn how to grow up living in a war that she called home." She later adds: "Bruises fade, father, but the pain remains the same and I still remember how you kept me so afraid. Strength is my mother for all the love she gave" and "to you it's just a memory, but for me it still lives on."

"How Come, How Long" by Stevie Wonder and Baby Face (5:05)

You will find several pages of various versions. The best one is Baby Face VEVO 2007, Sony BMI Music. This is the official music video version and is excellent. There is also another version that is used for Child Abuse Awareness.

This video tells the story of a woman who met the wrong man and died as a result of intimate partner violence. ("There's a girl I used to know, beautiful, she's not here anymore.") The lyrics demonstrate that intimate partner violence can affect anyone ("college degree … there wasn't enough education in this world to save this little girl.") The song also chastises people who know or suspect abuse but do nothing. ("She tried to give a cry for help, blamed herself, no one came to help.") It admonishes everyone to "look for the signs next time and save a life."

Additional Videos on Intimate Partner Violence

"Family Portrait" by Pink (3:44)

This video focuses on a child witness to family violence: "It ain't easy growing up in World War III" and the child's coping.

"Kim" by Eminem (3:25)

This video demonstrates abuse in a couple where the wife is having an affair.

"Black Eyes, Blue Tears" by Shania Twain (various versions)

The lyrics describe a woman who has been abused and makes the decision to leave: "black eyes, I don't need 'em; blue tears give me freedom" and later: "no more rollin' with the punches." Perhaps the most powerful of the music videos of this song is the one that incorporates graphic scenes of intimate partner violence from the movie: .45 (2006).

"Bowling Ball" by Superchick (4:30)

    The video takes place at a bowling alley and includes scenes of violence, statistics, facts, and more.

"Cry" by Danielle Staub (4:09)

    This video is sung by *Housewives of New Jersey* star Danielle Staub. It provides another example of the violence and abuse music video genre.

Child Abuse

"Concrete Angel" by Martina McBride (4:09)

    This is another powerful video by McBride. It focuses on a 7-year-old girl who is the victim of child abuse and neglect. She appears distracted in school ("sometimes she wishes she wasn't born"), wears the same clothes and often has to hide her bruises: "the teacher wonders but she doesn't ask." The only person who appears concerned and responds to her is the little boy next door. He sees her being abused through the bedroom window. The abuse can be heard: "the neighbors hear but they don't ask." The video ends with the death of the child. At the cemetery, the little boy leaves the gravesite and sees the little girl, now smiling. She is finally at peace.

"Alyssa Lies" by Jason Michael Carroll (4:42)

    Based on the true story of a girl named Alyssa, a victim of abuse, this music video is told from the perspective of the father of a classmate. This friend shares her concerns about Alyssa with her Dad and says: "Alyssa lies to the teachers; Alyssa lies to cover the bruises." The Dad hears his little girl praying: "God bless my Mom and Dad and my new friend Alyssa. I know she needs you bad." The video ends with the Dad having to tell his daughter that Alyssa won't be in school. She has died. Perhaps one of the most searing scenes is a closing view of the child-size casket holding Alyssa's body.

"Trying Not to Cry" by John Silvestry (4:24)

    This video has an underlying religious theme. It focuses on an African-American child who is the victim of child abuse who wants to "fly away to a place I'd be safe."

"Loaded Gun" by Dowell Band (3:57)

    This country music song offers very graphic photos of child abuse interspersed with the happy and healthy and "normal" photos of childhood. It contains statistics and facts related to this problem.

"Child Abuse" written and performed by Vince Royale (5:15)

This rap music video shows a child who is abused ("every day I am black and blue") by his father who is under the influence of alcohol. The child laments: "Everyone else had a great Dad. Am I the only one who got a face slap?"

"Daughter" by Pearl Jam (3:34)

The lyrics of this song allude to some type of child abuse: "Don't call me daughter, not fit to be. The picture kept will remind me." Other lyrics adding to the theme of abuse include "She holds the hand that holds her down."

Bullying

"Bully" by Six 8 (4:41)

This music video was filmed at Lincoln Elementary School in Fort Wayne, Indiana. It addresses bullying in school and online: "they do it in school and they do it online." The video shows children standing up to bullying.

"Without a Trace" by Wannabe (5:13)

The video scenes are taken from the television show *Without a Trace*, which featured an episode focused on bullying. This YouTube music video was made by David Berkeley for a film school project.

"The Way She Feels" by Between the Trees (4:03)

This is a powerful video of an overweight teenage girl who is bullied. She turns to cutting to cope with her feelings. She carved "alone" on her forearm. The cutting doesn't help her depression as she says: "the deeper I cut, it only gets worse." The video demonstrates the impact of parental love and family support. It has perhaps an unrealistic and overly happy resolution, but the focus on cutting and depression give merit to this video.

"You're Not Alone" by Rock4Youth (3:37)

This music video is written and performed by a UK club called Rock4Youth. It shows the perspective of a young girl who is the victim of bullying who doesn't know quite what to do: "Should I reveal what they have put me through?"

"Jeremy" by Pearl Jam (5:29)

The version by OUSO Marine includes some photos and Jeremy Wade Delle's yearbook photo at the start. This song is based on the true story of a boy who was bullied and committed suicide. The boy's sufferings appeared to have been ignored by his parents: "Daddy didn't give attention to the fact that Mommy didn't care."

"It Gets Better" created by Dan Savage and with thousands of other contributors from all walks of life.

The It Gets Better Project (www.itgetsbetter.org) was started in response to the startling number of lesbian, gay, bisexual. and transgender teen suicides. The messages, video-recorded by various celebrities and world figures, attempts to inspire hope to those who are bullied that no matter how bad things might be, life will improve after high school.

Public Health Videos

Public Service Announcements

- American Automobile Association, 1980s Flintstones Kids Seatbelt Safety PSA Commercial (Available at: www.youtube.com/watch?v=-XEfCwwAfEU).
- Stand Up to Cancer, CBS, ABC, NBC. (Available at: www.youtube.com/watch?v=hG1QGrFq4s8&feature=fvst; www.youtube.com/watch?v=756MiAuHItw).

Disease-Specific Videos: Gaucher Disease

- Emily's Journey with Gaucher Disease, Part 1 and 2 (Available at: www.youtube.com/watch?v=JGHQlHGNd84; www.youtube.com/watch?v=4qD2NQrAslY&feature=related).

- Little Miss Hannah: Our Fight Against Gaucher's Disease Type 2 or Type 3 (Available at: www.youtube.com/watch?v=qKEQHHNcBn8).
- Histopathology Spleen: Gaucher Disease (Available at: www.youtube.com/watch?v=0nX6QM5iVaU).
- Shire Announces FDA approval of VPRIV for Gaucher Disease (Available at: www.youtube.com/watch?v=RVAX4_Q-woE).

Dentistry: Dental Caries

- Tooth Decay (Dental Caries). ToothIQ.com.
  Link: www.youtube.com/watch?v=_oIlv59bTL4
- Cardiology Rap. University of the Pacific Dental School, 2007.
  Link: www.youtube.com/watch?v=BIXhIHUPyvo

Veterinary Medicine

Outbreaks of Zoonotic Diseases

- The Centers for Disease Control and Prevention. H1N1 (Swine Flu) (Available at: www.youtube.com/watch?v=85sD83aRUIQ).
- American Veterinary Medical Association. Role of the Veterinary Pathologist in Identifying the West Nile Virus (Available at: www.youtube.com/watch?v=xRAP8n6Z21Y&feature=related).

Wobbler Syndrome

- Wobbler's Syndrome: More Than just a Pain in the Neck! (Available at: www.youtube.com/watch?v=dK8QzGBCn_E).
- What to Look for if Your Dog has Wobblers (Available at: www.youtube.com/watch?v=2cKYXuot0Vo).
- Paint Horse with Wobbler's Syndrome (Available at: www.youtube.com/watch?v=XQSlN9tYudc&feature=related).

Discussion Questions

1 How can video-sharing websites such as YouTube help to educate health-care professionals and clients/patients about health-related issues?
2 How can video-sharing websites be used to educate a variety of different demographic groups and populations?
3 What role do celebrities have in promoting specific causes and charitable organizations?
4 Considering the examples provided for Gaucher disease, discuss how the different video clips and video formats serve to enhance the educational experience of the audience.
5 Discuss the utility of video as a tool for educating human patients or pet owners about neurological and orthopedic diseases.
6 What is the relationship between the entertainment value of a video and its potential to educate?
7 Can misinformation be conveyed when patients are turning to Internet resources for medical advice?
8 How can you and those you serve distinguish between credible vs. non-credible health information sources?
9 What are some ways to make an accurate, informative video stand out amongst numerous videos that contain misinformation?

References

1 Fealy GM, Newby M. Through the lens. In: Fealy GM, editor. *Care to Remember: nursing and midwifery in Ireland*. Cork: Mercier Press; 2005. pp. 69–88.
2 Kalisch BJ, Begeny S, Newman S. The image of the nurse on the Internet. *Nurs Outlook*. 2007; **55**(4): 182–8.

Further Reading

- Boucher JL. Technology and patient-provider interactions: improving quality of care, but is it improving communication and collaboration? *Diabetes Spectrum*. 2010; **23**(3): 142–4.

- Hawn C. Take two aspirin and tweet me in the morning: how Twitter, Facebook, and other social media are re-shaping health care. *Health Affairs*. 2009; **28**(2): 361–8.
- Hong T. Internet health information in the patient-provider dialogue. *Cyberpsychol Behav*. 2008; **1**(5): 587–8.
- Hou J, Shim M. The role of provider-patient communication and trust in online sources in Internet use for health-related activities. *J Health Commun*. 2010; **15**(3): 186–9.
- Iverson SA, Howard KB, Penney BK. Impact of Internet use in health-related behaviors and the patient-physician relationship: a survey-based study and review. *J Am Osteopath Assoc*. 2008; **108**(12): 699–711.
- Orsini M. Social media: how home health care agencies can join the chorus of empowered voices. *Home Health Care Manag Pract*. 2010; **22**(3): 213–17.
- Santana S, Lausen B, Bujnowska-Fedak M, *et al*. Informed citizen and empowered citizen in health: results from a European survey. *BMC Fam Pract*. 2011; **12**: 20.
- Santana S, Lausen B, Bujnowska-Fedak M, *et al*. Online communication between doctors and patients in Europe: status and perspectives. *J Med Internet Res*. 2010; **12**(2): e20.
- Thaker SI, Nowacki AS, Mehta NB, *et al*. How U.S. hospitals use social media. *Ann Intern Med*. 2011; **154**(10): 707–8.
- Wen-ying SC, Hunt YM, Burke-Beckjord E, *et al*. Social media use in the United States: implications for health communication. *J Med Internet Res*. 2009; **11**(4): e48.

49

Save the Last Chapter for Melody and Verse: Music Videos

Dennis J. Butler

Introduction

Medical educators routinely associate posttraumatic stress disorder with combat veterans, yet in medical school and residency, students and residents encounter many patients who have faced horrifying and traumatic events. Other populations at risk for disabling traumatic reactions include victims of crime, physical abuse and sexual trauma, and those who live through natural disasters.

Patients who survive motor vehicle crashes may also experience profound and prolonged traumatic reactions. Currently, over a quarter of the population of the United States have been in an automobile accident. Research suggests that up to 9% of those involved in a serious vehicular crash will develop posttraumatic stress disorder.[1] Although efforts to reduce vehicular mortality in the United States have resulted in decreased highway fatalities in recent years, traffic accidents in other countries, especially in Third World countries, continue to be a leading cause of death. Over 1.25 million people are killed in traffic-related events worldwide.

The Car Crash Songs

Car crash deaths in the United States were a significant public health problem in the 1950s and 1960s. Deaths from motor vehicle crashes among adolescents rose 41% between 1950 and 1967 to a rate of 48.5 per 100 000, the highest rate for any age group at any time in this nation's history and twice the rate for today's teens.[2] These numbers are even more telling when considering that the average number of vehicles per household in the United States in the early 1950s was less than one and the number of miles driven annually was a fraction of today's totals.

During that time, mechanical advances resulted in faster, more powerful automobiles. Engines increased in size from four to six, eight, and even ten cylinders, resulting in dramatic increases in horsepower. The characteristics most promoted and desired in new automobiles were speed and luxury and the automobile became a status symbol and proof of upward mobility.

But attention to safety features lagged. Vehicles lacked seat belts (known then as safety belts), were equipped with inadequate brakes, regular glass windows, and tires designed for lower speeds. The development of the first interstate highway system was intended to give the population faster access to far away destinations but roadway infrastructure lacked basic safety engineering and design. Adolescents' desire for independence, changing dating mores, increased use of alcohol, and tendencies toward impulsivity were increasingly and tragically acted out through the automobile.

Rock and roll emerged in the 1950s as the signature music of the adolescent generation and the genre reflected the attitudes, beliefs, fads, and experiences of it audience. Teens were enthralled with the automobile and songs with cars as the subject were prevalent and popular. To underscore this point it should be noted that most music historians consider the first recorded rock and roll song to be "Rocket 88," a song highlighting the introduction of the Oldsmobile 88, the first 8-cylinder production automobile. The lyrics capture the essential elements of cars and driving which were attractive to adolescents: popularity, speed, attracting the opposite sex, and having fun. Originally popular when recorded by Ike Turner, "Rocket 88" became even more popular when covered by teen idol Bill Haley and his band, The Comets. Other early iconic rock and roll car songs that idealized reckless driving were "Maybelline" by Chuck Berry and "Hot Rod Lincoln" by Charlie Ryan.

In the midst of the teen driving death epidemic, five highly successful rock and roll songs about car crash deaths were released within 6 years. Each charted in the Billboard Top Ten, the recording industry's list of the highest selling song (*see* Table 49.1).

TABLE 49.1 The Car Crash Songs

Title	Performers	Writers	Year
"Teen Angel"	Mark Dinning	Jean and Red Surrey	1958
"Tell Laura I Love Her"	Ray Peterson	Jeff Barry, Ben Raleigh	1960
"Last Kiss"	J. Frank Wilson and The Cavaliers	Wayne Cochran	1962
"Dead Man's Curve"	Jan and Dean	Jan Berry, Roger Christian, Artie Kornfield, Brian Wilson	1963
"Leader of the Pack"	The Shangri-Las	George Morton, Jeff Barry, Ellie Greenwich	1964

"Teen Angel" describes a tragedy nearly averted in a train-automobile wreck but the singer's girlfriend is killed when she returns to retrieve her boyfriend's ring. The lyrics portray the significant psychological conflict of the survivor over his responsibility for her death. "Tell Laura I Love Her" is a third-person ballad about the death of a teen who enters a stockcar race in hopes of winning $1000 to buy his girlfriend a wedding ring. His dying words haunt Laura as she tries to make sense of his death. "Last Kiss" describes how the singer found his dying girlfriend after a crash and his subsequent reactions. The lyrics of this song provide some of the more graphic descriptions of physical and psychological trauma. "Dead Man's Curve" by Jan and Dean is a first-person account of a fatal drag race, and, ironically, foretold the tragedy of Jan's subsequent car crash and consequent lifelong disability. The lyrics are set in the acute period immediately after the accident. "Leader of the Pack" is an eyewitness account of the death of the singer's boyfriend in a motorcycle crash. The lyrics describe a series of flashbacks and provide insight into the social and personal impact of losing a boyfriend who was considered a rebel by peers and parents.

Each of the car crash songs reflects individual reactions to trauma and death, yet each offers insight into distinct traumatic reactions including complicated and traumatic grief, acute stress disorder, and posttraumatic stress disorder. With the exception of "Dead Man's Curve," each individual who dies is involved in a romantic relationship, thus intensifying the reaction of the survivor.

Using the Car Crash Songs and Videos in Teaching

The car crash songs have been used to teach about the impact of traumatic events as part of the m-4 Medical Humanities course for the past 6 years. They have also been used in teaching sessions with residents, practicing physicians, and mental health professionals through interactive lectures and in small group sessions. The dramatic lyrics and emotional tone of these songs can be effectively used to develop participants' history taking skills, knowledge of traumatic reactions, empathy for survivors, and insight into the profound impact of motor vehicle crashes and other traumatic events. Because most participants are accustomed to traditional didactic approaches, it is very important to be clear about the educational objectives when using musical selections to teach.

Although each song can be individually presented for a teaching session, the advantage of presenting all five songs is in the variety of traumatic reactions they portray. "Dead Man's Curve" is set in the time frame immediately after a crash and provides insight into acute stress disorder. "Teen Angel" and "Tell Laura I Love Her" contain lyrics and bereavement themes and are excellent pieces to foster discussion of the characteristics of traumatic grief reactions. "Last Kiss" and "Leader of the Pack" contain descriptions of highly traumatic events and common reactions suggestive of posttraumatic stress disorder.

When using the car crash songs to teach about trauma, it is essential for the presenter to provide some context from the rock and roll era and to provide the audience with the song lyrics. In addition to interpreting the lyrics, participants can be asked to reflect on how the artists used melody, rhythm, inflection, tone, and sound effects in each song.

Participants may need to know about dating customs and become familiar with the language and terminology of the 1950s in order to fully understand the subject matter of each musical piece. It is especially helpful to play video clips of the original bands performing the selections or montage videos of the artists while the original song is being played. (A list of useful videos on YouTube is provided at the end of this chapter.) Despite the brevity of these songs, small groups are occasionally uncomfortable when only audio access is available. Showing video clips concurrent with the music provides a way for the audience to focus.

It has also been helpful to provide learners with historical background information about each song before listening to each selection. "Last Kiss" is based on an especially tragic teen car crash with multiple fatalities; "Dead Man's Curve" was inspired by the near-fatal crash of Mel Blanc (the voice of multiple Looney Toons cartoon characters) at Hollywood's actual deadman's curve. "Leader of the Pack" parallels the script of *The Wild One* (1953), a very popular movie starring Marlon Brando and based on the Hollister, California, motorcycle riot in 1947.

It has also been helpful to provide handouts to the audience with the formal diagnostic criteria for trauma-related disorders and have them identify symptoms as they occur in the lyrics. If the goals of the teaching session include improving trainee diagnostic abilities, having the diagnostic criteria can familiarize learners with how such symptoms manifest and help them differentiate various trauma-related disorders.

A challenge when using music for educational purposes is the tendency of students and residents to critique the characteristics of the musical piece rather than the content and context of the lyrics.[3] For example, "Tell Laura I Love Her" has elicited negative responses from some trainees who find its tone melodramatic. Others are distracted by amateurish sound effects in "Dead Man's Curve," or are unfamiliar with the adolescent dating customs of the 1950s described in "Leader of the Pack." Some trainees are more familiar with Pearl Jam's version of "Last Kiss" and find the original version amateurish. The inclusion of "Do Whop" background vocals on specific selections seems incongruous to some participants. Again, clarity of the educational objectives for the sessions is helpful to prevent participants from being distracted by such aspects and discourage off-task discussion.

The car crash songs contain traumatic and painful subject matter and some trainees have strong reactions based on personal experience or clinical exposure to trauma victims. Many have been in automobile crashes, and most can identify family, friends, and colleagues who also have been in crashes. Before playing the car crash songs, participants should be cautioned that discussion of trauma may precipitate distressing reactions, and it has been useful to engage participants in a discussion of their exposure to traumatic events. At times the campy nature or out-of-context content of these songs may produce some levity and distract from the serious nature of the topic. However, teaching sessions have unexpectedly produced distress in some vulnerable participants in the past. The presenter should monitor audience reactions during the session and offer to debrief with any participant who may experience unexpected reactions.

Because the car crash songs were written to entertain and not to teach, they are not diagnostically comprehensive and the presenter should be prepared to provide additionally didactic material about traumatic reactions. The lyrics were written well before the advent of diagnostic guidelines such as DSM-IV, and the artists were not concerned with providing accurate clinical descriptions. For example, the lyrics overemphasize intrusive recollections but fail to include common reactions such as hypervigilance, sleep disturbance, agitation, irritability, and withdrawal. These omissions should be addressed and discussed during the presentation along with other potential reactions.

Because these songs are brief, readily available on the Internet, and highly portable with today's technology, they can be very effective teaching tools. All are three minutes or less which allows them to be played in their entirety before the audience becomes distracted. Perhaps the most important advantage of using these songs to teach about traumatic reactions is that learners comprehend better when multiple sensory modalities are accessed. Participants read diagnostic criteria and lyrics, listen to music, watch videos of the performers, have a kinetic response while listening (e.g. toe tapping to the melodies), and engage in discussion. Despite the serious nature of the topic, audiences report this is a fun and enjoyable way to learn.

Many younger trainees are unfamiliar with the car crash songs because they were recorded 50 years ago. Despite their limitations, they capture the angst of adolescents, the tragedy of personal loss, and the deeper human impact of trauma. All five songs contain two of the universal themes associated with traumatic events: the intrusiveness of traumatic events in the lives of those affected and the need of human beings to process and make sense of tragedy. Using the car crash songs to teach about trauma also models two guiding principles for those who work with trauma victims; the process of adjustment and recovery begins when victims tell their stories (through the songs) and others listen.

References

1   Blanchard EB, Hickling EJ, editors. *After the Crash: assessment and treatment of motor vehicle accident survivors*. Washington, DC: American Psychological Association; 1997.

2   Department of Health, Education, and Welfare. *Motor Vehicle Accident Deaths in the United States, 1950–1967*. Vital and Health Statistics-Series 20, No. 9; December, 1970.

3   Newell GC, Hanes DJ. Listening to music: the case for its use in teaching medical humanism. *Acad Med*. 2003; **78**(7): 714–19.

Videos

The following videos are available on YouTube. Each provides either a montage or video of the band performing the identified song.

- "Dead Man's Curve," Jan and Dean (www.youtube.com/watch?v=pmw0wejzBvI)
- "Last Kiss," J. Frank Wilson and the Cavaliers (www.youtube.com/watch?v=bh4se9YMV3A)
- "Leader of the Pack," The Shangri-Las (www.youtube.com/watch?v=FGQt6GY8nKA)
- "Tell Laura I Love Her" Ray Peterson (www.youtube.com/watch?v=5B1C4nSUhw8)
- "Teen Angel," Mark Dinning (www.youtube.com/watch?v=KG_VIcoiCFA)

After the Injury (www.aftertheinjury.org) is a website sponsored by the Children's Hospital of Philadelphia. It provides information, educational material, rating scales, and advice for helping children who have been injured in vehicular crashes. The website contains five brief educational video clips about traumatic reactions in children: (1)What to expect after an injury, (2) You are not alone, (3) Reactions to injury, (4) What are traumatic stress reactions? and (5) How long do traumatic stress reactions last?

Appendices

Cinemeducation: Movie List

This list of films is meant to highlight many, but not all, of those cited in Volume 2 as well as other movies *not* included in this volume. Please note that several films are listed in multiple categories because of their varied content and applicability. At the end, we also include movies relevant to educational topics not included in this volume.

Lifespan and Developmental Issues

Couples
A Single Man
Baby Mama
Bloom
Blue Valentine
Boynton Beach Club
Brokeback Mountain
Charlotte Sometimes
Couples Retreat
Crazy Heart
Crazy Stupid Love
Father of the Bride 2
Fifty First Dates
It's Complicated
Lars and the Real Girl
Last Chance Harvey
Life as a House
Life Support
Love Actually
Love and Drugs
Match Point
Midnight in Paris
Motherhood
Old Dogs
One Week
Prague
Remember Me
Revolutionary Road
Taken
The Break-Up
The Ice Storm
The Notebook
The Painted Veil
The Secret Lives of Dentists
The Story of Us
Toy Story 3
We Don't Live Here Anymore

Family Dynamics
All or Nothing
Animal Kingdom
Happy Endings
How to Be
Joshua's Heart
Keeping Up with the Steins
Love Actually
Margot at the Wedding
Motherhood
Nil By Mouth
Nothing Like the Holidays
Remember Me
The Wrestler
Toy Story 3
Smart People
Snowcake
Surrender, Dorothy
The Clockmaker
The Family That Preys
The Secret Lives of Dentists
Then She Found Me
Tortilla Soup
We Don't Live Here Anymore

Appendices

Special Topics in Childhood and Adolescence

A Clockwork Orange
Adam
All the Little Animals
Animal Kingdom
Antonia's Line
A Simple Plan
Being There
Best Boy
Bill
Bill, On His Own
Bogus
Charley
Dad's in Heaven with Nixon
Dodes'ka-den
Dominick and Eugene
Forrest Gump
Homer and Eddie
House of Cards
I Stand Alone
Little Voice
Loving Lampposts
Mercury Rising
Mifune
Molly
Mozart and The Whale
Niagara, Niagara
Of Mice and Men
On The Outs
Precious
Rain Man
Rory O' Shea
Sling Blade
The Boy Who Could Fly
To Kill a Mockingbird
The Heart is a Lonely Hunter
The Other Sister
The Quiet Room
The Shower
The Wizard
Toe to Toe
What's Eating Gilbert Grape?
Winter's Bone

Bullying

About a Boy
A Christmas Story
Back to the Future
Big Bully
Bluebird (Netherlands)
Bully
Canvas
Diary of a Wimpy Kid
Elephant
Ferris Buehler's Day Off
Forrest Gump
Gran Torino
Max Kuble's Big Move
Mean Creek
Mean Girls
My Bodyguard
Napoleon Dynamite
Odd Girl Out
Revenge of the Nerds
Saint Ralph
School Ties
Speak
Stand By Me
The Benchwarmers
The Breakfast Club
The Karate Kid
The Tic Code
Thirteen
Thirteen Going on Thirty
Three O'Clock High

Documentaries on Bullying

Girls Can Sometimes Be Mean
Rats and Bullies
Teen Truth: An Inside Look at Bullying
    and School Violence
Trauma: Life and Death in the ER
Bullied

Adolescents Facing Challenges and Disappointments

Fish Tank (UK)
Flirting
Garden State
Heavenly Creatures
Joshua's Heart
On The Outs
Precious
Princes in Exile
Set Me Free

Sex Drive
The Dust Factory
The Education of Shelby Know
The Last Picture Show
The Man in the Moon
The Squid and the Whale

Teen Pregnancy
Daddy
Juno
On The Outs
Unwed Father

Families, Celebrations and Holidays
A Christmas Story
A Wonderful Christmas
Arranged
Bridal Fever
Bride and Prejudice
Bride Wars
Bridesmaids
Christmas in Connecticut
Christmas with the Kranks
Christmas Vacation
Cousins
Death at a Funeral
Dim Sum Funeral
First Morning
Four Christmases
Four Weddings and a Funeral
Holiday Heart
Holiday Inn
Home for the Holidays
Homeless for the Holidays
How About You?
It's a Wonderful Life
Jumping the Broom
Last Wedding
License to Wed
My Big Fat Greek Wedding
Monsoon Wedding
New Year's Eve
Nothing Like the Holidays
November Christmas
Our Family Wedding
Passover Fever
Pieces of April
Praying for Lior (Documentary)

Quinceanera
Sixty Six
The Family Holiday
The Family Stone
The Most Wonderful Time of the Year
White Christmas

Aging
A Gathering of Old Men
A Rather English Marriage
A Rumor of Angels
A Symphony for Martin
A Very Old Man with Enormous Wings
  (Cuba)
A Woman's Tale (Australia)
A Woman Under the Influence
About Schmidt
Afterlife (Japan)
An Empty Bed
Another Woman
Assisted Living
Away from Here
Babette's Feast (Denmark)
Bloom
Boynton Beach Club
Buena Vista Social Club (Documentary)
Camilla
Cemetery Club
Central Station (Brazil)
Cheri
Cinema Paradiso (France)
Cleopatra (Argentina)
Cocoon
Cocoon: The Return
Dad
Daughters of the Dust
Dim Sum
Driving Miss Daisy
Do You Remember Love?
Down in the Delta
El Cochecita (Spain)
El Milagro de P. Tinto (Spain)
Empties (Czech Republic)
Eternity and a Day
Evening
Firefly
Folks
Fried Green Tomatoes

Appendices

Gran Torino
Goodbye Solo
Grey Gardens
Grumpier Old Men
Grumpy Old Men
Harold and Maude
Harry and Tonto
How to Make An American Quilt
Hyenas (Senegal)
I'm Going Home (France/Portugal)
I'm Not Rappaport
I Never Sang for My Father
Innocence (Australia)
Intoxicating
Iris
Is Anybody There?
Kaas (Belgium)
King of California
Koza (Turkey)
Ladies in Lavender
Le Grande voyage
Letters to Juliet
Lovely, Still
Madadayo (Japan)
Martha and Ethel
Madea's Family Reunion
Monsieur Ibrahim
Mr. and Mrs. Bridge
Mrs. Dalloway
Mrs. Palfrey at the Claremont (UK)
Must Love Dogs
My Girl
My Failing Eyesight (Malaysia)
Nine Good Teeth
Nobody's Fool
Noel
Nostalgia (Italy)
On Golden Pond
One True Thing
Pushing Hands (China)
Racing Against the Clock (Documentary)
Saraband (Sweden/Norway)
Saving Our Parents (Documentary)
Secondhand Lions
Shadowlands
Shirley Valentine
Son of the Bride (Argentina)
Space Cowboys

Speed of Life
Spring Forward
Steel Magnolias
Strangers in Good Company (Canada)
Sunset Story
Tatie Danielle (France)
Terms of Endearment
That Evening Sun
To Dance with the White Dog
The Alzheimer Affair (Belgium/The
  Netherlands)
The Ballad of Narayama (Japan)
The Best Exotic Marigold Hotel
The Field
The First Grader
The Gin Game
The Golden Honeymoon
The Grandfather (Spain)
The Grass Harp
The Hours
The Lady Killers
The Last Station
The Old Woman's Step (Brazil)
The Notebook
The Personals
The Pumpkin Eaters
The Road Home
The Savages
The Son of the Bride (Argentina)
The Storekeeper (South Africa)
The Straight Story
The Trip to Bountiful
The Wash (Japan)
The Whales of August
The Winter Guest
This Old Cub
Travelling Companion
Traveling North (Australia)
Unforgiven
Unhook the Stars
United We Stand (Norway)
Up
Used People
Vernon, Florida
Waking Ned Devine
What About You?
Where's Poppa?
Widow's Peak

Wrestling Ernest Hemingway
Young at Heart (Documentary)

Mental Health
Alcohol and Drug Abuse
A Love Song for Bobby Long
A Scanner Darkly
Affliction
All Over Me
Altered States
American Heart
Angela's Ashes
Animal Kingdom (Australia)
Another Day in Paradise
Around Midnight
Arthur
Bad Lieutenant
Bad News Bears
Bad Santa
Barfly
Basquiet
Bastard Out of Carolina
Betty (French)
Berlin Calling
Beautiful Girls
Beautiful People
Beloved Infidel
Big Lebowski
Bird
Blindspot (TV movie)
Blow
Bob and Carol and Ted and Alice
Bongwater
Born on the Fourth of July
Bottle Shock
Boys on the Side
Bounce
Brainstorm
Breakfast of Champions
Bright Lights, Big City
Brokedown Palace
Bug
Bully
Candy
Can't Buy Me Love
Capote
Cat Ballou

Cat on a Hot Tin Roof
Chains of Gold
Changing Lanes
Chappaqua
Charlie Wilson's War
Chasing the White Dragon
Children of Men
Citizen Ruth
Clean (UK)
Clean and Sober
Cocaine Cowboys (documentary)
Coffee and Cigarettes
Crazy Heart
Curse of the Starving Class
Dark Obsession
Days of Wine and Roses
Daytime Drinking (Korea)
Detroit Rock City
Devdas
Dirty Habit
Disclosure
Divided Memories
Dogs in Space
Don't Come Knocking
Dopamine
Down in the Delta
Down to the Bone
Dr. T. and the Women
Drugstore Cowboy
Drunks
Duane Hopwood
Easy Rider
Educating Rita
El Cantante
Factotum
Fear and Loathing in Las Vegas
For One More Day
Fried Green Tomatoes
Full Blast
Gia
Go
Goodfellas
Grid Lock'd
Groove
Half Baked
Half Nelson
Hancock
Havoc

Appendices

Henry Fool
High Art
Homegrown
House of Sand and Fog
Huelepega: Glue Sniffer
Hustle and Flow
Idle Hands
I'll Cry Tomorrow
Illtown
Indebted
Intoxicating
Ironman
Ironweed
Jesus' Son
Karanja, The Suffering Alcoholic: Is There Hope? (Kenya, VHS)
Lady Sing the Blues
Leaving Las Vegas
Lenny
Long Day's Journey into Night
Lorna's Silence
Losing Isaiah
Love Liza
Luminous Motion
Luna
Maria, Full of Grace
Marine Life
Mariposas en el Estomago (Mexico)
Mask
My Beautiful Laundrette
My Favorite Year
My Name is Bill W. (TV movie)
My Name is Joe
Naked Lunch
National Lampoon's Animal House
New Jack City
Niagara Motel
Nil by Mouth
No Such Thing (Iceland)
Novocaine
One for the Road
Oxygen
Pay It Forward
Pinero
Platoon
Pollack
Postcard from the Edge
Pulp Fiction

Pusher (Denmark)
Pushing Tin
Quitting
Rabbit Proof Fence
Rachel Getting Married
Ratcatcher
Ray
Reefer Madness
Requiem for a Dream
Rush
Scarface
Shadow Hours
Shadrach
Shakes the Clown
She's So Lovely
Sid and Nancy
Sideways
Simpatico
Skin Deep
Solas
Sophie
Spun
Stardust
Strange Brew
Streamers
Sweet Nothing
Synanon
Tender Mercies
The Acid House (UK)
The Alcohol Years
The Aviator
The Basketball Diaries
The Boost
The Doors
The Hangover
The Fighter
The Legend of the Holy Drinker (Italy)
The Lonely Passion of Judith Hearne
The Lost Weekend
The Man with the Golden Arm
The Prize Winner of Defiance, Ohio
The Salton Sea
The Seven Percent Solution
The Wackness
The Wood
Traffic
Trainspotting
Twenty Four Seven

Under the Volcano
Viysl Dihnd
Wasted
We Children from Bahnhof Zoo
What's Love Go to Do with It?
When a Man Loves a Woman
Who'll Stop the Rain?
Winter's Bone
Withnail and I
Wonderland
Young Cesar
Youngster
16 Years of Alcohol (UK)
28 Days
35 Shots of Rum

Eating Disorders
Baby Fat
Disfigured
Eating
Fatboy: The Movie
Fat Girl (French)
Fat Girls
Feed
I Want Someone to Eat Cheese With
Life is Sweet
Love on a diet (Hong Kong)
Muffin Man (documentary)
Perfect Body
Run Fatboy Run
Seabiscuit
The Best Little Girl in the World

Nicotine-related Disorders
Bridget Jones's Diary
Cat's Eye
Coffee, Tea and Cigarettes
Love in a Puff

Problem Gambling
A Bronx Tale
A River Runs Through It
Bad Lieutenant
BINGO!
Black Cat, White Cat
Casino
Croupier
Deadly Bet

Deceiver
Desert Bloom
Diner
Dona Flor and Her Two Husbands
Duane Hopwood
Easy Money
Everybody's All-American
Face of a Stranger
Family Prayers
Fever Pitch
Frankie and Johnny
Get Shorty
Gladiator
Guys and Dolls
Hard Ball
Heat
High Stakes
Honeymoon in Vegas
Hoop Dreams
House of Games
Inside Out
Just the Ticket
Last Days of Frankie the Fly
Let it Ride
Maverick
Money Train
One Last Ride
Oscar and Lucinda
Out to Sea
Owning Mahoney
Parenthood
Queen of Hearts
Queen of Spades
Sgt. Bilko
Shade
Side Out
Sour Grapes
Suspicion
The Basket
The Big Payoff
The Break
The Champ
The Cheaters
The Color of Money
The Corrupter
The Gamble
The Hustler
The Linguini Incident

Appendices

The Seduction of Gina
The Squeeze
The Swindle
This is a Hijack
Vegas Vacation
Volunteers
White Men Can't Jump
Winner Take All
Wise Guys
21

Sex Addiction

Alfie
Autofocus
Burn after Reading
Easier with Practice
Mouth to Mouth
Shame
The Piano Teacher
Walk All Over Me

Loss and Bereavement

A Rumor of Angels
A Single Man
Always
An Unfinished Life
Angel in the Family
Angela's Ashes
Boynton Beach Club
Brian's Song
Brokeback Mountain
Catch and Release
City of Angels
Corrina, Corrina
Departures
Dragonfly
Eye of the Dolphin
Gates of Heaven
Ghost
In America
In Her Shoes
In the Bedroom
Marley and Me
Moonlight Mile
Mrs. Palfrey at the Claremont
Northfork
November Christmas
Philadelphia

Rabbit Hole
Ray
Reign Over Me
Remember Me
Snowcake
Straight from the Heart
Sunshine Cleaning
The Bucket List
The Grace Card
The Laramie Project
The Most Wonderful Time of the Year
The River Niger
The Savages
The Secret Life of Bees
The Space Between
The Way
The Winter Guest
Truly, Madly, Deeply
Tuesdays with Morrie
Up
Waking the Dead
Walk the Line
Wide Awake

Depression and Suicidal Behavior

A Dog's Dream
A Hole in One
A Little Crazy
A Single Man
About a Boy
Another Day in Paradise
Black Irish
Broken Flowers
Chapter Zero
Cry for Help (Documentary)
Dead Man on Campus
Devil's Playground (Documentary)
Does Your Soul Have a Cold?
Downloading Nancy
El Cantante
Goodbye, Solo
Kill Me Later
Letters from Iwo Jima
Little Miss Sunshine
Men Get Depression (Documentary)
Old Boy
On the Edge
One Week

Prozac Nation
Remember Me
Romulus, My Father (Australia)
Saviour Square (Poland)
Schultze Gets the Blues (Germany)
Set Me Free (Canada)
Seven Pounds
Stay
Suicide Club (Japan)
Sylvia, Set Me Free (UK)
The Bridge
The Girl on the Bridge (France)
The Hours
The Unsaid
The Virgin Suicides
They Shoot Horses, Don't They?
Two Lovers
What Dreams May Come
Wilbur (Wants to Kill Himself)

Self-injurious Behavior
Augusta Gone (TV)
Betty Blue
Black Swan
Bug
Cut
Dans Ma Peau
Girl Interrupted
Prozac Nation
Fucking Amal (Swedish)
Ik Ook Van Jou (Dutch)
Lady Vengeance
Manic
My First Mister
Old Boy
Stay
Strange Circus
The Piano Teacher
The Secretary
The Virgin Suicides
Thirteen
Whole
Wrist-cutters
28 Days

Trauma from Abuse and Violence
A Streetcar Named Desire
Affliction

American Beauty
Bastard out of Carolina
Beaten
Beautiful Creatures
Bhaji at the Beach
Bloom
Carousel
Crimes of the Heart
Dangerous Intentions
Diary of a Mad Housewife
Donovan's Reef
El Bola
Enough
Fried Green Tomatoes
Gaslight
Gone with the Wind
Honey and Ashes
In the Bedroom
John in the Sky
La Strada
Love Me or Leave Me
Madame Brouette
Mystic River
Nil By Mouth
Once Were Warriors
Othello
Personal Velocity
Petulia
Public Enemy
Radio Flyer
Sleeping with the Enemy
Smoke Signals
Solitaire
Solo Mio
Take My Eyes (Spain)
The Evening Sun
The Great Santini
The Joy Luck Club
The Night Listener
The Prize Winner of Defiance, Ohio
The Quiet Man
The Taming of the Shrew
Under the Skin of the City
Waitress
What's Love Got to Do with It?
Whatever Happened to Baby Jane?
Yellow Asphalt

Appendices

Sexual Abuse and Rape
Descent
Doubt
Hard Candy
Last Tango in Paris
My First Mister
Old Boy
Precious
Pretty Baby
Strange Circus
The Accused
The Last Picture Show
The Prince of Tides
Posttraumatic Stress Disorder
Blue
Crossroads (Iran)
Down Came a Blackbird
Fearless
K-Pax
Mine
Music in Exile
Rhapsody in August
Reign Over Me
Snowcake
The Axe in the Attic
The Fisher King
The Hurt Locker
The Waterdance
Trouble the Water
Walking on Dead Fish

The Workplace
A Brief Vacation
Disclosure
Everything Must Go
Glengarry Glen Ross
Homeless for the Holidays
Horrible Bosses
In Good Company
Kasak
Larry Crowne
Made in Dagenhan
North Country
Philadelphia
The Company Men
Two Weeks Notice
Up in the Air

Portrayals of Myers-Briggs Types
A Serious Man
Adaptation
Alexander
Amelie
Big Fish
Collateral
Doubt
Eternal Sunshine of the Spotless Mind
Fearless
Fight Club
Frost/Nixon
Good Night and Good Luck
In the Valley of Elah
Invictus
Jurassic Park
Lawrence of Arabia
Magnolia
Milk
Mr. Smith Goes to Washington
Revolutionary Road
Rushmore
Star Wars
Stranger Than Fiction
The Aviator
The Grapes of Wrath
The Good Shepherd
The Queen
The Social Network
The Station Agent
The Story of Us
The Wrestler

Specific Disease States and Health Care Issues
Cancer
A Brooklyn Family Tale
A Change of Heart
A Christmas Visitor
A Dedicated Life
A Family
A Gun, A Car, A Blonde
A Healthy Baby Girl
A Lion in the House (Documentary)
A Little Kiss
A Praise in the Valley
A Private Battle

A Shining Season
A Snake of June
A Thousand Acres
A Time for Dancing
A Walk to Remember
Aberdeen
Afterlife
Alchemy
Ali
Angel on My Shoulder
At Night
Bare Skyer
Beautiful Joe
Beveger Stjeenene
Bliss
Bloom
Blow
Blow Dry
Blue Vinyl
Breaking Away
Breaking Bad (TV Series)
Brian's Song
Burn the Bridges
C Me Dance
Caro Diario
C'est La Vie, Mon Cheri
Champions
Chernobyl Heart
Chocolate
Crazy Sexy Cancer
Crazy White Foreigner
Dad
Dah Be Alaveh Chahar
Death: A Love Story
Death Be Not Proud
Debutante
Der Himmel Kann Warten
Die Beunruhigung
Die Wunde
Doctor ZMack
Dying to Have Known
Dying Young
Eierdibe
Elegy
Evening
Extreme Honor
Familie
Family Pack

Flower Island
For Hire
Freeheld (Documentary)
Fubar
Full Moon
Funny People
Garden of Heaven
God said, Ha!
God's Army
Griffin and Phoenix
Hawks
Here on Earth
Hoxsey: When Healing Became a Crime
    (Documentary)
I'm with Cancer
I've Loved You So Long
Ikuru
In the Shadows
Jesus, Mary and Joey
Last Wish
Le Grand Role
Leap of Faith
Life as a House
Life is a Miracle
Les Corps Impatients
Living Proof
Look Both Ways
Love Lives on
Magnolia
Man on the Moon
Marvin's Room
Men Don't Cry: Prostate Cancer Stories
    (Documentary)
My Life without Me
My Sister's Keeper
No Higher Love
On the Edge
One Last Thing
Paris
Pieces of April
Pope Dreams
Princes in Exile
Rachel's Daughters
Stepmom
Shadowlands
Six Weeks
Southern Comfort
Space Cowboys

Appendices

Special Ed
Stepmom
Strapless
Sweet November
Terminal
Terminal City (Reality TV)
Terms of Endearment
The Big C (TV)
The Bucket List
The Bulls of Suburbia
The Bumblebee Flies Away
The Doctor
The Dream Chasers
The Good Fight
The Gospel according to Vic
The Guitar
The Last Dance
The Law of Enclosures
The Process
The Ride
The Setting Son
The Sleepy Time Gal
The Sunchaser
The Union Blue Project (Documentary)
The Whole of the Moon
Time to Leave
Treads of Destiny
Vaaranan (in Tamil)
Vernie
Vital Signs
Viva, Castro
When the Time Comes
Wit
3:19
50/50
57000 KM Entre Nous

Diabetes
Adventures for the Cure (Documentary)
Alma (documentary)
Bread and Roses
Big Nothing
Brokedown Palace
Chocolat
Click
Con Air
D4G
Derailed

Dog Day Afternoon
Gerbia
Gettin' Grown
Gunner Goes Comfortable
It Runs in the Family
Jerry and Tom
Kasak
La Debandade (France)
Mad Money
Meeting Daddy
Memento
Navajo Medicine
Nothing in Common
Panic Room
Poison
Promised a Miracle
Sleeping Dogs
Soul Food
Steel Magnolias
The Godfather III
This Old Cub
The Shaman's Apprentice

Disruptive Patients/ Disruptive Providers
Analyze This
Angels in America
Becker (TV)
Dogville
Dressed to Kill
Happiness
House (TV)
Intoxicating
Juno
Just Like Heaven
Little Shop of Horrors
M.A.S.H. (TV)
Novocaine
One Flew Over the Cuckoo's Nest
Quincy, M.E. (TV)
Reign Over Me
The English Patient
The Hospital
The House of God
The Neighbor
Where the Money Is

Emergency Medicine
Analyze This
Extreme Measures
John Q.
Just Like Heaven
Ocean of Pearls
Something's Gotta Give

Heart Disease
A Single Man
Beyond the Sea
Chernobyl Heart
Counting the Sheep
Heartbeat (Korea)
Heart Condition
Here on Earth
John Q.
Keep Coming Back
Last Holiday
Minor Mishaps
Open Hearted
Paris
Return to Me
Solitary Man
Something's Gotta Give
Son of the Bride
Sweet November
The Good Heart
The Man on the Train
The World's Fastest Indian
Untamed Heart

High Risk Obstetrics
Away We Go
Blindspot (TV movie)
Father of the Bride 2
Steel Magnolias
Waitress

Miscarriage
Bloom
Marley and Me

Vaginal Bleeding
Cries and Whispers

In Vitro Fertilization
Baby Mama

Bloom
Chutney Popcorn
Making Grace

Other Pregnancy-related Films
Arranged
What to Expect When you are Expecting
35 and Ticking

HIV/AIDS
A Mother's Prayer
An Early Frost (Made for TV)
And the Band Played On
Angels in America
Before Night Falls
Behind the Red Door
Breaking the Surface: The Greg Louganis
   Story
Carandiru
Day/Giorni (Italy)
El Cantante
It's My Party
Jeffrey
Life and Death on the A-List
   (Documentary)
Life Support
Long Time Companion
Love Valour Compassion
My Brother Nikhil (India)
My Own Country
Philadelphia
Phir Milenge (India)
On the Downlow
One Week
No One Sleeps
Rent
The Cure
The Fire Within (Documentary)
The Hours
Three Needles
World and Time Enough
Yesterday

International Medical Missions
Beyond Borders
City of Joy
Live and Become
Smile

Appendices

The Constant Gardener
The English Surgeon
The Last King of Scotland
The Nun's Story
Triage: Dr. James Orbinski's
    Humanitarian Dilemma

The Elephant Man
The English Patient
The Wacky Adventures of Dr. Boris and
    Nurse Shirley
Vera Drake
4 months, 3 weeks and 2 days

Marginalized Populations and Health Disparities
A Day without a Mexican
All of Us (Documentary)
Almost a Woman
Barrio Cuba
De Nadie
In America
Inch'Allah Dimarche
Innocent Voices
Life Support
One Week
Precious
Resurrecting the Champ
The First Grader
The Fisher King
The Help
The Pursuit of Happiness
The Saint of Fort Washington
The Soloist
Trouble the Water
Under the Same Moon
Yesterday

Medical Ethics
A Civil Action
Breast Men (Docudrama)
Dark Victory
Dirty Pretty Things
Dying Young
I've Loved You So Long
John Q.
Love and Other Drugs
Lovesick
Mar Adentro
Million Dollar Baby
My Life without Me
Southern Comfort
The Bone Collector
The Death of Mr. Lazarescu
The Diving Bell and the Butterfly

Medical Malpractice
Flatliners
Love and Other Drugs
Malice
Reign Over Me
Southern Comfort
The Fugitive
The Hand that Rocks the Cradle

Military Medicine/Psychology
Antwone Fisher
Apocalypse Now
Armadillo
Badland
Band of Brothers
Battle for Marjah
Blackhawk Down
Born on the Fourth of July
Boy in the Striped Pajamas
Casualties of War
Das Boot
D-Day
Forest Gump
Full Metal Jacket
Generation Kill (Documentary, HBO)
Grace is Gone
Guns of Navarone
Jarhead
Johnny Got His Gun
In Country
In the Valley of Elah
Ordinary People
Pearl Harbor
Platoon
Redacted
Saving Private Ryan
Sniper
Standard Operating Procedure
Stop-Loss
Streamers
Taking Chance

The Best Years of Our Lives
The Deer Hunter
The Great Santini
The Hurt Locker
The Lucky Ones
The Messenger
The Pacific
Tora Tora Tora
Windtalkers

Neurological Disorders
A Man Apart
Coma
Critical Care
Dead Zone
Dream Life of Angels
Face Off
Good-bye Lenin
Habla con Ella (Talk to Her)
Hard to Kill
Hilary and Jackie
Kill Bill I
Lorenzo's Oil
Lying in Wait
Monkey Bone
Regarding Henry
Reversal of Fortune
The Theory of Flight
While You Were Sleeping
28 Days Later

Palliative Care
A Wedding for Bella
Departures (Japan)
Evening
Ikiru (Japan)
L'Amour a Mort (France)
La Gueule Ouverte (France)
Maborosi (Japan)
My Sister's Keeper
The Basketball Diaries
The Bucket List
The Diving Bell and the Butterfly
   (France)
The English Patient
The Sea Inside (Spain)
Walking on Water

Rehabilitation Medicine
Born on the Fourth of July
The Theory of Flight
The Waterdance
Warm Springs

Sexuality and Health
American Pie
Black Swan
Bound
Couples Retreat
Kinsey
Knocked Up
Match Point
Sex and Death
Sex, Lies and Videotape
Something's Gotta Give
Teeth
The Oh in Ohio
There's Something about Mary

Sports Medicine and Sports Psychology
A League of Their Own
Ali
All the Right Moves
Any Given Sunday
Bad News Bears
Bend it Like Beckham
Big Fan
Billy Elliot
Black Cloud
Black Swan
Breaking Away
Brian's Song
Bull Durham
Champions
Chariots of Fire
Chasing 3000
Coach Carter
Cool Runnings
Eight Men Out
Fear Strikes Out
Field of Dreams
Friday Night Lights
For the Love of the Game
Gleaming the Cube
Glory Road

Goal!
Happy Gilmore
He Got Game
Hoop Dreams
Hoosiers
Hurricane
Invincible
Jerry Maguire
Jockeys
Love and Basketball
Major League I
Major League II
Million Dollar Baby
Miracle
Mr. Baseball
Murderball
Nacho Libre
Overseas
Over the Top
Peaceful Warrior
Ping Pong
Rad
Radio
Raging Bull
Rebound
Remember the Titans
Rollerball
Rounders
Rudy
Running Brave
Seabiscuit
Soul Surfer
Space Jam
Sugar
The Air Up There
The Basketball Diaries
The Blind Side
The Express
The Game Plan
The Greatest Game Ever Played
The Horsemasters
The Karate Kid
The Legend of Bagger Vance
The Long Green Line
The Lookout
The Natural
The Other Side of the Mountain
The Perfect Game

The Replacements
The Rookie
The Sandlot
The Wrestler
The Whole Nine Yards
The World's Fastest Indian
The Wrestler
This Old Cub
Tin Cup
We are Marshall
White Men Can't Jump
Wind
61

Surgical Interventions (plastic and reconstructive surgery)

A Thousand Acres
Absolutely Safe
America the Beautiful
Ash Wednesday
Breast Men (Docudrama)
Body Art (Documentary)
Chrysalis
Cleavage
Goodnight Vagina
Guinea Pig Club
Heartlift
Ki Rei: Terror of Beauty
La Ultima Noche
Lovely and Amazing
Models
Mouth to Mouth
Never Perfect
Perfect People
Smile
The Wacky Adventures of Dr. Boris and
    Nurse Shirley
Time
Vanilla Sky

Television, Medicine and Teaching

Autopsy Files
Becker
Ben Casey
Chicago Hope
China Beach
Combat Hospital
Dr. Kildare

Doc Martin
Grey's Anatomy
HawthoRNe
House
Off the Map
Out of Practice
Marcus Welby, M.D.
M.A.S.H.
Medic
Medical Center
Miami Medical
Quincy, M.E.
Royal Pains
St. Elsewhere

Documentaries and Docudramas
A Case of Valor
At the Kitchen Table
Body Art (Documentary)
Consider the Conversation
Fat, Sick and Nearly Dead
For Once in My Life
Forks over Knives
Killers at Large
Modify
Money Driven Medicine
Music in Exile
Never Perfect (documentary)
Return (documentary, Africa)
Salud
Sicko
The First Grader
The Vanishing Oath
Unforgotten
Waiting for Superman
Walking on Dead Fish
Whole

Reality TV
Addictions
Animal Hoarders
Celebrity Rehab
Dr. 90210
Hoarders
In Treatment
Intervention
Little People
Mental

Mystery Diagnosis
Mystery ER
Nip/Tuck
OCD
911: The Bronx

Traumatic Brain Injury
The Hurt Locker
The Lookout
Memento

Movie Portrayals of Health Care Professionals
Dentists
Bells are Ringing
Cactus Flower
Captives
Charlie and the Chocolate Factory (2005)
Compromising Positions
Eversmile, New Jersey
Finding Nemo
Ghost Town
Good Luck Chuck
Houseguest
Lethal Weapon 4
Little Shop of Horrors
Marathon Man
MASH
Novocaine
Reign Over Me
Serial Mom
Sidewalks of New York
Snow Dogs
The Dentist
The Hangover
The Hangover (2)
The In-Laws
The Whole Nine Yards
The Secret Lives of Dentists
The Secret Partner
Thumbsucker
Tombstone
Waiting for Guffman
Wild Hogs
10

Appendices

Group Therapists
Down Came a Blackbird
Drunks
Manic
Take My Eyes
28 Days

Nurses
Becker (TV)
Carry on Nurse
China Beach (TV)
Combat Hospital (TV)
Cry Havoc
Eastern Promises
Eating Raoul
ER (TV)
Florence Nightingale
Gifted Man (TV)
Grey's Anatomy (TV)
Hart of Dixie (TV)
HawthoRNe (TV)
House (TV)
Magnolia
Marcus Welby, M.D. (TV)
M.A.S.H.
Meet the Parents
Mercy (TV)
Miss Evers' Boys
Nurse Betty
Nurse Jackie (TV)
One Flew Over the Cuckoo's Nest
Precious
Prison Nurse
Private Practice (TV)
Requiem for a Dream
Royal Pains (TV)
Scrubs (TV)
So Proudly We Hail
Strong Medicine (TV)
The Bag of Knees
The English Patient
The Glades (TV)
The Fockers
The Nun's Story
The Nurse
The Nurses (TV)
The Sensuous Nurse
Scrubs (TV)

South Pacific
Why Me?
Wit
13 Weeks

Physicians
A Farewell to Arms
A Stranger's Heart
Adam Resurrected
Anatomy
Article 99
Back to You and Me
Bad Medicine
Bikini House Calls
Breast Men
Brittania Hospital
Carry on Doctor
Cider House Rules
City of Angels
Coma
Dead Ringers
Doctor at Large
Doctor at Sea
Doctor Bull
Doctor in the House
Doctor Zhivago
Extraordinary Measures
Flatliners
Garden State
Gifted Hands
House Calls
Interns Can't Take Money
Julie Walking Home
Just Like Heaven
Living Proof
Love and Other Drugs
Malice
M.A.S.H.
Near Death
Ocean of Pearls
Open Your Eyes
Rizzoli and Isles (TV)
So Proudly We Hail
Stella Dogs
Talk to Her
The Doctor
The Hospital
The Interns

The Last King of Scotland
The Painted Veil
The Savages
Whose Life is it Anyway?
Wit

Psychiatrists
Antwone Fisher
Benny and Joon
High Anxiety
Mr. Jones
Silence of the Lambs
The Sixth Sense

Psychologists and Psychotherapy
A Clockwork Orange
Analyze This
Antwone Fisher
Bloom
Conflict
Couples Retreat
Dead Man Out
Empathy
Good Will Hunting
Identity
Intimate Strangers
Ira and Abby
It's Complicated
Kiss the Girls
Mad Love
Manic
Mumford
Primal Fear
Prime
She's So Lovely
Solaris
The Dark Mirror
The Sixth Sense
The Unsaid

School Psychology
Leave it to Beaver
Parenthood
Parents

Social Workers
A Mother's Prayer

About Enormous Changes at the Last
   Minute
About Me and Veronica
Ann Vickers
Boyfriends
Cae 39
Chains of Gold
Crime in the Streets
Deuz Hommes Dans La Ville
East Side, West Side (TV)
Gambling House
Judging Amy (TV)
Kisses and Scratches
Last of the Great Survivors
Like Dandelion Dust
Losing Isaiah
Mr. Soft Touch
Niagara Motel
Paris
Pieces of Dreams
Precious
Punish Me
Raw Deal
Sammyville
Savage Messiah
Sunset Story
Take Me Away
The Golden Child
The Man Who Forgot
The Night Listener
Three Needles
Why Me?

TV Portrayals of Psychotherapists
Addiction
Hoarders
Intervention
Newhart
OCD
The Sopranos

Veterinary Medicine
Amores Perros
Harry and Tonto
K-9
Marley and Me
Mine
Seabiscuit

Appendices

Secretariat
Sleeping Dogs
The Nurses
The Savages
The Truth About Cats and Dogs
Turner and Hootch
Water for Elephants
Wendy and Lucy

Additional Topics Not Included in Volume 2

Editor's Note: The following list is meant to provide a brief overview of some of the many films, documentaries and television series that can provide material for other topics.

Please refer to Volume One for film clips on these topics.

Anxiety Disorders
Analyze This
As Good As it Gets
Batman Begins
Matchstick Men
Nobody's Child
The Aviator
The Dark Knight
The Sopranos
What About Bob?

Bipolar Disorders
A Fine Madness
Benny and Joon
Blue Sky
Bulworth
Cobb
David and Lisa
Don Juan de Marco
Frances
Lust for Life
Mad Love
Manic
Mr. Jones
The Gingerbread Man
The King of California
The Saint of Fort Washington
Through the Glass Darkly

Chronic Illness
A Brief Vacation
Garden State
Jack
Love and Other Drugs
My Name is Khan
Ray
Rory O' Shea
Sabine
The Life of a Child
Wretches and Jabberers

Cultural Diversity
A Day without a Mexican
Crossing Over
Invictus
Seven Soles
Slumdog Millionaire
The Blindside

Delusional and Dissociative Disorders
Dancer in the Dark
Nurse Betty
The Fan
The Story of Adele H.

Integrative Medicine
Doc Hollywood
Mystic Masseur
Return (documentary, Africa)

Interviewing Skills
An Unmarried Woman
Analyze This
Manic
What About Bob?

Lesbian, Gay, Bisexual, Transgender, Intersex, Questioning (LGBTIQ)
A Jihad for Love
A Single Man
Adventures of Felix (France)
Alabama
Boyfriends
Breakfast on Pluto
Capote
Fagbus
Far from Heaven

Fish Out of Water
Gendernauts
Get Your Stuff
Heavenly Creatures
Kissing Jessica Stein
Milk
Normal
Out of the Past
Prodigal Sons
Queens of Heart
Queer as Folk (Showtime TV)
River Was Over Me
Saving Face
Shortbus
Small Town Gay Bar
Southern Comfort
Streamers
The L Word (Showtime TV)
The Laramie Project
The Topp Twins
Transamerica
We Were Here

Mental Disabilities
Her Name is Sabine
I am Sam
My Name is Khan
Snowcake

Personality Disorders
Blue Sky
Fatal Attraction
Happy-go- Lucky
Heavy
Me Without You
Pollock
Punch Drunk Love
The Caine Mutiny
The Shipping News

The Squid and the Whale
2 Days
4 months, 3 weeks and 2 days

Physical Disability
Forrest Gump
Notting Hill
Rory O'Shea
The Keys to the House
The Man without a Face
The Waterdance
Vanilla Sky
Warmsprings

Schizophrenia
A Beautiful Mind
Clean, Shaven
Donnie Darko
Gothika
Mad Love
Manic
Secret Window
Stateside
The Soloist

Somatoform Disorders
Hannah and Her Sisters
Hollywood Ending

The Professional and Personal Self of the Physician
Critical Care
Gifted Hands
Something the Lord Made
The Locket

Useful Websites
www.lib.berkeley.edu/MRC
www.psychflix.com

Editors' Top Ten Cinemeducation Movie Picks

Matthew Alexander's Top Ten

A desire to understand and improve human relationships is the prime motivating factor of my professional life. Each of the movies cited in this list provides profound lessons about relationships. Each is compelling, beautifully acted and original in scope. Many of the scenes taken from these movies are seared into my consciousness and offer outstanding teaching material both for health-care learners and therapy clients, often couples.

Five of the movies (*Match Point*; *The Break-Up*; *Blue Valentine*; *Crazy Heart*; *Midnight in Paris*) deal directly with romantic relationships. Two of these films are directed by Woody Allen. *Match Point*, which has been cited by Allen as the favorite film in his oeuvre, reveals the passion and tragedy associated with extra-marital affairs while *Midnight in Paris* demonstrates how important value differences are often deal breakers in committed relationships. *Blue Valentine* and *Crazy Heart* both show the corrosive impact of alcohol abuse on relationships while *The Break-Up* illustrates how friends can inadvertently turn a fight over the dishes into permanent separation. The moral of that story is to be careful from whom you get your advice!

Another movie on my top ten, *Ira and Abby*, is an overlooked gem that showcases the dark side of the psychotherapeutic relationship, while *The Diving Bell and the Butterfly* reveals how a professional relationship between a speech therapist and a patient with locked-in syndrome can have a life-altering effect. *The Squid and the Whale* is a cautionary tale about how parents can wreak havoc on their children's lives by poor handling of a separation and divorce.

The Social Network is a memorable film that illustrates how individuals with variants of Asperger's syndrome are challenged in their relationships with others. Finally, *Slumdog Millionaire* is a brilliant movie about the transformative power of love. This film also stands as a testament to the pure emotional force of cinema. If you doubt me about this, please watch the closing scene when the two protagonists meet in the train station. I guarantee it will bring tears to your eyes.

1   *Match Point* (2005)
2   *Slumdog Millionaire* (2008)
3   *Ira and Abby* (2006)
4   *The Break-Up* (2006)
5   *Midnight in Paris* (2011)
6   *The Squid and the Whale* (2005)
7   *Blue Valentine* (2010)
8   *The Social Network* (2010)
9   *The Diving Bell and the Butterfly* (2007)
10 *Crazy Heart* (2009)

Patricia Lenahan's Top Ten

Movies have varying appeal to viewers depending on the "whys" of our watching them. My choices for the top ten movies for cinemeducation are different to those I would select for my top ten favorite movies that I watch for enjoyment, enlightenment, or escape. Also, it should be noted that my current list does not include my top five cinemeducation films cited in our first book, *Cinemeducation, Volume 1: a comprehensive guide to using film in medical education*, although these five do remain among my favorite teaching films. My choices here fall into three general categories: (1) aging, (2) chronic illness and diversity/health disparities, and (3) violence and abuse. Some of the films mentioned are not great films from the acting viewpoint. *Bloom* is an example of this; however, this film has multiple potential uses in teaching: violence and abuse, the therapeutic relationship, medical marriages, infertility and impotence, aging, and cancer.

Aging-Related Films

I have selected some lesser-known films here that I have been fortunate enough to discover. These include *Lovely, Still*; *Goodbye Solo*; and *How About You*. *The Savages*, which also makes my list, is a more widely seen film on Parkinson's dementia and family relationships.

Diversity/Health Disparities Films

Perhaps my favorite film used in *Cinemeducation, Volume 2* is a diversity- and cancer-related film, *Southern Comfort*, about a middle-aged female-to-male transgender individual who has terminal cancer. This documentary film follows Robert Eads and his "chosen family" during the last year of his life and his encounters with the health-care system. Other films in this category include *Yesterday* and *Life Support*, both films about HIV in minority populations. The final film in this category is *Love Actually*. One of my favorite scenes occurs during the opening and closing credits in which families of all races and ethnicities greet one another at Heathrow Airport in London. This film also provides a treasure trove of relationship issues including loss/bereavement, betrayal/infidelity, and first love.

Violence and Abuse

Two films: *Bloom*, which has been discussed already, and *Take My Eyes*, fall into the "violence and abuse" genre. *Take My Eyes* is a Spanish film that shows strong violent content. It deals with the treatment of batterers (both individual and group) in a way that I have not found in other films.

There are four films that make my "honorable mention" list. Two of these relate to substance abuse: *Animal Kingdom* and *Winter's Bone*. Both films focus on the impact of drug abuse and violence on the adolescents in the family. The third honorable mention goes to *The Hurt Locker*, which offers viewers a glimpse into the lives of the modern military and an exposure to the daily lives of those whose job it is to disarm bombs. The fourth honorable mention goes to *This Old Cub*, which chronicles the personal and professional life of major league baseball player Ron Santo, his struggle with diabetes, and his perceived need to keep the disease hidden.

The beauty of film is that various types of film and genre can appeal to us at different times and can serve to educate and offer moments of reflection as well as to entertain.

1	*Lovely, Still* (2008)
2	*Goodbye Solo* (2008)
3	*How About You* (2007)
4	*The Savages* (2007)
5	*Southern Comfort* (2001)
6	*Yesterday* (2004)
7	*Life Support* (2007)
8	*Love Actually* (2003)
9	*Bloom* (2003)
10	*Take My Eyes* (2003)

Anna Pavlov's Top Ten

My top ten list is an eclectic mix of drama ranging from life and relationship challenges to the death of a partner and suicidality. As a health psychologist teaching in a family medicine residency program, the films I have selected focus on individuals and families facing challenges in living with chronic problems and life-threatening illness, end of life, and tremendous loss. They also demonstrate the possibility of hope and personal growth at these times. These themes are present in *Elegy, The Bucket List, A Single Man, The Savages, Juno, Rabbit Hole*; and *Tree of Life*.

Black Swan is an intense film that demonstrates the pressures to be perfect and self-injurious behavior as a coping device. It is a stunning and courageous film. Few movies have made me laugh so much as *It's Complicated*, which astutely displays the confusion and messiness of postmodern divorce and redemption. *Lars and the Real Girl* is a tender look at individual difference and psychological barriers to real relationships. The film contains one of the best and most psychologically minded family doctor counseling scenes imaginable.

1	*It's Complicated* (2009)
2	*Elegy* (2008)
3	*The Bucket List* (2007)
4	*Lars and the Real Girl* (2007)
5	*The Savages* (2007)
6	*A Single Man* (2009)
7	*Black Swan* (2010)
8	*Rabbit Hole* (2010)
9	*Tree of Life* (2011)
10	*Juno* (2007)

Bibliography

Abramson PR, Mechanic MB. Sex and the media: three decades of best-selling books and major motion pictures. *Arch Sex Behav.* 1983; **12**(3): 185–206.

Adam MB. *On History, Literature, Media and the Arts in Medicine.* Available at: www.aap.org/sections/bioethics/Arts.cfm (last accessed 12/1/11)

Akram A, O'Brien A, O'Neill A, *et al.* Crossing the line: learning psychiatry at the movies. *Int Rev Psychiatry.* 2009; **21**(3): 267–8.

Alexander M. Cinemeducation: an innovative approach to teaching multi-cultural diversity in medicine. *Ann Behav Sci Med Educ.* 1995; **2**(1): 23–8.

——. The doctor: a seminal video for cinemeducation. *Fam Med.* 2002; **34**(2): 92–4.

——. Movies and medical education. *Fam Med.* 2008; **41**(3): 215. [Peer commentary on the movie *The Diving Bell and the Butterfly* by J. Schnabel].

——. The couple's odyssey: Hollywood's take on love relationships. *Int Rev Psychiatry.* 2009; **21**(3): 183–8.

Alexander M, Hall MN, Pettice YJ. Cinemeducation: an innovative approach to teaching psychosocial medical care. *Fam Med.* 1994; **26**(7): 430–3.

Alexander M, Pavlov A, Lenahan P. *Cinemeducation: a comprehensive guide to using film in medical education.* Oxford: Radcliffe Publishing; 2005.

——. Lights, camera, action: using film to teach the ACGME competencies. *Fam Med.* 2007; **39**(1): 20–3.

Alexander M, Waxman D. Cinemeducation: teaching family systems through the movies. *Fam Syst Health.* 2000; **18**(4): 455–66.

Alexander M, Waxman D, White P. *What's Eating Gilbert Grape?* a case study of illness. *J Learn Arts.* 2007; **2**(1): Article 13.

Anderson M. 'One flew over the psychiatric unit': mental illness and the media. *J Psychiatr Ment Health Nurs.* 2003; **10**(3): 297–306.

Aubert G. Aurthur Van Gehuchten takes neurology to the movies. *Neurology.* 2002; **59**(10): 1612–18.

Aulas JJ. [Madness in German cinema (1913–1933)]. *Ann Med Psychol (Paris).* 1980; **138**(8): 925–38. [French].

Banks JT. Moving pictures. Baltimore, MD: Johns Hopkins University Press, 1998.

Baños JE. How literature and popular movies can help in medical education: applications for teaching the doctor-patient relationship. *Med Educ.* 2007; **41**(9): 918.

Barinaga M. Biology goes to the movies. *Science.* 1990; **250**(4985): 1204–6.

Baxendale S. Memories aren't made of this: amnesia at the movies. *BMJ.* 2004; **329**(7480): 1480–3.

Bibliography

——. Wrestling fact from fiction. *Epilepsy Behav*. 2011; **22**(3): 420.

Bayles M. St. Elsewhere and the theater of the nearest-thing-to-reality. *Health Manage Q*. 1986; (4): 14–17.

Belling C. The "bad news scene" as clinical drama: Part I. Writing scenes. *Fam Med*. 2006; **38**(6): 390–2.

Bhugra D. *Exploring the Portrayal of Mental Illness in Conventional Hindi Cinema*. London; 2000. Available at: www.dineshbhugra.net/dbhindicinema.html (last accessed 12/1/11)

——. Teaching psychiatry through cinema. *Psychiatr Bull*. 2003; **27**(11): 429–30.

——. Using film and literature for cultural competence training. *Psychiatr Bull*. 2003; **27**(11): 427–8.

——. Mad tales from Bollywood: the impact of social, political, and economic climate on the portrayal of mental illness in Hindi films. *Acta Psychiatr Scand*. 2005; **112**(4): 250–6.

——. *Dinesh Bhugra: summary*. Dineshbhugra.net. Available at: www.dineshbhugra.net/dbsummary.html (last accessed 12/1/11)

Bhugra D, Gupta S. Psychoanalysis and the Hindi cinema. *Int Rev Psychiatry*. 2009; **21**(3): 234–40.

Blasco PG. Literature and movies for medical students. *Fam Med*. 2001; **33**(6): 426–8.

Blasco PG, Garcia DS, de Benedetto MA, *et al*. Cinema for education global doctors: from emotions to reflection, approaching the complexity of the human being. *Prim Care*. 2009; **10**(3): 45–7.

Blasco PG, Monaco CF, de Benedetto MA, *et al*. Teaching through movies in a multicultural scenario: overcoming cultural barriers through emotions and reflection. *Fam Med*. 2010; **42**(10): 22–4.

Blasco PG, Moreto G, Roncoletta AF, *et al*. Using movie clips to foster learners' reflection: improving education in the affective domain. *Fam Med*. 2006; **38**(2): 94–6.

Bonah C, Laukötter A. Moving pictures and medicine in the first half of the 20th century: some notes on international historical developments and the potential of medical film research. *Gesnerus*. 2009; **66**(1): 121–46.

Booth B. The softer side: women doctors on TV. *American Medical News*. Amednews.com. 2001 April 16. Available at: www.ama-assn.org/amednews/2001/04/16/prca0416.htm

Bowden FJ. The doctor is sick. *BMJ*. 2009; **339**: 4392.

Brett-MacLean P. Use of the arts in medical and health professional education. *University of Alberta Health Sciences Journal*. 2007; **4**(1): 26–9.

Bridges JM. Literature review on the images of the nurse and nursing in the media. *J Adv Nurs*. 1990; **15**(7): 850–4.

Brookes B. Health education film and the Maori: *Tuberculosis and the Maori People of the Wairoa District* (1952). *Health and Hist*. Health, Medicine and the Media. 2006; **8**(2): 45–68.

Brudenell K. Madness at the movies. *Ment Health Today*. 2003: 10–11.

Butler D. Teaching about the traumatic impact of vehicular crashes: rock 'n' roll never forgets. *Fam Med*. 2009; **41**(8): 549–51.

Butler JR, Hyler SE. Hollywood portrayals of child and adolescent mental health treatment: implications for clinical practice. *Child Adolesc Psychiatr Clin N Am*. 2005; **14**(3): 509–22.

Cantor D. Uncertain enthusiasm: the American Cancer Society, public education, and the problems of the movie, 1921–1960. *Bull Hist Med*. 2007; **81**(1): 39–69.

Cape G. Addiction, stigma and movies. *Acta Psychiatr Scand*. 2003; **107**(3): 163–9.

——. Movies as a vehicle to teach addiction medicine. *Int Rev Psychiatry*. 2009; **21**(3): 213–17.

Cartwright EF. *Physiological Modernism: cinematography as a medical research technology, 1895–1960*. New Haven, CT: Yale University Press; 1993.

Cartwright L. *Screening the Body: tracing medicine's visual culture*. Minneapolis: University of Minnesota Press; 1995.

Chan C, Wagner RF Jr. Dermatology at the movies. *Clin Dermatol*. 2009; **27**(4): 419–21.

Charles M. *The Hours*: between safety and servitude. *Am J Psychoanal*. 2004; **64**(3): 305–19.

Chez RA. Movies of human sexual response as learning aids for medical students. *J Med Educ*. 1971; **46**(11): 9977–81.

Chio A, Mutani R. Arthur Van Gehuchten takes neurology to the movies. *Neurology*. 2003; **61**(4): 587–8.

Chory-Assad RM, Tamborini R. Television doctors: an analysis of physicians in fictional and non-fictional television programs. *J Broadcast Electron*. 2001; **45**(3): 499–522.

——. Television exposure and the public's perception of physicians. *J Broadcast Electron*. 2003; **47**(3): 197–215.

Christen AG, Christen JA. Edgar Buchanan: dentist and popular character actor in movies and television. *J Hist Dent*. 2001; **49**(2): 57–61.

Clara A. The image of the psychiatrist in motion pictures. *Acta Psychiatr Belg*. 1995; **95**(1): 7–15.

Clothier JL, Freeman T, Snow L. Medical student attitudes and knowledge about ECT. *J ECT*. 2001; **17**(2): 99–101.

Colt H, Quadrelli S, Friedman L, editors. *The Picture of Health: medical ethics and the movies*. New York, NY: Oxford University Press; 2011.

Crawford TH. Visual knowledge in medicine and popular film. *Lit Med*. 1998; **17**(1): 24, 44.

Dakin P. Dr. Winkel's crucifix: moral ambiguity in *The Third Man*. *Clin Med*. 2010; **10**(4): 412–13.

Damjanović A, Vuković O, Jovanović AA, *et al*. Psychiatry and movies. *Psychiatr Danub*. 2009; **21**(2): 230–5.

Dans PE. The temple of healing: reflections from a physician at the movies. *Lit Med*. 1998; **17**(1): 114–25.

——. Women doctors in the movies. *Pharos Alpha Omega Alpha Honor Med Soc*. 1999; **62**(4): 13–14.

——. *Doctors in the Movies: boil the water and just say aah*. Bloomington, IL: Medi-Ed Press; 2000.

Bibliography

Datta V. Madness and the movies: an undergraduate module for medical students. *Int Rev Psychiatry*. 2009; **21**(3): 261–6.

Davin S. Healthy viewing: the reception of medical narratives. *Sociol Health Illn*. 2003; **25**(6): 662–79.

De Benedetti P, Beker E, Cimadoro A, *et al*. [Teamwork in teaching mental health in medical training]. *Vertex*. 2007; **18**(73): 215–20. [Spanish].

Dement JW. *Going for Broke: the depiction of compulsive gambling in film*. Lanham, MD: Scarecrow Press; 1999.

Dijck J. *The Transparent Body: a cultural analysis of medical imaging*. Seattle: University of Washington Press; 2005.

Dixon B. Medicine in the movies. *Br J Hosp Med*. 1978; **20**(6): 724.

Doron I. Bringing law to the gerontological stage: a different look at movies and old age. *Int J Aging Hum Dev*. 2006; **62**(3): 237–54.

Downey EP, Jackson RL, Puig ME, *et al*. Perceptions of efficacy in the use of contemporary film in social work education: an exploratory study. *Soc Work Educ*. 2003; **22**(4): 401–10.

Dudley M. Images of psychiatry in recent Australian and New Zealand fiction. *Aust N Z J Psychiatry*. 1994; **28**(4): 574–90.

Durkin P. Brainwashing: the power of the psychiatrist as portrayed in sixties visual media. *Med Humanit*. 2008; **34**(2): 80–3.

Ebert R. *The Great Movies*. New York, NY: Broadway Books; 2002.

Elder NC, Schwartzer A. Using the cinema to understand the family of the alcoholic. *Fam Med*. 2002; **34**(6): 426–7.

Elkamel F. The use of television series in health education. *Health Educ Res*. 1995; **10**(2): 225–32.

Engstrom F. *Movie Clips for Creative Mental Health Education*. New York, NY: Wellness Productions and Publishing; 2004.

Enns A, Smit CR, editors. *Screening Disability: essays on cinema and disability*. Lanham, MD: University Press of America; 2001.

Essex-Lopresti M. Centenary of the medical film. *Lancet*. 1997; **349**(9055): 819–20.

——. The medical film 1897–1997: Part I. The first half-century. *J Audiov Media Med*. 1998; **21**(1): 7–12.

Farré M, Bosch F, Roset PN, *et al*. Putting clinical pharmacology in context: the use of popular movies. *J Clin Pharmacol*. 2004; **44**(1): 30–6.

Fernández-Villanueva C, Revilla-Castro JC, Domínguez-Bilbao R, *et al*. Gender differences in the representation of violence on Spanish television: should women be more violent? *Sex Roles*. 2009; **61**(1–2): 85–100.

Ferns T, Chojnacka I. Angels and swingers, matrons, and sinners: nursing stereotypes. *Br J Nurs*. 2004; **14**(19): 1028–32.

Fetters M. The wizard of Osler: a brief educational intervention combining film and medical readers' theater to teach about power in medicine. *Fam Med*. 2006; **38**(5): 323–5.

Field AE, Camargo CA Jr., Taylor CB, *et al*. Relation of peer and media influences to the development of purging behaviors among preadolescent and adolescent girls. *Arch Pediatr Adolesc Med*. 1999; **153**(11): 1184–9.

Flores G. Mad scientists, compassionate healers, and greedy egotists: the portrayal of physicians in the movies. *J Natl Med Assoc*. 2002; **94**(7): 635–58.

——. Doctors in the movies. *Arch Dis Child*. 2004; **89**(12): 1084–8.

Footler. *The Pharmacist in the Movies*. Available at: www.pjonline.com (last accessed 12/1/11).

Freeman ML, Valentine DP. Through the eyes of Hollywood: images of social workers in film. *Soc Work*. 2004; **49**(2): 151–61.

Friedman L. *Cultural Sutures: medicine and media*. Durham, NC: Duke University Press; 2004.

Furman R, Negi N, Iwamoto D, *et al*. Social work practice with Latinos: key issues for social workers. *Soc Work*. 2009; **58**(2): 167–74.

Gabbard GO, Gabbard K. Countertransference in the movies. *Psychoanal Rev*. 1985; **72**(1): 171–84.

——. *Psychiatry and the Cinema*. 2nd ed. Washington, DC: American Psychiatric Press; 1999.

Gallagher P, Wilson N, Edwards R, Cowie R, Baker MG. A pilot study of medical student attitudes to, and use of, commercial movies that address public health issues. *BMC Research Notes*. 2011; **4**:111.

García-Sánchez JE, Fresnadillo MJ, García-Sánchez E. [Movies as a teaching resource for infectious diseases and clinical microbiology]. *Enferm Infecc Microbiol Clin*. 2002; **20**(8): 403–6. [Spanish].

Gharaibeh NM. The psychiatrist's image in commercially available American movies. *Acta Psychiatr Scand*. 2005; **111**(4): 316–19.

Girone JA. Medicine in the movies. *Postgrad Med*. 1985; **77**(8): 205, 208–9, 211.

Glantz SA. Smoking in movies: a major problem and a real solution. *Lancet*. 2003; **362**(938): 258–9.

Glantz SA, Kacirk KW, McCulloch C. Back to the future: smoking in the movies in 2002 compared with 1950 levels. *Am J Public Health*. 2004; **94**(2): 261–3.

Glasser B. *Medicinema: doctors in films*. Oxford: Radcliffe Publishing; 2010.

Golden G. The physician and the movies: *Master and Commander*. *Pharos Alpha Omega Alpha Honor Med Soc*. 2005; **68**(1): 51.

González J, Garcia Hernández E, Cibanal J, *et al*. [Nursing in the movies: its image during the Spanish Civil War]. *Reve Enferm*. 1998; **21**(244): 24–31. [Spanish].

González-Blasco P, Roncoletta AF, Moreto G, *et al*. [Family medicine and cinema: a humanist resource for educating affectivity?]. *Aten Primaria*. 2005; **36**(10): 566–72. [Spanish].

Gordon S, Johnson R. How Hollywood portrays nurses: report from the front row. *Revolution*. 2004 March/April: 15–21.

Green S, editor. *Leonard Maltin's Classic Movie Guide*. New York, NY: Penguin Group/ Plume; 2005.

Greenberg HR. A field guide to cinetherapy: on celluloid psychoanalysis and its practitioners. *Am J Psychoanal*. 2004; **60**(4): 329–39.

Bibliography

——. Caveat actor, caveat emptor: some notes on some hazards of Tinseltown teaching. *Int Rev Psychiatry*. 2009; **21**(3): 241–4.

Greenberg HR, Gabbard K. Reel significations: an anatomy of psychoanalytic film criticism. *Psychoanal Rev*. 1990; **77**(1): 89–110.

Gunasekera H, Chapman S, Campbell S. Sex and drugs in popular movies: an analysis of the top 200 films. *J R Soc Med*. 2005; **98**(10): 464–70.

Harper G, Moor A. *Signs of Life: cinema and medicine*. New York, NY: Wallflower Press; 2005.

Harris C. Health: the soap opera version. *IDRC Rep*. 1993; **20**(4): 24–5.

Harrison T. *Australian Film and TV Companion*. 2nd ed. Broadway, NSW: Citrus Press; 2007.

Henderson L, Franklin B. Sad not bad images of social care professionals in popular UK television drama. *Journal of Social Work*. 2007; 7(2): 133–53.

Heynick F. William T.G. Morton and "The Great Moment". *J Hist Dent*. 2003; **51**(1): 27–35.

Hicks G, Barragan M, Franco-Paredes C, *et al*. Health literacy is a predictor of HIV/ AIDS knowledge. *Fam Med*. 2006; **38**(10): 717–23.

Hill A. Psychiatric patients 'feel lost and unsafe'. *The Observer*. 2008 June 29. Available at: www.guardian.co.uk/society/2008/jun/29/mentalhealth.health3 (last accessed 4/15/12)

Hinton PR. *Stereotypes, Cognition, and Culture*. Philadelphia, PA: Psychology Press; 2000.

Hobson K. *How Hollywood Gets Medicine Right*. US News and World Report. 2007 Sep 19. Available at: http://health.usnews.com/health-news/articles/2007/09/19/ how-hollywood-gets-medicine-right (last accessed 4/15/12)

Hogg M (director). *Frankie Starlight* [motion picture]. USA: New Line Home Cinema; 1995.

Hyde NB, Fife E. Innovative instructional strategy using cinema films in an undergraduate nursing course. *ABNF J*. 2005; **16**(5): 95–7.

Hyler SE. DSM-III at the cinema, madness in the movies. *Compr Psychiatry*. 1988; **29**(2): 195–206.

Hyler SE, Gabbard GO, Schneider I. Homicidal maniacs and narcissistic parasites: stigmatization of mentally ill persons in the movies. *Hosp Community Psychiatry*. 1991; **42**(10): 1044–8.

Hyler SE, Schanzer B. Using commercially available films to teach about borderline personality disorder. *Bull Menninger Clin*. 1997; **61**(4): 458–68.

Ibáñez LMM. Editorial: medicine and cinema or cinema as therapy. *J Med Mov*. 2006; **2**: 77–9.

Jacobson S, Marcus EM. Movies on the brain. In: *Neuroanatomy for the Neuroscientist*. New York, NY: Springer; 2008. pp. 435–48.

Jones AH. Medicine and the movies: *Lorenzo's Oil* at Century's End. *Ann Intern Med*. 2000; **133**(7): 567–71.

Jones M. ER: *the unofficial guide*. New York, NY: Contender Entertainment Group; 2003.

Jukić V, Brečić P, Savić A. Movies in education of psychiatry residents. *Psychiatr Danub*. 2010; **22**(2): 304–7.

Kalisch BJ, Kalisch PA. The images of nurses in motion pictures. *Am J Nurs*. 1982; **82**(4): 605–11.

Kalisch BJ, Kalisch PA, McHugh ML. The nurse as a sex object in motion pictures, 1930 to 1980. *Res Nurs Health*. 1982; **5**(3): 147–54.

Kalra G. Teaching diagnostic approach to a patient through cinema. *Epilepsy Behav*. 2011; **22**(3): 571–3.

Karenberg A. Multiple sclerosis on-screen: from disaster to coping. *Mult Scler*. 2008; **14**(4): 530–40.

Kavaler-Adler S. Object relations perspectives on "Phantom of the Opera" and its demon lover theme: the modern film. *Am J Psychoanal*. 2009; **69**(2): 150–66.

Kerber CH, Clemens D, Medina W. Seeing is believing: learning about mental illness as portrayed in movie clips. *J Nurs Educ*. 2004; **43**(10): 479.

Kernberg OF. The erotic in film and in mass psychology. *Bull Menninger Clin*. 1994; **58**(1): 88–108.

Kerson JF, Kerson TS, Kerson LA. The depiction of seizures in film. *Epilepsia*. 2006; **40**(8): 1163–7.

Killen A. Psychiatry, cinema, and urban youth in early-twentieth-century Germany. *Harv Rev Psychiatry*. 2006; **14**(1): 38–43.

Koren G. *Awakenings*: using a popular movie to teach clinical pharmacology. *Clin Pharmacol Ther*. 1993; **53**(1): 3–5.

Kuhn A. *Cinema, Censorship and Sexuality, 1909–1925*. London: Routledge; 1988.

Kuppers P. *The Scar of Visibility: medical performances and contemporary art*. Minneapolis: University of Minnesota Press; 2007.

Lane SD. Television minidramas: social marketing and evaluation in Egypt. *Med Anthropol Q*. 1997; **11**(2): 164–82.

Lebas E. 'When every street became a cinema': the film work of Bermondsey Borough Council's Public Health Department, 1923–1953. *Hist Workshop J*. 1995; **39**(1): 42–66.

Lederer SE. *Subjected to Science: human experimentation in America before the Second World War*. Baltimore, MD: Johns Hopkins University Press; 1995.

——. Repellent subjects: Hollywood censorship and surgical images in the 1930s. *Lit Med*. 1998; **17**(1): 91–113.

——. Dark victory: cancer and popular Hollywood film. *Bull Hist Med*. 2007; **81**(1): 94–115.

Lenahan PM, Shapiro J. Facilitating the emotional education of medical students using literature and film in training about intimate partner violence. *Family Medicine*. 2005; **37**(8): 543–5.

Lenahan PM. Intimate partner violence and film: what do movies have to teach us? *International Review of Psychiatry*. 2009; **21**(3): 189–99.

Leventhal H, Kafes PN. The effectiveness of feararousing movies in motivating preventive health measures. *N Y State J Med*. 1963; **63**: 867–74.

Levine R. *A Summary of Films*. Omaha, NE: Association of Directors of Medical

Bibliography

Student Education in Psychiatry. Available at: www.dartmouth.edu/~admsep/resources/cinema.html (last accessed 12/1/11).

Lim RF, Diamond RJ, Chang JB, *et al*. Using non-feature films to teach diversity, cultural competence, and the DSM-IV-TR outline for cultural formulation. *Acad Psychiatry*. 2008; **32**(4): 291–8.

Loughlin K. The history of health and medicine in contemporary Britain: reflections on the role of audio-visual sources. *Soc Hist Med*. 2000; **13**(1): 131–45.

Lumlertgul N, Kijpaisalratana N, Pityaratstian N, *et al*. Cinemeducation: a pilot student project using movies to help students learn medical professionalism. *Med Teach*. 2009; **31**(7): 327–32.

Magala R, Thara R. Mental health in Tamil cinema. *Int Rev Psychiatry*. 2009; **21**(3): 224–8.

Maio G. [The presentation of disease and medicine in film: film stereotypes of epilepsy]. *Fortschr Neurol Psychiatr*. 2001; **69**(3): 138–45. [German].

Malmsheimer R. *"Doctors Only": the evolving image of the American physician*. New York, NY: Greenwood Press; 1988.

Mann B, Rossen EK. Media as a teaching tool in psychiatric nursing education. *Nurse Educ*. 2004; **29**(1): 36–40.

Marchessault J, Sawchuk K, editors. *Wild Science: reading feminism, medicine, and the media*. New York, NY: Routledge; 2000.

Masters JC. Hollywood in the classroom: using feature films to teach. *Nurse Educ*. 2005; **30**(3): 113–16.

Matusevich M, Matusevich D. [Pictures of autism in the American cinema]. *Vertex*. 2005; **16**(62): 301–5. [Spanish].

McArthur D, Peek-Asa C, Webb T, *et al*. Violence and its injury consequences in American movies: a public health perspective. *Inj Prev*. 2000; **6**(2): 120–4.

McCool JP, Cameron LD, Petrie KJ. Adolescent perceptions of smoking imagery in film. *Soc Sci Med*. 2001; **52**(10): 1577–87.

McDonald A, Walter G. The portrayal of ECT in American movies. *J ECT*. 2001; **17**(4): 264–74.

——. Hollywood and ECT. *Int Rev Psychiatry*. 2009; **21**(3): 200–6.

McNally G. Combating negative images of nursing: popular images of nurses in the media are largely inaccurate and usually negative. Kai Tiaki: *Nurs N Z*. 2009. Available at: www.thefreelibrary.com/Combatting+negative+images+of+nursing3A+popular+images+of+nurses+in…-a0213528326 (last accessed 4/15/12)

McNeilly DP, Wengel SP. The "ER" seminar: teaching psychotherapeutic techniques to medical students. *Acad Psychiatry*. 2001; **25**(4): 193–200.

Memel D, Raby P, Thompson T. Doctors in the movies: a user's guide to teaching about film and medicine. *Educ Prim Care*. 2009; **20**(4): 304–8.

Menon KV, Ranjith G. Malayalam cinema and mental health. *Int Rev Psychiatry*. 2009; **21**(3): 218–23.

Mensah MN. Screening bodies, assigning meaning: *ER* and the technology of HIV testing. In: Marchessault J, Sawchuk K, editors. *Wild Science: reading feminism, medicine, and the media*. New York, NY: Routledge; 2000. pp. 139–50.

Misch DA. Psychosocial formulation training using commercial films. *Acad Psychiatry*. 2000; **24**(2): 99–104.

Morton RL. Television comes to hospital leadership: managing conflict, change and quality fills a new time slot. *Healthc Exec*. 1989; **4**(3): 39–40.

Mosberg WH Jr. Trauma, television, movies, and misinformation. *Neurosurgery*. 1981; 8(6): 756–8.

Murphy-Shigematsu S, Grainger-Monsen M. The impact of film in teaching cultural medicine. *Fam Med*. 2010; **42**(3): 170–2.

Nakatani Y. [Dissociative disorders: from Janet to DSM-IV]. *Seishin Shinkeigaku Zasshi*. 2000; **102**(1): 1–12. [Japanese].

Neuendorf K, Gore T, Dalessandro A, *et al*. Shaken and stirred: a content analysis of women's portrayals in James Bond films. *Sex Roles*. 2009; **11**(12): 747–61.

Northington L, Wilkerson R, Fisher W, *et al*. (2005). Enhancing nursing students' clinical experiences using aesthetics. *J Prof Nurs*. 2005; **21**(1): 66–71.

O'Bannon T, Goldenberg M. *Teaching with Movies: recreation, sports, tourism, and physical education*. Champaign, IL: Human Kinetics; 2008.

Ochiai M (director). *Infection* [*Kansen*] [motion picture]. Japan: Lions Gate; 2004.

Ogando-Díaz B, García-Pérez C. [From Aristotle to Amenábar: narrative ethics, cinema, and medicine]. *Aten Primaria*. 2008; **40**(9): 469–72. [Spanish].

Olving P. [The physician in the movies … the mad, the good, the dirty]. *Lakartidningen*. 1994; **91**(10): 996–7. [Swedish].

O'Reilly KB. TV doctors' flaws become bioethics teaching moments. *American Medical News*. Amednews.com. 2009 January 26. Available at: www.ama-assn.org/amednews/2009/01/26/prl20126.htm (last accessed 4/15/12).

O'Shea JS. Motion pictures and the college: a history of learning by seeing. *Bull Am Coll Surg*. 2003; **88**(8): 16–23.

Osten P. [Affect, medicine and public enlightenment: the origin of the film genre "Deutscher Kulturfilm"]. *Gesnerus*. 2009; **66**(1): 67–102. [German].

Palmer J. The visible techno-foetus: ultrasound imagery and its non-medical significances in everyday contexts. *Dissertation Abstracts International. Section C: Worldwide*. 2007; **68**(3): 682.

Pavlov A, Dahlquist GE. Teaching communication and professionalism using a popular medical drama. *Fam Med*. 2010; **42**(1): 25–7.

Pernick MS. *The Black Stork: eugenics and the death of 'defective' babies in American medicine and motion pictures since 1915*. New York, NY: Oxford University Press; 1996.

Pfau M, Mullen LJ, Garrow K. The influence of television viewing on the public's perception of physicians. *J Broadcast Electron*. 1995; **39**(4): 441–58.

Pirkis J, Blood RW, Francis C, *et al*. On-screen portrayals of mental illness: extent, nature, and impacts. *J Health Commun*. 2006; **11**(5): 523–41.

Prasad CG, Babu GN, Chandra PS, *et al*. (2009). Chitrachanchala (pictures of an unstable mind): mental health themes in Kannada cinema. *Int Rev Psychiatry*. 2009; **21**(3): 229–33.

Psychflix.com. *Other Resources on Psychiatry in Film*. [Updated 2008 Apr 28]. Available at: www.psychflix.com/resources.html (last accessed 12/1/11)

Bibliography

Quadrelli S, Colt H, Semeniuk G. Appreciation of the aesthetic: a new dimension for a medicine and movies program. *Fam Med*. 2009; **41**(5): 316–18.

Quadrelli S, Sobrino E. Paul Eluard and a case of descriptive epidemiology. *Fam Med*. 2009; **41**(2): 96–8.

Raballo A, Larøi F, Bell V. Humanizing the clinical gaze: movies and the empathic understanding of psychosis. *Fam Med*. 2009; **41**(6): 387–8.

Rabkin LY. The movies' first psychiatrist. *Am J Psychiatry*. 1967; **124**(4): 545–7.

Raj YT. Medicine, myths, and the movies: Hollywood's misleading depictions affect physicians, patients alike. *Postgrad Med*. 2003; **113**(6): 9–10.

Rambor A, Kruse MH. [Hollywood movies and the production of meanings about nurses]. *Rev Gaucha Enferm*. 2007; **28**(1): 52–61. [Portuguese].

Reagan L, Tomes N, Treichler P. *Medicine's Moving Pictures: medicine, health, and bodies in American film and television*. Rochester, NY: University of Rochester Press; 2007.

Renshaw DC. Children and violence. *Compr Ther*. 2006; **32**(2): 106–10.

Ries P. Popularise and/or be damned: psychoanalysis and film at the crossroads in 1925. *Int J Psychoanal*. 1995; **76**(4): 759–91.

Roberts DF, Henriksen L, Christenson PG. *Substance Use in Popular Movies and Music*. Washington, DC: Office of National Drug Control Policy; Rockville, MD: Department of Health and Human Services; 1999.

Robinson DJ. *Reel Psychiatry: movie portrayals of psychiatric conditions*. Port Huron, MI: Rapid Psychler Press; 2003.

Rockwell C (director). *Holding Our Own: embracing the end of life* [motion picture]. USA: Fuzzy Slippers Productions; 2007.

Room R. Alcoholism and Alcoholics Anonymous in U.S. films, 1945–1962: the party ends for the "wet generations". *J Stud Alcohol*. 1989; **50**(4): 368–83.

Rose D. Television, madness and community care. *J Community Appl Soc*. 1998; **8**(3): 213–28.

Rosen A, Walter G. Way out of tune: lessons from *Shine* and its exposé. *Aust N Z J Psychiatry*. 2000; **34**(2): 237–44.

Rosen A, Walter G, Politis T, *et al*. From shunned to shining: doctors, madness and psychiatry in Australian and New Zealand cinema. *Med J Aust*. 1997; **167**(11–12): 640–4.

Rosendo LR. Fragile: a case of osteogenesis imperfect. Journal of Medicine and Movies. 2006; **2**(2): 51–5.

Ross AD, Gibbs H. *The Medicine of ER; or, How We Almost Die*. New York, NY: Basic Books; 1996.

Saab BR, Usta J. Communicating with terminal patients: lessons from "wit" and students. *Fam Med*. 2006; **38**(1): 18–20.

Salinsky J. Half a day at the movies: film studies in the VTS course. *Br J Gen Pract*. 2005; **55**(519): 806–9.

Sánchez JEG, Sánchez EG. Editorial: two years of the journal medicine and the cinema: an overview and the future. *J Med Mov*. 2006; **2**(4): 123–4.

Sargent JD, Wills TA, Stoolmiller M, *et al*. Alcohol use in motion pictures and its relation with early-onset teen drinking. *J Stud Alcohol*. 2006; **67**(1): 54–65.

Schiebinger L. *Nature's Body: gender in the making of modern science*. New Brunswick, NJ: Rutgers University Press; 2004.

Schmidt U. *Medical Films, Ethics, and Euthanasia in Nazi Germany: the history of medical research and teaching films of the Reich Office for Educational Films, Reich Institute for Films in Science and Education, 1933–1945*. Husum, Germany: Matthiesen; 2002.

Schneider I. Images of the mind: psychiatry in the commercial film. *Am J Psychiatry.* 1977; **134**(6): 613–20.

——. The theory and practice of movie psychiatry. *Am J Psychiatry.* 1987; **144**(8): 996–1002.

Schubert R, Pflesser B, Pommert A, *et al.* Interactive volume visualization using "intelligent movies". *Stud Health Technol Inform.* 1999; **62**: 321–7.

Scientists and Medical Doctors in the Movies. Berkley: University of California, Berkley, Media Resources Center; 2010. Available at: www.lib.berkeley.edu/MRC/sciencemovies.html (last accessed 12/1/11)

Segers K. Degenerative dementias and their medical care in the movies. *Alzheimer Dis Assoc Disord.* 2007; **21**(1): 55–9.

Shapiro J, Rucker L. The Don Quixote effect: why going to the movies can help develop empathy and altruism in medical students and residents. *Fam Syst Health.* 2004; **22**(4): 445–53.

Shapiro J, Rucker L, Beck J. Training the clinical eye and mind: using the arts to develop medical students' observational and pattern recognition skills. *Med Educ.* 2006; **40**(3): 263–8.

Shapshay S, editor. *Bioethics at the Movies*. Baltimore: The Johns Hopkins University Press; 2009.

Shimosa A. [Nurses in TV drama]. *Kango.* 1985; **37**(8): 84–8. [Japanese].

Shortland M. Screen memories: towards a history of psychiatry and psychoanalysis in the movies. *Br J Hist Sci.* 1987; **20**(67): 421–52.

Shortland M, Helfand W. *Medicine and Film: a checklist, survey and research resource.* Oxford: Wellcome Unit for the History of Medicine; 1989.

Shulga ID, Cherniakova IA. [Movies in teaching of a course in the propedeutics of internal disease]. *Ter Arkh.* 1974; **46**(12): 127–8. [Russian].

Siedlecky S. Sex education in New South Wales: the *Growing Up* film series. *Health and Hist.* 2006; **8**(2): 111–23.

Sierles FS. Using film as the basis of an American culture course for first-year psychiatry residents. *Acad Psychiatry.* 2005; **29**(1): 100–4.

Simon S. Greatest hits: domestic violence in American country music. *Or L Rev.* 2003; **82**(3): 1107–24.

Skårderud F. [Self-harm presentations in movies]. *Tidsskr Nor Laegeforen.* 2009; **129**(9): 896–9. [Norwegian].

Snyder S. Movies and juvenile delinquency: an overview. *Adolescence.* 1991; **26**(101): 121–32.

——. Movie portrayals of juvenile delinquency: Part 1. Epidemiology and criminology. *Adolescence.* 1995; **30**(117): 53–64.

Bibliography

——. Movie portrayals of juvenile delinquency: Part II. Sociology and psychology. *Adolescence*. 1995; **30**(118): 325–37.

Snyder WE. Medical movies: will results justify the expense and effort? *Vet Med Small Anim Clin*. 1970; **65**(5): 499–502.

Stanley DJ. Celluloid angels: a research study of nurses in feature films 1900–2007. *J Adv Nurs*. 2008; **64**(1): 84–95.

Stein EA. Colonial theatres of proof: representation and laughter in 1930s Rockefeller Foundation hygiene cinema in Java. *Health Hist* 2006; **8**(2): 14–44.

Stevenson J. *Addicted: the myth and menace of drugs in film*. Creation Books; 2000.

Strauman E, Goodier BC. Not your grandmother's doctor show: a review of *Grey's Anatomy, House,* and *Nip/Tuck. J Med Humanit*. 2008; **29**(2): 127–31.

Sukurov A (director). *Mother and Son* [motion picture]. Russia: Winstar; 1997.

Tarsitani L, Tarolla E, Pancheri P. [Psychiatry and psychiatrists in the U.S.A. cinema]. *Recenti Prog Med*. 2006; **97**(3): 165–72. [Italian].

Thibodeau E, Mentasti L. Who stole Nemo? *J Am Dent Assoc*. 2007; **138**(5): 656–60.

Thompson K, Yokota F. Depiction of alcohol, tobacco, and other substances in G-rated animated feature films. *Pediatrics*. 2001; **107**(6): 1369–74.

Tobier N. St. Elsewehere: is it St. Anywhere? *Resid Staff Physician*. 1983; **29**(4): 34–9, 43.

Toman SM, Rak CF. The use of cinema in the counselor education curriculum: strategies and outcomes. *American Counseling Association Counselor Education and Supervision*. 2000; **40**(2): 105–14.

Treichler PA, Cartwright L. *Camera Obscura*. Special issue: Imaging technologies, inscribing science. 1992; **28**.

Turner N. Movie review: *The Flintstones in Viva Rock Vegas* (2000). *J Gambling Iss*. 2001; (3). Available at: http://jgi.camh.net/doi/full/10.4309/jgi.2001.3.12?prevSearch=&searchHistoryKey (last accessed 4/15/12)

Turner NE, Fritz B, Zangeneh M. Images of gambling in film. *J Gambling Iss*. 2007; (20): 117–43.

Turrow J. *Playing Doctor: television, storytelling, and medical power*. New York, NY: Oxford University Press; 1996.

Valentine DP, Freeman M. Film portrayals of social workers doing child welfare work. *Child Adolesc Soc Work J*. 2002; **19**(6): 455–71.

Vanderford ML. Television and human values: a case study of "ER" and moral ambiguity. In: Eigo F, editor. *Religious Values at the Threshold of the Third Millennium*. Villanova, PA: Villanova University Press; 1999. pp. 33–73.

Ventura L, Uboldi P. [Pathology and the movies]. *Pathologica*. 1999; **91**(1): 63. [Italian].

Ventura S, Onsman A. The use of popular movies during lectures to aid the teaching and learning of undergraduate pharmacology. *Med Teach*. 2009; **31**(7): 662–4.

Vogel DL, Gentile DA, Kaplan SA. The influence of television on willingness to seek therapy. *J Clin Psychol*. 2008; **64**(3): 276–95.

Volandes A. Medical ethics on film: towards a reconstruction of the teaching of healthcare professionals. *J Med Ethics*. 2007; **33**(11): 678–80.

Wahl OF, Lefkowits JY. Impact of a television film on attitudes toward mental illness. *Am J Community Psychol*. 1989; **17**(4): 521–8.

Wakerlin RC. An overview of motion pictures in medical education. *J Med Educ*. 1971; **46**(7): 592–8.

Wall BM, Rossen EK. Media as a teaching tool in psychiatric nursing education. *Nurse Educ*. 2004; **29**(1): 36–40.

Walter G, McDonald A, Rey JM, *et al*. Medical student knowledge and attitudes regarding ECT prior to and after viewing ECT scenes from movies. *J ECT*. 2002; **18**(1): 43–6.

Walter G, Rosen A. Psychiatric stigma and the role of the psychiatrist. *Australas Psychiatry*. 1997; **5**(2): 72–4.

Want SC, Vickers K, Amos J. The influence of television programs on appearance satisfaction: making and mitigating social comparisons to "Friends". *Sex Roles*. 2008; **60**(9–10): 642–55.

Weber CM, Silk H. Movies and medicine: an elective using film to reflect on the patient, family, and illness. *Fam Med*. 2007; **39**(5): 317–19.

Wedding D, Boyd A. *Movies and Mental Illness: using films to understand psychology*. New York, NY: McGraw-Hill; 1999.

Welch M. *Shine*: still a glittering moment, or now a little bit tarnished? *Int J Ment Health Nurs*. 2007; **16**(3): 198–202.

Welsh CJ. OD's and DT's: using movies to teach intoxication and withdrawal syndromes to medical students. *Acad Psychiatry*. 2003; **27**(3): 182–6.

Welsh JM. Strong medicine at the movies: a review. *Lit Med*. 1993; **12**(1): 111–20.

Wijdicks EF, Wijdicks CA. The portrayal of coma in contemporary motion pictures. *Neurology*. 2006; **66**(9): 1300–3.

Wikipedia. *Cinemeducation*. http://en.wikipedia.org/wiki/Cinemeducation (accessed July 16, 2010).

Wilcox H (director). *Nurse Edith Cavell* [motion picture]. USA: RCA Victor; 1939.

Wingood GM, DiClemente RJ, Harrington K, *et al*. Exposure to X-rated movies and adolescents' sexual and contraceptive-related attitudes and behaviors. *Pediatrics*. 2001; **107**(5): 1116–19.

Winick G (director), Draper P (writer). *The Tic Code* [motion picture]. USA: Universal Studios; 1998.

Winter RO. The wizard in you. *Fam Med*. 2006; **38**(4): 241–3.

——. Your impossible dream. *Fam Med*. 2007; **39**(7): 470–2.

——. To save a mockingbird. *Fam Med*. 2008; **40**(8): 548–50.

Winter RO, Birnberg BA. Finding meaning in suffering and healing. *Fam Med*. 2006; **38**(9): 623–5.

——. Teaching professionalism artfully. *Fam Med*. 2006; **38**(3): 169–71.

——. Do you love me: teaching couple dynamics. *Fam Med*. 2007; **39**(2): 93–5.

——. Mistakes and disclosure. *Fam Med*. 2008; **40**(4): 245–7.

——. *Million Dollar Baby*: murder or mercy. *Fam Med*. 2009; **41**(3): 164–6.

Wolkenstein AS. Application of movies helpful for teaching. *Fam Med*. 2002; **34**(8): 563–4.

Bibliography

Wong RY, Saber SS, Ma I, *et al*. Using television shows to teach communication skills in internal medicine residency. *BMC Med Educ*. 2009; **9**: 9.

Yanof JA. *Hable con Ella (Talk to Her)* through the lens of gender. *Psychoanal Q*. 2008; **77**(2): 609–26.

Yates S. Finding your funny bone: incorporating humour into medical practice. *Aust Fam Physician*. 2001; **30**(1): 22–4.

Zagvazdin Y. Movies and emotional engagement: laughing matters in lecturing. *Fam Med*. 2007; **39**(4): 245–7.

Zaldivar SB. Health care personnel's critique on the Philippines' first movie on AIDS. *AIDS Care*. 1995; **7**(Suppl. 1): S95–8.

Zerby SA. Using the science fiction film invaders from Mars in a child psychiatry seminar. *Acad Psychiatry*. 2005; **29**(3): 316–21.

Zimmerman JN. *People Like Ourselves: portrayals of mental illness in the movies*. Lanham, MD: Scarecrow Press; 2003.

Index

Index

Index

Index

Index